NON-INVASIVE MANAGEMENT OF GYNECOLOGIC DISORDERS

Edited by

Aydin Arici MD
Yale University School of Medicine
New Haven, CT
USA

Emre Seli MD
Yale University School of Medicine
New Haven, CT
USA

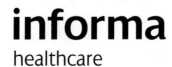

informa
healthcare

First published in the United Kingdom in 2008 by Informa Healthcare, Telephone House, 69-77 Paul Street, London EC2A 4LQ. Informa Healthcare is a trading division of Informa UK Ltd. Registered Office: 37/41 Mortimer Street, London W1T 3JH. Registered in England and Wales number 1072954.

Tel: +44 (0)20 7017 5000
Fax: +44 (0)20 7017 6699
Website: www.informahealthcare.com

A CIP record for this book is available from the British Library.

Library of Congress Cataloging-in-Publication Data

Data available on application

ISBN 10: 0 415 417 42 2
ISBN 13: 978 0 415 41742 6

Distributed in North and South America by
Taylor & Francis
6000 Broken Sound Parkway, NW, (Suite 300)
Boca Raton, FL 33487, USA
Within Continental USA
Tel: 1 (800) 272 7737; Fax: 1 (800) 374 3401
Outside Continental USA
Tel: (561) 994 0555; Fax: (561) 361 6018
Email: orders@crcpress.com

Book orders in the rest of the world:
Paul Abrahams
Tel: +44 207 017 4036
Email: bookorders@informa.com

Composition by C&M Digitals (P) Ltd, Chennai, India
Printed and bound in India by Replika Press Pvt Ltd

This book is dedicated to
My wife Meltem and my sons Devin and Deniz
My mentors Aydin Arici, and Joan A. Steitz
And to the loving memory of my father Kemal Seli (1917–2007) whose courage,
creativity, and integrity guides me…

Contents

Contributors

Annalisa Abbiati MD
University of Milan School of Medicine
Milan
Italy

Aydin Arici MD
Yale University School of Medicine
New Haven, CT
USA

Jonathan S Berek MD
Stanford University School of Medicine
Stanford, CA
USA

Sarah L Berga MD
Emory University School of Medicine
Atlanta, GA
USA

Bala Bhagavath MD
University of Texas Southwestern Medical Center
Dallas, TX
USA

Narender N Bhatia MD
Harbor-UCLA Medical Center
David Geffen School of Medicine UCLA
Los Angeles, CA
USA

Veronica Bianchi PhD
Yale University School of Medicine
New Haven, CT
USA

Karen D Bradshaw MD
University of Texas Southwestern Medical Center
Dallas, TX
USA

Jason G Bromer MD
Yale University School of Medicine
New Haven, CT
USA

John E Buster MD
Warren Alpert Medical School of Brown University
Providence, RI
USA

Maria Cerrillo MD
Instituto Valenciano de Infertilidad
Madrid and Valencia
Spain

Rafaella Daguati MD
University of Milan School of Medicine
Milan
Italy

Giuseppe Del Priore MD MPH
New York Downtown Hospital
New York, NY
USA

Antoni J Duleba MD
Reproductive Endocrinology and Infertility
UC Davis Fertility Center
Sacramento, CA
USA

Juan A Garcia-Velasco MD
Rey Juan Carlos Univerisity, and
Instituto Valenciano de Infertilidad
Madrid
Spain

Chad A Hamilton MD
Walter Reed Army Medical Center
Washington, DC
USA

Mat H Ho MD PhD
Harbor-UCLA Medical Center
David Geffen School of Medicine UCLA
Los Angeles, CA
USA

Bradley S Hurst MD
Carolinas Medical Center
Charlotte, NC
USA

Joshua Johnson PhD
Yale University School of Medicine
New Haven, CT
USA

Pinar H Kodaman MD PhD
Yale University School of Medicine
New Haven, CT
USA

Hetal Kothari MD
New York Downtown Hospital
New York, NY
USA

Stephan Krotz MD
Warren Alpert Medical School of Brown University
Providence, RI
USA

Charles J Lockwood MD
Yale University School of Medicine
New Haven, CT
USA

Jerry L Lowder MD MSc
University of Pittsburgh School of Medicine
Pittsburgh, PA
USA

Neal G Mahutte MD
Dartmouth Medical School
Lebanon, NH
USA

Paul B Marshburn MD
Carolinas Medical Center
Charlotte, NC
USA

Farzana Martin MD
New York Downtown Hospital
New York, NY
USA

Michelle L Matthews MD
Carolinas Medical Center
Charlotte, NC
USA

Genevieve Neal-Perry MD PhD
Albert Einstein College of Medicine
New York, NY
USA

Kunle Odunsi MD PhD
Roswell Park Cancer Institute
Buffalo, NY
USA

Lubna Pal MD
Yale University School of Medicine
New Haven, CT
USA

John K Park MD
Emory University School of Medicine
Atlanta, GA
USA

Beth W Rackow MD
Yale University School of Medicine
New Haven, CT
USA

Emre Seli MD
Yale University School of Medicine
New Haven, CT
USA

Carlos Simón MD PhD
Instituto Valenciano de Infertilidad, and
Valencia University
Valencia
Spain

Melissa A Simon MD MPH
Northwestern University
Feinberg School of Medicine
Chicago, IL
USA

Stacey A South MD
Roswell Park Cancer Institute
Buffalo, NY
USA

Rebecca S Usadi MD
Carolinas Medical Center
Charlotte, NC
USA

Paolo Vercellini MD
University of Milan School of Medicine
Milan
Italy

Anne M Weber MD MSc
National Institute of Child Health and
Development (NICHD)
National Institutes of Health (NIH)
Bethesda, MD
USA

Erin F Wolff MD
Yale University School of Medicine
New Haven, CT
USA

Introduction

Many of us entered the discipline of obstetrics and gynecology because we believed that it uniquely lent itself to a mix of medicine and surgery. This is certainly the most common attraction to the field cited by residency applicants to our institution. But how accurate is that assessment? It certainly applies to obstetrics and maternal fetal medicine where treatment of maternal medical conditions and obstetrical surgical treatments are seamlessly integrated on a daily basis. Moreover, in obstetrics there are many alternative medical and surgical treatments for dysfunctional labor, uterine atony, pregnancy termination, and certain fetal anomalies. But can medical and surgical treatments be viewed pari passu in gynecology? Increasingly the answer is yes. This unique textbook provides ample examples of alternative medical and surgical approaches to a host of common gynecologic conditions including ectopic pregnancy, abnormal uterine bleeding, endometriosis, myomas, and urinary incontinence. Particularly timely are its chapters on uterine artery embolization and fertility preservation in patients with early and reproductive tract malignancies and in women wishing to both delay and preserve fertility for social reasons.

The editors are truly gifted clinicians and scientists. Dr Aydin Arici has authored over 150 peer review publications, has garnered multiple National Institutes of Health (NIH) and sponsored grants, and is internationally recognized as an outstanding reproductive endocrinology and infertility (REI) specialist. He led the REI section at Yale for many years and established it as one of the top divisions in the United States. Having sent scores of patients to him over the years, I can personally attest to his clinical prowess. Dr Emre Seli is a brilliant young reproductive scientist who is conducting landmark research into oocyte biology and maternal age-associated infertility, as well as developing novel technologies for non-invasive assessment of embryo quality. He served his residency and REI fellowship at Yale and subsequently joined the faculty while conducting an NIH sponsored research program. Emre is also a truly gifted clinician. Drs Arici and Seli have assembled an 'All Star' cast of authors, each expert in the topics about which they write. The result is a concise, readable, and highly practicable resource. The goal of the text is to describe available medical treatments for common gynecologic conditions and compare them to surgical options using an 'evidenced-based' approach. This novel and exciting strategy produces a 'must read' for those interested in adding to their therapeutic armamentarium conservative treatments for many gynecologic conditions.

Charles J Lockwood MD
The Anita O'Keefe Young
Professor of Women's Health
Department of Obstetrics,
Gynecology, and Reproductive Sciences
Yale University School of Medicine
New Haven, CT
USA

1 Non-invasive management of ectopic pregnancy

Stephan Krotz and John E Buster

INCIDENCE

Over the past 60 years in the United States, the incidence of ectopic pregnancy has increased more than fivefold and now accounts for approximately 2% of all pregnancies.[1,2] Much of this increased incidence can be attributed to the increase in risk factors for ectopic pregnancy such as sexually transmitted infections,[3] surgical sterilization,[4] and the use of fertility enhancing drugs. During the past 30 years maternal mortality has decreased 11-fold, and currently results in one death in every 3135 patients[5] with an ectopic pregnancy. Although maternal mortality rates are significantly decreased and represent improvements in management, ectopic pregnancy is associated with a mortality risk that is four times higher than that of all other causes combined of pregnancy-related deaths.[5] Additionally, ectopic pregnancy remains the leading cause of death in the first trimester.[6]

RISK FACTORS

Despite advances in the diagnosis of ectopic pregnancy and reduced mortality rates, many cases of ectopic pregnancy are either misdiagnosed or missed during initial evaluation. One study of emergency rooms found that 45% of patients eventually diagnosed with an ectopic pregnancy were initially sent home without a correct diagnosis.[7] The old triad of amenorrhea, abdominal pain, and irregular vaginal bleeding occurs in less than half of patients with an ectopic pregnancy and serves more as an indicator for further evaluation than as diagnostic criteria. Therefore, careful consideration of specific risk factors, which are present in about 55% of patients with ectopic pregnancies, may lead to higher clinical suspicion and earlier detection. In general, risk factors can be stratified into three categories for ectopic pregnancy: *highly increased*, *moderately increased*, and *slightly increased* risk (Table 1.1).

Highly increased risk includes etiologies that result in fallopian tube damage including tubal surgery, tubal sterilization, history of previous ectopic pregnancies,

and history of surgery for ectopic pregnancies. The risk of recurrence of an ectopic pregnancy ranges 10–27%.[11] Although screening patients with a history of ectopic pregnancy would seem reasonable, the high false-positive rate of screening asymptomatic women leads to higher costs from unnecessary medical intervention.[12] Tubal pathology and infertility also significantly raise the odds of ectopic pregnancy, and may be secondary to impeded tubal motility or otherwise undocumented tubal obstruction leading to ectopic implantation.[8,9]

Moderately increased risk generally relates to tubal blockage via infectious etiologies. A history of pelvic inflammatory disease or gonorrhea or chlamydia infection, or a history of exposure to gonorrhea or chlamydia (as evidenced by circulating antibodies), moderately increases risk, presumably by causing intraluminal adhesions in the fallopian tubes which can prevent fertilized embryos from migrating to the uterus. Having more than one lifetime partner also has been shown to directly increase a patient's risk for ectopic pregnancy.[8] Surveys of US women show that with each additional sexual partner after the first, the risk of sexually transmitted bacterial infections increases, with nine times the risk for patients with more than five lifetime partners.[13] Cigarette smoking is an independent risk factor for ectopic pregnancy, and the risk correlates with the number of cigarettes. The odds ratio of ectopic pregnancy as it relates to smoking can range from 1.6 times the risk for five or fewer cigarettes per day to 3.5 times the risk for patients who smoke one pack or more per day.[14]

Slightly increased risk can be divided into behavioral factors and symptomatic factors. Certain methods of contraception such as birth control pills and the intrauterine device (IUD) are commonly believed to reduce the risk of ectopic pregnancy secondary to an overall reduction in pregnancy rates.[10] Once these methods fail, however, the risk for ectopic pregnancy is increased; in the case of birth control pills the mechanisms are unknown. Early age of intercourse also increases the risk, since younger women are often exposed to ascending infections.[14] Recently, several presenting symptoms and signs have been evaluated and their contribution to risk identified. These include

Table 1.1   Risk factors for ectopic pregnancy compared to all pregnant patients[8–10]

Risk	Odds ratio
Highly increased	
Previous tubal surgery[a]	21
Two prior ectopics[b]	16
Tubal sterilization[c]	9.3
Previous surgery for ectopic[a]	8.3
Tubal pathology[a]	3.5–25
One prior ectopic[b]	3.0
Infertility[a]	2.5–21
Moderately increased	
Chlamydia[a]	2.8–3.7
Gonorrhea[a]	2.9
Pelvic inflammatory disease[a,b]	1.5–2.5
Ever smoking[a]	2.5
Current smoking[a]	2.3
Lifetime sexual partners > 1[a]	2.1
Slightly increased	
Oral contraceptives[c]	1.8
hCG 501–2000 at presenation[b]	1.7
Primigravida[b]	1.6
Age at first intercourse < 18[a]	1.6
IUD in place[c]	1.6
Pain at presentation[b]	1.4
Moderate to severe vaginal bleeding[b]	1.4
Vaginal douching[a]	1.1–3.1

[a]From reference 8
[b]From reference 9
[c]From reference 10

β-human chorionic gonadotropin (hCG) levels between 500 and 2000 mIU/ml, first pregnancy, abdominal or pelvic pain, and moderate to severe bleeding.[9] While several of these may be subjective and consistent with intrauterine pregnancies or abortions, their additive presence may warrant closer patient monitoring.

Factors that have been cited but are not associated with an increased risk include previous non-tubal pelvic surgery, cesarean sections, and assisted reproductive technologies (ART). Previous association of ART procedures with ectopic pregnancy may be related to the initial cause of infertility such as tubal pathology. While zygote intrafallopian transfer (ZIFT) procedures are the only ART procedures associated with an increased risk (3.6%), in vitro fertilization (IVF) with embryo transfer has a significantly decreased risk of ectopic pregnancy (1.4%).[15] The decreased incidence of ectopic pregnancy associated with IVF and embryo transfer may be a result of bypassing the fallopian tubes, and would be consistent with the notion that tubal factor is solely responsible for a higher ectopic pregnancy rate in ART procedures. Other factors such as past IUD use and previous medical or spontaneous abortion remain disputed in the literature[8,9] as to whether they are protective or risk factors.

DIAGNOSIS

Presentation

Generally, any woman of reproductive age who presents with abdominal pain or vaginal bleeding should have a pregnancy test drawn upon initial evaluation, since 79–97% of patients with an ectopic pregnancy have these symptoms.[16] Once pregnancy has been confirmed with a urine or serum pregnancy test, the diagnosis of ectopic pregnancy relies on the combination of radiologic imaging, serum laboratory values, and, when needed, surgical diagnosis. The diagnosis of ectopic pregnancy should always be entertained until intrauterine pregnancy or miscarriage is confirmed. Heterotopic pregnancy is the only exception to this rule, since confirmation of intrauterine pregnancy does not result in proper evaluation or treatment planning for the ectopic portion of the pregnancy. The risk of heterotopic pregnancy is low, reported as 1 in 10 000 to 1 in 50 000 pregnant patients, except in patients who have a history of assisted reproduction for whom the risk has been reported as high, at 1 in 100.[17,18] If patients early in pregnancy present with tachycardia, hypotension, or rebound or cervical motion tenderness, immediate evaluation for ectopic pregnancy should occur, and surgical exploration for tubal or uterine rupture considered.

Confirming the location of an ectopic pregnancy is necessary to determine the course of management. Ninety-seven per cent of ectopic pregnancies are tubal, with 70–80% occurring in the ampullary segment, 12% in the isthmic segment, and 5–11% in the fimbria. The less common sites of ectopic implantation include interstitial or cornual (2%), abdominal (1.4%), ovarian (0.2–3.2%), and cervical (0.2%).[19,20] Rare implantation sites include previous cesarean scars or the abdomen.

Imaging

Pelvic ultrasound

Pelvic ultrasound should be the first diagnostic test performed after a thorough clinical evaluation (Figure 1.1). A diagnostic sequence beginning with a pelvic ultrasound scan misses the least number of ectopic pregnancies compared to various diagnostic sequences involving ultrasound, β-hCG level, and progesterone level.[21]

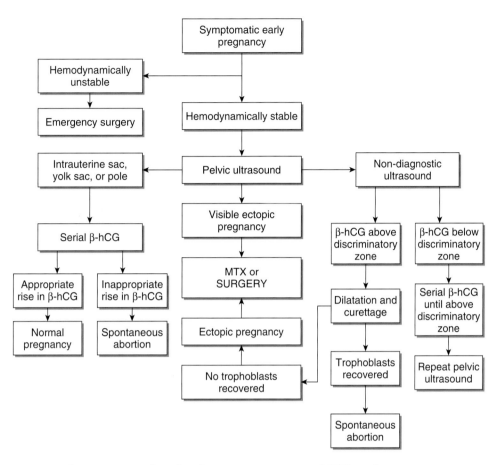

Figure 1.1   Diagnostic and management algorithm for ectopic pregnancies. MTX, methotrexate

Confirmation of an intrauterine pregnancy or miscarriage can occur as early as 4.5 weeks into the pregnancy by the identification of an intradecidual sign ('decidual reaction'), an echogenic rim in the endometrial cavity surrounding a fluid collection.[22] Since this finding can often be confused with a pseudosac in the uterus, which is a collection of blood from either an intrauterine or an ectopic pregnancy, it is advisable to rely on a double decidual sac sign ('double ring sign') or yolk sac, which occurs closer to 5 weeks of gestation.[23] The presence of a fetal pole with or without a heartbeat near 6 weeks confirms the presence of an intrauterine pregnancy.

Scanning the adnexa and pelvis for reliable signs of an ectopic pregnancy can be difficult, since the pathognomonic finding of an extrauterine fetal pole with a heartbeat is present only 8–26% of the time.[24] An extrauterine sac with a yolk sac is the next most reliable sign when imaging the adnexa, but care must be taken not to confuse this with a hemorrhagic cyst.[25] Use of Doppler ultrasound may locate a 'ring of fire' which characterizes the blood flow surrounding an ectopic pregnancy. This sign may be confused with luteal flow, which 90% of the time occurs on the same side as an ectopic pregnancy.[26] The finding of echogenic

fluid in the pelvis in the presence of a positive β-hCG has 86–93% positive predictive value for ectopic pregnancy,[25] and may yield information about the urgency of intervention.

Often the pelvic ultrasound scan is non-diagnostic, and a serum β-hCG must be taken to determine whether the ultrasound was performed above, below, or within the discriminatory zone. The discriminatory zone includes β-hCG values between 1500 and 2000 mIU/ml, which was determined by comparing β-hCG levels to ultrasound findings in normal intrauterine pregnancies. Below 1500 mIU/ml, the sensitivity in making the diagnosis of an intrauterine pregnancy is 29%, compared to 92% with values above 1500 mIU/ml. At a β-hCG level of 2000 mIU/ml, which corresponds to a pregnancy at 5.5 weeks' gestation, the sensitivity approaches 100%.[27–29] Failure to diagnose an intrauterine pregnancy with pelvic ultrasound above 2000 mIU/ml indicates an abnormal or non-viable pregnancy. A surgical approach to diagnosis using dilatation and curettage or manual vacuum aspiration should be undertaken to differentiate a spontaneous intrauterine abortion from an ectopic pregnancy. Patients with a β-hCG level below 1500 mIU/ml should be followed with serial β-hCG levels until it rises above the discriminatory zone, at which time the diagnosis can be confirmed.

The discriminatory zone is traditionally defined as a range of β-hCG values above which an intrauterine pregnancy will always be visualized. A range, instead of a threshold, allows for individual clinicians to determine their own threshold (β-hCG level) above which they expect to see an intrauterine pregnancy. The threshold chosen depends on a clinician's experience with the ultrasound equipment available, the sonographer's experience, and clinical preference. Choosing a threshold close to 1500 mIU/ml would have a high sensitivity and low specificity for an ectopic pregnancy, and risks defining a normal intrauterine pregnancy as abnormal. Choosing a threshold of 2000 mIU/ml or higher reduces the risk of classifying a normal intrauterine pregnancy as abnormal, but lowers the sensitivity for ectopic pregnancy and may delay its diagnosis.[21,30]

Magnetic resonance imaging

Pelvic ultrasound is considered first-line for diagnosis of ectopic pregnancy. When ultrasound is difficult or unclear, magnetic resonance imaging (MRI) can be useful, especially when imaging non-tubal ectopic pregnancies.[31–33] Failure to promptly diagnose an interstitial pregnancy[34] can lead to catastrophic uterine rupture and hemorrhage.

Serum tests

β-hCG

Serum β-hCG is the single most useful analyte used in the diagnosis of ectopic pregnancy. To use β-hCG values to differentiate normal from abnormal pregnancies, the expected rise and decline in both normal and abnormal pregnancies must be defined. Defining the expected rise and fall is especially useful for patients early in pregnancy requiring evaluation for vaginal bleeding or abdominal pain, since 75–80% presenting with these complaints have β-hCG values below the discriminatory zone.

In 1981, the minimum normal rise of serum β-hCG was first described as a 66% increase over 48 hours using the 85% confidence interval surrounding normal intrauterine pregnancies.[35] In 2006, the minimum normal rise for β-hCG was reduced to 35% in 48 hours with a 99.9% confidence interval surrounding normal intrauterine pregnancies.[36] This minimum rise is based on the management of over 1200 normal pregnancies with first trimester bleeding or pain. While this lower threshold may save many intrauterine pregnancies, it may also delay the diagnosis of ectopic pregnancy.

The minimum decline of β-hCG for a spontaneous abortion ranges from 21 to 35% at 2 days and 60 to 84% at 7 days for patients with a β-hCG value less than 10 000 mIU/ml.[37] The percentages of minimum decline were derived from the β-hCG levels of 700 patients experiencing spontaneous abortion. The higher is the initial β-hCG, the more rapid is the decline. A decline less than 21% at 2 days or 60% at 7 days suggests an ectopic pregnancy or retained trophoblasts. Seventy-one per cent of ectopic pregnancies exhibit an abnormal rise or fall. This indicates that 29% of ectopic pregnancies exhibit an expected rise or decline in β-hCG levels, which may lead to misdiagnosis of a normal intrauterine pregnancy or spontaneous abortion.[30] If an intrauterine or ectopic pregnancy cannot be identified by an abnormally rising or falling β-hCG above the discriminatory zone, dilatation and curettage or manual vacuum aspiration should be considered to determine whether there is a retained spontaneous abortion instead of an ectopic pregnancy.

Progesterone

Progesterone levels have frequently been incorporated into algorithms for ectopic pregnancy diagnosis.[38,39] More recently, their usefulness has been debated.[40] As progesterone levels rise, the probability of a normal intrauterine pregnancy increases while the probability of an ectopic pregnancy or spontaneous abortion[41] decreases. Unfortunately, only values at the ends of the spectrum yield definitive information. Thus, ectopic pregnancy incidence in patients with progesterone levels above 25 ng/ml is only 3%.[21] In contrast, the probability of a normal intrauterine pregnancy with progesterone below 5 ng/ml is only 0.16% or 1 in 625.[41] No normal intrauterine pregnancies have been documented below a progesterone level of 2.5 ng/ml. Also, low progesterone does not distinguish between ectopic pregnancies and spontaneous abortions,[41] and may only provide additional information in deciding to proceed with dilatation and curettage for an abnormal pregnancy. In one analysis of six approaches to evaluating patients, the use of progesterone prior to ultrasound or β-hCG levels was shown to increase the number of missed ectopic pregnancies,[21] and therefore may be detrimental when evaluating patients for an ectopic pregnancy.

Other serum tests

The use of other serum analytes in the diagnosis of ectopic pregnancy has been decreased. Glycoledin, human placental lactogen, leukemia inhibiting factor, pregnancy-associated plasma protein A (PAPP-A), and pregnancy specific B1-glycoledin have been looked at independently and are not useful in distinguishing an ectopic pregnancy from an intrauterine pregnancy or spontaneous abortion.[42,43] Vascular endothelial growth factor (VEGF) alone is the only individual marker shown to be significantly elevated in an ectopic pregnancy (median 227.2 pg/ml) versus an intrauterine pregnancy (median 107.2 pg/ml). When using a receiver operating characteristic (ROC) curve to differentiate an ectopic pregnancy from a spontaneous abortion, the use of 174.5 pg/ml as a threshold for diagnosis of an ectopic pregnancy yielded a sensitivity of 78% and a specificity of 100%.[42] When PAPP-A and progesterone levels were combined with VEGF as a 'triple marker analysis' (VEGF/(PAPP-A × progesterone)), it showed a sensitivity of 97.7% and specificity of 92.2%. The discriminatory value of this test decreases below 7 weeks of gestation, a time when most patients with ectopic pregnancies present, as the false-positive rate for ectopic pregnancy increases.[43] When considering the low sensitivity of VEGF individually or in combination with other markers at 7 weeks' gestation or less, and difficulties in attaining prompt results, VEGF has not become a clinically useful marker.

Operative diagnosis

Dilatation and curettage should be performed on patients in whom serial serum β-hCG measurements suggest an abnormal pregnancy, but an ectopic pregnancy cannot be identified on ultrasound. Confirming the presence of chorionic villi with dilatation and curettage is necessary to prevent the administration of methotrexate to patients who may have an abnormal intrauterine pregnancy. Up to 38% of patients with a presumed diagnosis of ectopic pregnancy based on β-hCG values and an empty uterus on pelvic ultrasound may be experiencing a spontaneous abortion.[44] Dilatation and curettage is the definitive treatment for those 38% of patients with a spontaneous abortion, the only exception being a heterotopic pregnancy. Alternatives to dilatation and curettage such as endometrial biopsy have variable sensitivity (30–63%) and specificity (80–100%), making them unreliable for diagnostic purposes.[45,46] Measurement of β-hCG should be performed immediately after dilatation and curettage and repeated 12–24 hours later, since chorionic villi are not identified on pathologic specimens in up to

20% of spontaneous abortions.[47] Expected decreases in β-hCG after dilatation and curettage are consistent with the diagnosis of a spontaneous abortion, while a plateau or rise suggests an ectopic pregnancy. While dilatation and curettage for diagnostic purposes is performed in the United States, the risk of interrupting a normal intrauterine pregnancy is considered too high in many countries, and is not practiced.[48]

EXPECTANT MANAGEMENT

Expectant management is not commonly practiced. Success rates nonetheless have been reported to average 68% in the evaluation of 15 studies.[49] While this number is high, currently there is no standard by which to determine those patients who will successfully experience resolution with expectant management alone. In one report, patients with a serum β-hCG of < 1000 mIU/ml had spontaneous resolution 88% of the time, while patients with a serum β-hCG > 1000 mIU/ml resolved only 48% of the time.[50] In most centers, methotrexate administration or surgery is preferred (Figure 1.2).

MEDICAL TREATMENT

Methotrexate: indications

The use of methotrexate to treat ectopic pregnancy was first described in 1982,[52] and was followed by the first case series in the mid-1980s establishing methotrexate as a viable medical option.[53,54] Methotrexate is a folic acid antagonist[55] that was originally used to treat choriocarcinoma.[56] Methotrexate acts by inhibiting dihydrofolate reductase (DHFR), an enzyme which reduces folate to tetrahydrofolate, a necessary cofactor in the synthesis of DNA and RNA. Methotrexate therefore targets rapidly dividing cells, and is a logical choice in the treatment of ectopic pregnancy, especially since no increased reproductive side-effects have been documented.[57] Leucovorin (folinic acid) is a methotrexate antagonist that is given during the administration of methotrexate, especially with high doses, to reduce some of the prohibitive adverse effects.[55,56] Comparisons between multidose methotrexate and laparoscopic salpingostomy show methotrexate to be equally successful in treating ectopic pregnancies[58] and allow patients a non-surgical, outpatient management option.

Candidates for methotrexate are hemodynamically stable, possess no contraindications to methotrexate,

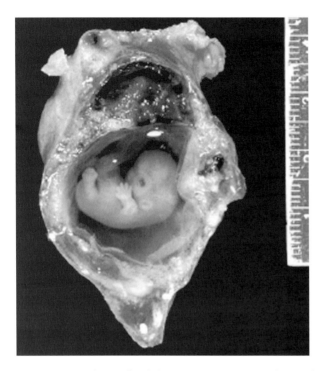

Figure 1.2 Advanced tubal ectopic pregnancy. Advanced ectopic pregnancies (formed limbs) should be treated with surgery. Reproduced with permission from reference 51

Table 1.2 Contraindications to methotrexate therapy. Adapted from reference 59

Absolute contraindications
- Intrauterine pregnancy
- Evidence of immunodeficiency
- Moderate to severe anemia, leukopenia, or thrombocytopenia
- Sensitivity to methotrexate
- Active pulmonary disease
- Active peptic ulcer disease
- Clinically important hepatic dysfunction
- Clinically important renal dysfunction
- Breastfeeding

Relative contraindications
- Embryonic cardiac activity detected by transvaginal ultrasonography
- High initial β-hCG concentration (>5000 mIU/ml)
- Ectopic pregnancy greater than 4 cm on transvaginal ultrasonography
- Refusal to accept blood transfusion
- Inability to participate in follow-up

and are willing to comply with the required follow-up. Relative contraindications for methotrexate include a gestational sac size greater than 4 cm (Figure 1.2), presence of fetal cardiac activity, and β-hCG levels ranging greater than 5000 mIU/ml.[59] Successful treatment of ectopic pregnancy with any of these relative contraindications is possible, but the risk of rupture is elevated. Absolute contraindications to treatment include hemodynamic instability and any of the pre-existing conditions listed in Table 1.2. Therefore, patients should be evaluated for methotrexate contraindications and have the appropriate screening laboratory examinations including complete blood count, liver function tests, an electrolyte panel including creatinine, and blood type including Rh factor. Patients with a history of lung disease should have a chest X-ray prior to methotrexate to evaluate for risk of interstitial pneumonitis.[30]

Methotrexate dosing: multidose or single-dose

Original protocols for methotrexate use were multidose, based on the treatment for gestational trophoblastic disease,[53,54] and are still followed today. Patients using the multidose regimen are given doses alternating every other day starting with methotrexate and followed by leucovorin (Table 1.3). Methotrexate is administered, up to four doses, until the serum β-hCG decreases by a minimum of 15% over 48 hours.[61] Serum β-hCG levels are drawn on day 1 and days 4–8 of the protocol, and are followed weekly until the serum β-hCG levels are negative. Laboratory values (complete blood count (CBC), platelets, liver function tests (LFTs), and creatinine levels) are repeated on day 8 and compared to the original values to evaluate for any adverse effects resulting from methotrexate administration. Additional courses of the multidose regimen can be given if deemed necessary and appropriate.

The individualization of methotrexate protocols[61] during initial studies with the multidose regimen led to development of the single-dose regimen (Table 1.3). Single-dose regimens were developed to increase compliance and lessen side-effects associated with multidose regimens. In single-dose, methotrexate is administered on day 1 of the protocol and again on day 7 if the serum β-hCG has not decreased by at least 15% since day 4. Serum β-hCG levels are drawn on day 1, checked again on days 4 and 7, and followed weekly until they are negative. In 85% of patients undergoing the single-dose regimen the serum β-hCG will rise between days 1 and 4, so following serum β-hCG values during this period will not yield clinically useful information.[62] Laboratory values (CBC, platelets, LFTs, and creatinine levels) are repeated on day 7 and compared to the original values to evaluate for adverse effects from methotrexate administration.

Table 1.3 Single- and multidose methotrexate regimens. Adapted from reference 60

Single dose			Multidose		
	Studies	**Treatment**		**Studies**	**Treatment**
Day 1	β-hCG CBC Platelet count LFTs RFTs	MTX 50 mg/m² IM	Day 1	β-hCG CBC Platelet count LFTs RFTs	MTX 1 mg/kg IM
Day 4	β-hCG		Day 2		Folinic acid 0.1 mg/kg IM
Day 7	β-hCG CBC Platelet count LFTs RFTs		Day 3	β-hCG	MTX 1 mg/kg IM
Weekly	β-hCG until negative		Day 4		Folinic acid 0.1 mg/kg IM
			Day 5	β-hCG	MTX 1 mg/kg IM
			Day 6		Folinic acid 0.1 mg/kg IM
			Day 7	β-hCG	MTX 1 mg/kg IM
			Day 8	CBC Platelet count LFTs RFTs	Folinic acid 0.1 mg/kg IM
			Weekly	β-hCG until negative	

hCG, human chorionic gonadotropin; CBC, complete blood count; LFTs, liver function tests; RFTs, renal function tests; MTX, methotrexate; IM, intramuscular

The decision to use single- or multidose is debated. Multiple studies evaluating the overall efficacy of both regimens over the past 20 years have demonstrated a success rate of 75–96%.[63] A recent meta-analysis of 1327 patients showed the success rates of the single-dose regimen and multidose regimen to be 88.1% and 92.7%, respectively.[64] The odds ratio for failure for single-dose compared to the multidose regimen for all data was 1.71. When serum β-hCG and embryonic cardiac activity were controlled for, the odds for failure of the single-dose regimen were 4.74 compared to the multidose regimen. While this meta-analysis represents the largest compiled data comparing the two regimens, it cannot control for all patient characteristics or variation in treatment protocols. When comparing laparoscopic salpingostomy to both regimens, the multidose regimen is equally efficacious[58] to laparoscopic salpingostomy while the single-dose regimen is significantly less efficacious (relative risk (RR) 0.83).[65] More recent data from a retrospective study of 643 patients[66] and a small randomized controlled trial of 108 patients, however, suggest that the single-dose regimen is as effective as the multidose regimen. Future tubal patency using both protocols is comparable to conservative surgical management with laparascopic salpingostomy.[58,65]

The number of methotrexate injections administered for each protocol are also associated with different outcomes. Almost 14% of patients undergoing the single-dose protocol received a second dose of methotrexate, and these demonstrated fewer treatment failures (odds ratio 0.64) compared to their single-dose counterparts.[64] Likewise, slightly fewer than 50% of patients undergoing the multidose regimen received four doses. If more than four doses (6.7% of patients) of methotrexate were required during the multidose regimen, the odds of failure were 4.9 times higher for those patients compared to those who received only four doses. The optimal number of doses remains to be determined, and may lie between one and four doses.

Methotrexate: predictors for success

Determining which patients can be successfully treated with methotrexate traditionally focused on selecting patients with specific criteria such as ectopic size less than 4 cm, no embryonic cardiac activity, no signs of hemoperitoneum, and β-hCG values below a threshold of 5000 mIU/ml.[59] Many of these criteria are based on older and smaller studies; serum β-hCG is the only predictive factor that can be considered reliable across many studies. One large study indicated that hemoperitoneum and size do not correlate with methotrexate success.[67] Data concerning fetal cardiac activity are conflicting, as some suggest it is a relative contraindication to methotrexate administration while others report success rates approaching 90%.[68] The percentage of ectopic pregnancies with fetal cardiac activity present usually coincides with the level of serum β-hCG.[67] Fetal cardiac activity is another measure of how advanced an ectopic pregnancy is, but is less useful than β-hCG since it cannot be measured on a continuum. Additionally, the presence of fetal cardiac activity also may be suggestive of a more advanced, cytogenetically normal ectopic pregnancy that would be more resistant to medical therapy with methotrexate.[69] In most of the larger studies in which serum β-hCG is identified as a reliable predictor of success, a specific β-hCG value is cited, above which the rate of treatment failure becomes unacceptable. This serum β-hCG level then becomes the chosen threshold above which ectopic pregnancies should be managed surgically, according to the study. In reality, the success of medical management compared to serum β-hCG is most likely a continuum[67] that varies with each physician, institution, patient population, and methotrexate treatment protocol. Increasing efficiency in diagnosis and earlier initiation of medical management may also skew these thresholds towards lower values, since many ectopic pregnancies that are bound to rupture will be detected earlier.[70]

Several additional factors that correspond with the clinical course of the ectopic pregnancy have been suggested as predictive of medical management failure. At presentation, patients with pelvic pain regardless of tenderness elicited on examination experience nine times the risk of methotrexate failure, while patients with vaginal bleeding experience six times the risk of methotrexate failure. The presence of a yolk sac on ultrasound is associated with a 71–88% methotrexate failure rate, with an odds ratio of 19.3 for failure.[71,72] A rise in β-hCG of 66% over 48 hours, prior to confirmation of the diagnosis of ectopic pregnancy, is associated with nine times the risk of tubal rupture.[70] A decline of less than 15% in the serum β-hCG levels between day 4 and day 7 after methotrexate therapy is associated with an odds ratio of 3.8 for medical failure. In summary, when evaluating patients for medical management, the initial β-hCG level should be taken into account with clinical progression and patient suitability for medical management.

Follow-up after methotrexate

After the administration of methotrexate, up to 60% of patients may experience increasing abdominal pain.[62]

The pain experienced after methotrexate administration is believed to be secondary to tubal abortion or more commonly hematoma formation in the tube, both of which are a normal part of the resolution process. One study using ultrasound to monitor patient progress showed that 63% of patients who were successfully treated with methotrexate experienced an increase in fallopian tube size with increased vascular flow.[73] Abdominal pain after methotrexate administration is usually self-limited and can be treated with non-steroidal anti-inflammatory drugs (NSAIDs). Approximately 20% of patients treated with methotrexate will experience severe pain and 13% will require hospitalization[74] for pain management. Serial ultrasound monitoring of patient response to methotrexate or for predicting rupture is generally not useful, since hemoperitoneum is present in 30–100% of patients with ectopic pregnancies, regardless of methotrexate success or failure.[67,74]

In the first 1–4 days after methotrexate administration, β-hCG levels will rise in the majority of patients[59,62,75,76] and should peak at the 4th day of injection. A decrease in β-hCG levels of 15% or more from day 4 to day 7 represents an adequate response to methotrexate.[59,62] If there is less than a 15% decline, then a second injection can be given on day 7 or the patient can undergo surgical management. If the levels plateau or increase in 7 days an additional dose may be given. The average time to resolution after methotrexate administration, when β-hCG reaches undetectable levels, is reported as 20–35 days,[62,68,75,76] but can take as long as 109 days.[68] The average time to rupture requiring surgery is reported as 14 days, but can take as long as 32 days.[68] Consideration to surgical management should be given if β-hCG levels plateau or rise after several doses of methotrexate with the single-dose regimen or four doses of methotrexate with the multidose regimen. Patients who experience significant increases in abdominal pain, hemodynamic instability, or decreases in hematocrit should be managed surgically.

Side-effects of methotrexate

In addition to pain, methotrexate has many potential side-effects. Since low doses of methotrexate are used, most patients do not experience severe side-effects. Thirty-six per cent of patients who receive methotrexate, though, will experience some side-effects. Most are minor, self-limited problems such as gastrointestinal upset, mild stomatitis, or mild elevations in liver transaminases.[66] While patients receiving the single-dose regimen of methotrexate may experience side-effects less frequently (odds risk 0.79), they experience abdominal pain and hospitalizations at roughly the same rates as in patients receiving the multidose regimen.

Since methotrexate is a folic acid antagonist, its greatest effect is on rapidly dividing cells.[55,59] Side-effects that are often cited but less commonly seen include nausea, vomiting, stomatitis, diarrhea, anorexia, hemorrhagic enteritis, and elevated liver enzymes. Methotrexate can also affect bone marrow, resulting in severe neutropenia, thrombocytopenia, granulocytopenia, and lymphopenia, although these side-effects are rare. Finally, methotrexate can cause nephrotoxicity, interstitial pneumonitis, and, rarely, reversible alopecia. Patients with pre-existing hepatic, renal, hematologic, pulmonary, or bone marrow disease, patients who are breastfeeding, and patients who suffer from alcoholism, therefore, should not be given methotrexate (Table 1.2).

SURGICAL MANAGEMENT

In the past, exploratory laparotomy with salpingectomy was the standard. With advances in surgical care and an emphasis on improving future reproductive outcomes and limiting costs, attention has shifted towards laparoscopy with salpingostomy when possible.[65] The decision to perform a salpingostomy versus salpingectomy depends on the patient's desire for future pregnancy and the degree to which the tube has been damaged. Patients who are hemodynamically unstable are preferably managed by laparotomy.

Initial studies done comparing laparoscopic salpingostomy to laparotomy for ectopic pregnancy individually showed no difference.[77–79] Postoperatively the patients managed by both methods demonstrated equivalent tubal patency and fertility rates.[77,80] However, these studies showed a significant decrease in blood loss, hospital stays, and convalescent periods postoperatively in patients undergoing laparoscopy. Additionally, patients who had undergone laparoscopy developed significantly fewer adhesions postoperatively.[80] A more recent meta-analysis[65] of these initial studies showed laparoscopy to be less effective than laparotomy (RR 0.90) due to a 3.6 times higher rate of persistent trophoblastic activity postoperatively. The persistence of trophoblastic tissue can be reduced by the administration of a single prophylactic dose of systemic methotrexate (1 mg/kg) postoperatively.[81,82] Prophylactic methotrexate significantly reduces the

percentage of patients who will experience tubal rupture and require reoperation. Side-effects are minimal (5.5%).

Tubal patency and fertility rates in patients who were treated by laparoscopic salpingostomy versus open salpingostomy are equivalent.[77–80,83] Reproductive potential in patients who have a salpingostomy compared to salpingectomy is substantially better regardless of laparoscopy or laparotomy, but carries a higher risk of ectopic recurrence. The rate of intrauterine pregnancy after salpingostomy is 61% vs 38% for salpingectomy, while the risk for recurrent ectopic pregnancy is 15% for salpingostomy vs 10% for salpingectomy.[84]

Economics of management

The opportunity to manage patients medically in an outpatient setting made methotrexate an attractive therapeutic option. Initial studies, though, suggested that methotrexate was more cost-effective than laparoscopy only for lower β-hCG values (<3000 mIU/ml) and more costly for higher values.[85–88] More recent studies show that methotrexate is significantly less expensive than laparoscopic surgery, resulting in an average saving of $3011 in the United States[89] and €1297 in Europe[90] per patient. When methotrexate follow-up was factored into the European study, the overall cost saving was 45%.

NON-TUBAL ECTOPIC PREGNANCIES

Abdominal pregnancies

Abdominal ectopic pregnancies account for 1.4% of ectopic pregnancies.[19,20] Of all ectopic pregnancies, they present the greatest risk for mother and fetus, with maternal mortality ranging between 0.5 and 18% and perinatal mortality ranging between 40 and 95%.[91] Compared to all ectopic pregnancies, the risk of death is 7.7 times higher and 90 times higher than associated with an intrauterine pregnancy.[91] Abdominal pregnancies result from primary implantation in the abdomen, or from secondary implantation in the abdomen as a result of tubal abortion or rupture. Presenting symptoms according to one series include abdominal pain (100%), nausea and vomiting (70%), general malaise (40%), and painful fetal movements (40%).[92] The most common physical examination findings include abdominal tenderness (100%), abnormal fetal lie (70%), and a displaced uterine cervix (40%).[92] The gold standard in diagnosis of abdominal pregnancies is laparoscopy. They can be diagnosed by ultrasound, although a high rate of error in diagnosis, up to 60%,[92] has led to increased usage of MRI for this purpose. Early abdominal pregnancies can be managed laparoscopically, while more advanced abdominal pregnancies should be managed with laparotomy. There is still much debate regarding placental management postoperatively. Recovery is most rapid if the placenta can be removed without causing injury to surrounding organs or structures. Other options include allowing placental reabsorption after the administration of methotrexate or preoperative embolization of the placenta and fetus[93] if the pregnancy is diagnosed early enough to warrant termination.

Cervical pregnancies

Cervical ectopic pregnancies are rare, and account for 0.2% of all ectopic pregnancies. After a cervical pregnancy is diagnosed, first-line treatment is systemic single- or multidose methotrexate with an overall success rate of 62%.[94] The success rate of primary methotrexate treatment can be as high as 92% if no fetal cardiac activity is present, or as low as 40% if fetal cardiac activity exists. Factors predisposing patients to an unsatisfactory result with primary methotrexate treatment alone include a gestational age ≥ 9 weeks, a serum β-hCG $\geq 10\,000$ mIU/ml, the presence of fetal cardiac activity, or a crown–rump length greater than 10 mm.[94] In patients in whom one of the above factors is present, localized treatment such as intra-amniotic injection of methotrexate, hyperosmolar glucose, or potassium chloride can reduce treatment failure with methotrexate.[94] Approximately 11% of patients treated with methotrexate may suffer from sudden massive bleeding, 4–28 days after methotrexate administration, secondary to failure of cervical involution after pregnancy termination or tissue necrosis from local methotrexate administration.[94] As a result, the need for surgical intervention including dilatation and curettage or hysterectomy after the administration of methotrexate can be as high as 43% in viable cervical pregnancies and 13% in non-viable cervical pregnancies.[95] Therefore, in patients who fail primary methotrexate treatment or a combination of primary systemic methotrexate and local medical treatment, prophylactic embolization of hypogastric arteries, vaginal ligation of cervical branches, or laparoscopy-assisted ligation of the uterine arteries may reduce the occurrence of massive bleeding.[96] If embolization or any other surgical intervention is the primary intervention, methotrexate should be given to eradicate any residual trophoblasts.[96]

Heterotopic pregnancies

The risk of heterotopic pregnancy is reported as 1 in 10 000 to 1 in 50 000, but can reach as high as 1 in 100 for patients undergoing in vitro fertilization.[18] Diagnosis is complicated by the coexistence of an intrauterine pregnancy, to which symptoms are often attributed;[97] β-hCG values are confounded by the intrauterine pregnancy. Pelvic ultrasound is the most sensitive diagnostic tool for indentifying heterotopic pregnancies.[98] Laparoscopy is the gold standard for heterotopic pregnancies;[99] otherwise, methotrexate can be a first-line agent. Treatment with ultrasound-guided transvaginal injection of KCl or hyperosmolar glucose has been described, but the risk of rupture in tubal heterotopic pregnancies and need for salpingectomy may be as high as 55%.[100] However, success rates in ultrasound-guided transvaginal injection of KCl or hyperosmolar glucose for unusual ectopic pregnancies such as cervical and cornual pregnancies have been described as high as 92%.[101] Injection of KCl or hyperosmolar glucose may be especially useful in interstitial (corneal) or cervical pregnancies when surgical management options could threaten to disrupt the intrauterine pregnancy.

Interstitial pregnancies

Interstitial (cornual) ectopic pregnancies represent 2% of all ectopic pregnancies[19,20] and exhibit a maternal mortality risk of 2–2.5%,[102] which is much higher than the 0.14% mortality rate for ectopic pregnancies overall. They result from implantation of the fertilized ovum in the proximal segment of the fallopian tube that is surrounded by the myometrium of the uterus. As a result of their location and the pliability of the myometrium, interstitial pregnancies can reach a greater gestational age and size before rupture compared to tubal ectopic pregnancies, and the related blood loss can be 2–2.5 times as much.[103] Risk factors are similar to those for any ectopic pregnancy, and include a history of ectopic pregnancy, salpingectomy, in vitro fertilization or ovulation induction, and sexually transmitted infections.[104] Pelvic ultrasound is the main diagnostic tool, and the following criteria on ultrasound can assist in making the diagnosis: an empty uterine cavity, a chorionic sac seen separately and located > 1 cm from the most lateral edge of the uterine cavity, and a thin myometrial layer less than 5 mm surrounding the chorionic sac.[105] In 1993, Ackerman and the other radiologists described the 'interstitial line sign' (an echogenic line extending into the cornual region and abutting the mid-portion of the interstitial mass), which is reported to be 80% sensitive and 98% specific in the diagnosis of interstitial pregnancy.[106] MRI can be used when the diagnosis is not clear from pelvic ultrasound. If neither modality provides a definite diagnosis, laparoscopy or hysteroscopy can be used. Medical management of interstitial pregnancies is possible, with local methotrexate injection exhibiting a higher success rate than systemic methotrexate (91% vs 79%).[107] Additionally, resolution of the β-hCG levels with local injection is three times faster (22±8 days vs 65±52 days).[107] Predicting who may be successfully treated with methotrexate prior to administration is difficult, since patients who are successfully treated and those who fail have similar β-hCG levels and ectopic gestational sac sizes.[107] Traditionally, cornual pregnancies were treated with laparotomy followed by cornual resection or hysterectomy. Now more conservative approaches such as laparoscopy and hysteroscopy have become the primary surgical approach in hemodynamically stable patients.[107] To date, no clear information exists as to the risk of uterine rupture in subsequent pregnancies after medical or surgical treatment of interstitial (cornual) pregnancies.[107]

Ovarian pregnancies

Ovarian pregnancies are uncommon, accounting for 0.2–3.2% of ectopic pregnancies.[19,20] In 1878, Spiegelberg established four pathologic criteria for the diagnosis of ovarian pregnancy: an intact ipsilateral tube separate from the ovary, a gestational sac occupying the position of the ovary, an ovary and gestational sac connected to the uterus by the utero-ovarian ligament, and histological presence of ovarian tissue in the gestational sac wall.[108] Risk factors for ovarian pregnancy include pelvic inflammatory disease, tubal surgery, and oophoritis. Most patients with ovarian pregnancies are younger and of higher parity than their counterparts with non-ovarian ectopic pregnancies, and the use of intrauterine devices is disproportionately high in patients who develop ovarian pregnancies.[109] Pelvic ultrasound is first-line in the diagnosis of ovarian pregnancy, although 75% of early ovarian pregnancies are misdiagnosed as a ruptured corpus luteum cyst.[110] More advanced ovarian pregnancies may present similarly to abdominal pregnancies. Primary treatment consists of laparoscopic ovarian wedge-resection or oophorectomy; an open approach may be used when surgically or clinically indicated. Successful treatment of ovarian pregnancies with systemic methotrexate has been reported in several cases[111] but is not yet widespread.

Cesarean scar pregnancies

Cesarean scar pregnancies, once considered the rarest form of ectopic pregnancy, are becoming increasingly common (1 in 2000 pregnancies).[112] Two out of three patients present with symptoms: most commonly painless vaginal bleeding, then painful vaginal bleeding, and least commonly abdominal pain alone. The sensitivity in diagnosis of cesarean scar pregnancy with pelvic ultrasound is 84.6%, with remaining cases incorrectly diagnosed as cervical pregnancies or spontaneous abortions. In 2000, Vial et al proposed the following ultrasound criteria for diagnosis of cesarean scar pregnancy: (1) the trophoblast is located between the bladder and the anterior uterine wall; (2) fetal parts are not present in the uterine cavity; and (3) on a sagittal uterine view that runs through the amniotic sac, no myometrium is seen between the gestational sac and the urinary bladder (lack of continuity of the anterior uterine wall).[113] Doppler ultrasound and MRI can be used adjunctively to clarify the diagnosis. Given that cesarean scar pregnancy is a relatively new entity in the literature, no standard of treatment has been defined. Expectant management is generally not recommended because of uterine rupture risk.[112] Systemic methotrexate has been successful in 50% of patients with cesarean scar pregnancy in whom it was attempted, and 100% successful in patients with an initial β-hCG less than 5000 mIU/ml.[112] Other medical options include local administration of methotrexate, KCl, or hyperosmolar glucose, and fine needle aspiration of the sac.[112] Laparotomy or laparoscopy with wedge resection, and hysteroscopic resection are all surgical approaches that have reasonable success rates.[112] Dilatation and curettage is often complicated by severe hemorrhage[112] and sequelae.

REPRODUCTION AFTER ECTOPIC PREGNANCY

In women with an unruptured ectopic pregnancy, future reproduction is a concern. Many papers have been published on the issue, but the data are contained only within small case series over the past 30 years; therefore, deriving any meaningful conclusion on the subject has been difficult. The effect of therapeutic

Table 1.4 Reproductive performance following four treatments for ectopic pregnancy: no difference in future reproductive outcome has been shown based on treatment regimen. Adapted from reference 49

Method	Number of Studies	Number of patients	Number with successful resolution	Tubal patency rate	Subsequent intrauterine pregnancy rate	Subsequent ectopic pregnancy rate
Laparoscopic salpingostomy	36	1750	1636 (93%)	170/233 (73%)	477/826 (58%)	105/866 (12%)
Variable-dose methotrexate	12	338	314 (93%)	136/182 (75%)	67/129 (52%)	10/129 (8%)
Single-dose methotrexate	7	393	340 (87%)	61/75 (81%)	39/64 (61%)	5/64 (8%)
Expectant management	15	717	488 (68%)	60/79 (75%)	388/681 (57%)	90/681 (13%)

approach, whether medical, surgical, or expectant, on future reproduction remains unknown. Patients undergoing emergency surgery for ruptured ectopic pregnancy cannot be included in these studies since their treatment options are limited by their clinical circumstance.

Comparison of the success rates of the four most common methods of treatment, laparoscopic salpingostomy (93%), multidose methotrexate (93%), single-dose methotrexate (87%), and expectant management (68%), demonstrates that resolution rates are all relatively equal except for expectant management in the studies containing information on reproductive performance (Table 1.4).[49] When comparing reproductive performance after ectopic pregnancy for the four management methods, all appear comparable. While selection criteria for medical and expectant management in these studies is comparable to those for laparoscopic salpingostomy (the gold standard), patients have never been randomized. Additionally, life-table analyses of pregnancy rates, birth rates, miscarriages, and repeated ectopic pregnancies following any of the four common treatments are not controlled for time, making comparison of these statistics difficult. Future reproductive performance should not factor in treatment selection.

CONCLUSION

The incidence of ectopic pregnancies has significantly increased over the past 60 years and now accounts for 2% of pregnancies. A history of previous ectopic pregnancies, tubal surgery, or infections in symptomatic patients in the first trimester should raise suspicion for ectopic pregnancy. Diagnosis should be performed with pelvic ultrasound first and then comparison to serum β-hCG levels should be undertaken. Patients with serum β-hCG less than 2000 mIU/ml should be followed until their levels exceed 2000 mIU/ml. Determination should then be made that the pregnancy is intrauterine or ectopic. It is suggested that patients with an abnormal rise in β-hCG levels should have a dilatation and curettage if an intrauterine gestation cannot be identified on ultrasound. Multidose intramuscular injection of methotrexate is the first-line treatment in patients who are hemodynamically stable and who have no medical contraindications. Surgical management should be reserved for patients who are hemodynamically unstable, refractory to methotrexate treatment, or unable to follow up appropriately for medical management. Unusual ectopic pregnancies are increasingly documented and their management remains controversial. No one method of management has been shown to enhance reproductive performance after an ectopic pregnancy better than another. Future reproductive performance should not be factored into management decisions.

REFERENCES

1. DeVoe RW, Pratt JH. Simultaneous intrauterine and extrauterine pregnancy. Am J Obstet Gynecol 1948; 56: 1119–26.
2. Current Trends Ectopic Pregnancy – United States, 1990–1992. MMWR Weekly January 27, 1995; 44: 46–8.
3. Centers for Disease Control. Sexually transmitted disease surveillance, 1992. Atlanta, GA: US Department of Health and Human Services, Public Health Service, CDC, July 1993.
4. Churgay CA, Apgar BS. Ectopic pregnancy: an update on technologic advances in diagnosis and treatment. Prim Care 1993; 20: 629–38.
5. Grimes DA. Estimation of pregnancy-related mortality risk by pregnancy outcome, United States, 1991 to 1999. Am J Obstet Gynecol 2006; 194: 92–4.
6. Goldner TE, Lawson HW. Surveillance for Ectopic Pregnancy – United States, 1970–1989. MMWR Weekly December 17, 1993; 42: 73–85.

7. Stovall TG, Kellerman AL, Ling FW, Buster JE. Emergency department diagnosis of ectopic pregnancy. Ann Emerg Med 1990; 19: 1098–103.
8. Ankum WM, Mol BW, Van der Veen F, Bossuyt PM. Risk factors for ectopic pregnancy: a meta-analysis. Fertil Steril 1996; 65: 1093–9.
9. Barnhart KT, Sammel MD, Gracia CR et al. Risk factors for ectopic pregnancy in women with symptomatic first trimester pregnancies. Fertil Steril 2006; 86: 37–43.
10. Mol BWJ, Ankum WM, Bossuyt PMM, Van der Veen F. Contraception and the risk of ectopic pregnancy: a meta-analysis. Contraception 1995; 52: 337–41.
11. Butts S, Sammel M, Hummel A, Chittams J, Barnhart K. Risk factors and clinical features of recurrent ectopic pregnancy: a case control study. Fertil Steril 2003; 80: 1340–4.
12. Mol BW, van der Veen F, Bossuyt PM. Symptom-free women at increased risk of ectopic pregnancy: should we screen? Acta Obstet Gynecol Scand 2002; 81: 661–72.
13. Miller HG, Cain VS, Rogers SM, Gribble JN, Turner CF. Correlates of sexually transmitted bacterial infections among US women in 1995. Fam Plann Perspect 1999; 31: 4–9.
14. Saraiya M, Berg CJ, Kendrick JS et al. Cigarrete smoking as a risk factor for ectopic pregnancy. Am J Obstet Gynecol 1998; 178: 493–8.
15. Clayton HB, Schieve LA, Peterson HB et al. Ectopic pregnancy risk with assisted reproductive technology procedures. Obstet Gynecol 2006; 107: 595–604.
16. Aboud E. A five-year review of ectopic pregnancy. Clin Exp Obstet Gynecol 1997; 24: 127–9.
17. Tal J, Haddad S, Gordon N, Timor- Tritsch I. Heterotopic pregnancy after ovulation induction and assisted reproductive technologies. A literature review from 1971 to 1993. Fertil Steril 1986; 66: 11–12.
18. Lemus JF. Ectopic pregnancy: an update. Curr Opin Obstet Gynecol 2000; 12: 369–75.
19. Breen JL. A 21 year survey of 654 ectopic pregnancies. Am J Obstet Gynecol 1970; 106: 1004–19.
20. Bouyer J, Coste J, Fernandez H, Pouly JL, Job-Spira N. Sites of ectopic pregnancy: a 10 year population-based study of 1800 cases. Hum Reprod 2002; 17: 3224–330.
21. Gracia C, Barnhart K. Diagnosing ectopic pregnancy: decision analysis comparing six strategies. Obstet Gynecol 2001; 97: 464–70.
22. Yeh HC, Goodman JD, Carr L, Rabinowitz JG. Intradecidual sign: a US criterion of early intrauterine pregnancy. Radiology 1986; 161: 463–7.
23. Bradley WG, Fiske CE, Filly RA. The double sac sign of early intrauterine pregnancy: use in exclusion of ectopic pregnancy. Radiology 1982; 143: 223–6.
24. Nyberg DA, Mack LA, Jeffrey RB Jr, Laing FC. Endovaginal sonographic evaluation of ectopic pregnancy: a prospective study. AJR Am J Roentgenol 1987; 149: 1181–6.
25. Russell SA, Filly RA, Damato N. Sonographic diagnosis of ectopic pregnancy with endovaginal probes: what really has changed? J Ultrasound Med 1993; 12: 145–51.
26. Taylor KJ, Meyer WR. New techniques in the diagnosis of ectopic pregnancy. Obstet Gynecol Clin North Am 1991; 18: 39–54.
27. Goldstein SR, Snyder JR, Watson C, Danon M. Very early pregnancy detection with endovaginal ultrasound. Obstet Gynecol 1988; 72: 200–4.
28. Timor-Tritsch IE, Yeh MN, Peisner DB, Lesser KB, Salvik BS. The use of transvaginal ultrasound in the diagnosis of ectopic pregnancy. Am J Obstet Gynecol 1988; 161: 157–61.
29. Barnhart KT, Kamelle SA, Simhan H. Diagnostic accuracy of ultrasound, above and below the beta-hCG discriminatory zone. Obstet Gynecol 1999; 94: 583–7.
30. Seeber BE, Barnhart KT. Suspected ectopic pregnancy. Obstet Gynecol 2006; 17: 399–413.
31. Nagayama M, Watanabe Y, Okumura A et al. Fast MR imaging in obstetrics. Radiographics 2002; 22: 563–80.
32. Ha HK, Jung JK, Kang SJ et al. MR imaging in the diagnosis of rare forms of ectopic pregnancy. AJR Am J Roentgenol 1993; 160: 1229–32.
33. Nishino M, Hayakawa K, Iwasaku K, Takasu K. Magnetic resonance imaging findings in gynecologic emergencies. J Comput Assist Tomogr 2003; 26: 756–61.
34. DeWitt C, Abbott J. Interstitial pregnancy: a potential for misdiagnosis of ectopic pregnancy with emergency department ultrasonography. Ann Emerg Med 2002; 40: 106–9.
35. Kadar N, Caldwell BV, Romero R. A method of screening for ectopic pregnancy and its indications. Obstet Gynecol 1981; 58: 162–6.
36. Seeber BE, Sammel MD, Guo W et al. Application of redefined human chorionic gonadotropin curves for the diagnosis of women at risk for ectopic pregnancy. Fertil Steril 2006; 86: 454–9.
37. Barnhart K, Sammel MD, Chung K et al. Decline of serum human chorionic gonadotropin and spontaneous complete abortion: defining the normal curve. Obstet Gynecol 2004; 104: 975–81.
38. Gelder MS, Boots LR, Younger JB. Use of a single random serum progesterone value as a diagnostic aid for ectopic pregnancy. Fertil Steril 1991; 55: 497–500.
39. Stovall TG, Ling FW, Cope J, Buster JE. Preventing ruptured ectopic pregnancy with a single serum progesterone. Am J Obstet Gynecol 1989; 160: 1425–8.
40. Mol BW, Lijmer JG, Ankum WM, van der Veen F, Bossuyt PM. The accuracy of single serum progesterone measurement in the diagnosis of ectopic pregnancy: a meta-analysis. Hum Reprod 1998; 13: 3220–7.
41. McCord ML, Arheart KL, Muram DM et al. Single serum progesterone as a screen for ectopic pregnancy: exchanging specificity and sensitivity to obtain optimal test performance. Fertil Steril 1996; 66: 513–16.
42. Daponte A, Pournaras S, Zintzaras E et al. The value of a single combined measurement of VEGF, glycodelin, progesterone, PAPP-A, HPL and LIF for differentiating between ectopic and abnormal intrauterine pregnancy. Hum Reprod 2005; 20: 3163–6.
43. Mueller MD, Raio L, Spoerri S et al. Novel placental and non-placental serum markers in ectopic versus normal intrauterine pregnancy. Fertil Steril 2004; 81: 1106–11.
44. Barnhart KT, Katz I, Hummel A, Gracia CR. Presumed diagnosis of ectopic pregnancy. Obstet Gynecol 2002; 100: 505–10.
45. Ries A, Singson P, Bidus M, Barnes JG. Use of the endometrial pipelle in the diagnosis of early abnormal gestations. Fertil Steril 2000; 74: 593–5.
46. Barnhart K, Gracia CR, Reindl B, Wheeler JE. Usefulness of pipelle endometrial biopsy in the diagnosis of women at risk for ectopic pregnancy. Am J Obstet Gynecol 2003; 188: 906–9.
47. Lindahl B, Ahlgren M. Identification of chorion villi in abortion specimens. Obstet Gynecol 1986; 67: 79–81.
48. Condous G, Kirk E, Lu C et al. There is no role for uterine curettage in the contemporary diagnostic workup of women with a pregnancy of unknown location. Hum Reprod 2006; 21: 2706–10.
49. Buster J, Krotz S. Reproductive performance after ectopic pregnancy. Semin Reprod 2007; 25: 131–3.
50. Trio D, Strobelt N, Picciolo C, Lapinski RH, Ghidini A. Prognostic factors for successful expectant management of ectopic pregnancy. Fertil Steril 1995; 63: 469–72.

51. Elvin JA, Crum CP, Genest DR. Complications of early pregnancy, including trophoblastic neoplasia. In: Crum CP, Lee KR, eds. Diagnostic Gynecologic and Obstetric Pathology, 1st edn. Philadelphia: Elsevier Saunders, 2006: 995–1040.

52. Tanaka T, Hayashi H, Kutsuzawa T, Fujimoto S, Ichinoe K. Treatment of interstitial ectopic pregnancy with methotrexate: report of a successful case. Fertil Steril 1982; 37: 851–2.

53. Rodi IA, Sauer MV, Gorrill MJ et al. The medical treatment of unruptured ectopic pregnancy with methotrexate and citrovorum rescue: preliminary experience. Fertil Steril 1986; 46: 811–13.

54. Ory SJ, Villanueva AL, Sand PK, Tamura RK. Conservative treatment of ectopic pregnancy with methotrexate. Am J Obstet Gynecol 1986; 154: 1299–306.

55. Calabresi P, Cahbner BA. Antineoplastic agents. In: Gilman A, Goodman LS, Goodman A, eds. The Pharmacologic Basis of Therapeutics, 8th edn. New York: Macmillan Publishing, 1990: 1275–6.

56. Berlin NI, Rall D, Mead JA et al. Folic acid antagonists: effects on the cell and the patient. Clinical staff conference at National Institutes of Health. Ann Intern Med 1963; 59: 931–56.

57. Walden PA, Bagshawe KD. Pregnancies after chemotherapy for gestational trophoblastic tumours. Lancet 1979; 2: 1241.

58. Hajenius PJ, Engelsbel S, Mol BW et al. Randomised trial of systemic methotrexate versus laparoscopic salpingostomy in tubal pregnancy. Lancet 1997; 350: 774–9.

59. ASRM Practice Committee. Treatment of ectopic pregnancy. Fertil Steril 2006; 86: S96–102.

60. Kovanci E, Buster JE. Ectopic pregnancy. In: Rakel RE, Bope ET, eds. Conn's Current Therapy, 1st edn. Philadelphia: Elsevier Saunders, 2005: 1157–9.

61. Stovall TG, Ling FW, Buster JE. Outpatient chemotherapy of unruptured ectopic pregnancy. Fertil Steril 1989; 51: 435–8.

62. Stovall TG, Ling FW. Single-dose methotrexate: an expanded clinical trial. Am J Obstet Gynecol 1993; 168: 1759–62.

63. Lipscomb GH, Stovall TG, Ling FW. Nonsurgical treatment of ectopic pregnancy. N Engl J Med 2000; 18: 1325–9.

64. Barnhart KT, Gosman G, Ashby R, Sammel M. The medical management of ectopic pregnancy: a meta-analysis comparing 'single dose' and 'multidose' regimens. Obstet Gynecol 2003; 101: 778–84.

65. Hajenius PJ, Mol BW, Bossuyt PM, Ankum WM, Van Der Veen F. Interventions for tubal ectopic pregnancy. Cochrane Database Syst Rev 2000; (2): CD000324.

66. Lipscomb GH, Givens VM, Meyer NL, Bran D. Comparison of multidose and single-dose methotrexate protocols for the treatment of ectopic pregnancy. Am J Obstet Gynecol 2005; 192: 1844–7.

67. Lipscomb GH, McCord ML, Stovall TG et al. Predictors of success of methotrexate treatment in women with tubal ectopic pregnancies. N Engl J Med 1999; 341: 1974–8.

68. Lipscomb GH, Bran D, McCord ML, Portera JC, Ling FW. Analysis of three hundred fifteen ectopic pregnancies treated with single-dose methotrexate. Am J Obstet Gynecol 1998; 178: 1354–8.

69. McKenzie LJ, El-Zimaity H, Krotz S et al. Comparative genomic hybridization of ectopic pregnancies that fail methotrexate therapy. Fertil Steril 2005; 84: 1517–19.

70. Dudley PS, Heard MJ, Sangi-Haghpeykar H, Carson SA, Buster JE. Fertil Steril 2004; 82: 1374–8.

71. Potter MB, Lepine LA, Jamieson DJ. Predictors of success with methotrexate treatment of tubal ectopic pregnancy at Grady Memorial Hospital. Am J Obstet Gynecol 2003; 188: 1192–4.

72. Bixby S, Tello R, Kuligowska E. Presence of a yolk sac on transvaginal sonography is the most reliable predictor of single-dose methotrexate treatment failure in ectopic pregnancy. J Ultrasound Med 2005; 24: 591–8.

73. Atri M, Bret PM, Tulandi T, Senterman MK. Ectopic pregnancy: evolution after treatment with transvaginal methotrexate. Radiology 1992; 185: 749–53.

74. Lipscomb GH, Puckett KJ, Bran D, Ling FW. Management of separation pain after single-dose methotrexate therapy for ectopic pregnancy. Obstet Gynecol 1999; 93: 590–3.

75. Saraj AJ, Wilcox JG, Najmabadi S et al. Resolution of hormonal markers of ectopic gestation: a randomized trial comparing single-dose intramuscular methotrexate with salpingostomy. Obstet Gynecol 1998; 92: 989–94.

76. Natale A, Busacca M, Candiani M et al. Human chorionic gonadotropin patterns after a single dose of methotrexate for ectopic pregnancy. Eur J Obstet Gynecol Reprod Biol 2002; 100: 227–30.

77. Vermesh M, Silva PD, Rosen GF et al. Management of unruptured ectopic gestation by linear salpingostomy: a prospective, randomized clinical trial of laparoscopy versus laparotomy. Obstet Gynecol 1989; 73: 400–4.

78. Lundorff P, Thorburn J, Hahlin M, Kallfelt B, Lindblom B. Laparoscopic surgery in ectopic pregnancy. A randomized trial versus laparotomy. Acta Obstet Gynecol Scand 1991; 70: 343–8.

79. Murphy AA, Nager CW, Wujek JJ et al. Operative laparoscopy versus laparotomy for the management of ectopic pregnancy: a prospective trial. Fertil Steril 1992; 57: 1180–5.

80. Lundorff P, Hahlin M, Kallfelt B, Thorburn J, Lindblom B. Adhesion formation after laparoscopic surgery in tubal pregnancy: a randomized trial versus laparotomy. Fertil Steril 1991; 55: 911–15.

81. Graczykowski JW, Mishell DR Jr. Methotrexate prophylaxis for persistent ectopic pregnancy after conservative treatment by salpingostomy. Obstet Gynecol 1997; 89: 118–22.

82. Gracia CR, Brown HA, Barnhart KT. Prophylactic methotrexate after linear salpingostomy: a decision analysis. Fertil Steril 2001; 76: 1191–5.

83. Vermesh M, Presser SC. Reproductive outcome after linear salpingostomy for ectopic gestation: a prospective 3-year follow-up. Fertil Steril 1992; 57: 682–4.

84. Yao M, Tulandi T. Current status of surgical and nonsurgical management of ectopic pregnancy. Fertil Steril 1997; 67: 421–33.

85. Mol BW, Hajenius PJ, Engelsbel S et al. Treatment of tubal pregnancy in the Netherlands: an economic comparison of systemic methotrexate administration and laparoscopic salpingectomy. Am J Obstet Gynecol 1999; 181: 945–51.

86. Sowter MC, Farquhar CM, Gudex G. An economic evaluation of single dose systemic methotrexate and laparoscopic surgery for the treatment of unruptured ectopic pregnancy. Br J Obstet Gynaecol 1999; 108: 204–12.

87. Nieuwkerk PT, Hajenius PJ, Ankum WM et al. Systemic methotrexate therapy versus laparoscopic salpingostomy in patients with tubal pregnancy. Part I. Impact on patients' health related quality of life. Fertil Steril 1998; 70: 511–17.

88. Nieuwkerk PT, Hajenius PJ, Van der Veen F et al. Systemic methotrexate therapy versus laparoscopic salpingostomy in tubal pregnancy. Part II. Patient preferences for systemic methotrexate. Fertil Steril 1998; 70: 518–22.

89. Morlock RJ, Lafata JE, Eisenstein D. Cost-effectiveness of single-dose methotrexate compared with laparoscopic treatment of ectopic pregnancy. Obstet Gynecol 2000; 95: 407–12.

90. Lecuru F, Robin F, Chasset S et al. Direct cost of single dose methotrexate for unruptured ectopic pregnancy. Prospective comparison with laparoscopy. Eur J Obstet Gynecol Reprod Biol 2000; 88: 1–6.

91. Atrash HK, Friede A, Hogue CJ. Abdominal pregnancy in the United States: frequency and maternal mortality. Obstet Gynecol 1987; 69: 333–7.

92. Rahman MS, Al-Suleiman SA, Rahman J, Al-Sibai MH. Advanced abdominal pregnancy–observations in 10 cases. Obstet Gynecol 1982; 59: 366–72.

93. Rahaman J, Berkowitz R, Mitty H et al. Minimally invasive management of an advanced abdominal pregnancy. Obstet Gynecol 2004; 103: 1064–8.

94. Hung TH, Shau WY, Hsieh TT et al. Prognostic factors for an unsatisfactory primary methotrexate treatment of cervical pregnancy: a quantitative review. Hum Reprod 1998; 13: 2636–42.

95. Kung FT, Chang SY. Efficacy of methotrexate treatment in viable and nonviable cervical pregnancies. Am J Obstet Gynecol 1999; 181: 1438–44.

96. Kung FT, Lin H, Hsu TY et al. Differential diagnosis of suspected cervical pregnancy and conservative treatment with the combination of laparoscopy-assisted uterine artery ligation and hysteroscopic endocervical resection. Fertil Steril 2004; 81: 1642–9.

97. Botta G, Fortunato N, Merlino G. Heterotopic pregnancy following administration of human menopausal gonadotropin and following in vitro fertilisation and embryo transfer: two case reports and a review of the literature. Eur J Obstet Gynaecol Reprod Biol 1995; 59: 211–15.

98. Em F, Gersovich EO. High resolution ultrasound in thediagnosis of heterotopic pregnancy combined transabdominal and transvaginal approach. BJOG 1993; 100: 871–2.

99. Wang PH, Chao HT, Tseng JY. Laparoscopic surgery for heterotopic pregnancies: a case report and a brief review. Eur J Obstet Gynaecol Reprod Biol 1998; 80: 267–71.

100. Goldstein JS, Ratts VS, Philpott T, Dahan MH. Risk of surgery after use of potassium chloride for treatment of tubal heterotopic pregnancy. Obstet Gynecol 2006; 107: 506–8.

101. Doubilet PM, Benson CB, Frates MC, Ginsburg E. Sonographically guided minimally invasive treatment of unusual ectopic pregnancies. J Ultrasound Med 2004; 23: 359–70.

102. Rock JA, Thompson JD. TeLinde's Operative Gynecology, 8th edn. Philadelphia: Lippincott-Raven, 1997.

103. Felmus LB, Pedowitz P. Interstitial pregnancy: a survey of 45 cases. Am J Obstet Gynecol 1953; 66: 1271–9.

104. Tulandi T, Al-Jaroudi D. Interstitial pregnancy: results generated from the Society of Reproductive Surgeons Registry. Obstet Gynecol 2004; 103: 47–50.

105. Timor-Tritsch IE, Monteagudo A, Matera C, Veit CR. Sonographic evolution of cornual pregnancies treated without surgery. Obstet Gynecol 1992; 79: 1044–9.

106. Ackerman TE, Levi CS, Dashefsky SM, Holt SC, Lindsay DJ. Interstitial line: sonographic finding in interstitial (cornual) ectopic pregnancy. Radiology 1993; 189: 83–7.

107. Lau S, Tulandi T. Conservative medical and surgical management of interstitial ectopic pregnancy. Fertil Steril 1999; 72: 207–15.

108. Spiegelberg O. Zur Casuistik der Ovarialschwangerschaft. Arch Gynaekol 1878; 13: 73–9.

109. Hallatt JG. Primary ovarian pregnancy: a report of twenty-five cases. Am J Obstet Gynecol 1982;143: 55–60.

110. Jonathan S, Adashi BE, Hillard PA. Novak's Textbook of Gynaecology, 12th edn. Baltimore: Williams & Wilkins, 1999: 512–13.

111. Mittal S, Dadhwal V, Baurasi P. Successful medical management of ovarian pregnancy. Int J Gynaecol Obstet 2003; 80: 309–10.

112. Rotas MA, Haberman S, Levgur M. Cesarean scar ectopic pregnancies: etiology, diagnosis, and management. Obstet Gynecol 2006; 107: 1373–81.

113. Vial Y, Petignat P, Hohlfeld P. Pregnancy in a cesarean scar. Ultrasound Obstet Gynecol 2000; 16: 592–3.

2 Pregnancy loss and termination

Melissa A Simon

INTRODUCTION

The approach to management of abnormal pregnancies is important to master. The techniques of medical or surgical uterine evacuation are similar regardless of the indication for the procedure. The indications for uterine evacuation or pregnancy termination can be divided into four categories: elective/therapeutic, fetal indications (diagnosis of genetic/structural abnormalities), fetal demise (failure of development), maternal indications (e.g. Eisenmenger syndrome), or ectopic location of pregnancy.

This chapter aims to outline the management of abnormal pregnancies and methods of pregnancy termination. Management of ectopic pregnancy is reviewed in Chapter 1.

PREGNANCY LOSS

Spontaneous abortion (SAB), also known as miscarriage, refers to a pregnancy that ends spontaneously before the 20th week of gestation.[1] The World Health Organization defines it as expulsion or extraction of an embryo or fetus weighing 500 g or less from its mother. The frequency of non-viable or non-continuous intrauterine pregnancies is higher than initially estimated, with reported rates ranging from 20 to 62%.[2]

Epidemiology

SAB is the most common complication of early pregnancy.[1] Eight to 20% of clinically recognized pregnancies less than 20 weeks' gestation will result in a spontaneous abortion; 80% of these occur in the first trimester.[3,4] The risk of SAB after 15 weeks is approximately 0.6% for chromosomally and structurally normal fetuses.[5] These statistics vary according to maternal age and ethnicity.

Numerous factors are associated with an increased risk of pregnancy loss: age, previous spontaneous abortion, smoking, alcohol, gravidity, cocaine, non-steroidal anti-inflammatory drugs, fever, caffeine, prolonged ovulation to implantation interval, prolonged time to pregnancy, and low folate level.

Two per cent of pregnant women lose two consecutive pregnancies. Only 0.4–1% of women have three consecutive losses.[6] The recurrence rate of miscarriage is about 20% after one miscarriage, 28% after two miscarriages, and 43% after three or more.[7] When a woman has repeated miscarriages of three or more clinically recognized pregnancies (or two or more in some instances such as advanced maternal age) a workup is warranted. Recurrent pregnancy loss is an important condition; however, the cause of it can only be determined in about 50% of patients.[8] Chromosomal anomalies are the most common reason for recurrent pregnancy loss. Other etiologies of recurrent pregnancy loss include genetic, uterine, endocrine, immunologic, thrombophilic, and environmental factors. Further in depth discussion is outside the scope of this chapter.

Etiology of spontaneous abortion

One-third of the products of conception from spontaneous abortions occurring at or before 8 weeks are 'blighted' or anembryonic. When an embryo is found, about one-half are abnormal, dysmorphic, stunted, or too macerated for examination.[9]

Chromosomal abnormalities account for about one-half of miscarriages (Table 2.1) Most of these are aneuploidies, and arise de novo. Structural abnormalities, mosaicism, and single gene defects are responsible for relatively few abortions. Cytogenetic defects are more common in earlier-age abortions. Abnormal fetal karyotype is 50% at 8–11 weeks' gestation and is 30% at 16–19 weeks.[10] The most frequent types of abnormalities are: autosomal trisomies (52%); monosomy X (19%); polyploides (22%); other (7%).

Spontaneous abortion may also be caused by host factors such as congenital or acquired uterine abnormalities (septum, submucosal leiomyoma, intrauterine adhesions) that interfere with optimal implantation and growth of the embryo. Maternal infection such as with *Listeria monocytogenes*, *Toxoplasma gondii*, parvovirus B19, rubella, herpes simplex, cytomegalovirus, or lymphocytic chroriomeningitis virus can also lead to abortion. Maternal endocrinopathies (thyroid dysfunction, Cushing's syndrome, polycystic ovarian syndrome) can also contribute to suboptimal host environment.

Table 2.1   Etiology of spontaneous abortion

Etiology	Comment
Chromosomal abnormalities	50–60% of SABs are associated with chromosomal anomalies: autosomal trisomy is the most common finding, monosomy X is the next most common
Maternal factors	Medical disorders (e.g. diabetes mellitus, infections) Drug use (e.g. tobacco and alcohol use) Environmental conditions (small studies: arsenic, lead, formaldehyde, benzene, ethylene oxide) Immunological factors (autoimmune or alloimmune) Inherited thrombophilia (e.g. factor V Leiden mutation) Aging gametes Uterine abnormalities (including location of fibroids; in utero exposure to diethylstilbestrol (DES); some uterine septa; incompetent cervix)
Paternal factors	Little is known: chromosomal translocations in sperm can lead to SAB

Table 2.2   Categories of spontaneous abortion

Term	Contents of uterus	Cervical os
Threatened abortion	Vaginal bleeding only	Closed
Missed abortion	Fetus and products of conception retained	Closed
Incomplete abortion	Retained products of conception	Open
Inevitable abortion	Uterine contractions, ± fluid, ± bleeding	Open

A hypercoaguable state due to inherited or acquired thrombophilia and abnormalities of the immune system that lead to immunological rejection or placental damage are under investigation.

Diagnosis

Vaginal bleeding is common in the first trimester of pregnancy (up to 20–40% of pregnant women).[11] It is also the most predictive sign of an impending pregnancy loss. Bleeding in the first trimester may be light, heavy, intermittent, or constant. It may be painless or painful.

The differential diagnosis of pregnancy loss includes: physiologic; ectopic pregnancy; impending miscarriage; cervical, vaginal or, uterine pathology.

Physical examination can help reveal the source of bleeding (trauma, polyp, cervicitis, neoplasia). Direct visualization of a cervix which is dilated or products of conception lead the differential towards inevitable, incomplete, or complete abortion (Table 2.2). Ultrasound examination can provide additional, sometimes unexpected, information such as multiple gestations, heterotopic pregnancy, or retained products of conception. A definitive diagnosis of a missed abortion or non-viable intrauterine pregnancy is made upon either of the following: absence of fetal cardiac activity in an embryo with crown–rump length greater than 5 mm; or absence

of a fetal pole when the mean sac diameter is greater than 25 mm measured transabdominally or greater than 18 mm by transvaginal ultrasound.[12,13]

Differentiation of normal and abnormal pregnancies

Transvaginal ultrasonography is the cornerstone of evaluation of bleeding in early pregnancy. It is used for distinguishing intrauterine from extrauterine (ectopic) and viable from non-viable pregnancies.

Measurement of human chorionic gonadotropin (hCG) concentration in the serum is helpful especially in the case where ultrasound is non-diagnostic (meaning the site and viability of pregnancy are not evident). A single hCG measurement is never diagnostic; serial measurements are necessary. Serial hCG measurements showing declining βhCG concentrations are consistent with both a non-viable intrauterine pregnancy or an ectopic pregnancy. However, these serial serum hCG measurements alone cannot distinguish between an intrauterine and an ectopic pregnancy.

Management

Pregnant women at less than 20 weeks' gestation with vaginal bleeding are managed expectantly until resolution of their symptoms, a definitive diagnosis of non-viable pregnancy is made, or there is progression to an inevitable, incomplete, or complete abortion.

There are no therapeutic interventions that prevent pregnancy loss in the first trimester. There is no evidence from a randomized controlled trial that bed rest is beneficial.[14] Hormonal supplements such as progesterone, although promising, are currently still under investigation for their effectiveness in preventing early pregnancy loss.[15]

Suspected septic abortion should be managed by stabilizing the patient, obtaining blood and endometrial cultures, and administering parenteral broad-spectrum

Table 2.3 Selected broad-spectrum parenteral antibiotic regimens

Single agent regimens	Multiagent regimens
Ticarcillin clavulanate 3.1 g every 4 hours	Clindamycin 900 mg every 8 hours, gentamicin 5 mg/kg/day with or without ampicillin 2 g every 4 hours
Piperacillin tazobactam 4.5 g every 6 hours	Ampicillin and gentamicin and metronidazole 500 mg every 8 hours
Imipenem 500 mg every 6 hours	Levofloxacin 500 mg daily and metronidazole 500 mg every 8 hours

antibiotics (Table 2.3). The uterine contents should be surgically evacuated. Delay in evacuation and treatment may cause morbidity and mortality. Failure to treat a septic abortion could result in a pelvic abscess or clostridial necrotizing myonecrosis (gas gangrene). Such a complications may result in a laparotomy and possible hysterectomy. Nevertheless, it is important to distinguish such a condition from mild endometritis, which is usually marked by a low grade fever and mild uterine tenderness. Mild infection can be managed with oral broad-spectrum antibiotics.

Tissue that is passed should be examined to confirm whether or not it is a product of conception. Placental villi can be difficult to tell apart from some clots. One way to distinguish villi is to place the products in water and see if they 'float'.

Intervention should not be necessary following a complete spontaneous abortion. However, complete abortions are sometimes difficult to distinguish from incomplete abortions. As a result, some providers will perform aspiration/curettage in all of these patients, although there is no evidence of benefit from these interventions.

Women with incomplete, inevitable, or missed abortions can be managed expectantly, medically, or surgically. Systematic reviews of randomized trials of all three of these management modalities concluded that all therapies were effective.[16,17] The risk of infection is not an important variable in choosing the therapeutic approach as evidenced by the MIST (miscarriage treatment) trial which compared surgical, medical, and expectant management of failed pregnancy in 1200 women and reported that the incidence of infection was 2–3% for all three groups.[18]

Expectant management

Expectant management is a viable alternative for women with early pregnancy failure with stable vital signs and no signs of infection or hemorrhage. A systematic review from the Cochrane database concluded from five randomized trials that expectant management was associated with a higher risk of incomplete miscarriage, need for unplanned surgical emptying of the uterus, and bleeding.[17] Nevertheless, this review concluded that it is not an unreasonable approach, especially with respect to patient preference.

The majority of expulsions occur in the first 2 weeks after diagnosis; however, some women may require more prolonged follow-up.[19] An interval of up to 3–4 weeks is not uncommon. Many women are willing to wait, depending on the counseling they receive and how well they are prepared for what to expect.[20]

Medical or surgical treatment can be administered if expectant management does not result in expulsion of the products of conception. There are no universally defined criteria for an empty uterus. Some providers proceed with surgical uterine evacuation if retained tissue with a diameter of more than 15 mm is present,[21] while there is no evidence that increased endometrial thickness is predictive of morbidity in asymptomatic women.[22] If the ultrasound reveals retained tissue and the patient is asymptomatic, then surgical evacuation or expectant management for another 2 weeks is an acceptable form of management.

The largest series evaluating expectant management outcomes involved 1096 patients with suspected first trimester miscarriage followed for up to 4 weeks.[23] Each pregnancy was diagnosed by transvaginal ultrasound. Women who did not have a complete miscarriage were offered expectant management or surgical evacuation. Successful spontaneous abortion occurred in 81% of all expectantly managed patients, 91% of those with incomplete miscarriages, 76% of those with missed abortions, and 66% of those with anembryonic pregnancies. Complications (such as infection and excessive pain or bleeding) occurred in 1% of expectantly and 2% of surgically managed patients.

Medical management

Effective medical therapies for inducing abortion have created new options for women who want or need to avoid surgery. Although not approved by the United States Food and Drug Administration for treatment of early pregnancy failure, misoprostol (Cytotec®) is the most commonly used agent. The advantages of misoprostol are cost-effectiveness, low incidence of side-effects when given intravaginally, stability at room temperature, and availability.[24]

The efficacy of misoprostol for medical management of pregnancy failure in the first trimester has been recently illustrated in a large, well-designed trial. A total of 652 women with missed, incomplete, or inevitable abortions were randomly assigned 3:1 to receive 800 μg of misoprostol intravaginally or undergo vacuum aspiration.[25] Misoprostol was repeated on day 3 if expulsion was incomplete by ultrasound; vacuum aspiration was performed on day 8 if expulsion was still incomplete. In medically managed patients, complete expulsion occurred in 71% by day 3 and 84% by day 8. Pregnancy duration did not affect the rate of successful expulsion, but successful expulsion was lower with anembryonic gestations compared to incomplete or inevitable abortions (81 vs 93%). Most importantly, both medical and surgical therapies were safe, effective, and acceptable to patients.

A combination of mifepristone (progesterone antagonist) and misoprostol has also been used. One prospective cross-over trial reported complete expulsion of missed abortion in almost 75% of patients with either misoprostol alone or a combination of misoprostol and mifepristone.[26] The long-term conception rate and pregnancy outcome are similar for women who undergo medical or surgical evacuation for early pregnancy failure.[27]

Surgical management

Surgery is necessary for women who have excessive bleeding, unstable vital signs, or obvious signs of infection. Whether the uterus should be evacuated in uncomplicated cases needs to be determined by comparative studies that juxtapose different treatment approaches and consider the type of miscarriage (incomplete or complete), the gestational age, the clinical status, and preferences of the mother. If the ultrasound shows an empty uterus and the bleeding is minimal, no further action is needed.

The traditional surgical treatment of first or early second trimester failed pregnancy is dilatation and curettage (D&C) or dilatation and evacuation (D&E). The immediate purpose of surgical management is to prevent potential hemorrhagic and infectious complications from the retained products of conception.[28] Risks of anesthesia, uterine perforation, infection, and bleeding are the most common. Less common risks of surgical management include intrauterine adhesions and cervical trauma. Surgical management is appropriate for women who do not want to wait for spontaneous or medically induced abortion. If the patient is unstable, such as with hemorrhage or sepsis, surgical management should not be delayed. Suction aspiration is the preferred method of D&C rather than sharp curettage since it holds greater morbidity potential.[29] Doxycycline is the preferred antibiotic to be administered for surgical abortion management.

Recommended regimens include 100 mg 12 hours apart for two doses, or 100 mg 12 hours apart for six doses. A meta-analysis showed that peri-abortal antibiotics reduce infection rates by 42%.[30]

FETAL DEMISE: SECOND AND THIRD TRIMESTERS

For fetal demise (traditionally defined as a demise that is ≥ 20 weeks' gestation), D&E has multiple advantages over labor induction. Such benefits range from improved safety to efficiency to patient satisfaction. Moreover, a D&E is marked by a significantly shorter operating time as opposed to a potentially prolonged labor induction method. Most patients find D&E less stressful physically and emotionally.[31] Although some women elect to have labor induction to avoid surgery, the need for surgical aspiration or curettage to treat incomplete abortion is 15–30% or higher.

From a patient perspective, the choice between D&E and labor induction is dependent on multiple factors. Patients with anomalous fetuses may find much anguish in the prospect of a long induction, or they may decide that their grieving process would best be aided by holding the fetus after an induction. From a provider perspective, D&E places a greater emotional burden on the surgeon and support staff.[32] Moreover, many physicians who provide obstetric and gynecologic services are not trained or not willing to perform this procedure.[33]

In terms of pathological diagnosis, data indicate that D&E does not interfere with such diagnosis except for a few rare anomalies.[34] Thus, choosing the best way to manage uterine evacuation depends on the availability of skilled personnel, the indication for uterine evacuation, patient and provider preference, and other factors. Softening of the cortical bone after a fetal demise may make the uterine evacuation technically easier. With labor induction, intervals from induction to abortion tend to be shorter in these cases (however, still longer than a D&E). Regardless of the evacuation method used, a coagulopathy evaluation is recommended since fetuses that have been demised for 4 or more weeks may cause consumptive coagulopathies.[35]

PREGNANCY TERMINATION

With the recent Food and Drug Administration (FDA) approval of an implantable contraceptive device, chewable contraceptive pills, limited approval of emergency contraception over the counter, and with numerous other contraceptives in clinical trials, contraception is currently the most effective and convenient that it has ever been. Nevertheless, the available methods are not perfect. Even the most conscientious contraceptive users can experience contraceptive failure.

Epidemiology

In the mid-20th century, vacuum aspiration led to much safer abortion and, beginning in Asia, induced abortion was gradually legalized in developed countries. In the late 1960s, California, New York, and other states rewrote their abortion laws. The US Supreme Court in 1973 in the 'Roe versus Wade' decision limited the circumstances under which 'the right to privacy' could be restricted by local abortion laws. By 1980, legal abortion became the most common surgical procedure performed in the USA.

Half of all pregnancies in American women are unintended: four in 10 unintended pregnancies end in abortion.[36] About half of American women have experienced an unintended pregnancy, and at current rates, 35% will have had an abortion by age 45.[37] Overall, unintended pregnancy rates have been stagnant over the last 10 years, yet unintended pregnancy increased by 29% among poor women while decreasing 20% among higher-income women.[38] There were 1.29 million abortions in 2002 down from 1.36 million abortions in 1996.[38] This is partly because the number of pregnancies in the USA has been decreasing and the proportion of reproductive-age women under age 30 is also decreasing.

Nine in 10 abortions occur in the first trimester of pregnancy.[37] The proportion of abortions performed in hospitals has steadily declined. According to a recent study, 56% of women have abortions in their 20s; 61% have one or more children; 67% have never married; 57% are economically disadvantaged; 88% live in a metropolitan area; and 78% report a religious affiliation.[39] The most common reasons for choosing abortion are that having a baby would interfere with work, school, or other responsibilities; inability to afford a child; and not wanting to be a single parent or having problems with a husband or partner.[40]

Epidemiologic and public health research has consistently demonstrated that the legalization of abortion reduced maternal morbidity and mortality more than any single development since the advent of antibiotics to treat puerperal infections and blood banking to treat hemorrhage. The number of American women reported as dying from abortion declined from nearly 300 deaths in 1961 to only about 11 in 1991 or, rather, 0.8 deaths for every 100 000 legal abortions.[41] The most important determinants of mortality related to abortion are gestational age and type of anesthesia administered; that is, more advanced gestational ages and general anesthesia are more prone to complications.[42,43]

As with mortality, morbidity rates vary primarily with gestational age of the pregnancy, but other factors are important as well, including: type of operation, age of patient, type of anesthesia, surgeon's skill, and method of cervical dilatation. More experienced surgeons and younger, healthier women are less likely to have complications.

The possibility that abortion can result in longer-term complications has been examined in numerous studies. There is no evidence suggesting that vacuum aspiration adversely affects fertility[44] or pregnancies,[45] or increases the risk for ectopic pregnancy.[46] The psychological sequelae of elective abortion have been studied and debated. Unequivocal evidence indicates that depression is less frequent among women post-abortion compared with postpartum.[47] In studies that avoid recall bias, the risk of breast cancer is identical in women with and without induced abortions.[48]

Pre-management workup

The care of the patient who has decided to terminate a pregnancy begins with the diagnosis of an intrauterine pregnancy and an accurate estimation of gestational age. Most women who want to terminate their pregnancy in the first trimester are good candidates for local anesthesia and the procedure done in an outpatient setting.

Preoperative considerations include location; laboratory tests; imaging; antibiotic prophylaxis; and anesthesia. Uterine evacuation can be performed safely in freestanding clinics or office-based settings.[40] A comprehensive patient history and complete physical examination with a special focus on the uterine size and position are important starting points. Then, there should be confirmation of pregnancy via urine or serum hCG, and sonographic visualization of an intrauterine pregnancy. Together with menstrual history, the bimanual uterine examination should help the provider conclude the gestational age. Preoperative ultrasonography is especially useful if there is a discrepancy between uterine size and gestational age, there is uncertain fetal viability, or the diagnosis is in doubt (e.g. ectopic or hydatidiform mole).

The patient's hematocrit/hemoglobin and Rh(D) status are the two most important laboratory tests to obtain. Many providers screen for sexually transmitted infections at the time of examination prior to the procedure and treat accordingly.

Pregnancy options counseling

Counseling has a key role in pregnancy termination care. No matter where the pregnancy termination is performed, there must be someone available for adequate and accurate counseling. A counselor should be available to help facilitate decision making, as well as provision of accurate information about the procedure, obtaining informed consent, provision of emotional support before, during, and after the procedure, and provision of information about contraception. A non-directive discussion of alternatives including continuing the pregnancy or adoption is also important.[49] Informed consent should include the possibilities of common adverse outcomes: incomplete abortion, infection, uterine perforation, the need for laparotomy, ectopic pregnancy, and failed abortion.

Some states have mandatory waiting times between when the patient is counseled and the actual procedure, and some states require parental notification for pregnancy terminations in minors. Minors have a right to seek a court order authorizing the pregnancy termination. Other states mandate that specific subjects be covered in the counseling session. It is important that abortion providers are informed about the local and federal laws covering their practice.

Possible management options

Uterine evacuation is an integral part of obstetric and gynecologic care. The choice of technique for uterine evacuation depends more upon uterine volume and operator experience than the underlying indication for the procedure. The most commonly used technique for first trimester pregnancy termination is vacuum aspiration.

Hysterectomy and hysterotomy are rarely performed for pregnancy termination and are less safe than extraction procedures or medical management.

Medical management

Vacuum aspiration is a safe and effective method for pregnancy termination but is not available everywhere. Some women find it hard to undergo a surgical procedure or to go to a clinic where they may be subject to loss of privacy or harassment. Medical options help make pregnancy termination available to more

Table 2.4 Eligibility criteria for medical termination of pregnancy (according to manufacturer Danco Laboratories)

Pregnancy up to 49 days' gestation
Agreement to undergo surgical abortion if the procedure fails
Absence of a contraindication to surgical abortion
Agreement to complete therapy and all clinic visits
A means of reaching an emergency facility within 1 hour if problems occur
Legal competence to sign a consent form for obtaining an abortion

women and improve the circumstances under which pregnancies are terminated (Tables 2.4 and 2.5).

The progesterone antagonist mifepristone (RU 486) and the antimetabolite methotrexate have both been demonstrated to induce abortion early in pregnancy when combined with a prostaglandin.

Mifepristone's major action is its blockade of progesterone receptors in the endometrium. This leads to a disruption of the embryo and the production of prostaglandins. The disruption of the embryo and perhaps a direct action on the trophoblast lead to a decrease in hCG and a withdrawal of support from the corpus luteum. The success rate is dependent on the length of pregnancy – the more dependent is the pregnancy on progesterone from the corpus luteum, the more likely is the progesterone antagonist, mifepristone, to result in abortion.

The FDA-approved regimen of medication abortion with mifepristone includes a single 600-mg oral dose of mifepristone followed 2 days later by the oral administration of 400 μg of misoprostol (a stable, orally active synthetic analogue of prostaglandin E1, available commercially for the treatment of peptic ulcer). The patient is then required to follow-up 14 days later. This regimen is approved up through 49 days of gestation. In the large US trial of 600 mg of mifepristone followed by 400 μg of misoprostol, given orally, there was a 1% failure rate under 7 weeks of pregnancy and 9% at 8–9 weeks.[50]

Many studies have shown that alternative regimens to this FDA-approved protocol are equally safe and effective. The most common regimen modification decreases the dose of mifepristone to 200 mg and misoprostol is then taken 1, 2, or 3 days later.[51] Based on worldwide experience, the regimen with the fewest side-effects and least cost, but equally good efficacy, is a combination of a lower dose of oral mifepristone (200 mg) and, 36–48 hours later, the vaginal administration of 800 μg misoprostol.[52] Other studies have demonstrated that this modified protocol is effective up to 63 days of gestation.[53]

Table 2.5 Advantages and disadvantages of medication versus surgical approaches to pregnancy termination

Method	Advantages	Disadvantages
Medication abortion	Used early during pregnancy	Often requires at least two clinic visits
	Resembles a natural miscarriage	Takes days to complete
	Often considered more private	Efficacy decreases at later gestational ages
	Usually avoids aspiration intervention	Women may see blood clots and the products of conception
	Anesthesia not required	Mifepristone and/or methotrexate may not be available
	High success rates (for mifepristone/ misoprostol and methotrexate/ misoprostol regimens)	Mifepristone can be expensive
Aspiration abortion	High success rate (>99%)	Involves an invasive procedure
	May require only one clinic visit	May not be available very early in pregnancy
	Procedure completed within minutes	Often considered to be 'less private'
	Sedation is available	

To date, there is no FDA-approved protocol for the use of methotrexate and misoprostol to terminate an early pregnancy. However, many clinical trials have shown that the methotrexate/misoprostol regimen is approximately 95% effective in terminating pregnancies $\leq$49 days' gestation.[54] The most common evidence-based regimen is with intramuscular injection (50 mg/m^2) or oral administration (50 mg) of methotrexate. Three to 7 days later 800 μg of misoprostol is administered vaginally. Follow-up with the provider is 7 days after administration of the methotrexate, and misoprostol is repeated once if no abortion has occurred. Aspiration abortion is performed if the abortion is not complete after repeat misoprostol.

A final alternative medication abortion regimen uses misoprostol only. Research throughout Latin America and East Asia has explored vaginal and sublingual regimens, different dosing schedules, and different doses. These studies have shown that misoprostol alone is effective (72% after one dose, 86% after two doses, 88% after three doses), and the most commonly used regimen is vaginal administration of 800 μg every 24 hours for up to three doses in gestational ages up to 56 days.[55]

For medical uterine evacuation at >15 weeks of gestation, systemic or intra-amniotic abortifacients such as intravaginal prostaglandins, intra-amniotic saline, or prostaglandin F2α are administered to induce labor. Although the optimal regimen has not been determined, it appears that 200–600 μg of misoprostol administered vaginally every 12 hours or 400 μg of misoprostol given vaginally every 3 hours (maximum five doses) successfully induces labor in the second trimester.[56] A misoprostol dose of 100 μg every 12 hours results in success rates that approach 100% in the third trimester induction of a fetal demise.[57] For fetal death near term, a dose of 50 μg of misoprostol every 12 hours may be adequate for induction of labor.

It is important to emphasize that providers who use non-surgical methods of termination must be prepared to utilize surgical techniques of uterine evacuation when there are retained products of conception.

Surgical management

Suction aspiration is the safest technique of surgical uterine evacuation. Prior to aspiration, the cornerstone to sound surgical management is proper cervical management. Dilatation of the cervix is usually necessary prior to surgical abortion to allow atraumatic insertion of instruments and removal of uterine contents. Very early pregnancies may not require cervical dilatation (up to 7 weeks). Between 7 and 13 weeks, either the cervical canal can be manually dilated or osmotic dilators can be used to gradually dilate the cervix. Osmotic dilators are recommended for all second trimester surgical procedures.

Mechanical dilatation is performed using instrument sets with progressively increasing diameters (Pratt; Denniston; Hegars: less preferred because they are not tapered). Mechanical dilatation is believed to be more traumatic to the cervix than other methods.[58]

Some surgeons recommend the preoperative insertion of cervical tents. These are osmotic dilators of dried seaweed (*Laminaria japonica*) or synthetic hydrophilic substances (Dilapan™, Lamicel®) that are left in place from a few hours to overnight. Osmotic dilators function by absorbing moisture from the cervix, gradually enlarging the endocervical canal, and softening the cervix. Utilization of osmotic dilators results in a fivefold reduction in cervical trauma – especially lacerations – when compared to manual dilatation.[58]

As the cervix dilates with osmotic dilators, endogenous prostaglandins are released.[59] These also facilitate the dilatation process.

Despite reduced trauma, osmotic dilators must be placed several hours prior to the procedure to effect adequate cervical change. The diameter of *Laminaria* increases by 25% if left in place for 4 hours and by 90% if left in place overnight.[60] Synthetic dilators achieve optimal dilatation in 6–8 hours. Manual dilatation is performed immediately before evacuation of the uterus.

Laminaria is usually placed with a paracervical block, and the cervix may be held with an Allis clamp, tenaculum, or ring forceps. *Laminaria* is inserted into the endocervical canal after preparing with povidone-iodine. Some cramping is common. The *Laminaria* should then be packed in place with 1–2 gauze sponges. The patient should avoid both intercourse and submerging her pelvis in water. Failure to remove the *Laminaria* within 48 hours can result in severe infection.

Misoprostol can also be used to help prepare the cervix prior to aspiration.[61] A dose of misoprostol 400 μg given vaginally 3–4 hours prior to the procedure has been found to be effective in ripening the cervix to the equivalent of one medium-sized *Laminaria* placed for 4 hours.[62,63] Randomized trial data suggest that *Laminaria* is more effective than misoprostol alone in achieving cervical dilatation in second trimester procedures.[64] *Laminaria* placement in second trimester procedures resulted in greater mean initial dilatation, less need for additional dilatation, and faster procedure times in nulliparous women. Nevertheless, patients preferred same-day misoprostol for both convenience and comfort over *Laminaria* placement.

Other agents used in cervical preparation include isosorbide dinitrate and mifepristone. Isosorbide dinitrate has had mixed results compared with prostaglandins.[65] The use of mifepristone as an agent in promoting cervical dilatation has been shown to be somewhat effective, but is off-label and should only be recommended in the case of clinical investigations.[66]

In the case of an anomaly of the cervix or uterus, or abnormal uterine contents such as a molar pregnancy, concurrent sonography can be performed during the actual uterine evacuation.

Dilatation and evacuation (D&E) is the term used for the surgical procedure for second trimester terminations. The medical termination of second trimester pregnancies includes vaginal, intramuscular, or intra-amniotic administration of prostaglandins (as discussed earlier in this chapter) and intra-amniotic injection of hypertonic saline or urea. D&E is safer and less expensive than the medical methods and is better tolerated and preferred by patients.[67] Training, experience, and skill of the surgeon are the primary factors that limit the gestational age at which surgical abortion can be safely performed. Advanced gestational age by itself incurs risks for all types of complications. These are multiplied when the duration of pregnancy is discovered after beginning uterine evacuation to be beyond the experience and skill of the surgeon or capacity of the equipment.

Anesthesia

Anesthesia for the procedure ranges from a paracervical block to conscious sedation.[68] Local anesthesia with or without conscious sedation is adequate for most first trimester procedures. Most second trimester uterine evacuations require some sedation. Fentanyl and/or midazolam are viable options for conscious sedation because of their rapid onset and short duration. There is evidence from histological and neurophysiological studies that the fetus does not feel pain prior to the third trimester.[69] Moreover, there are no proven regimens to provide fetal analgesia or anesthesia directly or transplacentally.

The administration of NSAIDs (non-steroidal anti-inflammatory drugs) 1 hour prior to the procedure can reduce discomfort.[70,71] Paracervical block is placed by injecting about 10–20 ml of anesthetic agent (1% lidocaine) at 4 and 8 o'clock (some providers have different variations of placement including the 12 and 6 o'clock positions; it is also important to note the use of negative pressure prior to injection of the anesthetic agent to prevent intravascular administration). If using lidocaine, the maximum dose is 4.5 mg/kg body weight or 20 ml for a 50-kg woman). Ten milliliters of 1% lidocaine reach peak plasma level at about 10–15 minutes post-injection.[72] A vasovagal reaction can occur following cervical manipulation, especially after the administration of a paracervical block. Such an episode is marked by bradycardia, rapid recovery, and no post-ictal state. (Atropine can be used to treat such episodes.)

Some providers add synthetic vasopressin (Pitressin®) to the injectable anesthetic to reduce blood loss intraoperatively.[73]

Spinal, epidural, or general anesthesia may be used if the patient desires or if required because of probable extensive uterine manipulation. These types of anesthesia are considered, in general, to be not as safe as local anesthesia, but modern advances have overall decreased anesthesia-related morbidity. The CDC (Centers for Disease Control and Prevention) reported that over 1972–1991, anesthesia accounted for 35% of first trimester abortion-related deaths, while hemorrhage, infection, and thromboembolism accounted for only 15%.[74]

Postoperative care

Patients should be observed for at least 30 minutes to 1 hour after the surgical evacuation. Women who are Rh negative and unsensitized should receive Rh(D) immunoglobulin following the procedure. Some providers administer agents (such as Methergine® and Pitressin) prophylactically to prevent uterine atony and hemorrhage after the procedure.

Women should be informed that they will have cramping and vaginal bleeding comparable to that with menstrual flow. All patients should be able to contact someone on a 24-hour basis. Most complications occur within the first week of the procedure. Pelvic rest is recommended for 2 weeks post-procedure. The provider should be contacted if menses has not returned by about 6 weeks after the termination. Light vaginal bleeding can persist for approximately 2 weeks after the evacuation of uterine contents. Serum hCG values return to normal within 2–4 weeks.

It is usually advised that trials to become pregnant should resume after the first normal menses or 2–3 months post-uterine evacuation. Many studies have shown no risk of adverse outcomes with a shorter interpregnancy interval.[75]

Importantly, any type of contraception including an intrauterine device may be started immediately post-abortion completion.[76]

Complications

Postoperative complications (Table 2.6) of elective terminations are classified as either immediate or delayed. Uterine perforation and uterine atony are immediate complications. Delayed complications can occur several hours to several weeks after operation. These usually present with bleeding, pain, and continuing symptoms of pregnancy.

Perforation   The procedure should stop if a perforation is suspected and evaluation should proceed via either laparoscopy or laparotomy. The location of uterine perforation tends to determine the extent of hemorrhage and the patient's symptoms. Most (two-thirds) perforations occur in the fundal area and are undetected

Table 2.6   Complications of pregnancy termination[77]

Complication	Per 100 000 induced abortions
Major complications (hospitalization required)	
Retained tissue	27.7
Sepsis	21.2
Uterine perforation	9.4
Hemorrhage	7.1
Inability to complete procedure	3.5
Intrauterine + tubal pregnancy	2.4
Minor complications (managed in clinic or office)	
Mild infection	462
Re-aspiration same day	180.8
Re-aspiration later	167.8
Cervical stenosis	16.5
Cervical laceration	10.6
Underestimated gestation	6.5
Convulsive seizure	4.0

since bleeding is often minimal. A lateral perforation may result in profound hemorrhage and possibly a broad ligament hematoma. Performance of the procedure by an experienced surgeon and use of preoperative cervical dilatation with osmotic dilators are two factors associated with decreased risk of perforation.[78]

Bleeding   The most common cause of unusually heavy post-abortion bleeding is retained products of conception. Rates in large series vary from 0.2 to 6%.[77] Patients with retained products of conception occasionally present several weeks after an abortion, but most report excessive bleeding within 1 week. Severe pain or pelvic tenderness suggests that infection is also present. Treatment is prompt aspiration of the uterus with the largest cannula that will pass through the cervix.

Infection   Infection is sometimes marked by uterine bleeding. Fever and uterine tenderness are the most common signs of post-abortal endometritis, occurring in about 0.5% of cases. Some studies indicate that prophylactic antibiotics reduce the risk of post-abortal infection.[79] Most clinicians agree that women at risk of pelvic infection benefit from the use of prophylactic antibiotics prior to induced abortion. A meta-analysis of antibiotics at the time of induced abortion unequivocally concluded that prophylactic antibiotics should be routinely used without exceptions.[80] Because gonorrhea and chlamydia as well as other diseases can cause post-abortion infection, a tetracycline such as doxycycline is the best drug for prophylaxis. There is no consensus on the optimal duration of post-procedure antibiotic prophylaxis. In some randomized trials, 3 days appeared to be as effective as 7, and 1 day was more effective than placebo.[81,82] Metronidazole has been tested and is effective treatment for patients with bacterial vaginosis detected at the time of abortion.

Patients who present with uterine tenderness, fever, and bleeding require uterine aspiration as well as antibiotic treatment. Patients who have fevers above 38°C (101°F) and signs of peritoneal inflammation, as well as uterine tenderness, require hospitalization and intravenous antibiotics active against anaerobes, gonorrhea, and chlamydia. Outpatient treatment with doxycycline twice a day for 14 days should be given to those patients with localized tenderness to the uterus.

Dysfunctional uterine bleeding following abortion
Women may present with uterine bleeding without signs of retained products of conception or infection. The bleeding itself can be treated hormonally; aspiration/curettage is rarely necessary unless bleeding is extensive.

Ectopic pregnancy   Failure to diagnose ectopic pregnancy at the time of induced abortion can cause a patient to return with complaints of persistent bleeding with or without pelvic pain. Careful examination of the uterine aspirate for villi at the time of abortion should make a missed ectopic pregnancy an unusual cause of delayed bleeding. If, however, a patient presents with this possibility, quantitative measurement of hCG and vaginal ultrasonograpy should be performed for accurate diagnosis and management.

Cervical stenosis (hematometra)   Patients who experience amenorrhea or hypomenorrhea and cyclic uterine pain after first trimester abortion may have stenosis of the internal cervical os. Usually there is immediate postoperative pain without any vaginal bleeding. Examination reveals a large globular uterus. This occurs in about 0.02% of cases and is more common among those carried out early in the first trimester with minimal cervical dilatation. This condition is treated with cervical dilatation with Pratt dilators under paracervical block.

Other late complications   Amenorrhea without pain can also be caused by Asherman's syndrome, destruction and scarring of the endometrium. This condition is very rare and usually follows endometrial infection. This problem is best diagnosed and treated at hysteroscopy.

Rh sensitization   Sensitization of Rh negative women should be prevented. About 4% of these women become sensitized following induced abortion (the later the

Table 2.7   Maternal mortality. Adapted from reference 84

Type of pregnancy	Death rate
Legal pregnancy termination	0.567 per 100 000 terminations
Miscarriage	1.19 per 100 000 miscarriages
Live birth	7.06 per 100 000 live births
Ectopic pregnancy	31.9 per 100 000 ectopic pregnancies

abortion, the higher the proportion). Subsequent hemolytic disease of the newborn can be prevented by administering Rh immunoglobulin to all Rh negative, Du negative women undergoing early abortion.

Despite these complications, surgical abortion is a safe procedure. Elective abortion at any gestational age is safer for the mother than carrying a pregnancy to term (Table 2.7). First trimester abortions are safer than second trimester procedures (0.1–0.4 deaths per 100 000 first trimester procedures versus 1.7–8.9 deaths per 100 000 procedures).[83] Deaths in developing countries where abortion is illegal account for a significant percentage of maternal deaths worldwide. The World Health Organization reports that one out of eight maternal deaths is due to abortion-related complications.

CONCLUSION AND KEY POINTS

There is good evidence from randomized trials that surgical, medical, and expectant management of incomplete, inevitable, or missed abortion all result in evacuation of products of conception in most patients. Surgical management is a more successful primary therapy over medical or expectant management. The effectiveness of expectant or medical management is dependent on the time allowed before secondary surgical intervention and upon the type of non-viable pregnancy. Patients with septic abortions should be stabilized, be administered broad-spectrum antibiotics, and undergo surgical evacuation of uterine contents.

Post-abortal infection rates are low for all three treatment modalities, and the frequency of other complications is low. Therefore, the choice of treatment, as long as the patient is stable and not septic, should be placed in the hands of the patient.

A review of 10 studies of the long-term impact of uterine evacuation by suction aspiration in the first trimester found that women whose first pregnancy, ended in induced abortion had no greater risk of bearing low birth weight babies, delivering prematurely, or suffering spontaneous abortions in subsequent pregnancies than women who carried their first pregnancy to term.[85] Two series addressing future pregnancy in women who had undergone a prior second trimester uterine evacuation using *Laminaria* to dilate the cervix did not report any cases of spontaneous mid-trimester loss or an increased risk of spontaneous preterm birth.[86,87]

Relief, transient guilt, sadness, and a sense of loss are the most common emotional reactions after pregnancy termination.[88] There is no good evidence from large surveys that choosing to terminate over full term delivery of an unwanted first pregnancy places women at higher risk of subsequent depression.[89]

Safe abortion is still unavailable to many women in the developing world. Therefore, many women resort to clandestine, unsafe abortions, accounting for about one-fifth of the world's maternal mortality. These deaths are preventable. Family planning services that provide effective contraceptive choices as well as access to safe abortion early in pregnancy are essential in order for societies to achieve desired fertility rates and a healthy female population.

REFERENCES

1. Regan L, Rai R. Epidemiology and the medical causes of miscarriage. Baillieres Best Pract Res Clin Obstet Gynaecol 2000; 14: 839–54.
2. Zinaman MJ, Clegg ED, Brown CC et al. Estimates of human fertility and pregnancy loss. Fertil Steril 1996; 65: 503–9.
3. Wilcox AJ, Weinberg CR, O'Connor JF et al. Incidence of early loss of pregnancy. N Engl J Med 1988; 319: 189–94.
4. Wang X, Chen C, Wang L et al. Conception, early pregnancy loss, and time to clinical pregnancy: a population based prospective study. Fertil Steril 2003; 79: 577–84.
5. Wyatt PR, Owolabi T, Meier C, Huang T. Age-specific risk of fetal loss observed in a second trimester serum screening population. Am J Obstet Gynecol 2005; 192: 240–6.
6. Salat-Baroux J. Recurrent spontaneous abortions. Reprod Nutr Dev 1988; 28: 1555–68. [in French]
7. Regan L, Braude PR, Trembath PL. Influence of past reproductive performance on risk of spontaneous abortion. BMJ 1989; 299 (6698): 541–5.
8. Cook CL, Pridham DD. Recurrent pregnancy loss. Curr Opin Obstet Gynecol 1995; 7: 357–66.
9. Fantel AG, Shepard TH. Morphological analysis of spontaneous abortuses. In: Bennett MJ, Edmonds DK, eds. Spontaneous and Recurrent Abortion. Oxford: Blackwell Scientific Publications, 1987: 8–28.
10. Hsu LYF. Prenatal diagnosis of chromosomal abnormalities through amniocentesis. In: Milunsky A, ed. Genetic Disorders and the Fetus, 4th edn. Baltimore: The Johns Hopkins University Press, 1998: 179–248.
11. Strobino B, Pantel-Silverman J. Gestational vaginal bleeding and pregnancy outcome. Am J Epidemiol 1989; 129: 806–15.
12. Goldstein SR. Significance of cardiac activity on endovaginal ultrasound in very early embryos. Obstet Gynecol 1992; 80: 670–2.
13. Filly RA. Ultrasound evaluation during the first trimester. In: Callen PW, ed. Ultrasonography in Obstetrics and Gynecology, 3rd edn. Philadelphia: WB Saunders Co, 1998: 63–85.
14. Aleman A, Althabe F, Belizan J, Bergel E. Bed rest during pregnancy for preventing miscarriage. Cochrane Database Syst Rev 2005; (2): CD003576.
15. Oates-Whitehead RM, Hass DM, Carrier JA. Progestogen for preventing miscarriage. Cochrane Database Syst Rev 2003; (4): CD003511.
16. Sotiriadis A, Makrydimas G, Papatheodorou S, Ioannidis JP. Expectant, medical or surgical management of first trimester miscarriage: a meta-analysis. Obstet Gynecol 2005; 105: 1104–13.
17. Nanda K, Peloggia A, Grimes DA et al. Expectant care versus surgical treatment of miscarriage. Cochrane Database Syst Rev 2006; (2): CD003518.
18. Trinder J, Brockelhurst P, Porter R et al. Management of miscarriage: expectant, medical or surgical? Results of randomized controlled trial (miscarriage treatment (MIST) trial). BMJ 2006; 332: 1235–40.
19. Banerjee S, Aslam N, Woelfer B et al. Expectant management of early pregnancies of unknown location: a prospective evaluation of methods to predict spontaneous resolution of pregnancy. BJOG 2001; 108: 158–63.
20. Creinin MD, Schwartz JI, Guido RS, Pymar HC. Early pregnancy failure – current management concepts. Obstet Gynecol Surv 2001; 56: 105–13.
21. Nielsen S, Hahlin M. Expectant management of first trimester spontaneous abortion. Lancet 1995; 345: 84–6.
22. Creinin MD, Harwood B, Guido RS et al. Endometrial thickness after misoprostol use for early pregnancy failure. Int J Gynaecol Obstet 2004; 86: 22–6.
23. Luise C, Jermy K, May C et al. Outcome of expectant management of spontaneous first trimester miscarriage: observational study. BMJ 2002; 324: 873–5.
24. Graziosi GC, van der Steeg JW, Reuwer PH et al. Economic evaluation of misoprostol in the treatment of early pregnancy failure compared to curettage after an expectant management. Hum Reprod 2005; 20: 1067–71.
25. Zhang J, Gilles JM, Barnhart K et al. A comparison of medical management with misoprostol and surgical management of early pregnancy failure. N Engl J Med 2005; 353: 761–9.
26. Gronlund A, Gronlund L, Clevin L et al. Management of missed abortion: comparison of medical treatment with either mifepristone + misoprostol or misoprostol alone with surgical evacuation. A multi-center trial in Copenhagen county, Denmark. Acta Obstet Gynecol Scand 2002; 81: 1060–5.
27. Tam WH, Tsui MH, Lok IH et al. Long-term reproductive outcome subsequent to medical versus surgical treatment for miscarriage. Hum Reprod 2005; 20: 3355–9.
28. Hemminki E. Treatment of miscarriage: current practice and rationale. Obstet Gynecol 1998; 91: 247–53.
29. Grimes DA. Unsafe abortion: the silent scourge. Br Med Bull 2003; 67: 99–113.
30. Sawaya GF, Grady D, Kerlikowske K, Grimes DA. Antibiotics at the time of induced abortion: the case of universal prophylaxis based on a meta-analysis. Obstet Gynecol 1996; 87: 884–90.
31. Freeman EW. Abortion: subjective attitudes and feelings. Fam Plann Perspect 1978; 10: 150–5.
32. Kaltreider NB, Goldsmith S, Margolis AJ. The impact of midtrimester abortion techniques on patients and staff. Am J Obstet Gynecol 1979; 135: 235–8.
33. Stubblefield PG. Pregnancy termination. In: Gabbe SG, Nieble JR, Simpson JL, eds. Obstetrics: Normal and Problem Pregnancies. New York: Churchill-Livingstone, 1996: 1249–78.
34. Shulman LP, Ling FW, Meyers CM et al. Dilation and evacuation for second-trimester genetic pregnancy termination. Obstet Gynecol 1990; 75: 1037–40.
35. Mishell DR Jr. Spontaneous and recurrent abortion: etiology, diagnosis and treatment. In: Mishell DR Jr, Stenchever MA,

Droegemueller W et al, eds. Comprehensive Gynecology, 3rd edn. St Louis: Mosby, 1997: 403–30.

36. www.agi-usa.org/pubs/fb_induced_abortion.html. accessed 12/15/06.

37. Finer LB, Henshaw SK. Abortion incidence and services in the United States in 2000. Perspect Sex Reprod Health 2003; 35: 6–15.

38. Boonstra HD, Benson-Gold R, Richards CL, Finer LB. Abortion in Women's Lives. New York: Guttmacher Institute, 2006.

39. Jones RK, Darroch JE, Henshaw SK. Patterns in the socio-economic characteristics of women obtaining abortions in 2000–01. Perspect Sex Reprod Health 2002; 34: 226–35.

40. Grimes DA, Cates W Jr, Selik RM. Abortion facilities and the risk of death. Fam Plann Perspect 1981; 13: 30–2.

41. Lawson H, Frye A, Atrash H et al. Abortion mortality, United States, 1972 through 1987. Am J Obstet Gynecol 1994; 171: 1365–72.

42. Buehler J, Schulz K, Grimes D, Mogue C. The risk of serious complications from induced abortion: do personal characteristics make a difference? Am J Obstet Gynecol 1985; 153: 14–20.

43. Grimes DA, Schulz KF, Cates W Jr, Tyler CW Jr. Local versus general anesthesia: which is safer for performing suction curettage abortions? Am J Obstet Gynecol 1979; 135: 1030–5.

44. Stubblefield P, Monson R, Schoenbaum S et al. Fertility after induced abortion: a prospective follow-up study. Obstet Gynecol 1984; 63: 186–93.

45. Frank PI, McNamee R, Hannaford PC et al. The effect of induced abortion on subsequent pregnancy outcome. Br J Obstet Gynaecol 1991; 98: 1015–24.

46. Atrash HK, Strauss LT, Kendrick JS et al. The relation between induced abortion and ectopic pregnancy. Obstet Gynecol 1997; 89: 512–18.

47. Dagg PK. The psychological sequelae of therapeutic abortion-denied and completed. Am J Pscyhiatry 1991; 148: 578–85.

48. Melbye M, Wohlfahrt J, Olsen JH et al. Induced abortion and the risk of breast cancer. N Engl J Med 1997: 336: 81–5.

49. Chervenak FA, McCullough LB. Ethics in fetal medicine. Baillieres Best Pract Res Clin Obstet Gynaecol 1999; 13: 491–502.

50. Spitz IM, Bardin CW, Benton L et al. Early pregnancy termination with mifepristone and misoprostol in the United States. N Engl J Med 1998; 338: 1241–7.

51. Schaff E, Fielding SL, Westhoff C et al. Vaginal misoprostol administered 1, 2, or 3 days after mifepristone for early medical abortion: a randomized trial. JAMA 200; 284: 1948–53.

52. Ashok PW, Penney GC, Flett CM, Templeton A. An effective regimen for early medical abortion: a report of 2000 consecutive cases. Hum Reprod 1998; 13: 2962–5.

53. Newhall E, Winikoff B. Abortion with mifepristone and misoprostol: regimens, efficacy, acceptability and future directions. Obstet Gynecol 2000; 183: S44–53.

54. Pymar H, Creinin M. Alternatives to mifepristone regimens for medical abortion. Am J Obstet Gynecol 2000; 183: S54–64.

55. Jain JK, Dutton C, Harwood B et al. A prospective randomized, double-blinded, placebo-controlled trial comparing mifepristone and vaginal misoprostol to vaginal misoprostol alone for elective termination of early pregnancy. Hum Reprod 2002; 17: 1477–82.

56. Goldberg AG, Greenberg MB, Darney PD. Misoprostol and pregnancy. N Engl J Med 2001; 344: 38–47.

57. Bugalho A, Bique C, Machungo F, Faaundes A. Induction of labor with intravaginal misoprostol in intrauterine fetal death. Am J Obstet Gynecol 1994; 171: 538–41.

58. Schulz KF, Grimes DA, Cates W Jr. Measures to prevent cervical injury during suction curettage abortion. Lancet 1983; 1: 1182–5.

59. Uldberg N, Ulmsten U. The physiology of cervical ripening and cervical dilation and the effect of abortifacient drugs. Baillieres Clin Obstet Gynaecol 1990; 4: 263–82.

60. Krammer J, O'Brien WF. Mechanical methods of cervical ripening. Clin Obstet Gynecol 1995; 38: 280–6.

61. Sharma S, Refaey H, Stafford M et al. Oral versus vaginal misoprostol administered one hour before surgical termination of pregnancy: a randomized controlled trial. BJOG 2005; 112: 456–60.

62. Singh K, Fong YF, Prasad RN, Dong F. Randomized trial to determine optimal dose of vaginal misoprostol for preabortion cervical priming. Obstet Gynecol 1998; 92: 795–8.

63. MacIsaac L, Grossman D, Balistreri E, Darney PA. A randomized controlled trial of laminaria, oral misoprostol, and vaginal misoprostol before abortion. Obstet Gynecol 1999; 93: 766–70.

64. Goldberg AB, Drey EA, Whitaker AK et al. Misoprostol compared with laminaria before early second-trimester surgical abortion: a randomized trial. Obstet Gynecol 2005; 106: 234–41.

65. Arteaga-Troncoso G, Villegas-Alvarado A, Belmont-Gomez A et al. Intracervical application of nitric oxide donor isosorbide dinitrate for induction of cervical ripening: a randomized controlled trial to determine clinical efficacy and safety prior to first trimester surgical evacuation of retained products of conception. BJOG 2005; 112: 1615–19.

66. Ashok PW, Flett GM, Templeton A. Mifepristone versus vaginally administered misoprostol for cervical priming before first trimester termination of pregnancy: a randomized, controlled study. Am J Obstet Gynecol 2000; 183: 998–1002.

67. Peterson WF, Berry FN, Grace MR, Gulbranson CL. Second trimester abortion by dilation and evacuation: an analysis of 11 747 cases. Obstet Gynecol 1983; 62: 185–90.

68. Stubblefield PB, Carr-Ellis S, Borgatta L. Methods for induced abortion. Obstet Gynecol 2004; 104: 174–85.

69. Lee SJ, Ralston HJ, Drey EA et al. Fetal pain: a systematic multidisciplinary review of the evidence. JAMA 2005; 294: 947–54.

70. Li CF, Wong CY, Chan CP, Ho PC. A study of co-treatment of nonsteroidal anti-inflammatory drugs (NSAIDs) with misoprostol for cervical priming before suction termination of first trimester pregnancy. Contraception 2003; 67: 101–5.

71. Creinin MD, Shulman T. Effect of non-steroidal anti-inflammatory drugs on the action of misoprostol in a regimen for early abortion. Contraception 1997; 56: 165–8.

72. Blanco LJ, Reid PR, King TM. Plasma lidocaine levels following paracervical infiltration for aspiration abortion. Obstet Gynecol 1982; 60: 506–8.

73. Keder LM. Best practices in surgical abortion. Am J Obstet Gynecol 2003; 189: 418–22.

74. Koonin LM, Smith JC, Ramick M et al. Abortion Surveillance – United States, 1993 and 1994. MMWR CDC Surveill Summ 1997; 46 (SS-4): 37–98.

75. Goldstein RR, Croughan MS, Robertson PA. Neonatal outcomes in immediate versus delayed conceptions after spontaneous abortion: a retrospective case series. Am J Obstet Gynecol 2002; 186: 1230–4.

76. Grimes DA, Shulz KA, Stanwood N. Immediate post-abortal insertion of intrauterine devices. Cochrane Database Syst Rev 2000; (2): CD001777.

77. Hakim-Elahi E, Tovell H, Burnhill M. Complications of first trimester abortions: a report of 170 000 cases. Obstet Gynecol 1990; 76: 129–35.

78. Grimes DA, Schulz KF, Cates WJ Jr. Prevention of uterine perforation during curettage abortion. JAMA 1984; 251: 2108–11.

79. Park TX, Flock M, Schulz KF, Grimes DA. Preventing febrile complications of suction curettage abortion. Am J Obstet Gynecol 1985; 152: 252–5.

80. Sawaya GF, Grady D, Kerlikowske K, Grimes DA. Antibiotics at the time of induced abortion: the case of universal prophylaxis based on a meta-analysis. Obstet Gynecol 1996; 87: 884–90.

81. Lichtenberg ES, Schott S. A randomized clinical trial of prophylaxis for vacuum abortion: 3 versus 7 days of doxycycline. Obstet Gynecol 2003; 101: 726–31.

82. Levallois P, Rioux JE. Prophylactic antibiotics for suction curettage abortion: results of a clinical controlled trial. Am J Obstet Gynecol 1988; 158: 100–5.
83. Bartlett LA, Berg CJ, Shulman HB et al. Risk factors for legal induced abortion-related mortality in the United States. Obstet Gynecol 2004; 103: 729–37.
84. Grimes DA. Estimation of pregnancy-related mortality risk by pregnancy outcome, United States, 1991 to 1999. Am J Obstet Gynecol 2006; 194: 92–4.
85. Hogue CJ, Cates W Jr, Tietze C. The effects of induced abortion on subsequent reproduction. Epidemiol Rev 1982; 4: 66–94.
86. Kalish RB, Chasen ST, Rosenzwig LB, Rashbaum WK. Impact of midtrimester dilation and evacuation on subsequent pregnancy outcome. Am J Obstet Gynecol 2002; 187: 882–5.
87. Schneider D, Halperin R, Langer R, Caspi E. Abortion at 18–22 weeks by laminaria dilation and evacuation. Obstet Gynecol 1996; 88: 412–14.
88. Stotland NL. Psychosocial aspects of induced abortion. Clin Obstet Gynecol 1997; 40: 673–86.
89. Korenromp MJ, Christiaens GC, van den Bout J et al. Long-term psychological consequences of pregnancy termination for fetal abnormality: a cross-sectional study. Prenat Diagn 2005; 25: 253–60.

3 Chronic pelvic pain

Paolo Vercellini, Raffaella Daguati, and Annalisa Abbiati

INTRODUCTION

Chronic pelvic pain (CPP) is a frequent and important disorder of both women and men that may negatively affect health-related quality of life. Whereas in men the etiology is usually referable to bacterial or non-bacterial chronic prostatytis,[1,2] in women several causes are recognized, although in a not neglibile proportion of patients a definite diagnosis cannot be made.[3]

Prevalence figures of CPP in the general female population differ greatly according to several variables, including definition, country, and socioeconomic status[4]. Several definitions have been adopted based on duration of symptoms, cyclicity, location of pain, type of discomfort, and negative physical or laparoscopic findings.[5,6]

Six months of pain is a common standard for chronic diseases and, therefore, could be used to define CPP.[7] In fact it is approximately at this time that the behavioral and emotional changes seen in patients with CPP become clinically important.[5] However, even a 3-month period has been adopted.[8] Both cut-off limits are arbitrary and not validated. Most investigators prefer to include only non-cyclic symptoms in the definition, since pain which has exquisitely cyclic characteristics, such as dysmenorrhea, is generally caused by a specific disease (e.g. endometriosis). A further discrimination should be made between spontaneous and elicited pain. Women who describe symptoms which are solely related to sexual intercourse (i.e. dyspareunia) are usually excluded. With regard to location and comorbidity, the American College of Obstetricians and Gynecologists has endorsed the following detailed definition of CPP: 'noncyclic pain of 6 or more months' duration that localizes to the anatomic pelvis, anterior abdominal wall at or below the umbilicus, the lumbosacral back, or the buttocks and is of sufficient severity to cause functional disability or lead to medical care'.[9]

Based on 40 high quality studies with representative samples, the reported rate of non-cyclical pelvic pain varies from 2.1 to 24% in least, less, and developed countries.[4] The variation in geographical distribution may be related to study characteristics and quality, age groups included, and definitions used, rather than intrinsic differences in the prevalence of CPP between the different populations. Alternatively, the variable findings may be explained by differences in prevalence of sexually transmitted infections, availability of medical or other resources, or cultural differences.[4]

According to a recent systematic literature review, [10] several risk factors are associated with CPP, including drug or alcohol abuse, miscarriage, heavy menstrual flow, pelvic inflammatory disease, previous cesarean section, pelvic pathology, abuse, and psychological comorbidity.

Overall, CPP is a common gynecologic problem with an estimated prevalence of 38 per 1000 in women aged 15–73, a rate higher than that of migraine 21/1000 and comparable to that of asthma (37/1000) and chronic back pain (41/1000).[11] CPP is the single most common indication for referrals to gynecology clinics, accounting for 20% of all appointments in secondary care, and constiues the indication for 12% of all hysterectomies and over 40% of gynecologic diagnostic laparoscopies.[12] In a Gallup poll of 5325 US women, 16% reported CPP, 11% limited their home activity, 12% limited their sexual activity, 16% took medications, and 4% missed at least 1 day of work per month.[13] An estimated 274 million dollars is spent annually on the management of this condition in the UK National Health System[14] and 881 million a year on its outpatient management in the USA.[13] Direct and indirect costs may total over 2 billion dollars per year.[13] CPP may cause prolonged suffering and disability, with consequent loss of employment, family conflicts, repetitive unsuccessful treatments, and serial ineffective surgical procedures.

CPP is frustrating not only for patients but also for physicians, who are usually in desperate search for some pathologic lesion in order to clarify the clinical condition and avoid admitting their incapability to explain the very cause of symptoms. However, even when anything 'abnormal' is finally found, it does not necessarily mean that it is the source of the complaints referred by the woman. On the other hand, many subjects with inconclusive diagnostic investigations are too often erroneously labeled with a psychogenic cause of their pain, thus further increasing the patient's disappointment.

A rational approach to the differential diagnosis and management of CPP may limit the number of investigations, referrals to various specialists, and undue surgical procedures, and may avoid prolonged suffering and limit the cost of management.

PATHOPHYSIOLOGY

Different neurophysiological mechanisms are involved in the pathophysiology of CPP. Pain may be classified as nociceptive or non-nociceptive. In the first case the symptom originates from stimulation of a pain-sensitive structure, whereas in the second, pain is considered neuropathic or psychogenic.[15,16] Nociceptive pain may be further subclassified into somatic or visceral subtypes. Somatic pain originates from the abdominal wall as well as pelvic muscles, bones, and joints, and is transmitted along sensory fibers. This type of pain is usually well localized and generally described as sharp. Visceral pain originates from intraperitoneal organs and is transmitted through the sympathetic fibers of the autonomic nervous system. It is usually described as poorly localized, dull, or crampy, and is frequently associated with autonomic phenomena such as nausea, vomiting, and sweating.[15,16] Moreover, in many patients the message within the cord may undergo diffuse dispersal, such that the subject experiences the pain over several dermatomes and not only from the one at which the signal originated. Complex interactions occur between reproductive organs, the urinary tract, and the bowel. Inflammation or congestion of the genital organs could enhance pain in viscera, skin, or muscle that share common spinal cord segments, resulting in the so-called viscerovisceral hyperalgesia.[15] This may explain catamenial excerbations of CPP not to be confused with dysmenorrhea.

Neuropathic pain is caused by damage to the central or peripheral nervous system, and usually generates burning, lancinating pain and paresthesias. Allodynia (an exacerbation of pain when a non-painful stimulation is generated) and hyperalgesia (a pain sensation that is out of proportion with the intensity of nociceptor stimulation) are the major manifestations of neuropathic pain. They are characterized by a deplacement to the left of the stimulus/response curve which induces an increase in the pain sensation associated with a lower threshold of pain perception and an increased sensitivity of nociceptors.[17,18] Inflammatory processes may lead to an increase in synthesis of molecules such as nerve growth factor (NGF), its receptor subunit NGFRp75, and the tyrosine kinase receptor Trk-A, which induce

growth of new nerve fibers (neurotropism), as well as induce degranulation of mast cells with release of prostaglandins, interleukins, tumor necrosis factor, transforming growth factor α1, histamine (H), and seratonin and consequent sensitization/activation of sensory nerve fibers. These concomitant mechanisms may cause visceral hyperalgesia, an exaggerated pain response to nociceptive stimuli. Finally, estrogens themselves may have an impact on neurogenic inflammation as well as on peripheral transmission and central delivery and modulation of sensory impulses.[16] This could explain the female predominance in chronic pain disorders in general.

If no possible explanations for the patient's pain are identified, psychogenic origin of the symptom might be considered. When contemplating such diagnosis of exclusion, the definite effect on pain experience of psychologic aspects such as premorbid personality, depression, and behavioral disturbances should be considered.[15,19] It is known that psychologic and behavioral factors may contribute to pain experience.[20] If the patient lacks the capacity to promote the experiences that fascilitate development of emotional expression and healthy interpersonal relationships, she may learn to express both physical and emotional pain in physical terms. The prevalence of depression is high among patients with CPP, with estimates of 30–54% as compared to baseline rates of 5–17% in the general population.[15] It is unclear whether the pain–depression relationship is related to the specific diagnosis of pain or if it correlates better to the presence of a chronic illness, because elevated rates of depression are also related to other severe chronic medical conditions. Personality disorders have an important impact on behavioral response to pain and are negative predictors for response to therapy and return to functionality.[15]

ETIOLOGY

Many disorders of the reproductive tract, urological organs, and gastrointestinal, musculoskeletal, and psychoneurological systems may be associated with CPP (Table 3.1). Occasionally only one of these disorders is present, and treatment is curative. Commonly pain is associated with several diagnoses and a number of contributing factors need to be considered. Frequently, treatment is not curative in these cases. Often the etiology of CPP is not discernible.[21]

Reviewing all the potential causes of CPP is out of the scope of the present chapter. Five disorders are indicated as the most frequent cause of CPP: endometriosis, postoperative adhesions, pelvic varices,

Table 3.1 Benign causes of chronic pelvic pain

Gynecologic conditions

Endometriosis
Chronic pelvic infection
Pelvic varicosities
Ovarian remnant/retention

Urologic conditions

Interstitial cystitis/painful bladder
Detrusor dyssynergia
Urethral syndrome

Gastrointestinal conditions

Irritable bowel syndrome
Inflammatory bowel diseases
Diverticular disease
Celiac disease
Post-surgical dense adhesions

Musculoskeletal disorders

Abdominal wall myofascial pain (trigger points)
Fibromyalgia
Pelvic floor myalgia (levator ani or piriformis syndrome)
Neuralgia of iliohypogastric, ilioinguinal, or
  genitofemoral nerve
Coccygeal or lumbosacral back pain
Peripartum pelvic pain syndrome

Other

Depression
Visceral hyperalgesia
Somatization disorders
Psychosexual dysfunction (including previous or
  current sexual abuse)
Porphyria

interstitial cystitis (IC), and irritable bowel syndrome (IBS). Endometriosis is addressed in Chapter 7 and will not be delt with here except for its inclusion in the differential diagnostic process of CPP.

Postoperative adhesions

Pelvic adhesions may be caused by acute or chronic inflammatory disorders (i.e. tubo-ovarian infections and endometriosis), or a physicochemical trauma (surgery). The specific role of adhesions associated with chronic pelvic infection and endometriosis in causing CPP is hard to define, since many variables of these two conditions determine the frequency and severity of the symptoms perceived. Accordingly, when addressing adhesions as a potential cause of CPP, postoperative adhesions only will be considered. The economic impact of adhesions is impressive, as in the USA adhesiolysis was the indication for 303836 hospital admissions in a single year,[22] mainly for procedures on the digestive and female reproductive systems, which accounted for 846 415 days of inpatient care and 1.3 billion dollars in hospitalization and surgeon costs.

Adhesions are found in 25–50% of women with CPP, but their role as a cause of pain remains controversial. A review of over 3000 women with CPP and over 2000 controls demonstrated that adhesions are present in 36% of the former and 15% of the latter patients.[23] However, these findings do not explain whether the association is causal or casual. There is still no consensus on the role of postoperative adhesions in generating chronic pain, also because they constitute a very common finding at repetitive surgery in women without CPP.[24] It has been proposed that intraperitoneal adhesions cause pain when they modify the normal anatomic relationships, and when activities such as running or sexual intercourse cause stretching of the peritoneum or visceral serosa at the adhesion's attachment sites.[25] Moreover, adhesions that are dense and vascular are more likely to result in pain.[26]

The peritoneum, when under traction and tension, produces pain as a result of the activation of nociceptors in the adhesion tissue and viscera. Interestingly, it has been shown that adhesions contain nerve fibers. However, pain perception requires a complete and complex neural linking network with the central nervous system, and the mere presence of nerve fibers in some adhesions cannot be taken as direct proof of a causative role. In fact, Kligman et al[27] proved that neural tissue was equally present in patients with adhesions who had pain and in those who were pain free.

Pelvic varices

The pelvic congestion syndrome (PCS) is a cluster of pain symptoms associated with the presence of ovarian and pelvic (internal iliac) varices associated with venous incompetence and reduced venous clearance in the pelvis.[28] The exact pathophysiology is unknown, and links with psychological, sexual, and genetic–biological factors have been hypothesized.[29] According to several studies, up to 30% of patients with CPP have pelvic varices as the sole etiology of their symptoms, and an additional 12% in combination with another pelvic pathology. Soysal et al[30] performed transabdominal and transvaginal ultrasonography, per-uterine phlebography, and laparoscopy in 148 women with CPP and in 30 asymptomatic, sexually active women undergoing tubal sterilization. In 47 patients (31%) with CPP, pelvic congestion was the only abnormality identified. No case of severe pelvic congestion was observed in the control group.

Significant between-group differences in favor of subjects undergoing tubal ligations were observed not only in perceived pain levels, but also in anxiety and depression indicators, as well as in sexual satisfaction descriptors.

The primary problem of pelvic congestion is thought to be incompetence and reflux of pelvic veins secondary to anatomic and hormonal factors.[31] The cause of pain due to pelvic congestion is still unclear, but the most likely explanation is that increased dilatation, concomitant with stasis, leads to the release of local pain-producing substances.[32–34]

Interstitial cystitis

Interstitial cystitis (IC) is a poorly understood chronic inflammatory condition of the bladder whose causes are substantially unknown.[35] Prevalence estimates of IC in the USA range from 10 to 67/100 000 with a female/male ratio of 10:1.[36] IC is characterized by chronic pelvic, suprapubic, perineal, vulvovaginal pain and pressure with urinary urgency, diurnal frequency, and nocturia in the absence of a well-defined cause.[37] Exacerbations of pain can be experienced during or after sexual intercourse.[38] Patients void 8–15 times per day, with an average volume of 70–90 ml. Voiding can occur once or twice per night.[36] IC can affect women of all ages, is predominantly diagnosed among women between 42 and 46 years, and usually becomes symptomatic in women in their mid-30s.[39] Symptoms of IC may resemble a low urinary tract infection, but cultures are usually negative. About 10–15% of patients with IC also have an overactive bladder. Recently, coexistence of IC with endometriosis has been observed.[36,40,41] However, the possible presence of bladder detrusor endometriosis, which shares several symptoms with IC, should not be forgotten.

Irritable bowel syndrome

Irritable bowel syndrome (IBS) is a common functional dysmotility disorder of the bowel which affects up to 15% of adults, and twice as many women as men.[36] The etiology is uncertain, and multifactorial pathophysiologic causes have been suggested, including altered bowel motility, visceral hypersensitivity, and psychosocial factors.[36] Symptoms likely result from overdistension of the colon wall by bowel content and gas, leading to the stimulation of stretch receptors. Patients present with abdominal pain and

Table 3.2 Differential diagnosis of 'organic' versus 'functional' pain based on clinical characteristics. Adapted from reference 42

Organic pain	Functional pain
Recent onset	Present for months before seeking medical attention
Consistently localized	Variable location, periumbilical or diffuse
Awakens patient from sleep	Exacerbated by stress
Precipitated by eating	Work absence/functional
Involuntary weight loss	impairment seems out of proportion to findings
Systemic symptoms are consistent with a single disease process	Systemic symptoms are not consistent with a single disease process

discomfort, bloating, and disturbed bowel habits (diarrhea, constipation, or both). Symptoms suggesting IBS are referred in a large proportion of patients presenting with CPP, and many of them consult a gynecologist instead of a gastroenterologist. Gynecologic diseases can also be misdiagnosed as IBS, which indicates a symptomatologic overlap between gynecologic and intestinal disorders. IBS can be associated with dyspareunia, and bowel symptoms worsen during menstruation in about half of the affected subjects.

HISTORY

Patient history is generally of the utmost importance for a correct diagnosis, sometimes being more indicative than several diagnostic investigations. The main contributing factors in women with CPP can still be identified by history and physical examination in most cases. Patients should be specifically questioned about the location and character of pain, exacerbating and relieving factors, the temporal course, and the relationship with the menstrual cycle. Pain both ventrally and dorsally often suggests intrapelvic pathology, whereas only dorsal lower back pain suggests an orthopedic or musculoskeletal origin. When a patient indicates precisely the location of pain, an organic cause of symptoms should be strongly suspected. In fact, usually, women with psychogenic CPP do not precisely localize the site of their pain and when asked to indicate where it hurts, they often move their hand around along all the abdominal quadrants (Table 3.2).

Information should be obtained about previous medical therapies, their effect on pain, and associated side-effects, as well as previous surgical procedures.

Reproductive history is important because pregnancy and childbirth are traumatic to the musculoskeletal system, especially the pelvis and back, and may lead to CPP. Difficult delivery, delivery of a large infant, and use of vacuum or forceps are relevant diagnostic hints if CPP began in the postpartum period.[21] The peripartum syndrome is probably caused by strain of the pelvic and lower spine ligaments due to a combination of factors, including hormonal changes, mechanical damage, muscle weakness, and weight of the fetus as well as the gravid uterus.[43]

Cyclicity related to pain usually suggests a gynecologic origin, although also other non-genital conditions such as IC and IBS may worsen in the perimenstrual period. Severe dysmenorrhea might be more predictive of endometriosis as compared with milder forms of the symptom. Dyspareunia might be associated with endometriosis, pelvic floor dysfunction, interstitial cystitis (deep-thrust dyspareunia), and vulvodynia-vulvovestibulitis (superficial or introital dyspareunia). In a woman with dyspareunia and infertility, a history of previous sexually transmitted infection and pelvic pain associated with low-grade fever is usually indicative of chronic pelvic infection.

The common symptoms associated with pelvic varices are: a changing location of pain, congestive dysmenorrhea, deep dyspareunia and postcoital pain, and a dull chronic pain with exacerbations after prolonged standing and triggered by postural changes. Pain can usually be reduced by lying down and elevating the legs. The pain of PCS is typically aggravated by states of pelvic venous engorgement such as prolonged standing, working for many hours in a sitting position, and after coitus. Pain from PCS usually disappears after the menopause.[30]

Dysuria, urgency, frequency, nocturia, and repetitive culture-negative urinary tract infections in a patient with pelvic pain are strongly suggestive of IC.[44] The IC symptom index is a validated questionnaire that reliably predicts the diagnosis of IC and may be used to discriminate patients in whom cystoscopy is indicated.[44,45]

The prevalence of IBS in women with CPP might be as high as 65–79%.[46] Alternating constipation and diarrhea, abdominal distension, mucus per rectum, improvement in pain after a bowel movement, and the sensation of incomplete evacuation after defecation indicate the presence of IBS. At the moment, the diagnosis of IBS is based on the Rome II criteria.[47] Attention should be paid not to underestimate a neoplasm or a bowel stenosis secondary to an endometriotic lesion.

The patient's social history enables the clinician to assess support systems and to investigate abuse or domestic violence. Women who have suffered from prolonged abuse may develop somatization and post-traumatic stress disorders, although research has not substantiated a psychological causal link between abuse and CPP. A history of abuse, which often makes it more difficult for a woman to deal with her symptoms, should be investigated with a delicate and sympathetic approach. Victims of abuse and domestic violence have a higher prevalence of chronic somatic complaints, exacerbations of chronic medical conditions, chronic pain, non-compliance with medical treatment, substance abuse, anxiety, depression, and suicide.[48]

Gynecologists and family physicians cannot be expected to conduct a thorough psychological evaluation. However, they have an important role in identifying patients who may benefit from psychosocial assessment and treatment. Depression, a predictor of pain severity and an indicator of responsiveness to treatment, should always be investigated. Women identified as affected by considerable psychosocial impact from their CPP can be referred to a mental health practitioner with specific training and experience in chronic health conditions.[36]

PHYSICAL EXAMINATION

The physical examination, which is often painful and emotionally stressful for the patient with CPP, should be performed gently and meticulously, so as to establish trust and confidence.[21] The abdominal examination should include inspection for scars and palpation to rule out masses. The precise location of pain should be defined to verify correspondence with the distribution of the ilioinguinal and genitofemoral nerves. In patients with functional pain, the abdominal examination typically reveals mild-to-moderate tenderness that is diffuse or periumbilical, while a more severe, localized tenderness with guarding should raise suspicion of organic pathology. Musculoskeletal causes of CPP are easily overlooked if the clinician does not explicitly investigate this possibility. Hernias should be noted. Tender points (pain with pressure) and trigger points (localized areas of deep muscle tenderness in a tight band of a muscle) are distinct, hyperirritable areas that are locally tender with palpation and cause referred pain that is often visceral. They may be located in the abdominal wall, low back, or vaginal areas. Abdominal wall trigger points should be localized by means of single-digit palpation and mapped with a pen. When an area of abdominal tenderness is palpated, the patient should be asked to voluntarily tense the muscles by raising her head or legs. An increase in pain while maintaining palpation suggests a myofascial origin, whereas a decrease or no change suggests a visceral cause. Identified abdominal wall trigger points should be blocked with a local anesthetic before performing the pelvic examination. Poor posture (exaggerated lumbar lordosis and thoracic kyphosis) or body mechanics may cause chronic repetitive stress and strain on these structures, leading to CPP. In fact, faulty posture may cause muscle weakness and deconditioning, which may result in pelvic imbalances with development of trigger points and hypertonicity. Other causes of low back pain, including leg length discrepancy and lumbar vertebral or disc disease, may similarly cause referred pelvic pain.

Examination of the external genitalia should be performed for lesions and vulvar, vestibular, and urethral point tenderness. Pain in this area in the absence of visible pathologies may be indicative of vulvodynia, a condition detected frequently in patients with CPP. Vaginal examination should begin with insertion of the index finger only, without using the palpating abdominal hand. Pelvic floor muscles, including the levator ani, obturator, pubococcygeus, and deep transverse perineal muscles, should be assessed for painful spasm and trigger points. Pelvic floor pain may be a primary problem or secondary to other diseases such as IC or endometriosis. Eliciting an excruciating pain when palpating the anterior vaginal wall is suggestive of IC or urethral syndrome. With deeper palpation of the cervix and vaginal fornices, painful areas suggestive of endometriosis or chronic pelvic infection can be detected. Uterine tenderness may be consistent with adenomyosis, PCS, or chronic pelvic infection. A fixed, retroflexed uterus is suggestive of endometriosis or adhesions. At this point, the traditional bimanual examination can be carried out. However, this modality may be less sensitive and discriminating since it involves stimulation of all abdominal wall structures including the parietal peritoneum, in addition to the palpated organs. Subsequently, a rectal or rectovaginal examination should be performed allowing more precise appreciation of endometriotic lesions. In subjects with a suspected pudendal nerve injury, the perineum should be evaluated for areas of hypoesthesia or paresthesia and the anal sphincter tone should also be assessed. At speculum examination, bacteriological specimens can be obtained, and cervical as well as paracervical tissues should be evaluated for tenderness

with a cotton-tipped applicator. In a case of previous hysterectomy, the vaginal cuff should be carefully assessed, and areas of tenderness that may be indicative of trigger points, neuromas, or visceral referral should be identified with the same technique.

INVESTIGATIONS

The investigations performed for women presenting with CPP will be based upon the history and physical examination findings. However, it is reasonable to support the use of the following basic laboratory studies in most women presenting with CPP: complete blood count, serum chemistry, sedimentation rate, urine microscopy and culture, and vaginal and endocervical swabs for microscopy, culture, and chlamydia detection. A test for occult blood in the stool is reasonable also to screen for inflammatory bowel disease. If diarrhea is a prominent symptom, stool may be cultured and evaluated for ova and parasites. Antinuclear antibodies, rheumatoid factor, and other tests for autoantibodies should be requested in selected circumstances.

Imaging studies such as abdominopelvic ultrasound scans, sigmoidoscopy and/or colonoscopy, and laparoscopy may be necessary.[49,50] Abdominal computed tomography (CT) or a small bowel radiographic series may be performed if pain is consistent and localized, or if there is a strong suspicion of Crohn's disease.[51]

Current evidence from randomized controlled trials (RCTs) provides support for the use of ultrasound scanning as an aid to counseling and reassurance.[52] Pelvic sonography may easily demonstrate ovarian masses, ovarian remnants, tubal dilatation (sactosalpinx), adenomyosis, bladder detrusor endometriosis, and, with the use of a transrectal probe, endometriotic rectovaginal plaques. Combined transabdominal and transvaginal ultrasound are also a potentially useful non-invasive screening technique in the evaluation of patients with PCS, and characteristic sonographic findings such as pelvic varices, reversed caudal flow in dilated ovarian veins, dilated arcuate veins crossing the uterine myometrium, and variable duplex waveform during the Valsalva maneuver may be demonstrated.[53] Adnexal varices are found more frequently on the left side, because the absence of ovarian vein valves is more common with respect to the right side (15% vs 6%, respectively).[31] Pelvic varices can also be demonstrated by helical CT, magnetic resonance imaging (MRI), or laparoscopy. However, during laparoscopy, both Trendelenburg positioning and increased intraabdominal pressure caused by pneumoperitoneum may induce venous decompression, leading to false-negative results. Definite but invasive and scarcely used diagnostic modalities for PCS include selective ovarian and internal iliac phlebography via the basilic, femoral, or internal jugular vein, or, alternatively, per-uterine phlebography.

Patients with IC have increased epithelial permeability.[54,55] Accordingly, the intravescicle potassium (KCl) sensitivity test has been proposed as a minimally invassive diagnostic modality. Pain and urgency are evaluated after intravesical instillation of 40 ml of KCl (0.4 mEq/ml) compared with symptoms after instillation of 40 ml of water. For some women this procedure is very distressing, but can be useful in detecting patients with altered epithelial permeability who might respond to sodium pentosan polysulfate. However, the diagnostic validity of the intravesical KCl sensitivity test for IC, flawed by low specificity, is still controversial.

When IC is suspected cystoscopy may be performed. Cystoscopic criteria for IC are the presence of glomerulations, submucosal hemorrhages, or ulcers, with bladder distension of 80–100 cmH2O pressure under anesthesia and decreased bladder capacity (less than 350 ml) without anesthesia. Again, the specificity and overall reliability of the above cystoscopic findings in the diagnosis of IC have been questioned.[56]

Laparoscopy is indicated in the presence of a pelvic mass of unknown etiology, whereas performance of the procedure in the absence of preoperative abnormal findings is based on the tenet that only direct visual inspection can identify the cause of CPP when physical examination and imaging techniques are undiagnostic.[57] The objective is to find and simultaneously treat a disorder causally linked to the symptoms reported in order to substantially improve health-related quality of life. However, this is not always possible, and laparoscopy should never be substituted for careful clinical evaluation. Watching appears easier than reasoning, and it is tempting to suggest surgery based on the belief that even the patient would understand that this is the maximum and most effective diagnostic effort that can be made.[58] Forty percent of diagnostic laparoscopies are performed for CPP, and 40% of these reveal a normal pelvis. Of those revealing abnormalities, around 85% show endometriosis or adhesions.[12] However, it does not automatically follow that an identified pathology is causally related to pain. Moreover, negative results of laparoscopy do not exclude disease or mean that there is no organic basis for the patient's pain. Several disorders that contribute to CPP cannot be identified with the laparoscope.

Microlaparoscopic pain mapping, or patient-assisted laparoscopy, is a technique involving conscious sedation and local analgesia that is used to identify sources of CPP by reproducing the patient's symptoms with probing or traction of pelvic tissues and structures. Howard[21] found no difference in outcome between 50 subjects treated after microlaparoscopic pain mapping and a historical cohort of 65 women who underwent traditional laparoscopy. Most studies involved small groups of patients and have not reported medium- and long-term outcomes after surgery.[59] Moreover, it is unclear how referred pain and hyperalgesia affect laparoscopic pain mapping. No RCT has compared pain mapping with standard laparoscopy. Patient-assisted microlaparoscopy under conscious sedation remains an experimental procedure.

Laparoscopy should be indicated in selected clinical conditions, and even when suspecting endometriosis a trial of a gonadotropin releasing hormone (GnRH) agonist or a continuous oral contraceptive must be prescribed. In fact, there is no definitive demonstration that staging the disease is useful for therapeutic or prognostic purposes,[60,61] and delaying surgery is not deleterious if a prolonged, effective medical therapy is used and if no pelvic masses are present. This clinical approach is approved by some of the most influential gynecologic associations.[9,62–65]

DIAGNOSTIC STRATEGY

A pragmatic and clinically sound approach for women with CPP has been suggested in order to identify two distinct categories of patients with potentially different causes of symptoms, and in whom diverse diagnostic and therapeutic options should be initially offered.[8] This strategy seems very practical and, in spite of some limitations that will be discussed, greatly simplifies an issue that appears rather intricate to most gynecologists and general practitioners. The rationale is based on the demonstration that endometriosis accounts for about two-thirds of the diagnoses made in women with CPP.[66] Moreover, endometriosis may affect other organ systems, causing intestinal motility disorders, bladder dysfunction, and pain.[8,67] Different from other causes of CPP, endometriosis can be treated effectively with drugs, surgery, or both. Hence, a sensible aim for the clinician should be identifying in a simple and non-invasive manner those women whose pain is probably caused by endometriosis. The definition of this group of patients with a 90% likelihood of having endometriosis[68] will leave a remaining

Table 3.3   Selected medical management options for chronic pelvic pain

Class	Drug	Dosage
Analgesics	Naproxen sodium	275–550 mg 2 times daily
	Sodium diclofenac	100 mg once daily (sustained release)
	Acetaminofen	500 mg 2–3 times daily
	Tramadol	100 mg 2 times daily (sustained release)
Tricyclic antidepressants	Amitriptyline	10–25 mg at bedtime
Antiepileptics	Gabapentin	300 mg 3 times daily
	Pregabalin	75 mg 2 times daily
Benzodiazepines	Diazepam	2 mg 2 times daily
Anticholinergics	Oxybutynin	5 mg 2 times daily
	Tolterodine	2–4 mg once daily
Antispasmodics	Pinaverium	50 mg 2–3 times daily
	Dicyclomine	20–40 mg 4 times daily
	Clidinium/chlordiazepoxide	1–2 caplets 3–4 times daily
	Propantheline/bromazepam	1 caplet 3–4 times daily
Ovarian cycle inhibitors	20-μg ethinylestradiol pills	Cyclic or continuous use
	Norethisterone acetate	2.5 mg daily, continuous use
	Medoxyprogesterone acetate	150 mg every 3 months IM
Various	Pentosan polysulfate	100 mg 3 times daily

IM, intramuscularly

cohort of subjects who most probably have causes of pain other than endometriosis. Only in these latter women should the diagnostic process proceed in order to identify different, often non-gynecologic, origins of symptoms.

The use of a GnRH agonist has been proposed to identify women with CPP caused by endometriosis without resorting to laparoscopy.[68] The empiric use of GnRH agonists is based on the presupposition that the induced hypoestrogenic state will result in a dramatic improvement in symptoms in nearly all women with endometriosis.[8] Accordingly, the response of a patient with CPP to a trial of 2–3 months of a GnRH agonist is strongly supportive of a diagnosis of endometriosis (or adenomyosis). However, a favorable reaction to these hypoestrogenizing drugs is observed not only when endometriosis is present, but also in case of pelvic varicosities, IBS, and IC, which usually have temporal exacerbations associated with the menstrual cycle. Furthermore, the placebo response rate may be substantial, at least in the short term. Nonetheless, all patients with a cyclic component to their pain should be offered a trial of menstrual suppression. Empiric treatment with GnRH agonists without first performing laparoscopy is deemed an acceptable approach to treatment.[9,69] If a 3-month trial is successful, long-term therapy with a continuous, low-dose, monophasic oral contraceptive or with a progestogen (e.g. oral norethisterone acetate, 2.5 mg/day, used continuously) should then be taken into adequate consideration.[70–73]

MANAGEMENT

Unfortunately, there are very few RCTs on treatment of CPP. In a Cochrane systematic review of treatments for CPP,[52] only medroxyprogesterone acetate (50 mg once daily), counseling (after negative ultrasonography), a multidisciplinary approach, and lysis of deep adhesions were found to be of proven benefit.[52] The multidisciplinary approach for reducing pain included physiotherapy, psychotherapy, and attention to dietary and environmental factors.[26,74]

Eventually, the management of CPP can focus on treating the pain itself, on treating the underlying cause, or on both.[21] Treatment of chronic pain, different from that of acute pain, generally requires acceptance of the concept of managing rather than curing pain.[21]

Treatment of pain

Pharmacologic approach

Analgesics are the mainstay of pharmacological treatment (Table 3.3). Therapy directed to the peripheral nerves (pain reception) involves the use of prostaglandin synthesis inhibitors, such as non-steroidal anti-inflammatory drugs (NSAIDs) as well as disruptors of sodium channel activity, such as carbamazepine[36] with a starting dose of 100 mg/day, which can be increased up to 100 mg thrice daily. Diclofenac can be prescribed in an oral, once-a-day, sustained-release preparation of 100 mg. Naproxen is among the preferred NSAIDs due to its efficacy and plasma half-life of 14 hours that allows consumption of 500 mg only once or twice daily. These first-line drugs are generally effective, but individual variation in response to different NSAIDs is frequent, so different medications should be tried in case of limited efficacy. Chronic use of NSAIDs is associated with major adverse effects. In the case of long-term treatment, patients should undergo careful observation and, in selected circumstances, H_2-receptor antagonist therapy. When acetylsalicylic acid and NSAIDs are contraindicated, acetaminophen (paracetamol, 500 mg twice or thrice daily) can be used. Its mechanism of action is still unclear, but may include a weak anti-inflammatory action and a major inhibiting action in the central nervous system. The most serious adverse effect of acute overdosage of paracetamol is a dose-dependent, potentially fatal hepatic necrosis. Chronic abuse of paracetamol may cause nephrotoxicity.

Novel neuroleptics, such as gabapentin, inhibit excessive stimulation of the secondary neurons in the spinal cord (pain transmission), as do carbamazepine, phenytoin, and clonazepam.[36] Gabapentin may be more tolerable than carbamazepin, and equally effective. The usual starting dose in a case of neuropathic pain is 300 mg thrice daily and can be increased, if necessary, based on the patient's response. Pregabalin is a strictly related compound that has been specifically developed for neuropathic pain and is generally prescribed at the dose of 75 mg twice daily.

Therapy directed at the central processing of pain with modulation and inhibition of unbearable stimuli (pain perception) includes the use of opiates that act on the dorsal horns of the spinal cord and agents that inhibit serotonin uptake, thereby increasing its availability (amitriptyline and paroxetine).

The use of opioid analgesics in the treatment of chronic pain is controversial, and, although opioid therapy may allow the return of normal function in those who have failed other treatments, the possibilty of addiction, especially in subjects with major psychological distress, is of utmost concern. Furthermore, even when addiction is deemed improbable, tolerance and dependence may still constitute important problems. Opioid maintainance therapy for CPP should generally be discouraged, and considered only after all other reasonable attempts at pain control have failed and when persistent pain is the major obstacle to improved function. If this therapeutic option is chosen, the patient should be referred to a tertiary care center with experience in pain therapy.

Tramadol may constitute an alternative to classic opiods. It is active per os, inhibits serotonin and norepinephrine reuptake, and displays mild opioid as well as non-opioid action. It binds to μ receptors responsible for subspinal analgesia, and is antagonized only partly by naloxone. Sustained-release preparations of 100, 150, and 200 mg are available. The suggested starting dose should be 100 mg twice daily. Tramadol is generally well-tolerated, has only minor respiratory depression activity and does not cause constipation.

Tricyclic antidepressants have been used to treat several chronic pain syndromes, as they have been demonstrated to improve pain tolerance, restore sleep, and reduce depressive symptoms. Amitriptyline is generally efficacious in the treatment of chronic pain at dosages inferior to those used for therapy of depression. It can be prescribed at the dose of 10–25 mg to be taken at bedtime. In the single published trial on a tricyclic antidepressant for CPP without obvious pathology, nortriptyline proved of some efficacy in a small group of 14 women.[75] Six subjects were pain free at 1-year follow-up, but another seven dropped out of the study because of side-effects. Sertraline (50 mg twice daily) has not been demonstrated to be more effective than placebo in a small, double-blind, crossover trial in women with CPP. Further studies are needed to evaluate the efficacy of selective serotonin reuptake inhibitors such as fluoxetine and sertraline. Independent of analgesic efficacy, antidepressants have the added advantage of ameliorating the often poor psychological status of patients with CPP.

As suggested by Howard,[21] combination drug therapy with medications with different mechanisms of action may improve therapeutic results. If inflammation is a major component of the pain syndrome, a NSAID (e.g. diclofenac or naproxen) can be combined with tramadol. In selected patients, the combination of two centrally acting drugs, but with different mechanisms, may also be appropriate, such as a trycyclic antidepressant (e.g. amitriptyline) and tramadol. If muscle spasm or tension contributes substantially to pain, a benzodiazepine with muscle-relaxant properties (e.g. diazepam, 2 mg twice daily) could be combined with a NSAID in order to enhance efficacy.

As a general rule in chronic pain management, analgesics should be given on a scheduled basis, improving effectiveness because the drug is taken before severe symptom insurgence, thus avoiding the amplified focus on pain that may actually exacerbate with an 'as needed' dosing. A preplanned scheduled modality avoids a pain-contingent approach that has the tendency to use medication as a reinforcer of pain behaviors.[21]

Surgical approach

Denervating procedures   Sensory innervation of the pelvic organs is from the superior hypogastric plexus or presacral nerve, the nervi erigentes or pelvic nerves, and the ovarian plexuses.[76] The segmental derivation of the presacral nerve is T11–L2. Sympathetic effector fibers and most sensory fibers from the pelvic organs enter the superior hypogastric plexus. The latter usually consists of interlaced nerve bundles lying on the L4 and L5 bodies and the sacral promontory, extending over most of the interiliac triangle.[76–78] The nervi erigentes originate from S2–S4, and consist of parasympathetic effector and sensory fibers.

Both sympathetic and parasympathetic fibers run in and around the uterosacral folds and reach the parametrium, posterolateral to the uterine cervix, where they unite to form the plexuses of Frankenhauser. The latter may be considered a 'clearing station' for these fibers, which enter the plexuses, intermingle, and then proceed together to innervate the upper part of the vagina, uterus, proximal portion of the tubes, bladder, urethra, and rectum.[77,78] Innervation of the tubal ampullae and ovaries is instead from the ovarian plexus, which is formed mainly of sympathetic fibers of T9–T10 derivation that run along the vessels of the infundibulopelvic ligament. Although the uterine body is innervated mainly by fibers of the hypogastric plexus, the fundus receives fibers also from the ovarian plexuses.[77,78]

Severe, disabling dysmenorrhea is by far the most frequent problem in women with endometriosis.[79] Accordingly, the addition of uterine denervation to lesion destruction has been suggested to improve long-term antalgic results.[80] Two types of pelvic denervating procedures have been proposed in women with CPP, namely presacral neurectomy (PSN) and uterosacral ligament resection (i.e. laparoscopic uterosacral nerve ablation (LUNA)). The efficacy of both interventions has been assessed in a few RCTs.[81]

The results of the three published RCTs on PSN in women with endometriosis are inconsistent. Tjaden et al[82] recruited eight subjects who were randomly allocated to presacral neurectomy in addition to conservative surgery (n=4) or to conservative surgery only (n=4) for moderate or severe midline dysmenorrhea associated with stage III–IV endometriosis. Eighteen other women wanting (n=13) or refusing (n=5) presacral neurectomy were included in the evaluation. At the 6-month follow-up, 15/17 subjects who underwent presacral neurectomy experienced dysmenorrhea relief (four randomized and 11/13 non-randomized),

whereas all the subjects who underwent conservative surgery only remained symptomatic. This led the monitoring committee to stop the study, because it was considered unethical to continue to deprive patients of the evident benefit of presacral neurectomy. In the second RCT by Candiani et al,[83] 71 women with moderate or severe midline dysmenorrhea were allocated to conservative surgery at laparotomy and presacral neurectomy (n=35) or conservative surgery only (n=36). Recurrence of moderate or severe dysmenorrhea at the 1-year follow-up was observed in 6/35 (17%) in the experimental group and 9/36 (25%) in the control group according to a linear analog scale, and, respectively, 5/35 (14%) and 7/36 (19%) according to a multidimensional verbal rating scale, the differences not being statistically significant. In the presacral neurectomy group, constipation developed or worsened in 13 patients and urinary urgency occurred in three. In the third, more recent, RCT,[84] 141 subjects with severe dysmenorrhea were allocated to laparoscopic surgery for endometriosis plus PSN or laparoscopic surgery only. Sixty-three women in each study group were included in the efficacy analysis. At the 6- and 12-month follow-ups, the cure rate in terms of dysmenorrhea relief was significantly higher in the PSN group than in the surgery only group (respectively, 87% vs 60% and 86% vs 57%). At the end of the study period, also the frequency and severity of deep dyspareunia and non-menstrual pain were significantly lower in women in the former group with respect to those in the latter.

The efficacy of LUNA has been evaluated in RCTs conducted in women with pain associated with endometriosis as well as in those without obvious pathology.

In the study by Sutton et al,[85] 27 subjects were randomly allocated to laparoscopic surgery for endometriosis plus LUNA and 24 to laparoscopic surgery only. Significant differences in favor of the surgery only group were observed in dysmenorrhea as well as in non-menstrual pain scores at the 3- and 6-month follow-ups. Results were similar with regard to deep dyspareunia.

The largest RCT on the efficacy of LUNA for endometriosis-associated moderate-to-severe dysmenorrhea was conducted on Milan in 180 women undergoing first-line surgery for stage I–IV disease.[86] Among the patients who were evaluable 1 year after operative laparoscopy, 23 of 78 (29%) women who had LUNA and 21 of 78 (27%) women who had conservative surgery only reported recurrent dysmenorrhea. The corresponding numbers of patients at 3 years were 21 of 59 (36%) and 18 of 57 (32%) women, respectively. Pain was substantially reduced, and subjects in both groups experienced similar and significant improvements in health-related quality of life, psychiatric conditions, and sexual satisfaction. Overall, 68 of 90 (75%) patients in the LUNA group and 67 of 90 (75%) patients in the conservative surgery only group were satisfied at 1 year.

Johnson et al[87] designed a double-blind RCT recruiting 67 women with and 56 without endometriosis. The addition of LUNA to laparoscopic surgical treatment of endometriosis was not associated with a significant difference in any pain outcome. However, significantly greater relief from dysmenorrhea was observed at the 12-month follow-up in women without endometriosis who underwent LUNA, 42% vs 14% experiencing a successful treatment defined as a 50% or greater reduction in visual analog scale (VAS) score. No significant between-group difference was observed in relief from non-menstrual pelvic pain, deep dyspareunia, or dyschezia.

The results of Johnson et al[87] confirm the findings of Lichten and Bombard,[88] who were the first to conduct a randomized trial, albeit small, on the effect of LUNA in 21 subjects with no demonstrable pelvic pathology at laparoscopy performed because of severe dysmenorrhea. Nine of the 11 patients (81%) allocated to LUNA reported postoperative relief of menstrual pain, compared with none in the control arm.

Yen et al[89] evaluated the efficacy of LUNA in 85 women with dysmenorrhea associated with fibroids treated by laparoscopic bipolar coagulation of uterine vessels. At the 6-month follow-up, 92% of subjects allocated to LUNA referred improvement of dysmenorrhea compared with 74% of those who underwent bipolar coagulation of uterine vessels only.

Recently, Palomba et al[90] compared the efficacy of LUNA and vaginal uterosacral ligament resection in 80 postmenopausal women with intractable midline CPP. The cure rate at the 12-month follow-up was similar in the two groups (27/36, 75% vs 28/38, 74%). However, the mean cost of LUNA was significantly higher than that of the vaginal procedure.

Two RCTs compared the efficacy of PSN and LUNA in women with primary dysmenorrhea, with contradictory results.[91,92]

Latthe et al[93] recently published the results of a meta-analysis conducted by the Cochrane Menstrual Disorders and Subfertility Group. After pooling the results of the above-considered RCTs, the authors concluded that for the treatment of primary dysmenorrhea, LUNA was better than control or no treatment

at 12 months after surgery (odds ratio (OR) 6.12, 95% confidence interval (CI) 1.78–21.03). The comparison of LUNA with PSN for primary dysmenorrhea showed that, at the 12-month follow-up, PNS was more effective (OR 0.10, 95% CI 0.03–0.32). In secondary dysmenorrhea, along with laparoscopic surgical treatment of endometriosis, the addition of LUNA did not improve the pain relief (OR 0.77, 95% CI 0.43–1.39), whereas PNS did (OR 3.14, 95% CI 1.59–6.21). The authors conclude that the evidence for nerve interruption in the management of dysmenorrhea is limited, and that more, methodologically adequate RCTs are needed. A further meta-analysis on the effectiveness of LUNA is currently being performed by collecting individual patient data from the existing trials.[94]

Several women who underwent PNS experienced complications and side-effects, postoperative constipation being the most frequent disturbance.[93,95] It cannot be excluded that in some trials side-effects were considered only if sufficiently severe to cause withdrawal of the patient, or that only spontaneously reported and not regularly assessed side-effects were included. The inconveniences caused by uterosacral ligament resection are rare and of limited severity; this may be the result of more selective uterine denervation or, alternatively, indirect proof that such a localized neurotomy does not affect the overall innervation and function of pelvic organs.

Presacral neurectomy is carried out in a complex anatomic area, and great care must be taken to avoid damaging major as well as midsacral vessels and also the right ureter. Fatal venous sacral hemorrhages have been reported, and postoperative bowel and bladder dysfunctions are not infrequent. Presacral neurectomy should be performed only by expert surgeons in highly selected women who specifically report midline, hypogastric pain without lateral components.

Performance of laparoscopic uterosacral ligament resection appears simple and quick, and gives the impression that everything that is surgically feasible has been done, including an intervention on the peripheral nervous system. This may be gratifying for both gynecologists and patients, but it is not possible to exclude that this type of neurotomy is of little or no benefit. Contrary to the case of presacral neurectomy, almost all laparoscopic surgeons feel that they are able to carry out uterosacral ligament resection safely. However, complications have been reported also after this apparently easy operation, including hemorrhages, ureteral damage, and pelvic support disorders.[83,96–101]

Although the main anatomic pathways through which pelvic pain impulses are transmitted are known, precise relations between site of pain sensation, area of corresponding innervation, and afferent fibers are difficult to define.[76,79,102,103] The old clinical tenet that lateral, adnexal pain cannot be influenced by pelvic denervations and that only central, hypogastric pain may be reduced or abolished must clearly be borne in mind. However, also uterine sensory innervation may be neither simple nor schematic. Nerve fibers may be distributed more widely or have more complex interconnections than previously thought. Finally, a chronic inflammatory status, such as that associated with endometriosis, may cause stimulation of pain sensory fibers innervating a vast area of the pelvic peritoneum.[79,103,104] This incomplete knowledge makes surgical treatment of pelvic pain by denervations empirical.

Although the results of conservative surgery only for endometriosis are suboptimal in terms of long-term pain relief, routine complementary performance of denervating procedures cannot be recommended based on the quality of the available information.

Hysterectomy for CPP of different etiology   Approximately 10–18% of hysterectomies are performed because of CPP.[105] In a recent survey by Learman et al,[106] the presence of multiple pelvic symptoms, previous use of a GnRH agonist, and absence of symptom resolution predicted the likelihood of subsequent hysterectomy, which reached 95% if all three predictors were simultaneously present.

Histology studies on patterns of uterine innervation in women with CPP provide a pathophysiological rationale in support of hysterectomy.[107,108] Atwal et al[108] demonstrated that in uteri removed from women with CPP without endometriosis there were increased numbers of nerve fibers compared with control specimens from patients with painless gynecologic conditions. Two distinctive patterns of reinnervation were observed, namely, disruption of nerve bundles (collateral sprouting with microneuroma formation) and ingrowth around blood vessels (perivascular nerve fiber proliferation). No differences were observed in nerve fiber distribution and reinnervation patterns in women with CPP with or without associated endometriosis.

However, definitive surgery in women with chronic pain of various origins is a controversial procedure, especially in young women (less than 35 years) and in the absence of obvious pathologies.[109,110] Patient self-reported outcomes of hysterectomy have generally revealed high levels of satisfaction in various clinical conditions. Nonetheless, a careful preoperative assessment and the detailed discussion of alternative therapeutic choices with examination of risk–benefit ratios are mandatory, and the patient's preference regarding treatment alternatives must be considered carefully.[111]

Stovall et al[112] reviewed the long-term outcome in 99 women who underwent hysterectomy for chronic pelvic pain of presumed uterine origin. Histology revealed leiomyomata in 12 subjects, adenomyosis in 20, and both anomalies in two. After a mean follow-up of 22 months, 77 women reported the absence of notable symptoms. The remaining 22 had persistent pelvic pain, which was however improved in five of them.

The findings of the study by Beard et al[113] on the effect of hysterectomy in patients with CPP associated with pelvic varicosities are described in the section on PCS.

Carlson et al[105] reported the results of the Maine Women's Health Study, a prospective cohort study of 418 patients aged 25–50 years undergoing hysterectomy for non-malignant conditions. A total of 199 of 355 evaluated subjects experienced very frequent pelvic pain at baseline; of those, only 11 (6%) claimed that symptoms persisted 12 months after surgery. The women operated for pelvic pain referred a marked improvement in physical as well as psychological symptoms and sexual dysfunction. Significant improvements in mental, as well as in general health and activity index scores were also observed. Only half of these women had a specific diagnosis, such as endometriosis, fibroids, or adhesions.

The same authors published the results of a prospective, comparative study of women undergoing non-surgical management ($n=380$) or hysterectomy ($n=311$) for leiomyomas, abnormal uterine bleeding, or chronic pelvic pain.[114] One year after enrolment, 24/50 (49%) women receiving non-surgical management still experienced high symptom levels, whereas only 2/68 (3%) who underwent hysterectomy reported pain as a persistent and considerable problem. Almost one-quarter of patients initially treated non-surgically subsequently underwent hysterectomy. Operated women scored consistently better at quality of life assessment by the Mental Health, General Health, and Activity Indices.

Hillis et al[115] assessed variations in symptoms 1 year after hysterectomy for chronic pelvic pain of at least 6 months' duration. Of the 279 evaluated subjects, 206 (74%) reported no pain, 58 (21%) decreased, and 15 (5%) unchanged or increased pain. An increased probability of persistent pain was observed among women who had no identified pelvic disease. In this group, complete symptom relief was achieved in 62% of the cases.

Tay and Bromwich[116] studied retrospectively 228 women who underwent hysterectomy for pelvic pain associated with mixed conditions (leiomyomas, 74%; adenomyosis, 40%; ovarian cysts, 19%; endometriosis, 8%). Almost half of the patients had multiple disease. Of the 98 subjects with pain as the only or main indication for hysterectomy, 71 responded to an outcome survey 12 or more months after surgery, which showed that 62 of them (87%) were satisfied with the intervention, eight (11%) were unsure, and one (1%) was dissatisfied; 68 (96%) women reported relief from their symptoms.

The results of the Maryland Women's Health Study, a prospective cohort study conducted in 1299 women who underwent hysterectomy in 28 hospitals,[117] demonstrated that symptom severity, depression, and anxiety levels decreased significantly after surgery and quality of life improved. A total of 657 patients out of the 745 who referred CPP before hysterectomy (88%) were relieved from symptoms at the 1-year follow-up. The proportion did not vary at the 2-year assessment (644/720, 89.4%). The percentage of subjects who developed new clinical problems after surgery was, respectively, 3.6% and 2.8%. Therapy for emotional or psychologic problems, depression, and low income were associated with lack of symptom relief.

Hartmann et al[118] examined differences in quality of life and sexual function after hysterectomy among the women enrolled in the Maryland Women's Health Study who had preoperative pain and depression. At 24 months, women with pain and depression had reduced prevalence of pelvic pain (from 97% to 19%), limited physical function (66% to 34%), impaired mental health (93% to 38%), and limited social function (41% to 15%). Women with pelvic pain only improved in pelvic pain (95% to 9%) and limited activity level (74% to 24%). The group with depression only had improvement in impaired mental health (85% to 33%). Dyspareunia decreased in all groups. In the authors' experience, women with pelvic pain and depression fare less well 24 months after hysterectomy than women who have either disorder alone or neither. Nevertheless, these women improve substantially over their preoperative baseline in all the quality of life and sexual function areas assessed.

Traditionally, it is deemed that in patients with chronic pelvic pain without obvious disease or with pelvic varicosities, definitive surgery should be avoided or deferred as long as possible, because psychoaffective disturbances may be the real cause of the syndrome.[109,110,119,120] Supporters of this belief maintain that different types of psychiatric disorder are often diagnosed in these women, that a history of sexual abuse or depression is frequently elicited, and that hysterectomy will not cure pelvic pain or will only induce its 'migration' to another organ or apparatus.[77,78,110,121] The information available suggests that the outcome at the 1- to 2-year follow-up is consistently satisfactory (Table 3.4). However, in several studies, the definition of CPP is somewhat vague, including dysmenorrhea, pain and pressure from pelvic floor relaxation, and pain from uterine fibroids. Limiting the analysis to young women with a normal pelvis (the subgroup at highest risk of treatment failure), substantial pain relief can be achieved in no more than 60% of cases.[115] Preoperative patient assessment must obviously be complete, including testing for bowel dysmotility, urologic disorders, muskuloskeletal lesions, and psychosocioenvironmental factors.[26,102,121] When no other possible cause of pain is identified and the woman has completed her family, hysterectomy can be considered as an alternative with the hypothesis that this will improve health-related quality of life. This is particularly true when the uterus is exquisitely tender, its palpation or mobilization causes excruciating pain, and several courses of medical therapies have failed. However, women should be adequately informed on the expected probability of success, and should specifically be aware that in the absence of obvious pathology almost 40% of subjects will have persistent pain after hysterectomy. This percentage is reduced (10–20%) when pelvic lesions are present. Nevertheless, as women with CPP are often hyperalgesic, the possibility of unrecognized comorbid disorders should not be disregarded even in the presence of documented organic pathology. A minority of patients (3–5%) will experience worsening of pain or will develop new symptoms after surgery. This should be specifically included in the preoperative informed consent form.

According to the results of a Danish nationwide survey on risk factors for CPP after hysterectomy for benign indications, 32% of women experienced pain at the 1-year assessment, and 14% had pain on more than 2 days a week.[122] Pain was not present before surgery in 15% of subjects with chronic post-surgical pain. Risk factors for CPP were preoperative pelvic pain (OR 3.25, 95% CI 2.40–4.41), previous cesarean delivery (OR 1.54, 95% CI 1.06–2.26), pain as the main indication for surgery (OR 2.98, 95% CI 1.54–5.77), and pain problems elsewhere (OR 3.19, 95% CI 2.29–4.44). Interestingly, spinal anesthesia was associated with a lower frequency of chronic pain compared with general anesthesia (OR 0.42, 95% CI 0.21–0.85).

Table 3.4   Results of studies on outcome of hysterectomy for chronic pelvic pain of presumed uterine origin

Source	Year	Type of study	Pelvic anomaly	Duration of follow-up (months)	Subjects experiencing pain relief or improvement		
					n	%	95% CI
Stovall et al[112]	1990	Retr	None except small myomas or adenomyosis	≥12	82/99	83	74–90
Beard et al[113]	1991	Prosp	Pelvic congestion	12	35/36	97	85–100
Carlson et al[105]	1994	Prosp	Mixed conditions	12	188/199	94	90–97
Hillis et al[115]	1995	Prosp	Mixed conditions	12	264/279	95	91–97
Tay and Bromwich[116]	1998	Retr	Mixed conditions	12	68/71	96	88–99
Kjerulff et al[117]	2000	Prosp	Mixed conditions	24	644/720	89	87–92
Hartmann et al[118a]	2004	Prosp	Mixed conditions	24			
			pain only		193/213	91	86–94
			depressed only		89/100	89	81–94
			pain and depression		119/146	81	74–87

[a]Subjects included in Hartmann et al's study are a subset of those enrolled in Kjerulff et al's study (the Maryland Women's Health Study)

Retr, retrospective; Prosp, prospective

The most common histopathologic findings at laparoscopy in women with CPP after hysterectomy and bilateral salpingo-oophorectomy include adhesions, endometriosis, and adnexal remnants.[123] This confirms the need for radical removal of ovaries when adnexectomy is indicated because, if gonadal tissue is left, the ovarian remnant syndrome may ensue. The condition is characterized by pelvic pain, development of functional and peritoneal cysts, dense adhesions in the adnexal regions, and normal estradiol and follicle stimulating hormone (FSH) levels. Treatment consists of gonadal suppression (e.g. depo-medroxyprogesterone acetate, 150 mg intramuscularly every 3 months) or repetitive extirpative surgery.

TREATMENT OF SPECIFIC CONDITIONS

Postoperative adhesions

Although it is rarely clarified, the treatment of adhesions associated with chronic pelvic infection and endometriosis constitutes an integral part of the overall management of these two conditions, and the specific effect of adhesiolysis cannot be extrapolated.

There are only two published RCTs evaluating the role of adhesiolysis in the treatment of CPP. Peters et al[26] enrolled 48 symptomatic patients with laparoscopically diagnosed pelvic adhesions. Main outcome measures were pain assessed by the McGill questionnaire, subjective pain evaluation, and interference with daily activities. After 9–12 months there were no significant differences between the 24 women allocated to adhesiolysis and the 24 receiving non-surgical management. A subgroup of 15 women with severe, vascularized, and dense adhesions involving the bowel had significantly less pain after adhesiolysis according to two of the three assessment methods.

A more recent, blinded RCT[124] of laparoscopic adhesiolysis versus diagnostic laparoscopy alone conducted in 87 women and 13 men with chronic abdominal pain found that, at 12 months after treatment allocation, the same proportion (27%) of subjects in the two study arms reported resolution or substantial reduction of pain. There were no complications in the diagnostic laparoscopy group, but five of the 52 patients in the adhesiolysis group had complications, including small bowel perforation, hemorrhage necessitating blood transfusion, abdominal abscess, rectovaginal fistula, and protracted paralytic ileus.

A comprehensive review of the available data confirmed contradictory findings on the relation between adhesions and CPP, as well as highly variable effects of adhesiolysis.[25]

At present, adhesiolysis cannot be recommended as a standard procedure in women with CPP.[24] Patient counseling in this particular situation is not easy, and it must be emphasized that resolution of pain after surgery cannot be assured. Women should be informed that pelvic adhesions are frequently found in asymptomatic subjects, and a thorough evaluation including psychological assessment is advisable before choosing surgical management. It must also be clarified that 'normalization' of pelvic anatomy at the end of the procedure does not necessarily mean that the surgical results will be maintained in the future, as it has been demonstrated that adhesion reformation is disappointingly frequent.[125] The perplexities that exist concerning adhesiolysis for women with CPP are also based on the consideration that it has still not been definitively demonstrated that pain is caused by mild and moderate adhesions, which are probably more frequent than the severe ones. Before surgery is suggested, the patient's expectations should be tempered, and detailed counseling with alternative treatment options offered.

Pelvic varices

A variety of medical and surgical approaches are available to treat PCS. Pharmacological agents to suppress ovarian function such as medroxyprogesterone acetate (MPA) or GnRH agonists have been proved to significantly reduce pain in the short term. In fact it has been suggested that, as estrogens are venous dilators, inducing a hypoestrogenic milieu may result in the resolution of symptoms.[33,126] Farquhar et al[126] assessed the effect of MPA and of psychotherapy in the treatment of lower abdominal pain due to pelvic congestion. Eighty-four women with abnormal pelvic venography were randomized to 4-month management with MPA alone at the dose of 30 mg/day, MPA plus psychotherapy, placebo alone, and placebo plus psychotherapy. During treatment, 73% of subjects allocated to MPA reported at least 50% improvement, compared with 33% of those allocated to placebo. At the 9-month follow-up no overall effect of MPA or psychotherapy was demonstrated, but an interaction between MPA and psychotherapy was observed in 71% of women allocated to the combined treatment, showing ≥50% reduction in pain score.

More recently, Soysal et al[30] formally compared a subcutaneous depot GnRH agonist formulation (goserelin, 3.6 mg/month) with oral MPA (30 mg/day).

Both during the 6-month therapy period and 1 year after treatment, goserelin proved significantly superior to MPA in terms of pelvic venographic improvements, symptoms and signs relief, sexual functioning amelioration, and anxiety and depression reduction.

Percutaneous transcatheter embolotherapy of ovarian and pelvic varices has been shown to be a feasible technique, leading to relief of pain in 50–80% of patients.[127–129] Laparoscopic ligation of the ovarian veins is of anecdotal evidence.[130] The long-term impact of the above treatment modalities on CPP needs further and more robust evaluation.

Hysterectomy and bilateral salpingo-oophorectomy has been suggested to be an effective treatment for CPP due to pelvic varices which has failed to respond to medical therapy. Beard et al[113] enrolled 36 patients with CPP associated with objectively demonstrated pelvic varicosities in a prospective non-comparative study on the effect of hysterectomy with bilateral oophorectomy. One year after surgery, 24 women were completely asymptomatic, 11 reported greatly reduced pain, and in only one patient did pain still affect quality of life. The median frequency of sexual intercourse increased from once per month preoperatively to eight times per month at follow-up evaluation.

Interstitial cystitis

Hydrodistension of the bladder has been considered for a long time to be the traditional treatment of IC. However, general or spinal anesthesia is needed, and no more than 30% of patients experience relief for 3–6 months. Dimethylsulfoxide administered intravesically may result in remission but not definitive cure of the disease. Treatments are generally repeated 4–8 times at 1–2-week intervals. However, a recent systematic review by the Cochrane Collaboration did not demonstrate apparent differences from placebo.[131]

Sodium pentosan polysulfate is polyanionic analog of heparin. This polysaccharide is one of the glycosaminoglycans in the bladder surface mucin, and it is hypothesized to work by repairing the altered permeability of the bladder surface.[15] One placebo-controlled, double-blind study of pentosan polysulfate (100 mg per os thrice a day) demonstrated a 50% response rate compared with 23% in the placebo group. In particular, a decrease in pelvic pain was observed in, respectively, 45% vs 18% of the subjects in the two study groups.[132] It could take up to 6 months for the maximal effect.

GnRH analogs and oral contraceptives have been used with similar efficacy as post-hydrodistension therapy in a small series of patients with IC associated with bladder symptoms that fluctuated with the menstrual cycle.[133] Other medical treatments reported to be effective in limited case-series include cyclosporine, L-arginine, nifedipine, antihistamines such as hydroxyzine, and anticholinergics.[21] Tricyclic antidepressants, in particular amitriptyline, are also used to treat IC. Non-comparative studies suggest improvement in about two-thirds of subjects treated with 25–75 mg/day of amitriptyline at bedtime.[134] A systematic review on medical treatments for IC is being conducted by the Cochrane Collaboration.[135]

Irritable bowel syndrome

Functional bowel disorders, including IBS, are amenable to a variety of treatment approaches such as dietary management, medical therapy, and, in specific traumatic or stressful conditions, even psychotherapy. Elimination of dietary lactose, sorbitol, and fructose is advised.[36] Lactose intolerance can mimic IBS and contribute to symptomatology. Caffeinated products such as coffee, tea, cola, carbonated products, and gas-producing foods should be avoided.

In patients with predominantly pain, gas, and bloating, an anticholinergic such as dicyclomine hydrochloride or hyoscyamine sulfate and an antispasmodic such as chlordiazepoxide with clidinium may be tried.[136] If constipation is the main complaint (hypomotile patients), oral fiber supplementation in the form of psyllium powder should be prescribed, in order to increase stool bulk and water content and decrease transit time; oral fiber also decreases the frequency of bowel movements and facilitates formed stools in subjects with an overactive colon. Positive results require consistent long-term psyllium supplementation in adequate dosage of at least 6 g (one tablespoon) daily.[121] Loperamide is the most commonly used agent in patients with hypermotile patterns of diarrhea.[36]

ALTERNATIVE TREATMENTS

Several non-invasive treatments have been proposed for women with CPP, including exercise programs, cognitive and behavioral medicine, physical therapy, dietary modification, massage, and acupuncture.[74] Very few of these approaches have been evaluated in formal clinical trials. In particular, there are no data on the efficacy of exercise for relief of CPP. However, suggesting physical activity may be important not only in terms of antalgic results but also for psychological purposes: women with CPP should be encouraged to live as normally as possible, limiting the feeling of being handicapped by ill-health. Internal manual therapy for myofascial trigger points in the pelvic floor have shown improvements in two-thirds of subjects.[137]

Acupuncture, acupressure, and transcutaneous nerve stimulation therapy have been shown to be better than placebo in women with dysmenorrhea, but data on treatment of non-menstrual CPP are lacking.[9] Acupuncture is of benefit in back pain and and in lumbar and pelvic pain in pregnancy. Moreover, acupuncture has a demonstrated long-lasting efficacy for symptom relief in men with chronic prostatitis and CPP syndrome,[138] as well as for the relief of chronic pain in oncologic patients. The precise mechanisms of action of acupuncture are not completely clear, but include gate control of pain pathways, increased endogenous opioid release, and altered sympathetic tone.[138]

Modulation of γ-aminobutyric acid receptors may be inhibited by electric stimulation. Neurostimulation at the third sacral nerve root (sacral nerve stimulation) is an implantable technology for urinary urgency and frequency and for IC. It is hypothesized to work by modulating afferent impulses, and it may reduce pain and improve voiding dysfuction in subjects with IC and pelvic floor dysfunction. Neuromodulation should be offered only in selected conditions when all other treatments have failed. However, for some women with intractable CPP, sacral nerve stimulation might allow for a return to functioning and a reduction in medications.[139]

Myofascial pain might respond to injections of trigger points with a long-acting local anesthetic such as bupivacaine. Botulinum toxin A can also be used for abdominal wall trigger point injections with long-term pain reduction. This toxin induces local, temporary muscle paralysis, and it possibly diminishes mediators of neurogenic inflammation.[15]

Nerve blocks with a long-acting local anesthetic might be both diagnostic and therapeutic in several conditions, including post-hysterectomy groin pain due to genitofemoral or ilioinguinal nerve injury as well as pudendal nerve damage after delivery or vaginal surgery.

Psychosomatic factors appear to have an important role in CPP,[46,140] and psychiatric evaluation should be taken into adequate consideration. Moreover, the data generated by the psychological assessment are useful for selecting appropriate psychosocial interventions, directed towards alleviating the psychological and behavioral sequelae of CPP through lifestyle modification and alteration in pain coping style. The objectives of psychiatric interventions are treatment of primary or secondary mental health disorders, when present,

and the reduction of psychosocial stress, which may moderate pain experience. Psychological treatment and support may decrease suffering and disability in women with CPP independent of the effect on pain symptoms. For patients with severe pain, these interventions may be very important especially when integrated within the framework of a comprehensive healthcare plan.[141]

Physical abuse, conjugal conflicts, borderline personality disorders, difficulty in maintaining relationships, or distressed family origin may render patients more vulnerable to nociceptive stimuli, and may reduce their capability to deal with painful somatic sensations associated with disease processes.[21,38,142–144] Referral to a mental healthcare provider can be of major benefit in such circumstances.

CONCLUSION

Chronic pelvic pain is not a diagnosis but a description of a clinical condition. The modern definition of pain acknowledges both sensory and affective aspects of the experience. Furthermore, particularly when moderate or severe, CPP can have a negative impact on the woman's capacity to function in family, sexual, social, and occupational roles. This condition is called chronic pain syndrome.

CPP is a symptom, not a disease, and rarely reflects a single pathologic process. When multiple factors are present, treatment of only some of them will lead to incomplete relief and frustration for both patient and clinician.[145] A RCT conducted in women with CPP without obvious pathology demonstrated that the results obtained with a multidisciplinary approach are significantly better than those observed after traditional treatment by gynecology alone.[26] Nevertheless, it has been reported that women with CPP generally experience modest improvements in pain and depression after recommended surgical or non-surgical therapies.[146] The long-term outcome of women with CPP has been defined in a prospective observational cohort study of 370 patients evaluated in a tertiary care pelvic pain clinic who underwent a primarily medical (pharmacotherapy, psychotherapy, physical therapy, or combination of the three) or surgical (hysterectomy, resection or ablative procedures, oophorectomy, diagnostic surgery, pain mapping) treatment. One year after the initial evaluation, 46% reported improvement in pain and 32% improvement in depression. Outcomes were similar in both treatment groups even after adjusting for background characteristics, psychosocial comorbidity, and previous treatments.[146]

Accordingly, patients should be persuaded that the most reasonable aim of treatment is not definitive cure, but achievement of a clinical condition that allows restoration of normal activities and a good enough health-related quality of life. In this regard, long-term rehabilitation strategies are probably as important as first-line therapies. Achievement of higher function in life in spite of some persisting pain should be regarded as a reasonable goal of management.

Finally, as reported by Price et al,[147] improvements are needed in the outpatient care of women presenting with CPP. According to the authors, patients want: personal care, which they often do not receive; to feel understood and to be taken seriously, although they often feel dismissed; explanation, which is often not provided, as much as cure; to be reassured, which often they are not. Changes in management should focus on providing more personal care, so that presenting problems are seen to be taken seriously, findings and treatments are appropriately explained, and women are more effectively reassured. Gaining women's trust and developing a strong patient–physician relationship may be no less important than drugs or surgery.

REFERENCES

1. Hakenberg OW, Wirth PA. Chronic pelvic pain in men. Urol Int 2002; 68: 138–43.
2. Zermann D, Ishigooka M, Doggwiler-Wiygul R et al. The male chronic pelvic pain syndrome. World J Urol 2001; 19: 173–9.
3. Bordman R, Jackson B. Below the belt. Can Fam Phys 2006; 52: 1556–62.
4. Latthe P, Latthe M, Say L et al. WHO systematic review of prevalence of chronic pelvic pain: a neglected reproductive health morbidity. BMC Public Health 2006; 6: 177–84.
5. Williams RE, Hartmann KE, Steege JF. Documenting the current definitions of chronic pelvic pain: implications for research. Obstet Gynecol 2004; 103: 686–91.
6. Leserman J, Zolnoun D, Meltzer-Brody S et al. Identification of diagnostic subtypes of chronic pelvic pain and how subtypes differ in health status and trauma history. Am J Obstet Gynecol 2006; 195: 554–61.
7. Zondervan K, Yudkin P, Vessey MP et al. The community prevalence of chronic pelvic pain in women and associated illness behaviour. Br J Gen Pract 2001; 51: 541–7.
8. Scialli AR. Evaluating chronic pelvic pain. A consensus recommendation. Pelvic pain expert working group. J Reprod Med 1999; 44: 945–52.
9. ACOG Committee on Practice Bulletins. ACOG Practice Bulletin No. 51. Chronic pelvic pain. Obstet Gynecol 2004; 103: 589–605.
10. Latthe P, Mignini L, Gray R et al. Factors predisposing women to chronic pelvic pain: systematic review. BMJ 2006; 332: 749–55.
11. Zondervan K, Yudkin P, Vessey MP et al. Chronic pelvic pain in the community – symptoms, investigations, and diagnoses. Am J Ostet Gynecol 2001; 184: 1149–55.
12. Howard FM. Laparoscopic evaluation and treatment of women with chronic pelvic pain. J Am Assoc Gynecol Laparosc 1994; 1: 325–31.
13. Mathias SD, Kupperman M, Liberman RF et al. Chronic pelvic pain: prevalence, health-related quality of life, and economic correlates. Obstet Gynecol 1996; 87: 321–7.
14. Davies L, Gangar KF, Drummond M et al. The economic burden of intractable gynaecological pain. J Obstet Gynecol 1992; 12: S54–6.
15. Gunter J. Chronic pelvic pain: an integrated approach to diagnosis and treatment. Obstet Gynecol Surv 2003; 58: 615–23.
16. Lamvu G, Steege MP, Steege JF. The anatomy and neurophysiology of pelvic pain. J Minim Invasive Gynecol 2006; 13: 516–22.
17. Anaf V, Simon P, El Nakadi I et al. Hyperalgesia, nerve infiltration and nerve growth factor expression in deep adenomyotic nodules, peritoneal and ovarian endometriosis. Hum Reprod 2002; 17: 1895–900.
18. Anaf V, Chapron C, El Nakadi I et al. Pain, mast cells, and nerves in peritoneal, ovarian, and deep infiltrating endometriosis. Fertil Steril 2006; 86: 1336–43.
19. Walker E, Katon W, Harrop-Griffiths J. Relationship of chronic pelvic pain to psychiatric diagnoses and childhood sexual abuse. Am J Psychiatry 1988; 145: 75–80.
20. Fry RP, Crisp AH, Beard RW. Sociopsychological factors in chronic pelvic pain: a review. J Psychosom Res 1997; 42: 1–5.
21. Howard FM. Chronic pelvic pain. Obstet Gynecol 2003; 101: 594–611.
22. Ray NF, Denton WG, Thamer M et al. Abdominal adhesiolysis: inpatient care and expenditures in the United States in 1994. J Am Coll Surg 1998; 186: 1–9.
23. Saravelos H, Cooke I. Adhesions and chronic pelvic pain. Cont Rev Obstet Gynecol 1995; 7: 172–7.
24. Alexander-Williams J. Do adhesions cause pain? BMJ 1987; 294: 659–60.
25. Hammoud A, Gago LA, Diamond MP. Adhesions in patients with chronic pelvic pain: a role for adhesiolysis? Fertil Steril 2004; 825: 1483–91.
26. Peters AA, van Dorst E, Jellis B et al. A randomized clinical trial to compare two different approaches in women with chronic pelvic pain. Obstet Gynecol 1991; 77: 740–4.
27. Kligman I, Drachenberg C, Papadimitriou J et al. Immunohistochemical demonstration of nerve fibers in pelvic adhesions. Obstet Gynecol 1993; 82: 566–8.
28. Beard RW, Higham JH, Pearce S et al. Diagnosis of pelvic varicosities in women with pelvic pain. Lancet 1984; 2: 946–9.
29. Cheong Y, Stones RW. Chronic pelvic pain: aetiology and therapy. Best Pract Res Clin Obstet Gynecol 2006; 20: 695–711.
30. Soysal ME, Soysal S, Vicdan K et al. A randomized controlled trial of goserelin and medroxyprogesterone acetate in the treatment of pelvic congestion. Hum Reprod 2001; 16: 931–6.
31. Fassiadis N. Treatment for pelvic congestion syndrome cuasing pelvic and vulvar varices. Int Angiol 2006; 25: 1–3.
32. Beard R, Reginald PW, Pearce S. Pelvic pain in women. Br Med J 1986; 283: 160–2.
33. Reginald PW, Adams J, Franks S et al. Medroxyprogesterone acetate in the treatment of pelvic pain due to venous congestion. Br J Obstet Gynaecol 1989; 96: 1148–52.
34. Porpora MG, Gomel V. The role of laparoscopy in the management of pelvic pain in women of reproductive age. Fertil Steril 1997; 68: 765–79.
35. Burkman RT. Chronic pelvic pain of bladder origin. Epidemiology, pathogenesis and quality of life. J Reprod Med 2004; 49: 225–9.

36. Jarrell JF, Vilos GA, Allaire C et al. Consensus guidelines for the management of chronic pelvic pain. J Obstet Gynecol Can 2005; 164: 781–826.

37. Stanford EJ, Koziol J, Feng A. The prevalence of interstitial cystitis, endometriosis, adhesions, and vulvar pain in women with chronic pelvic pain. J Minim Invasive Gynecol 2005; 12: 43–9.

38. Whitmore K, Siegel JF, Kellog-Spadt S. Interstitial cystitis/painful bladder syndrome as a cause of sexual pain in women: a diagnosis to consider. J Sex Med 2007; 4: 720–7.

39. Sand PK. Chronic pain syndromes of gynecologic origin. J Reprod Med 2004; 49: 230–4.

40. Butrick CW. Patients with chronic pelvic pain: endometriosis or interstitial cystitis/painful bladder syndrome? JSLS 2007; 11: 182–9.

41. Paulson JD, Delgado M. The relationship between interstitial cystitis and endometriosis in patients with chronic pelvic pain. JSLS 2007; 11: 175–81.

42. Holland-Hall CM, Brown RT. Evaluation of the adolescent with chronic abdominal or pelvic pain. J Pediatr Adolesc Gynecol 2004; 17: 23–7.

43. Mens JM, Vleeming A, Stoeckart R et al. Understanding peripartum pelvic pain. Implications of a patient survey. Spine 1996; 21: 1363–9.

44. Clemons JL, Arya LA, Myers DL. Diagnosing interstitial cystitis in women with chronic pelvic pain. Obstet Gynecol 2002; 100: 337–41.

45. O'Leary MP, Sant GR, Fowler JF et al. The interstitial cystitis symptom index and problem index. Urology 1997; 49: 58–63.

46. Walker EA, Gelfand AN, Green C et al. Chronic pelvic pain and gynaecological symptoms in women with irritable bowel syndrome. J Psychosom Obstet Gynecol 1996; 17: 39–46.

47. Drossman DA. The functional gastrointestinal disorders and the Rome II process. Gut 1999; 45: 1–5.

48. Eisenstat SA, Bankroft L. Domestic violence. N Engl J Med 1999; 341: 886–92.

49. Cody RF, Ascher SM. Diagnostic value of radiological tests in chronic pelvic pain. Best Pract Res Clin Obstet Gynecol 2000; 14: 433–66.

50. Moore J, Copley S, Morris J et al. A systematic review of the accuracy of ultrasound in the diagnosis of endometriosis. Ultrasound Obstet Gynecol 2002; 76: 588–94.

51. Kalish GM, Patel MD, Gunn ML et al. Computed tomographic and magnetic resonance features of gynaecologic abnormalities in women presenting with acute or chronic abdominal pain. Ultrasound Q 2007; 23: 167–75.

52. Stones W, Cheong YC, Howard FM. Interventions for treating chronic pelvic pain in women. Cochrane Database Syst Rev 2005; (2): CD000387.

53. Park SJ, Lim JW, Ko YT et al. Diagnosis of pelvic congestion syndrome using transabdominal and transvaginal sonography. AJR Am J Roentgenol 2004; 182: 683–8.

54. Parsons CL, Greenberg M, Gabal L et al. The role of urinary potassium in the pathogenesis and diagnosis of interstitial cystitis. J Urol 1998; 159: 1862–6.

55. Parsons CL. Diagnosing chronic pelvic pain of bladder origin. J Reprod Med 2004; 49: 235–42.

56. Waxman JA, Sulak PG, Kuhel TJ. Cystoscopic findings consistent with interstitial cystitis in normal women undergoing tubal ligation. J Urol 1998; 160: 1663–7.

57. Howard FM. The role of laparoscopy as a diagnostic tool in chronic pelvic pain. Best Pract Res Clin Obstet Gynecol 2000; 14: 467–94.

58. Elcombe S, Gath D, Day A. The psychological effects of laparoscopy on women with chronic pelvic pain. Psychol Med 1997; 27: 1041–50.

59. Swanton A, Iyer L, Reginald PW. Diagnosis, treatment and follow up of women undergoing conscious pain mapping for chronic pelvic pain: a prospective study. BJOG 2006; 102: 792–6.

60. Vercellini P, Fedele L, Aimi G et al. Reproductive performance, pain recurrence and disease relapse after conservative surgical treatment for endometriosis: the predictive value of the current system. Hum Reprod 2006; 21: 2679–85.

61. Vercellini P, Fedele L, Aimi G et al. Association between endometriosis stage, lesion type, patient characteristics and severity of pelvic pain symptoms: a multivariate analysis of over 1000 patients. Hum Reprod 2007; 22: 266–71.

62. Gambone JC, Mittman BS, Munro MG et al. Consensus statement for the management of chronic pelvic pain and endometriosis: proceedings of an expert-panel consensus process. Fertil Steril 2002; 78: 961–72.

63. Royal College of Obstetricians and Gynaecologists. The initial management of chronic pelvic pain. RCOG Guideline No. 41. London: RCOG Press, April 2005.

64. Kennedy S, Bergqvist A, Chapron C et al. ESHRE guidelines for the diagnosis and treatment of endometriosis. Hum Reprod 2005; 20: 2698–704.

65. The Practice Committee of the Society for Reproductive Medicine. Treatment of pelvic pain associated with endometriosis. Fertil Steril 2006; 86: S18–27.

66. Koninckx PR, Meuleman C, Demeyere S et al. Suggestive evidence that pelvic endometriosis is a progressive disease, whereas deeply infiltrating endometriosis is associated with pelvic pain. Fertil Steril 1991; 55: 759–65.

67. Williams RE, Hartmann KE, Sandler RS et al. Recognition and treatment of irritable bowel syndrome among women with chronic pelvic pain. Am J Obstet Gynecol 2005; 152: 761–7.

68. Ling FW. Randomized controlled trial of depot leuprolide in patients with chronic pelvic pain and clinically suspected endometriosis. Pelvic Pain Study Group. Obstet Gynecol 1999; 93: 51–8.

69. Barbieri RL. Primary gonadotropin-releasing hormone agonist therapy for suspected endometriosis: a nonsurgical approach to the diagnosis and treatment of chronic pelvic pain. Am J Manag Care 1997; 3: 285–90.

70. Vercellini P, Trespidi L, Colombo A et al. A gonadotropin-releasing hormone agonist versus a low-dose oral contraceptive for pelvic pain associated with endometriosis. Fertil Steril 1993; 60: 75–9.

71. Vercellini P, Frontino G, De Giorgi O et al. Continuous use of an oral contraceptive for endometriosis-associated recurrent dysmenorrhea that does not respond to a cyclic pill regimen. Fertil Steril 2003; 80: 560–3.

72. Vercellini P, Pietropaolo G, De Giorgi O et al. Treatment of symptomatic rectovaginal endometriosis with an estrogen-progestogen combination versus low-dose norethindrone acetate. Fertil Steril 2005; 84: 1375–87.

73. Vercellini P, Somigliana E, Vigano P et al. Endometriosis: current and future medical therapies. Best Pract Res Clin Obstet Gynecol 2007 Nov 22 [Epub ahead of print]

74. Jarrell JF, Vilos GA, Allaire C et al. Chronic Pelvic Pain Working Group; SOGC. Consensus guidelines for the management of chronic pelvic pain. J Obstet Gynecol Can 2005; 27: 869–87.

75. Onghena P, Van Houdenhove BV. Antidepressant-induced analgesia in chronic non-malignant pain: a metanalysis of 39 placebo controlled studies. Pain 1992; 49: 205–19.

76. Bonica JJ. General considerations of pain in the pelvis and perineum. In: Bonica JJ, Loeser JD, Chapman CR, Fordyce WE eds. The Management of Pain, 2nd edn. Malvern, PA: Lea & Febiger, 1990: 1283–312.

77. Renaer M. Chronic Pelvic Pain in Women. Berlin: Springer-Verlag, 1981.

78. Rocker I. Pelvic Pain in Women. Diagnosis and Management. London: Springer-Verlag, 1990.

79. Vercellini P, Trespidi L, De Giorgi O et al. Endometriosis and pelvic pain: relation to disease stage and localization. Fertil Steril 1996; 65: 299–304.

80. Vercellini P, Fedele L, Bianchi S et al. Pelvic denervation for chronic pain associated with endometriosis: fact or fancy? Am J Obstet Gynecol 1991; 165: 745–9.

81. Proctor ML, Latthe PM, Farquhar CM et al. Surgical interruption of pelvic nerve pathways for primary and secondary dysmenorrohea. Cochrane Database Syst Rev 2005; (4): CD001896.

82. Tjaden B, Schlaff WD, Kimball A et al. The efficacy of presacral neurectomy for the relief of midline dysmenorrhea. Obstet Gynecol 1990; 76: 89–91.

83. Candiani GB, Fedele L, Vercellini P et al. Presacral neurectomy for the treatment of pelvic pain associated with endometriosis: a controlled study. Am J Obstet Gynecol 1992: 167: 100–3.

84. Zullo F, Palomba S, Zupi E et al. Effectiveness of presacral neurectomy in women with severe dysmenorrhea caused by endometriosis who were treated with laparoscopic conservative surgery: a 1-year prospective randomized double-blind controlled trial. Am J Obstet Gynecol 2003; 189: 5–10.

85. Sutton C, Pooley AS, Jones KD et al. A prospective, randomized, double-blind controlled trial of laparoscopic uterine nerve ablation in the treatment of pelvic pain associated with endometriosis. Gynecol Endosc 2001; 10: 217–22.

86. Vercellini P, Aimi G, Busacca M et al. Laparoscopic uterosacral ligament resection for dysmenorrhea associated with endometriosis: results of a randomized, controlled trial. Fertil Steril 2003; 80: 310–19.

87. Johnson NP, Farquhar CM, Crossley S et al. A double-blind randomized controlled trial of laparoscopic uterine nerve ablation for women with chronic pelvic pain. BJOG 2004; 111: 950–9.

88. Lichten EM, Bombard J. Surgical treatment of primary dysmenorrhea with laparoscopic uterine nerve ablation. J Reprod Med 1987; 32: 37–41.

89. Yen YK, Liu MW, Yuan CC et al. Addition of laparoscopic uterine nerve ablation to laparoscopic bipolar coagulation of uterine vessels for women with uterine myomas and dysmenorrhea. J Am Assoc Gynecol Laparosc 2001; 8: 573–8.

90. Palomba S, Russo T, Falbo A et al. Laparoscopic uterine nerve ablation versus uterosacral ligament resection in postmenopausal women with intractable midline chronic pelvic pain: a randomized study. Eur J Obstet Gynecol Reprod Biol 2006; 129: 84–91.

91. Chen FP, Chang SD, Chu KK et al. Comparison of laparoscopic presacral neurectomy and laparoscopic uterine nerve ablation for primary dysmenorrhea. J Reprod Med 1996; 41: 463–6.

92. Juang CM, Chou P, Yen MS et al. Laparoscopic uteroscacral uterine nerve ablation with and without presacral neurectomy in the treatment of primary dysmenorrhea: a prospective efficacy analysis. J Reprod Med 2007; 52: 591–6.

93. Latthe P, Proctor ML, Farquhar CM et al. Surgical interruption of pelvic nerve pathways in dysmenorrhea: a systematic review of effectiveness. Acta Obstet Gynecol 2007; 86: 4–15.

94. Xiong T, Daniels J, Middleton L et al. Meta-analysis using individual patient data from randomised trials to assess the effectiveness of laparoscopic uterosacral nerve ablation in the treatment of chronic pelvic pain: a proposed protocol. BJOG 2007; 114: 1580, e1–7.

95. Vercellini P, De Giorgi O, Pisacreta A et al. Surgical management of endometriosis. Baillieres Best Pract Res Clin Obstet Gynecol 2000; 14: 501–23.

96. Daniell JF. Fiberoptic laser laparoscopy. Baillieres Clin Obstet Gynaecol 1989; 3: 545–62.

97 Grainger DA, Soderstrom RM, Schiff SF et al. Ureteral injuries at laparoscopy: insights into diagnosis, management, and prevention. Obstet Gynecol 1990; 75: 839–43.

98. Good MC, Copas PR, Doody MC. Uterine prolapse after laparoscopic uterosacral transection. J Reprod Med 1992; 37: 995–6.

99. Davis GD. Uterine prolapse after laparoscopic uterosacral transection in nulliparous airborne trainees. A report of three cases. J Reprod Med 1996; 41: 279–82.

100. Chen FP, Lo TS, Soong YK. Management of chylous ascites following laparoscopic presacral neurectomy. Hum Reprod 1998; 13: 880–3.

101. Lo TS, Chen FP, Chu KK et al. Successful management of chylous ascites after laparoscopic presacral neurectomy. J Am Assoc Gynecol Laparosc 1998; 5: 431–3.

102. Guzinski GM, Bonica JJ, McDonald JS. Gynecologic pain. In: Bonica JJ, Loeser JD, Chapman CR, Fordyce WE, eds. The Management of Pain, 2nd edn. Malvern, PA: Lea & Febiger, 1990: 1344–67.

103. Vercellini P. Endometriosis: what a pain it is. Semin Reprod Endocrinol 1997; 15: 251–61.

104. Vercellini P, Boccciolone L, Vendola N et al. Peritoneal endometriosis: morphologic appearance in women with chronic pelvic pain. J Reprod Med 1991; 36: 533–6.

105. Carlson KJ, Miller BA, Fowler FJ Jr. The Maine Women's Health Study: I. Outcome of hysterectomy. Obstet Gynecol 1994; 83: 556–65.

106. Learman LA, Kuppermann M, Gates E et al. Predictors of hysterectomy in women with common pelvic problems: a uterine survival analysis. J Am Coll Surg 2007; 204: 633–41.

107. Quinn MJ, Kirk N. Differences in uterine innervation at hysterectomy. Am J Obstet Gynecol 2002; 187: 1515–19.

108. Atwal G, du Plessis D, Armstrong G et al. Uterine innervation after hysterectomy for chronic pelvic pain with, and without, endometriosis. Am J Obstet Gynecol 2005; 193: 1650–5.

109. Chamberlain A, LaFerla JJ. The gynecologist's approach to chronic pelvic pain. In: Burrows JD, Elton D, Stanley GV, eds. Handbook of Chronic Pain Management. Amsterdam: Elsevier, 1987: 371–82.

110. Crosignani PG, Aimo G, Vercellini P et al. Hysterectomy for benign gynecologic disorders: when and why. Postgrad Med 1996; 100: 133–40.

111. Lefebvre G, Allaire C, Jeffrey J et al. Clinical Practice Gynecology Committee and Executive Committee and Council, Society of Obstetricians and Gynecologists of Canada. SOCG clinical guidelines. Hysterectomy. J Obstet Gynecol Can 2002; 24: 37–61.

112. Stovall TG, Ling FW, Crawford DA. Hysterectomy for chronic pelvic pain of presumed uterine etiology. Obstet Gynecol 1990; 75: 676–9.

113. Beard RW, Kennedy RG, Gangar KF et al. Bilateral oophorectomy and hysterectomy in the treatment of intractable pelvic pain associated with pelvic congestion. Br J Obstet Gynaecol 1991; 98: 988–92.

114. Carlson KJ, Miller BA, Fowler FJ. The Maine Women's Health Study: II. Outcomes of nonsurgical management of leiomyomas, abnormal bleeding, and chronic pelvic pain. Obstet Gynecol 1994; 83: 566–72.

115. Hillis SD, Marchbanks PA, Peterson HB. The effectiveness of hysterectomy for chronic pelvic pain. Obstet Gynecol 1995; 86: 941–5.

116. Tay SK, Bromwich N. Outcome of hysterectomy for pelvic pain in premenopausal women. Aus NZ J Obstet Gynaecol 1998; 38: 72–6.

117. Kjerulff KH, Lagenberg PW, Rhodes JC et al. Effectiveness of hysterectomy. Obstet Gynecol 2000; 3: 319–26.

118. Hartmann KE, Cindy MA, Lamvu GM et al. Quality of life and sexual function after hysterectomy in women with preoperative pain and depression. Obstet Gynecol 2004; 104: 701–9.

119. Parsons LH, Stovall TG. Surgical management of chronic pelvic pain. Obstet Gynecol Clin North Am 1993; 20: 765–78.

120. Sharp HT. Surgical management of pelvic pain. In: Blackwell RE, Olive DL, eds. Chronic Pelvic Pain. New York: Springer, 1998: 153–66.

121. Reiter RC. Evidence-based management of chronic pelvic pain. Clin Obstet Gynecol 1998: 41: 422–35.

122. Brandsborg B, Nikolajsen L, Hansen CT et al. Risk factors for chronic pelvic pain after hysterectomy. Anesthesiology 2007; 106: 1003–12.

123. Behera M, Vilos GA, Hollett-Caines J et al. Laparoscopic findings, histopathologic evaluation, and clinical outcomes in women with chronic pelvic pain after hysterectomy and bilateral salpingo-oophrectomy. J Minim Invasive Gynecol 2006; 13: 431–5.

124. Swank DJ, Swank-Bordewijk SC, Hop WC et al. Laparoscopic adhesiolysis in patients with chronic abdominal pain: a blinded randomised controlled multi-centre trial. Lancet 2003; 361: 1247–51.

125. Diamond MP, Daniell JF, Feste J et al. Adhesion reformation and de novo adhesion formation after reproductive pelvic surgery. Fertil Steril 1987; 47: 864–6.

126. Farquhar CM, Rogers V, Franks S et al. A randomized controlled trial of medroxyprogesterone acetate and psychotherapy for the treatment of pelvic congestion. Br J Obstet Gynaecol 1989; 96: 1153–62.

127. Venbroux AC, Chang AH, Kim HS et al. Pelvic congestion syndrome (pelvic venous incompetence): impact of ovarian and internal iliac vein embolotherapy on menstrual cycle and chronic pelvic pain. J Vasc Interv Radiol 2002; 13: 171–8.

128. Kim HS, Malhotra AD, Rowe PC et al. Embolotherapy for pelvic congestion syndrome: long-term results. J Vasc Intern Radiol 2006; 17: 289–97.

129. Kwon SH, Oh JH, Ko KR et al. Transcatheter ovarian vein embolization using coils for the treatment of pelvic congestion syndrome. Cardiovasc Intervent Radiol 2007; 30: 655–61.

130. Takeuchi K, Mochizuki M, Kitagaki S. Laparoscopic varicocele ligation for pelvic congestion syndrome. Int J Gynecol Obstet 1996; 55: 177–8.

131. Dawson TE, Jamison J. Intravesical treatments for painful bladder syndrome/interstitial cystitis. Cochrane Database Syst Rev 2007; (4): CD006113.

132. Mulholland SG, Hanno P, Parsons Cl et al. Pentosan polysulfate sodium therapy of interstitial cystitis. A double-blind placebo-controlled clinical study. Urology 1990; 35: 552–8.

133. Lentz GM, Bavendam T, Stenchever MA et al. Hormonal manipulation in women with chronic, cyclic irritable bladder symptoms and pelvic pain. Am J Obstet Gynecol 2002; 186: 1268–71.

134. Kirkemo AK, Miles BJ, Peters JM. Use of amitriptyline in the treatment of interstitial cystitis. J Urol 1989; 141: 846–8.

135. Jamison J, Dawson TE, Helfand M. Medical treatments for painful bladder syndrome (interstitial cystitis). Cochrane Database Syst Rev 2007; (3): CD006730.

136. Quartero AO, Meineche-Schimdt V, Muris J et al. Bulking agents, antispasmodic and antidepressant medication for the treatment of irritable bowel syndrome. Cochrane Database Syst Rev 2005; (2): CD003460.

137. Weiss JM. Pelvic floor myofascial trigger points: manual therapy for interstitial cystitis and the urgency-frequency syndrome. J Urol 2001; 166: 2226–31.

138. Chen R, Nickel JC. Acupuncture ameliorates symptoms in men with chronic prostatitis/chronic pelvic pain syndrome. Urology 2003; 61: 1156–93.

139. Siegel S, Paszkiewicz E, Kirkpatrick C et al. Sacral nerve stimulation in patients with chronic intractable pelvic pain. J Urol 2001; 166: 1742–5.

140. Renaer M, Vertommen H, Nijs P et al. Psychological aspects of chronic pelvic pain in women. Am J Obstet Gynecol 1979; 134: 75–80.

141. Lifford KL, Barbieri RL. Diagnosis and management of chronic pelvic pain. Urol Clin North Am 2002; 29: 637–47.

142. Reed BD, Haefner HK, Punch MR et al. Psychosocial and sexual functioning in women with vulvodynia and chronic pelvic pain. A comparative evaluation. J Reprod Med 2000; 45: 624–32.

143. Randolph ME, Reddy DM. Sexual functioning in women with chronic pelvic pain: the impact of depression, support, and abuse. J Sex Res 2006; 43: 38–45.

144. Meltzer-Brody S, Leserman J, Zolnoun D et al. Trauma and post-traumatic stress disorder in women with chronic pelvic pain. Obstet Gynecol 2007; 109: 902–8.

145. Kamm MA. Chronic pelvic pain in women – gastroenterological or psychological? Int J Colorectal Dis 1997; 12: 57–62.

146. Lamvu G, Williams R, Zolnoun D et al. Long-term outcomes after surgical and nonsurgical management of chronic pelvic pain: one year after evaluation in a pelvic pain specialty clinic. Am J Obstet Gynecol 2006; 195: 591–8.

147. Price J, Farmer G, Harris J et al. Attitudes of women with chronic pelvic pain to the gynaecological consultation: a qualitative study. BJOG 2006; 113: 446–52.

4 Adnexal masses

Genevieve Neal-Perry and Lubna Pal

OVERVIEW

The purpose of this chapter is to equip providers of gynecologic care with guidelines, from a 'conservationist's' perspective, to utilize non-surgical methodologies to evaluate and manage a newly diagnosed adnexal mass. The overall aim is to help the clinician minimize inherent risks of non-essential and non-requisite invasive interventions, thereby maintaining the paradigm of 'do no harm' as principle supreme.

INTRODUCTION

The term 'adnexal mass' often evokes great fear in patient and clinician alike, being perceived as synonymous with the leading cause of gynecologic mortality, i.e. ovarian cancer.[1] The incidence of ovarian cancer increases with advancing reproductive age. It is estimated that during their lifetime, 5–10% of women in the USA alone will undergo a surgical procedure for a suspected ovarian neoplasm,[1] with 13–21% being diagnosed with an ovarian malignancy. The poor survival rates associated with ovarian cancer are attributed, in part, to vague symptomatology and non-specific complaints, leading to a delayed diagnosis;[2,3] indeed at the time of diagnosis, 70% of patients will have advanced disease.[4] Given the poor prognosis attributed to diagnostic delay, the medical community is charged with the responsibility of differentiating between benign and malignant processes. Moreover, clinicians need to identify strategies that unmask ovarian cancer while it is in the early and curable stages as well as to develop sensitive and specific methods for evaluating adnexal masses with a potential for malignancy.[2,5]

Although ovarian cancer is the leading cause of gynecologic mortality, it is important to appreciate that the likelihood of an incidental adnexal mass being ovarian cancer is relatively small and that the vast majority of adnexal pathology is secondary to benign processes.[6,7] Consistent with this fact, a substantial proportion of adnexal masses spontaneously resolve when given the 'tincture of time'. Nonetheless, it is imperative that the possibility of inadvertently dismissing a sinister pathology such as ovarian cancer be seriously entertained and

systematically excluded prior to a decision to pursue a conservative management approach.[3]

The demonstrated reluctance for subspecialty referrals[5] for the evaluation of adnexal masses with perceived malignant potential appears to stem from concerns regarding instigation of 'unnecessary alarm'. While the primary providers are more likely to offer reassurance to a patient diagnosed with a pelvic mass, it must be appreciated that only 42–48% of women with ovarian cancer are actually referred to a gynecologic oncologist at any time point in their clinical care.[8] Although attempts to conserve and preserve ovarian function underlie the principles of reproductive endocrinology,[9] we vehemently acknowledge the need for extirpative intervention for adnexal masses posing a health risk for any individual woman; we herein outline non-invasive diagnostic approaches for ruling out a malignant ovarian neoplasm and identify 'red flags' that should be recognized as an indication for referring the patient to an appropriate subspecialist, as well as present approaches for conservative and non-invasive management of adnexal masses deemed as benign.

EVALUATION OF THE ADNEXAL MASS

While an adnexal mass is considered synonymous with 'of ovarian origin', it is important to appreciate the anatomical contributors to the 'adnexa', i.e. the ovary, fallopian tube, the broad ligament, and other embryologic remnants. The picture may be further complicated by processes occurring within neighboring non-gynecologic organs, i.e. the bowel, omentum, the renal–urinary system, and the uterus, all of which have the potential to give rise to eccentrically placed masses that may appear to be of adnexal origin.[10,11] Additionally, an adnexal mass that is likely of ovarian origin merits interpretation within the context of dynamics of ovarian physiology across the reproductive age spectrum. Consequently, when developing a list of plausible differential diagnoses during evaluation of an adnexal mass, one must consider not just the age of the patient, but also symptomatology pertinent to the various anatomic structures that may potentially contribute to the adnexal mass (Table 4.1).

Table 4.1   Differential diagnosis of an adnexal mass according to organ of origin

Ovary

Functional
Developmental
Endometriosis
Neoplasm
   appearance
   size
   interval change
   age
Inflammatory

Fallopian tube

Developmental
Inflammatory
Neoplasm

Para-tubal

Developmental

Uterus

Pregnancy
Developmental
Leiomyoma – broad ligament

Bowel

Neoplasm
Inflammatory
   diverticulitis/appendicitis/IBD
Developmental

Renal

Pelvic kidney
Urachal cyst
Bladder distension

IBD, inflammatory bowel disease

The management schema for any pathology, including a newly diagnosed adnexal mass, begins with history and physical examination, identification of personal/family risk factors,[12] and other relevant characteristics that may guide the clinician's analysis along the differential diagnostic maze. While a number of investigative tools that will help to reinforce or refute the clinical impressions exist, and may provide critical prognostic information regarding the presentation, these modalities are no replacement for an astute clinical assessment!

History

The spectrum of differential diagnoses while evaluating an adnexal mass is heavily weighted by family history and the patient's age at presentation.[6,13–15] Adnexal masses are much more likely to be benign and amenable to

spontaneous resolution when discovered in women of reproductive ages (i.e. beyond menarche and before menopause), whereas there is a greater likelihood of malignancy at either extreme of the reproductive spectrum, i.e. in pre-menarchal and postmenopausal women (Table 4.2). From a practical perspective, realizing the potential for morbidity and mortality, and the relatively common prevalence, the possibility of an ectopic pregnancy must be entertained when evaluating an adnexal mass, irrespective of the patient's age, barring the postmenopausal period that is remote from menopause.

A detailed family history is critical when selecting appropriate management plans for an adnexal mass.[12,16–19] A personal or family history of breast or ovarian cancer in a first degree relative,[18] particularly when cancer occurred at an age < 50 years, should heighten the clinician's concern regarding the possibility of an underlying genetic predisposition to malignant processes, and hence appropriate triage to a relevant subspecialist.

Symptomatology

The American College of Obstetricians and Gynecologists/Society of Gynecologic Oncologists (ACOG/SGO) Committee opinion[20] acknowledges that the symptoms of ovarian cancer are subtle and non-specific. Diagnosis of an adnexal mass is likely to be incidental in the majority of patients. A variety of non-specific gastrointestinal symptoms, however, may be primarily attributable to adnexal pathology and may dictate the acuity of intervention. For example, constitutional symptoms such as generalized malaise and weight loss in the background of rectal pressure, dischezia, abdominal distension, altered bowel habits, ascites, or early satiety may be suggestive of pelvic–abdominal mass effect. Gynecologic symptoms such as chronic pelvic pain, dyspareunia, menstrual irregularity, or pre-menarchal or postmenopausal vaginal bleeding should alert a clinician regarding the possibility of adnexal pathology. Additionally, new onset acne and hirsutism, male pattern hair loss, breast atrophy, voice changes, and even increased libido may be indicative of an androgen producing ovarian lesion. Clinicians must be alert to the spectrum of symptomatology[21,22] so as to initiate timely intervention, if indeed the mass is not benign.

Clinical examination

An evolving list of 'state of the art' diagnostic modalities cannot and should not substitute for a keen clinical

Table 4.2 Differential diagnoses of an adnexal mass according to age at presentation

Pre-menarchal	Reproductive age	Postmenopausal
Developmental		
Dermoid (rare)	Dermoid (common)	Dermoid (very rare)
Para-ovarian remnants	Para-ovarian cyst	Para-ovarian cyst
Mullerian abnormality non-communicating	Mullerian abnormality non-communicating	
Pelvic kidney	Pelvic kidney	Pelvic kidney
Pregnancy (common)	Pregnancy (most common)	
Inflammatory		
Tubo-ovarian abscess	Tubo-ovarian abscess	Tubo-ovarian abscess
Peri-appendiceal abscess	Peri-appendiceal abscess	Diverticulitis (rare)
Appendiceal mucocele	Inflammatory bowel disease	Peri-appendiceal abscess
		Inflammatory bowel disease
Functional		
Precocious puberty	Follicular cyst	
McCune–Albright syndrome	Hemorrhagic cyst	
Endometrioma	Endometrioma	
Neoplasm		
Primary ovarian		
Germ cell (rare)	Germ cell (common)	Germ cell (rare)
Epithelial (rare)	Epithelial (rare)	Epithelial (very common)
Fibroma (very rare)	Fibroma (common)	Fibroma
Secondary breast/bowel/lymphoma		
Rare	Uncommon	Common

evaluation. Identifiable stigmata that suggest a sinister underlying pathology, and hence a need for prompt onward referral, include cachexia, lymphadenopathy, and clinically appreciable ascites. In contrast, features of androgenization in an otherwise healthy young woman should initiate a diagnostic workup aiming to unmask the underlying pathophysiological mechanism. In a patient diagnosed with an adnexal mass, the examination should thus encompass the general appearance and overall well-being, as well as specific features of the mass, as outlined in Table 4.3.

INVESTIGATIONS IN THE MANAGEMENT OF AN ADNEXAL MASS

Poor sensitivity of a pelvic examination in terms of identifying malignant from benign pelvic processes is recognized.[2] The ACOG and SGO joint opinion supports the use of investigative modalities to further elucidate the nature of adnexal pathology, including the use of transvaginal ultrasound and the utilization of serum biomarkers, specifically CA125.[23] The interpretation of accrued data, however, may be markedly influenced by the clinician's index of suspicion, patient's age, and the related *normal* physiology. More important, a diagnosis must be achieved while keeping the entire patient in context!

Diagnostic imaging

Transvaginal ultrasonographic (TVUS) assessment of the pelvis provides reliable diagnostic as well as prognostic information regarding an adnexal mass; the superiority of TVUS over a transabdominal approach in this regard is well established.[24] Sonographic evaluation of an adnexal mass has demonstrated sensitivity ranging from 88 to 100% and specificity from 62 to 96% in discriminating between benign versus malignant adnexal processes.[25] An influence of the sonographer's experience in the diagnostic accuracy of an ultrasound study, however, needs to be appreciated.[26] A number of sonographic features in an adnexal mass are of proven prognostic value,[25] leading to the concept of a 'morphological index' or 'pattern recognition' for evaluating the likelihood of identifying a malignant adnexal mass (Table 4.4). For example, the presence of

Table 4.3 Assessment of adnexal mass

1. History

Age and symptomatology
Gynecologic history: parity, menstrual irregularity, androgenization, history of use of hormonal contraceptives or IUD, sexual history including history of and risk for STDs, history of dyspareunia or pelvic discomfort
Family history of cancer: breast, bowel, ovary, uterus, pancreas and age at diagnosis
Review of systems
    weight loss
    fatigue
    anemia

2. Examination

General
    appearance/cachexia/anemia/thyroid/pulse
    cutaneous striae suggestive of significant weight loss
    lymphadenopathy: supraclavicular/inguinal
    hair growth pattern
    secondary sexual characteristics, especially if pre-pubertal
Breast examination
    mass/nipple discharge
Abdomen
    Caput medusa
    peri-umbilical nodules
    distension
    visceromegaly
    ascites
Pelvic
    evidence of clitoromegaly
    bimanual examination:
        size
        location – central versus eccentric
        solid versus cystic
        mobility
        tenderness
    rectovaginal examination:
        size
        location
        solid versus cystic
        tenderness
        mobility
        stool guaiac

IUD, intrauterine device; STD, sexually transmitted disease

Table 4.4 Sonographic assessment of an adnexal mass: features distinguishing benign from sinister pathologies

Feature	Benign	Of concern
Size	<5 cm	Variable according to age
Translucency	Cystic	Complex with solid areas
Wall	Thin and uniform	Thick and nodular
Septum	Absent	Present
Papillations	Absent	Present

imaging to morphological ultrasound evaluation has somewhat, albeit arguably, enhanced the specificity of sonographic assessments.[27] More sophisticated diagnostic modalities including three-dimensional (3D) ultrasound,[27,28] pelvic computed tomography (CT),[29] magnetic resonance imaging (MRI),[30] and radio-immunoscintography[31] have additionally been evaluated in attempts to enhance the predictive values for diagnosis of ovarian cancer. One or more of these diagnostic modalities may provide additional information beyond that gleaned with routine TVUS; however, with exorbitant costs in the background of relatively little additional gain, these diagnostic tests cannot be, at present, purported as a first-line screening tool.

Biomarkers

The concept of a simple blood test to define an individual's risk for a disease process underlies the quest for biomarkers reflecting risk of ovarian cancer (Table 4.5). CA125 is probably the most widely utilized of all ovarian biomarkers.[2] First described in 1981,[32] serum levels of CA125 have demonstrated an acceptable degree of predictive value for the diagnosis of preclinical epithelial ovarian cancer,[33,34] especially in the postmenopausal population.[35] By utilizing age-specific/population cut-off levels, a gain in sensitivity for ovarian malignancy is achieved. Moreover, an improved survival benefit is suggested when CA125 is used as a first-line screening test.[36]

In the context of benign adnexal pathology, it is important to appreciate confounding influences, especially in the premenopausal patient population, of a variety of non-malignant processes that result in increased CA125. Gynecologic and non-gynecologic entities that may contribute to elevated serum levels of CA125 can include: normal menses, endometriosis, pelvic inflammatory disease, pancreatitis, colitis, peritonitis, pleuritis and ascites, and systemic lupus erythematosus.[2,37] The potential for these various pathological and non-pathological processes to contribute to elevated CA125 levels and a 'false-positive' screening test for

solid areas, irregularities, and papillary projections within an adnexal mass presumed to have ovarian origin begs an oncologic referral, whereas if a clinical evaluation is unremarkable and a simple appearing, thin, and smooth walled cyst is found, especially if unilocular, conservative management may be an option.

Within the context of benign ovarian pathologies, certain adnexal masses exhibit sonographic characteristics that may help direct the clinical management, e.g. endometriomas, hemorrhagic cyst, dermoid, and hydrosalpinx. The addition of color flow Doppler

Table 4.5 Serum biomarkers and associated adnexal pathology

Biomarker	Relevance
CA125 – serous	Epithelial ovarian tumor
LDH	Germ cell tumor
CEA	Bowel
AFP	Endodermal sinus tumor/ bowel/liver
CA19–9	Mucinous epithelial
Inhibin B	Granulosa cell tumor
Mullerian inhibitory substance	Granulosa cell tumor
βhCG	Choriocarcinoma

LDH, lactate dehydrogenase; CEA, carcinoembryonic antigen; AFP, α-fetoprotein

ovarian malignancy must be appreciated. Indeed, this latter understanding has led to a concept of 'variable thresholds' for CA125 levels based on the patient's age.[37] The CA125 threshold level frequently used in clinical practice is 30 U/ml[2,38] in the postmenopausal population and 200 U/ml[2] in the reproductive aged woman.

Recently, an appreciation of the rate of change in serum levels, rather than absolute cut-offs, has been shown to be of prognostic relevance.[15] Skates et al provided evidence of rising levels of CA125 in association with ovarian cancer, whereas static or even falling levels are associated with benign adnexal pathologies. A retrospective study utilizing a 'risk of ovarian cancer' algorithm that incorporates patient's age and a rate of change in CA125 levels demonstrated a sensitivity and specificity of 83% and 99.7%, respectively, for a diagnosis of ovarian cancer; these latter findings have subsequently been substantiated prospectively.[39]

While both TVUS and biomarkers[40] are of proven value in the evaluation of an adnexal pathology and discrimination between benign and malignant ovarian processes, a combination of the two techniques, i.e. multimodal screening, has been shown to improve the positive predictive value of diagnosing ovarian cancer. For example, significantly increased sensitivity and specificity of ovarian cancer diagnosis is afforded by using CA125 as a first-line test, and if abnormal, the inclusion of TVUS is recommended for a more complete evaluation of the adnexae.[37] Preliminary results from studies designed to assess the respective sensitivities of CA125 and ultrasound as first-line screening tests for early stage ovarian cancer suggest that, when compared to CA125 or TVUS alone, the combination of CA125 and TVUS increases the positive predictive value of ovarian cancer diagnosis more than sevenfold.[41] Depending upon your index of suspicion for sex cord, embryonal, and/or germ cell tumor and the history of present illness, it may also be appropriate to

check β human chorionic gonadotropin (βhCG), follicle stimulating hormone (FSH), luteinizing hormone (LH), estradiol, androgen profile, and insulin or thyroid stimulating hormone (TSH) levels.

The use of a panel of biomarkers such as macrophage-colony stimulating factor (M-CSF), OVX1, prostacin, osteopontin, kallikrein, lysophosphatidic acid (LPA), and CA72-4 has also been proposed to improve the sensitivity and specificity for the diagnosis of ovarian cancer. These markers may be more useful when evaluating tumors such as mucinous cystadenomas, which often may not be associated with CA125 elevations. More recently, gene arrays, proteomics, and bioinformatics have been utilized to catalog 'biomarker profiles' in women with ovarian cancer as compared to healthy controls[42] as potential screening tools for ovarian cancer. As of yet, pending availability of data from ongoing trials, this approach to ovarian cancer screening has not been validated for routine clinical use.[42]

Decision algorithm for non-surgical management

Once all parameters that could suggest the existence of an ovarian malignancy are systematically excluded, options for conservative management should be entertained and discussed with the patient (Table 4.6). When choosing the appropriate patient for a conservative management plan, it is important to ensure that the patient is able to comply with the periodic follow-up necessitated by such a decision, until recognizable resolution or evolution of the pathology. Should clinical evidence suggest progression of a pathological process, then a prompt decision for onward referral to an appropriate subspecialist for an exploratory approach is warranted.

Non-surgical approach to management of an adnexal mass

Having assessed the probability of malignancy being remote in the workup of an adnexal mass and depending upon the most plausible diagnoses, one can choose from a variety of non-surgical approaches (Table 4.6).

Simple ovarian cysts

Expectant management The least invasive approach in the management of a presumably benign adnexal mass is 'patient observation'. This approach is ideal in premenopausal or postmenopausal women diagnosed with a simple ovarian cyst less than 5 cm and without a family or personal history of malignancy. Most

Table 4.6 Conservative and non-invasive approaches in managing an adnexal mass deemed to be of low-risk potential

Non-invasive approach	Indication
Observation	Premenopausal patient
	Postmenopausal patient with simple cyst
Ovarian suppression	
OCP	Functional ovarian cyst
GnRH agonist	Endometrioma
	Precocious puberty
Insulin sensitizing agents	PCOS/ovarian thecosis
metformin	
thiozolidinediones	
Progestogenic agents	Endometrioma
danazol	
provera®	
Antiprogestogenic	Leiomyoma
mifepristone	
Aromatase inhibitor	Precocious puberty
letrozole	
Thyroid replacement	Hypothyroidism
Antibiotics	PID/tubo-ovarian abscess

PCOS, polycystic ovarian syndrome; PID, pelvic inflammatory disease

functional ovarian cysts will resolve spontaneously within 6–8 weeks.

Oral contraceptives (OCPs)   The use of the combined oral contraceptive pill in an attempt to suppress functional ovarian cysts is well documented,[43] albeit with equivocal success. The rationale proposed for the use of combined OCPs in this setting is an attempt to achieve hypothalamic–pituitary quiescence, thereby affording spontaneous resolution of an existing and gonadotropin responsive functional ovarian cyst. While the efficacy of OCPs in facilitating regression of existing functional ovarian cysts is debatable,[44] the role of OCPs in minimizing the formation of new ovarian cysts is well established.[45]

Gonadotropin releasing hormone (GnRH) agonists The use of GnRH agonists to desensitize the pituitary and decrease gonadotropin release for acute management of simple ovarian cysts is debatable. Indeed, the induction of functional ovarian cysts attributable to a 'flare effect' of GnRH agonists is well described, and attributed in part to the GnRH activity that is independent of pituitary release of gonadotropins, and possibly a direct effect of GnRH agonists on ovarian steroidogenesis.[46]

GnRH antagonists   While suppression of the hypothalamic–pituitary–ovarian axis can successfully be achieved with GnRH antagonists, and theoretically

may facilitate regression of a functional ovarian cyst, the use of a GnRH antagonist in this context has not been reported.

Thyroxine   The development of ovarian cysts in the setting of primary hypothyroidism is well described, as is their regression following appropriate thyroxine replacement.[47-50]

Inflammatory process

An adnexal mass deemed to be of an 'inflammatory and infected' nature merits prompt treatment with appropriate antibiotics.[51] Special consideration should be given to the postmenopausal woman in this setting as a primarily infectious process at this age is an unlikely event, and the possibility of an occult malignancy with focal necrosis and potential involvement of the bowel must be entertained.[52]

Adnexal masses and endometriosis

Afflicting 1–5% of reproductive aged women, endometriosis is a commonly underlying etiology in women presenting with chronic pelvic pain and/or infertility. Although several pathophysiological mechanisms are proposed to underlie the evolution of this process, the exact mechanisms are still under investigation.[53]

In addition to chronic pelvic pain and infertility, endometriosis often makes its clinical debut as an adnexal mass, i.e. an endometrioma.[54] While surgical resection/ablation remains the definitive management for endometriosis and an endometrioma,[55] concerns regarding iatrogenic reduction in ovarian reserve and the potential for reduced future fertility secondary to the surgical intervention are emerging. A more conservative approach utilizing medical management along with serial ultrasonography[56] and surveillance of a suspected endometrioma has been proposed for women with surgically confirmed endometriosis.[55] The therapeutic armamentarium available for the medical management of endometriosis includes progestins such as Depo-Provera®, antiprogestins, danazol, GnRH agonists, GnRH antagonists, and more recently, aromatase inhibitors.[57,58]

Uterine leiomyomas presenting as an adnexal mass

Uterine leiomyomas are not uncommon contributors to an adnexal mass.[59] In the asymptomatic woman in whom the uterine leiomyomas were diagnosed incidentally, conservative management with serial radiological assessment[60-62] and/or medical management are reasonable options.

Estradiol is important for the growth, development, and sustenance of leiomyomas. The ability of aromatase inhibitors,[63] GnRH agonists, or GnRH antagonists[64] to downregulate estradiol production has been appreciated, and as a consequence these agents have been used with modest success to medically manage symptomatic uterine leiomyomas.[65] Because progesterone has been proposed to modulate mitosis, growth factors, and their respective receptors, progestins have also been utilized with success in the medical management of uterine leiomyomas.[66,67] Other potential therapies to consider include antiprogestins,[68,69] danazol,[70] several experimental non-hormonal regimens,[71] and selective estrogen receptor modulators.[72,73]

SUMMARY

The diagnosis of an adnexal mass warrants a thorough evaluation. The role of surgery in the case of suspected malignancy is unambiguous. However, when the likelihood of malignancy is low, the risk/benefit ratio of a surgical intervention must be evaluated and subsequent management individualized. Non-invasive management may offer a high benefit/low risk approach for an individual patient diagnosed with an adnexal mass that is deemed 'non-malicious' by the various assessment modalities discussed earlier; in this context, resolution of the adnexal mass may be achieved, much to the patient's and provider's relief, in a significant proportion of cases.

REFERENCES

1. Jemal A, Siegel R, Ward E et al. Cancer statistics, 2006. CA Cancer J Clin 2006; 56: 106–30.
2. Rosenthal AN, Menon U, Jacobs IJ. Screening for ovarian cancer. Clin Obstet Gynecol 2006; 49: 433–47.
3. Barrenetxea G, Schneider J, Rodriguez-Escudero FJ. Abdominal mass in a young woman. Pitfalls and delayed diagnosis. Case report. Eur J Gynaecol Oncol 1996; 17: 507–9.
4. Dunleavey R. Importance of early diagnosis in managing ovarian cancer. Nurs Times 2006; 102: 28–9.
5. Murta EF, Nomelini RS. Early diagnosis and predictors of malignancy of adnexal masses. Curr Opin Obstet Gynecol 2006; 18: 14–19.
6. Jermy K, Luise C, Bourne T. The characterization of common ovarian cysts in premenopausal women. Ultrasound Obstet Gynecol 2001; 17: 140–4.
7. Heinemann K, Thiel C, Mohner S et al. Benign gynecological tumors: estimated incidence. Results of the German Cohort Study on Women's Health. Eur J Obstet Gynecol Reprod Biol 2003; 107: 78–80.
8. Gostout BS, Brewer MA. Guidelines for referral of the patient with an adnexal mass. Clin Obstet Gynecol 2006; 49: 448–58.
9. Maltaris T, Seufert R, Fischl F et al. The effect of cancer treatment on female fertility and strategies for preserving fertility. Eur J Obstet Gynecol Reprod Biol 2007; 130: 148–55.
10. Husain S, Thompson D, Thomas L, Donaldson B, Sabbagh R. Adnexal mass: an unusual presentation of small-bowel adenocarcinoma. J Nat Med Assoc 2006; 98: 799–802.
11. Spencer JR, Eriksen B, Garnett JE. Metastatic renal tumor presenting as ovarian clear cell carcinoma. Urology 1993; 41: 582–4.
12. Figueiredo JC, Ennis M, Knight JA et al. Influence of young age at diagnosis and family history of breast or ovarian cancer on breast cancer outcomes in a population-based cohort study. Breast Cancer Res Treat 2007; 105: 69–80.
13. Reimer T, Gerber B, Muller H et al. Differential diagnosis of peri- and postmenopausal ovarian cysts. Maturitas 1999; 31: 123–32.
14. Schultz KA, Ness KK, Nagarajan R, Steiner ME. Adnexal masses in infancy and childhood. Clin Obstet Gynecol 2006; 49: 464–79.
15. Skates SJ, Menon U, MacDonald N et al. Calculation of the risk of ovarian cancer from serial CA-125 values for preclinical detection in postmenopausal women. J Clin Oncol 2003; 21 (Suppl): 206–10.
16. Andrykowski MA, Zhang M, Pavlik EJ, Kryscio RJ. Factors associated with return for routine annual screening in an ovarian cancer screening program. Gynecol Oncol 2007; 104: 695–701.
17. Lacey JV Jr, Greene MH, Buys SS et al. Ovarian cancer screening in women with a family history of breast or ovarian cancer. Obstet Gynecol 2006; 108: 1176–84.
18. Malone KE, Daling JR, Doody DR et al. Prevalence and predictors of BRCA1 and BRCA2 mutations in a population-based study of breast cancer in white and black American women ages 35 to 64 years. Cancer Res 2006; 66: 8297–308.
19. Trentham-Dietz A, Newcomb PA, Nichols HB, Hampton JM. Breast cancer risk factors and second primary malignancies among women with breast cancer. Breast Cancer Res Treat 2007; 105: 195–207.
20. American College of Obstetricians and Gynecologists. ACOG Committee Opinion: number 280, December 2002. The role of the generalist obstetrician-gynecologist in the early detection of ovarian cancer. Obstet Gynecol 2002; 100: 1413–16.
21. Goff BA, Mandel LS, Drescher CW et al. Development of an ovarian cancer symptom index: possibilities for earlier detection. Cancer 2007; 109: 221–7.
22. Lataifeh I, Marsden DE, Robertson G, Gebski V, Hacker NF. Presenting symptoms of epithelial ovarian cancer. Aust NZ J Obstet Gynaecol 2005; 45: 211–14.
23. Im SS, Gordon AN, Buttin BM et al. Validation of referral guidelines for women with pelvic masses. Obstet Gynecol 2005; 105: 35–41.
24. Ferrazzi E, Lissoni AA, Dordoni D et al. Differentiation of small adnexal masses based on morphologic characteristics of transvaginal sonographic imaging: a multicenter study. J Ultrasound Med 2005; 24: 1467–73; quiz 1475–6.
25. Valentin L, Ameye L, Testa A et al. Ultrasound characteristics of different types of adnexal malignancies. Gynecol Oncol 2006; 102: 41–8.
26. Timmerman D, Bourne TH, Tailor A et al. A comparison of methods for preoperative discrimination between malignant and benign adnexal masses: the development of a new logistic regression model. Am J Obstet Gynecol 1999; 181: 57–65.
27. Kurjak A, Prka M, Arenas JM et al. Three-dimensional ultrasonography and power Doppler in ovarian cancer screening of asymptomatic peri- and postmenopausal women. Croatian Med J 2005; 46: 757–64.
28. Geomini PM, Kluivers KB, Moret E et al. Evaluation of adnexal masses with three-dimensional ultrasonography. Obstet Gynecol 2006; 108: 1167–75.
29. Balan P. Ultrasonography, computed tomography and magnetic resonance imaging in the assessment of pelvic pathology. Eur J Radiol 2006; 58: 147–55.

30. Hauth EA, Wolfgarten B, Kimmig R, Forsting M. [MR imaging of the pelvis in characterization of adnexal masses]. Zentralbl Gynakol 2005; 127: 373–9.

31. Maughan TS, Haylock B, Hayward M et al. OC125 immunoscintigraphy in ovarian carcinoma: a comparison with alternative methods of assessment. Clinical Oncol (R Coll Radiol). 1990; 2: 199–205.

32. Bast RC Jr, Xu FJ, Yu YH et al. CA 125: the past and the future. Int J Biol Markers 1998; 13: 179–87.

33. Berek JS, Bast RC Jr. Ovarian cancer screening. The use of serial complementary tumor markers to improve sensitivity and specificity for early detection. Cancer 1995; 76 (Suppl): 2092–6.

34. Kabawat SE, Bast RC Jr, Bhan AK et al. Tissue distribution of a coelomic-epithelium-related antigen recognized by the monoclonal antibody OC125. Int J Gynecol Pathol 1983; 2: 275–85.

35. Fritsche HA, Bast RC. CA 125 in ovarian cancer: advances and controversy. Clin Chem 1998; 44: 1379–80.

36. Jacobs IJ, Skates SJ, MacDonald N et al. Screening for ovarian cancer: a pilot randomised controlled trial. Lancet 1999; 353: 1207–10.

37. McDonald JM, Modesitt SC. The incidental postmenopausal adnexal mass. Clin Obstet Gynecol 2006; 49: 506–16.

38. Roupa Z, Faros E, Raftopoulos V et al. Serum CA 125 combined with transvaginal ultrasonography for ovarian cancer screening. In Vivo 2004; 18: 831–6.

39. Menon U, Skates SJ, Lewis S et al. Prospective study using the risk of ovarian cancer algorithm to screen for ovarian cancer. J Clin Oncol 2005; 23: 7919–26.

40. Menon U, Talaat A, Jeyarajah AR et al. Ultrasound assessment of ovarian cancer risk in postmenopausal women with CA125 elevation. Br J Cancer 1999; 80: 1644–7.

41. Buys SS, Partridge E, Greene MH et al. Ovarian cancer screening in the Prostate, Lung, Colorectal and Ovarian (PLCO) cancer screening trial: findings from the initial screen of a randomized trial. Am J Obstet Gynecol 2005; 193: 1630–9.

42. Gogoi R, Srinivasan S, Fishman DA. Progress in biomarker discovery for diagnostic testing in epithelial ovarian cancer. Expert review of molecular diagnostics 2006; 6: 627–37.

43. Grimes DA, Jones LB, Lopez LM, Schulz KF. Oral contraceptives for functional ovarian cysts. Cochrane Database Syst Rev 2006; (4): CD006134.

44. MacKenna A, Fabres C, Alam V, Morales V. Clinical management of functional ovarian cysts: a prospective and randomized study. Hum Reprod 2000; 15: 2567–9.

45. Should OCs be prescribed to prevent adnexal masses? Contracept Technol Update 1982; 3: 116–18.

46. Mehta RH, Anand Kumar TC. Can GnRH agonists act directly on the ovary and contribute to cyst formation? Hum Reprod 2000; 15: 505–7.

47. de Lima GR, Grabert H, Zaroni AA, Reis LC, Lippi UG. Ovarian lutein cysts associated with normal single pregnancy and primary hypothyroidism. Matern Infanc (Sao Paulo) 1970; 39: 357–9.

48. Evers JL, Rolland R. Primary hypothyroidism and ovarian activity evidence for an overlap in the synthesis of pituitary glycoproteins. Case report. Br J Obstet Gynaecol 1981; 88: 195–202.

49. Pongpipat D, Anumanrajadhon Y, Suvatte A. Cretinism with ovarian cyst causing precocious puberty. J Med Assoc Thai 1972; 55: 57–61.

50. Wood LC, Olichney M, Locke H et al. Syndrome of juvenile hypothyroidism associated with advanced sexual development: report of two new cases and comment on the management of an associated ovarian mass. J Clin Endocrinol Metab 1965; 25: 1289–95.

51. Beigi RH, Wiesenfeld HC. Pelvic inflammatory disease: new diagnostic criteria and treatment. Obstet Gynecol Clin North Am 2003; 30: 777–93.

52. Ben-Baruch G, Menashe Y, Leibovitz S, Schiff E, Menczer J. Pelvic malignancy presenting as a pelvic inflammatory process in pre- and postmenopausal women. Eur J Gynaecol Oncol 1991; 12: 347–9.

53. Einspanier A, Lieder K, Bruns A et al. Induction of endometriosis in the marmoset monkey (Callithrix jacchus). Mol Hum Reprod 2006; 12: 291–9.

54. Practice Committee of the American Society for Reproductive Medicine. Endometriosis and infertility. Fertil Steril 2006; 86 (Suppl): S156–60.

55. Barbieri RL. Endometriosis 1990. Current treatment approaches. Drugs 1990; 39: 502–10.

56. Fleischer AC, Cullinan JA, Jones HW 3rd et al. Serial assessment of adnexal masses with transvaginal color Doppler sonography. Ultrasound Med Biol 1995; 21: 435–41.

57. Crosignani P, Olive D, Bergqvist A, Luciano A. Advances in the management of endometriosis: an update for clinicians. Hum Reprod Update 2006; 12: 179–89.

58. Garcia-Velasco JA, Quea G. Medical treatment of endometriosis. Minerva Ginecol 2005; 57: 249–55.

59. Killackey MA, Neuwirth RS. Evaluation and management of the pelvic mass: a review of 540 cases. Obstet Gynecol 1988; 71: 319–22.

60. Caoili EM, Hertzberg BS, Kliewer MA, DeLong D, Bowie JD. Refractory shadowing from pelvic masses on sonography: a useful diagnostic sign for uterine leiomyomas. AJR Am J Roentgenol 2000; 174: 97–101.

61. Kim JC, Kim SS, Park JY. 'Bridging vascular sign' in the MR diagnosis of exophytic uterine leiomyoma. J Comput Assist Tomogr 2000; 24: 57–60.

62. Murase E, Siegelman ES, Outwater EK, Perez-Jaffe LA, Tureck RW. Uterine leiomyomas: histopathologic features, MR imaging findings, differential diagnosis, and treatment. Radiographics 1999; 19: 1179–97.

63. Shozu M, Murakami K, Inoue M. Aromatase and leiomyoma of the uterus. Semin Reprod Med 2004; 22: 51–60.

64. De Falco M, Pollio F, Pontillo M et al. GnRH agonists and antagonists in the preoperative therapy of uterine fibroids: literature review. Minerva Ginecol 2006; 58: 553–60.

65. Gao Z, Matsuo H, Nakago S, Kurachi O, Maruo T. p53 Tumor suppressor protein content in human uterine leiomyomas and its down-regulation by 17 beta-estradiol. J Clin Endocrinol Metab 2002; 87: 3915–20.

66. Schweppe KW. Progestins and uterine leiomyoma. Gynecol Endocrinol 1999; 13 (Suppl 4): 21–4.

67. van de Ven J, Sprong M, Donker GH et al. Levels of estrogen and progesterone receptors in the myometrium and leiomyoma tissue after suppression of estrogens with gonadotropin releasing hormone analogs. Gynecol Endocrinol 2001; 15 (Suppl 6): 61–8.

68. Chegini N, Ma C, Tang XM, Williams RS. Effects of GnRH analogues, 'add-back' steroid therapy, antiestrogen and antiprogestins on leiomyoma and myometrial smooth muscle cell growth and transforming growth factor-beta expression. Mol Hum Reprod 2002; 8: 1071–8.

69. De Leo V, Morgante G, La Marca A et al. A benefit-risk assessment of medical treatment for uterine leiomyomas. Drug Saf 2002; 25: 759–79.

70. Olive DL, Lindheim SR, Pritts EA. Non-surgical management of leiomyoma: impact on fertility. Curr Opin Obstet Gynecol 2004; 16: 239–43.

71. Young SL, Al-Hendy A, Copland JA. Potential nonhormonal therapeutics for medical treatment of leiomyomas. Semin Reprod Med 2004; 22: 121–30.

72. Cook JD, Walker CL. Treatment strategies for uterine leiomyoma: the role of hormonal modulation. Semin Reprod Med 2004; 22: 105–11.

73. Palomba S, Orio F Jr, Morelli M et al. Raloxifene administration in women treated with gonadotropin-releasing hormone agonist for uterine leiomyomas: effects on bone metabolism. J Clin Endocrinol Metab 2002; 87: 4476–81.

5 Dysfunctional uterine bleeding

Juan A Garcia-Velasco, Maria Cerrillo, and Carlos Simón

INTRODUCTION

Bleeding from the genital tract can be a physiologic process – normal menstruation – or can be a consequence of a pathologic process. Dysfunctional uterine bleeding (DUB) is included in a group of disorders known as abnormal uterine bleeding, in which frequency and/or quantity differ from normal menstrual bleeding.

Concept DUB could be defined as a variation in bleeding without existing disease or pathologic condition or pregnancy.[1] To study DUB, we distinguish ovulatory and non-ovulatory bleeding. If regular menstrual bleeding exists (i.e. every 21–35 days), cycles are usually ovulatory, but if bleeding is irregular or non-cyclic, anovulation or oligo-ovulation is occurring.

Frequency It is difficult to establish DUB incidence, but estimates are that it corresponds to around 10–15% of all gynecologic consultations.[2] It may vary with age, being more frequent at the reproductive age extremes, and 70% of these cases are anovulatory. Ovulatory DUB usually occurs in women between 20 and 40 years of age (Table 5.1).

It is relevant to establish what a normal menstrual cycle is because it varies among women. The only way to address this issue is to define it according to duration: 2–8 days. Normal menstrual cycles last between 21 and 35 days, and the volume of blood lost is 30 ml on average and less than 80 ml.

Because DUB is so frequent in outpatient gynecologic clinics, and 1 in 4 women surveyed state that they have experienced at least one abnormally intense bleeding episode in their lives,[3] there is strong interest in identifying less aggressive, lower-cost therapeutic alternatives to hysterectomy, which has been the traditional and definitive treatment for DUB. Thus, in the last few years there has been a focus on better understanding of the physiologic causes underlying DUB and the development of effective drugs for treatment.

PATHOPHYSIOLOGY

To completely understand the pathophysiology of DUB, it is relevant to review the physiology of normal menstruation and the different factors involved.

Table 5.1 Frequency of dysfunctional uterine bleeding (DUB)

<20 years	25%
20–40 years	30%
>40 years	40%

Menstruation is regulated by *vascular factors*: both the vasoconstriction and vasodilatation that precede menstruation are regulated by vasoconstrictor prostaglandins (PGs) (PGF2α and endothelin 1) and/or vasodilator PGs (PGE2 and prostacyclins). Lysosome membrane desensitization facilitates proteolytic enzyme entrance into the cytoplasm, resulting in cell degradation. Also playing a relevant role are *hemostatic factors*: a delicate balance between the coagulation system and fibrinolysis is necessary so that bleeding is not excessive and is self-regulated. Thus, systemic or intraendometrial anomalies in the fibrinolytic system, plaque defects, or coagulation factor problems all may cause DUB.[1] Any alteration in these factors or in the secretion of ovarian sex steroids may cause DUB.

Dysregulation of cellular and vascular factors causing DUB

One of the most-studied DUB causes is the exaggerated production of intraendometrial PGs. As mentioned above, normal menstruation is preceded by a sequence of vasospasm and vasodilatation of spiral arteries, with a final dominance of vasoconstriction, leading to ischemia. This ischemia increases capillary permeability and breakage of arteriolar walls, creating hemorrhagic foci. These vascular changes are PG mediated, involving vasoconstriction by PGF2α and endothelin 1 and vasodilatation by PGE2 and prostacyclin. Patients with DUB have shown an imbalance in PG production that favors vasodilating PGs.[1]

Another route of DUB pathophysiology that has been investigated is lysosome membrane desensitization. Lysosome membranes are stabilized by the estrogen/progesterone equilibrium. With an imbalance, microruptures will occur, allowing passage of enzymes into the cytoplasm, inducing cell lysis. Recently, it has been shown that in 70% of DUB, matrix metalloproteinases are upregulated (MMPs 1, 2, 3, and 9). Not only are

MMPs upregulated in the bleeding endometrium, but also their tissue inhibitors (TIMP-1) are downregulated in these patients. Extracellular matrix destruction induces destabilization of basal membranes and vessels, causing endometrium breakdown.[4]

Certain growth factors are also involved. In a recent publication, menstrual bleeding of women with menorrhagia was associated with lower amounts of vascular endothelial growth factor type-A (VEGF-A), which may influence the deregulation of endometrial vessels occurring at menstruation.

Anomalies in the endometrial or systemic coagulation systems causing DUB

In a normal menstrual period, the amount of blood loss is controlled by local coagulation and fibrinolytic mechanisms.[1] Tissue factor (TF) and plasminogen activator inhibitor (PAI-1) change at the endometrial level, modulating the amount of blood loss. Excessive bleeding is observed when fibrinolytic activity is increased because of a reduction in PAI-1 that elicits an increase in plasminogen activator[5] (Figure 5.1).

Excessive menstrual bleeding may also be caused by systemic alteration of the coagulation/fibrinolytic system. For instance, von Willebrand disease, inherited deficiency of factor X, factor XI, or vitamin K, platelet function alterations, and therapeutic anticoagulation are all causes of hemorrhage. This etiology should be considered mainly in adolescent DUB because it represents 11–17% of the cases in this age group.[6]

Inappropriate secretion of ovarian sex steroids causing DUB

Persistent corpus luteum   Disruption of progestins induces irregular menstrual bleeding, and the patient presents with persistent hemorrhage. In the endometrial biopsy, both secretory endometrium from the previous cycle as well as proliferative endometrium from the following cycle are found.

Estrogen deprivation hemorrhage   In this subgroup, all anovulatory DUB as well as endometrial hyperplasia DUB is included. Bleeding is caused by disruption of estradiol, and it will be heavier when estrogen concentration is higher, such as occurs in polycystic ovarian syndrome (PCOS) and/or obese patients or in patients with an immature hypothalamic–pituitary–ovarian axis.[1] The cause behind the symptoms is an absent luteinizing hormone (LH) peak together with continuous follicle

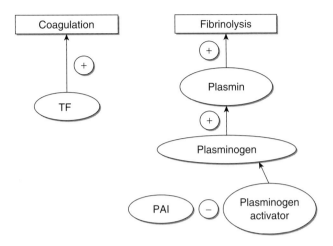

Figure 5.1   Diagram of coagulation–fibrinolvsis. TF, tissue factor; PAI, plasminogen activator inhibitor

stimulating hormone (FSH) stimulation of ovarian follicle growth (up to 3 cm or more), which increases estradiol concentrations. Estradiol will stimulate endometrial growth, and if it is unopposed by progestins, will alter normal endometrial morphology.

Bleeding in these cases occurs because of disruption: local asynchronic stromal development foci will appear, vessels will curve, and necrosis will start. If anovulation is prolonged, endometrial growth can be exaggerated, originating different stages of endometrial hyperplasia. This is an organic pathology that can be diagnosed with the usual techniques.

DIAGNOSIS

First of all, we should clarify whether the bleeding is DUB or not because there is some difficulty in objectively evaluating what could be considered a 'normal' amount of blood loss. Menstrual blood loss evaluation is routinely performed by detailed anamnesis, but there are some objective and semi-objective methods for quantifying it.

Among subjective methods, patient perception is the reference, even though most of the time this is not accurate. One survey showed that 14% of women who lost less than 20 ml during their menstrual period considered it to be an intense hemorrhage, 49% of women who thought similarly lost less than 80 ml, and 34% of women who lost more than 80 ml considered their menstrual blood loss 'normal'.[7] Frequently, during the anamnesis, indirect indicators could be helpful; these include blood clots with the menstrual effluent and/or ferropenic anemia without any other causative condition.

Table 5.2   Differential diagnosis of DUB

Pregnancy bleeding	Anatomic defects	Systemic diseases	Coagulopathies	Neoplasm	Not uterine	Infectious
Miscarriage	Endometrial polyp	Thyroid disease	von Willebrand	Cervical cancer	Genital injury	STD
Trophoblastic disease	Fibroids	Renal insufficiency	Factor X, XI $\downarrow$		Foreign body	
Ectopic pregnancy	Cervical polyp	Cirrhosis		Endometrial cancer		
Placental polyp				Tubal cancer		

STD, sexually transmitted disease

To correctly diagnose DUB, we should perform:

- Anamnesis: truly fundamental, it can guide us regarding which complementary tests to order.
- Clinical examination: both a general and a pelvic examination, including visualization of the cervix and vagina and bimanual palpation.
- Blood tests:
  - hemogram
  - pregnancy test (to rule out any early pregnancy complications causing bleeding)
  - hepatic and renal function tests (if we suspect liver or kidneys to be affected based on anamnesis citing similar cases in the family or alcoholism, jaundice, etc.)
  - thyroid function tests (not routinely, only when anamnesis suggests an alteration in function)
  - hemostasis profile: if menstrual abnormalities began with menarche, when there are familial cases of hemorrhagic diathesis, or in women not responding to conventional treatments.
- Transvaginal ultrasound (TVUS): most authors agree that TVUS should be performed at the initial evaluation of DUB.[8] With TVUS, we can evaluate endometrial growth and organic lesions, such as polyps, submucosal myomas, and adenomyosis, and also ovarian lesions such as persistent corpus luteum that may cause the abnormal bleeding. When intracavitary lesions are suspected, hysterosonography may be of great value in the differential diagnosis.
- Cervicovaginal cytology (Pap smear): this test is required to rule out bleeding from a cervical cause.
- Endometrial biopsy: this assessment is the standard technique for evaluating the endometrium, with a sensitivity of 85–90% and specificity of 95%.[9] Generally speaking, it is not required at the initial evaluation of DUB. It may be indicated in patients over 35–40 years old, in the case of failed previous therapies, prior to any surgical treatment, or if risk factors for endometrial cancer are present.
- Hysteroscopy: this is the gold standard technique to evaluate the endometrium and any abnormal uterine

bleeding. It is not required in all women with abnormal uterine bleeding[10] but only when intracavitary lesions are suspected or in patients with recurrent DUB.

Differential diagnosis

As indicated in Table 5.2, different diagnoses can be made to rule out any organic cause of bleeding, to adequately diagnose DUB cases.

MEDICAL TREATMENT OF DYSFUNCTIONAL UTERINE BLEEDING

Before selecting the best treatment of DUB for any specific patient, the clinician must consider whether cycles are ovulatory or not, whether the patient requires contraception, the patient's choice, and treatment contraindications.

Non hormonal treatment options

Medical treatment can be *hormonal* or *non-hormonal*. In ovulatory DUB, non-hormonal treatments are the first approach, with antifibrinolytics and non-steroidal anti-inflammatory drugs (NSAIDs).[11]

Non-steroidal anti-inflammatory drugs

These drugs exert their action by inhibiting the enzyme cyclooxygenase; in doing so, they block the conversion of arachidonic acid into PGs. They inhibit all PGs, both vasoconstrictors (PGF2α and TX A2) and vasodilators (PGE2 and prostacyclin). The ideal NSAID for the treatment of DUB would be a selective inhibitor of vasodilating PGs, permitting the vasoconstrictor PGs to inhibit the excessive menstrual blood loss, but such a selective inhibitor is not yet available. However, there is enough evidence to support that NSAIDs reduce menstrual blood loss in women with ovulatory cycles, as well as improving dysmenorrhea in most of these women.[12]

NSAIDs used in women with DUB reduce blood loss by 20–35%.[11,13] Not all women respond similarly to treatment, but approximately 40–50% improve.[1]

Lethaby et al, in a Cochrane review[12] evaluating 16 randomized controlled trials, concluded that NSAIDs are more effective than placebo in DUB, but less than tranexamic acid (an antifibrinolytic). No differences were found between the two NSAIDs evaluated (naproxen and mefenamic acid) in hemorrhage reduction.

The most commonly used protocols in the clinic are mefenamic acid (500 mg/8 h) taken orally during the days of the menstrual period, and naproxen (500 mg/12 h) taken orally 3–5 days during menstruation.

Antifibrinolytics

It is known that in women with excessive menstrual bleeding, plasminogen activators are overexpressed in the endometrium when compared to women with normal menstrual periods. These drugs inhibit the activation of plasminogen into plasmin, inducing hemostasis. Results from a recent randomized trial indicated that that tranexamic acid given during menstruation was an effective treatment for menorrhagia.[11,14]

In the same Cochrane review,[14] it was clear that antifibrinolytic therapy reduces blood loss more effectively than placebo and other treatment options such as NSAIDs, luteal phase administration of progestins, or etamsylate. Although the frequency of secondary effects seems to be similar to that with other treatments, there are no cost–benefit studies or available data from randomized trials about thromboembolic phenomena.

Tranexamic acid reduces excessive blood loss in 50% of women with DUB and an ovulatory cycle.[11,13] To have a therapeutic effect, it must be administered in high doses, which may increase secondary effects, although different studies showed that adverse reactions to this drug were mild and rare.[14,15] The therapeutic dose is 1g/6 h for 3–5 days.

Some clinicians are reluctant to use tranexamic acid because of the hypothetical risk of thrombogenic disorders. However, studies have shown that the incidence of thrombosis in women treated with this drug is comparable to that in the general female population.[14]

Other non-hormonal treatment options

Other non-hormonal treatments are drugs that protect the vascular wall. Etamsylate (aminocaproic acid or EACA) seems to exert its effect by fortifying the capillary wall and thus reducing capillary bleeding. A randomized, controlled trial showed that tranexamic acid reduces excessive blood loss more effectively than etamsylate.[15] In the Cochrane review mentioned above, no significant differences were found in menstrual blood loss when two NSAIDs were compared with etamsylate,

but there was an unfavorable trend. Therapeutic doses are 2–4 g/6 h taken orally for 3–5 days.

Hormonal treatment options

Hormonal treatment is mainly indicated in anovulatory DUB. Traditionally, the most-used drugs have been progestins, given during the luteal phase of the cycle or continuously for 21 days throughout the cycle; when administered in this way, they may act as a contraceptive, although they are not a first choice for contraception. For a woman with DUB who also desires contraception, the best option would be oral contraceptive pills (OCPs) because they regulate menstrual cycles much better. Thus, there are on the market progesterones for daily use such as norethisterone, medroxyprogesterone acetate (MPA), or micronized natural progesterone, as well as depot preparations for longer action. Recently, a levonorgestrel-releasing intrauterine device (IUD) has been developed.

Combined OCPs

Among many other effects, they reduce menstrual bleeding because endometrial thickness is less than in a natural cycle, resulting in reduced menstrual blood loss.[16] The published evidence supports that OCPs reduce the amount of bleeding with menstruation, increase hemoglobin concentration, and reduce anemia due to iron deficiency.[13] Most studies used tablets containing 30–35 µg of ethinyl estradiol (EE) together with a second-generation progestin. Compounds with less than 30 µg of EE have a higher incidence of intermenstrual bleeding for the first 3 months of treatment, so they are not the first choice for DUB treatment.[17]

Similar to other indications, OCPs should be prescribed for DUB treatment only after considering the need for contraception, patient age, smoking habits, and cardiovascular risk factors.

In the case of acute anovulatory DUB, OCPs can be prescribed in a high, intense dose of two tablets every 8 h for 7 days; if hemorrhage ceases, treatment is maintained with one tablet/24 h for another 14 days to prepare the endometrium for the next withdrawal bleeding. Treatment should be restarted on the fifth day of the period on the usual dose and continued for a minimum of two or three additional cycles.[1]

Progestins

Many studies have shown that progestins are ineffective for the treatment of ovulatory DUB when compared with NSAIDs and tranexamic acid.[18] However, in anovulatory DUB there is no progesterone deprivation in the endometrium and cycles are thus irregular. Continuous estrogenic stimulation will produce a bleeding endometrium due to shedding. This is the rationale for progesterone treatment during the second half of the menstrual cycle so that there will be a regular cycle induced through withdrawal bleeding. Continuous progestin administration will induce endometrial atrophy[19] as well as anovulation and thus it can be used as a contraceptive method.

Oral progestins   When given during the second phase of the cycle (days 15–26), they offer no advantage over treatments described for ovulatory women; they would only be beneficial in women with anovulatory cycles, although very high doses (norethisterone or MPA 5–10 mg three times a day) for 21 days will reduce excessive blood loss but can elicit side-effects, such as headache or weight gain, reducing compliance.[13]

Depot progestins   *MPA* can be given every 3 months in a single 150-mg injection. Irregular bleeding may occur during the first months of use, and after prolonged administration, the patient will enter amenorrhea (44% after 1-year administration).[16] There are several *subcutaneous implants* on the market, releasing 150–216 mg of levonorgestrel; by continuous liberation of progestin, they suppress ovulation. Once placed subcutaneously, they are effective for 3–5 years. They may produce mild, irregular bleeding, so they are not the first-choice treatment for DUB.

Progestin-releasing IUD   The levonorgestrel-releasing IUD (L-IUD) is a new approach in progestin administration. Not only is it an effective contraceptive method but also it is a useful alternative for DUB.[20] The only product available on the market is a T-shaped IUD loaded with 52 mg of levonorgestrel, releasing 20 μg of the drug to the uterine cavity for 5 years.[20] Studies show that the L-IUD reduces menstrual blood loss from 79 to 97%.[20,21] The mechanism of action, other than reaction against a foreign body, is based on endometrial atrophy induced by the locally released levonorgestrel, which modifies endometrial morphology causing stromal decidualization and glandular atrophy.[22] During the first few months after L-IUD insertion, women suffer intermenstrual bleeding, but after the first year, most will bleed just 1 day a month, and 15% will be amenorrheic.[20,23] Side-effects are headache, weight gain, and swelling. A recent study showed that the L-IUD does not alter lipid and hepatic metabolism or blood pressure but that it does increase fasting plasma glucose, so patients with glucose intolerance should be advised before insertion, but more studies are necessary to confirm this.[21] There are no data on the long-term implications of this issue. In a Cochrane review comparing different medical and surgical treatments of excessive menstrual blood loss,

the L-IUD achieved a better reduction in bleeding than norethisterone, NSAIDs, or tranexamic acid.[24] The L-IUD is an alternative to classical medical and surgical treatment of DUB. When compared to endometrial resection, the L-IUD has a lower efficiency but similar satisfaction rates. If compared to hysterectomy its efficiency is lower, but infertility can be reversed if it is removed, and cost-effectiveness is much higher with the L-IUD.[25]

Other hormones

The other two hormonal treatments that may be effective in reducing menstrual blood loss are danazol and gonadotropin releasing hormone (GnRH) analog, but their side-effects limit their administration to a few months;[13] they are usually given prior to endometrial surgery.[26]

Danazol   This is an androgen-like synthetic steroid that inhibits ovarian steroidogenesis, reducing estrogen concentration and thus inducing endometrial atrophy. Doses ranging between 100 and 200 mg per day for 3 months reduce menstrual bleeding, but there are noticeable side-effects (including weight gain, acne, oily skin, hirsutism, voice modifications, irritability, and bone mineral density loss). Because its use during pregnancy carries the risk of virilization of a female fetus, additional contraceptive methods are required with danazol.[27]

GnRH analog   By binding to the GnRH receptor, GnRH analog desensitizes pituitary cells, inducing hypoestrogenism and endometrial atrophy.[13] Depot preparations require only a single monthly injection and are the preferred choice. The most frequent side-effects are a consequence of the hypoestrogenism (e.g. hot flashes, amenorrhea, osteopenia). GnRH analog may be used to thin the endometrium prior to hysteroscopic surgery.[26]

SURGICAL TREATMENT OF DYSFUNCTIONAL UTERINE BLEEDING

Only when medical treatment has failed or when it is contraindicated for any reason will surgical treatment for DUB be discussed.

Dilatation and curettage   D&C is not the first-choice treatment and is only indicated when acute hemorrhage requires immediate treatment.

Endometrial ablation/resection   EAR is the first option after failed medical treatment and before considering hysterectomy because it is cheaper, carries fewer risks, is less invasive, and allows the patient to retain her uterus. Gold standard techniques – also called first-generation techniques – are laser, loop, or roller ball ablation.[13] All of these approaches require uterine visualization through hysteroscopy. More recent, second-generation techniques – such as microwave or radiofrequency endometrial destruction or endometrial cryoablation – require less operating time because hysteroscopy is not required, and they are simpler to perform. Although these new techniques are easier than hysteroscopy-based methods, they must include 1–3 mm of myometrium to be able to destroy the basal endometrial layer.[28] The most severe complication of EAR is uterine perforation, which cannot be ruled out without direct hysteroscopic visualization of the endometrial cavity.

Hysterectomy   This is the ultimate method to definitively solve the problem, but it is an aggressive treatment. Before choosing hysterectomy, many conditions have to be taken into consideration (e.g. age, associated disorders, patient's wish to have a child). A total of 58% of hysterectomies in the USA are performed because of abnormal uterine bleeding.[29] It may be done through classical laparotomy, vaginal surgery, or translaparoscopically, offering with the last a shorter recovery time and a better post-surgical condition. A recent Cochrane review covering randomized trials comparing EAR with hysterectomy for abnormal uterine bleeding treatment concluded that hysterectomy is the best method for inducing amenorrhea, with a very high satisfaction rate among patients, although satisfaction was also high after EAR; in fact, EAR reduced hospital stay length, post-surgical complications, and recovery time.[30]

REFERENCES

1. Speroff L, Glass RH, Kase Na. Dysfunctional uterine bleeding. In: Clinical Gynecologic Endocrinology and Fertility. Philadelphia: Lippincott Williams & Wilkins, 1999: 575–93.
2. James M, Shwayder MD. Pathophysiology of abnormal uterine bleeding. Contemporary management of abnormal uterine bleeding. Obstet Gynecol Clin North Am 2000; 27: 219–34.
3. Carlson KJ, Schiff I. Alternatives to hysterectomy for menorrhagia. N Engl J Med 1996; 335: 198–9.
4. Galant C, Berliere M, Dubois D et al. Focal expression and final activity of matrix metalloproteinases may explain irregular dysfunctional endometrial bleeding. Am J Pathol 2004; 165: 83–94.
5. Lockwood C, Krikun G, Papp C et al. The role of progestionally regulated stromal cell tissue factor and type 1 plasminogen activator inhibitor (PAI 1) in endometrial hemostasis and menstruation. Ann NY Acad Sci 1994; 734: 57–9.
6. Kadir RA, Economides DL, Sabin CA, Owens D, Lee CA. Frequency of inherited bleeding disorders in women with menorrhagia. Lancet 1998; 351: 485–9.
7. Halberg L, Nilsson L. Determination of menstrual blood loss. Scand J Clin Lab Invest 1964; 16: 244–8.
8. Higham J, O'Brien P, Shaw R. Assessment of menstrual blood loss using a pictorial chart. Br J Obstet Gynaecol 1990; 97: 734–9.
9. Bayer S, de Cherney A. Clinical manifestations and treatment of dysfunctional uterine bleeding. JAMA 1993; 269: 1823–8.
10. Matorras R, Ocerin I. Menorragias: estado actual de conocimientos. Folia Clin Obstet Ginecol 2001; 25: 9–31.
11. Prentice A. Medical management of menorrhagia. Br Med J 1999; 319: 1343–5.
12. Lethaby A, Augood C, Duckitt K. Nonsteroidal anti-inflammatory drugs for heavy menstrual bleeding. Cochrane Database Syst Rev 2002; (1): CD000400.
13. Bongers MY, Mol BW, Brolmann HA. Current treatment of dysfunctional uterine bleeding. Maturitas 2004; 47: 159–74.
14. Lethaby A, Farquhar C, Cooke I. Antifibrinolytics for heavy menstrual bleeding Cochrane Database Syst Rev 2000; (4): CD000249.
15. Bonnar J, Sheppard BL. Treatment of menorrhagia during menstruation: randomised controlled trial of ethamsylate, mefenamic acid, and tanexamic acid. Br Med J 1996; 313: 579–82.
16. Royal College of Obstetricians and Gynaecologists. The Initial Management of Menorrhagia. National Evidence-Based Clinical Guideline No. 1. London: RCOG, 1998.
17. ESHRE Capri Workshop Group. Ovarian and endometrial function during hormonal contraception. Hum Reprod 2001; 7: 1427–34.
18. Vilos GA, Lefebvre G, Graves GR et al. Guidelines for the management of abnormal uterine bleeding. SOCG Clinical Practice Guidelines No. 106. J Obstet Gynaecol Can 2001; 23: 704–9.
19. Hickey M, Highman J, Fraser IS. Progestogens versus oestrogens and progestogens for irregular uterine bleeding associated with anovulation. Cochrane Database Syst Rev 2000; (2): CD001895.
20. Varma R, Sinha D, Gupta JK. Non-contraceptive uses of levonorgestrel-releasing hormone system (LNG/IUS) – a systematic enquiry and overview. Eur J Obstet Gynecol Reprod Biol 2006; 125: 9–28.
21. Andersson JK, Rybo G. Levonorgestrel releasing intrauterine device in the treatment of menorrhagia. Br J Obstet Gynaecol 1990; 97: 690–4.
22. Pakarinen P, Tovivonen J, Luukkainen T. Therapeutic use of LNG IUS and counseling. Semin Reprod Med 2001; 19: 364–72.
23. Kayikcioglu F, Gunes M, Ozdegirmenci O, Haberal A. Effects of levonorgestrel-releasing system on glucose and lipid metabolism: a 1-year follow-up study. Contraception 2006; 75: 528–31.
24. Lethaby AE, Cooke I, Rees M. Progesterone or progestogen-releasing intrauterine systems for heavy menstrual bleeding. Cochrane Database Syst Rev 2005; (4): CD002126.
25. Jou JH, Sahota DS, Mo Yuen P. A cost/utility analysis of hysterectomy, endometrial resection and ablation and medical therapy for menorrhagia. Hum Reprod 2006; 21: 1878–83.
26. Higham JM, Shaw RW. A comparative study of danazol, a regimen of decreasing doses of danazol and norethisterone in the treatment of objectively proven unexplained menorrhagia. Am J Obstet Gynecol 1993; 169: 1134–9.
27. Pre-operative endometrial thinning agents before endometrial destruction for heavy menstrual bleeding. Cochrane Database Syst Rev 2002; (3): CD001124.
28. Lethaby A, Hickey M, Garry R. Endometrial destruction techniques for heavy menstrual bleeding. Cochrane Database Syst Rev 2005; (4): CD001501.
29. Farquhar CM, Steiner CA. Hysterectomy rates in the United States, 1990–1997. Obstet Gynecol 2002; 99: 229–34.
30. Lethaby A, Shepperd S, Cooke I, Farquhar C. Endometrial resection and ablation versus hysterectomy for heavy menstrual bleeding. Cochrane Database Syst Rev 2000; (2): CD000329.

6 Endometrial ablation

Erin F Wolff and Antoni J Duleba

INTRODUCTION

Abnormal uterine bleeding (AUB) is one of the most common gynecologic problems. Up to 1 in 5 women of reproductive age suffer from menorrhagia, generating 2.7 million office visits in the USA each year.[1] Ultimately, AUB contributes to at least 40% of the over 600 000 hysterectomies performed each year,[2] making hysterectomies one of the most common surgeries performed in the USA. AUB is often difficult to treat medically, which leads many patients and physicians to 'definitive management', i.e. hysterectomy.

However, recent advances in less invasive surgical techniques have prompted patients as well as physicians to reexamine the risks and benefits of this common surgery and consider alternatives. Hysterectomy is a major operation, usually requiring general anesthesia and several weeks of recovery and lost work time. Risks of significant complications from hysterectomy are in the range of 2–32%[3,4] and include significant blood loss from damage to pelvic vessels and injury of ureters, bladder, and bowel, as well as infections, pelvic adhesions, and chronic pain. These risks are heightened by the rise in obesity, diabetes, and cesarean section rate. In an increasingly litigious, as well as cost conscious environment, there is growing pressure to ensure that the least invasive, least risky, and least costly treatment options are used.

ABNORMAL UTERINE BLEEDING

To understand abnormal uterine bleeding, we must first understand normal menstrual bleeding. The normal menstrual cycle is defined as 21–35 days in duration, with menstrual flow lasting 7 days or less.[5] AUB occurs at unexpected times or is of abnormal duration or amount. Heavy menstrual bleeding, or menorrhagia, is clinically defined as greater than or equal to 80 ml of blood loss per menstrual cycle.[6,7] Dysfunctional uterine bleeding (DUB) is a term often used when AUB cannot be attributed to organic systemic, iatrogenic, or anatomic causes. It is often, but not exclusively, a result of anovulatory, non-cyclic bleeding associated with disordered steroid hormone action. DUB is common after menarche due to an immature hypothalamic–pituitary–ovarian axis and in perimenopause due to declining ovarian function.

The standard of care for treating AUB is to first try medical therapy. While many options for medical treatment exist, most practitioners start with oral contraceptive pills (OCPs). Interestingly, most medical treatments are similar in efficacy. OCPs have been evaluated in one small randomized controlled trial, where they appear to have a comparable efficacy to mefenamic acid, naproxen, and low dose danazol; the average impact of these therapies was a reduction in menstrual blood loss by 43%.[8] Progestin-only therapies are another option, and should be considered particularly for patients at risk for endometrial hyperplasia, including those with polycystic ovarian syndrome (PCOS), obesity, or diabetes. However, in a Cochrane review, low dose luteal phase progestins were found to be less effective in controlling bleeding than tranexamic acid, danazol, or the progesterone-releasing intrauterine system (IUS).[9] Although effective, danazol is rarely used because of androgenic side-effects.

SURGICAL THERAPY FOR CHRONIC MENORRHAGIA

Many practitioners find AUB difficult to successfully treat medically. Patients are often not satisfied with the results or unable to tolerate the side-effects. These factors often lead patients and physicians to select surgical management. When medical therapy fails or is not acceptable to the patient, many surgical options exist. Dilatation and curettage is commonly performed, but usually offers only temporary relief. It is best used as an acute treatment of severe bleeding or as a diagnostic procedure to evaluate for possible endometrial hyperplasia or neoplasm.

Given the prevalence of AUB and the risks associated with hysterectomy, less invasive alternatives to hysterectomy to treat menorrhagia have been developed. Endometrial ablation works by destroying the full thickness of the endometrial lining of the uterus. Since the endometrium has tenacious regenerative abilities, it is essential for tissue destruction to reach the basal gland layer, where the regenerative potential of the endometrium is believed to reside. However, even destruction of the entire basal layer of endometrium may not assure permanent amenorrhea; recent evidence indicates that stem cells from the bone marrow travel to the endometrium where they can differentiate into endometrial cells.[10]

In general, there are two categories of ablative methods. First generation methods are considered the gold standard or 'standard' endometrial ablation techniques. These procedures include transcervical resection of the endometrium (TCRE or endomyoresection) with a wire loop, laser ablation, and rollerball ablation. Standard endometrial ablation requires direct visualization using a large operative hysteroscope, usually under general anesthesia.

The newer, second generation techniques or 'global' ablation procedures differ in that they are largely automated and designed to be easier, faster, and safer. For most of these new procedures (except for hydrothermal ablation) the hysteroscope is not necessary and the procedures are performed blindly. The second generation ablations are more suited to outpatient use, and include cryoablation,[11] hot saline solution irrigation,[12] diode laser hyperthermy (heating),[13] microwave ablation,[14] a heated balloon system,[15] radiofrequency,[16,17] and photodynamic therapy (intrauterine light delivery).[18] Only a few randomized controlled trials have been undertaken to assess their efficacy, safety, and acceptability.

PREOPERATIVE ASSESSMENT AND CARE

Preoperative endometrial thinning with gonadotropin releasing hormone (GnRH) agonists have been associated with a shorter duration of surgery, greater ease of surgery, and a higher rate of postoperative amenorrhea at 12 months with hysteroscopic resection or ablation, as well as reduced postoperative dysmenorrhea compared to no treatment. GnRH agonists appear to produce slightly more consistent results than danazol.[19] Progestins have also been used as preoperative thinning agents, but are less well studied.

Endometrial ablation is typically reserved for premenopausal patients with DUB who have no future fertility plans and who have failed medical management, do not want to take medications, or have contraindications to medical therapy. Women with structural lesions including large fibroids and polyps as a cause of their bleeding or suspected neoplastic processes, in general, are not good candidates.

An endometrial biopsy to rule out neoplastic disease should be performed. A transvaginal ultrasound scan can

Table 6.1 Endometrial ablation preoperative patient assessment

- No future fertility plans
- Benign endometrial sampling; no history of endometrial hyperplasia/atypia
- Normal Pap smear
- Sonographic assessment (uterine size, cavity shape, fibroids)
- Possible preoperative endometrial preparation:
  - GnRH analogs
  - OCPs
  - progestins
  - preoperative D&C
  - timing of procedure to the early proliferative phase
- Reliable contraception postoperatively

be used to assess the endometrial stripe in women with postmenopausal bleeding to screen for endometrial hyperplasia or cancer. Many different imaging modalities can be used to assess pelvic anatomy for structural causes (fibroids, polyps, adnexal masses) contributing to AUB, including transvaginal ultrasound, sonohysterography, hysterosalpingography, and hysteroscopy.

Table 6.1 summarizes key preoperative considerations relevant to any of the endometrial ablation procedures.

FIRST GENERATION ABLATION METHODS

Advantages of standard ablative procedures using laser, rollerball desiccation, or endomyoresection with a wire loop include direct visualization permitting immediate assessment of structural anomalies and the detection of complications such as uterine perforation or bleeding. Standard endometrial ablation may be performed in approximately 10 minutes by an experienced operator. Disadvantages include the necessity of performing the procedure in an operating room because of discomfort of the electroablation and because the large operative hysteroscope requires significant dilatation of the cervix usually under general anesthesia. Furthermore, these procedures require considerable operator skill and strict monitoring of the 'ins and outs' of the volume of distension fluid to avoid complications related to volume overload and hyponatremia.

Laser

Laser ablation was one of the first described methods for endometrial ablation. It is performed via an operative hysteroscope under direct visualization. It was first introduced by Goldrath et al using a neodymium–yttrium aluminum garnet (Nd:YAG) laser,[20] and later using an argon laser. In the original study, patients were pretreated with danazol to achieve a hypoestrogenic state.[20] The concept was that Asherman's syndrome almost exclusively occurred in the puerperal state, and the authors attempted to recreate such an endocrine environment. Under general anesthesia, the cervix was dilated to 20Fr, which allows egress of intrauterine fluid around the hysteroscope to clear blood and bubbles. Yoon tubal rings were applied to prevent tubal spill into the peritoneal cavity if sterilization had not previously been done. Five per cent dextrose in normal saline was used initially; later normal saline was used without dextrose. A 0.6-mm laser fiber was inserted through the operating channel of an operative hysteroscope. (Protective eye equipment is required for anyone in a room where laser equipment is being used.) Under direct hysteroscopic visualization, the laser tip was placed in close contact with the endometrium and dragged over the surface starting at the fundus and working down the anterior and posterior walls of the uterus. To avoid treating the endocervix, Goldrath et al described marking the cervical length on the hysteroscope. Treated areas turned from white-pink to brown-black from carbonization of the underlying myometrium.

Repeated examinations often reveal skipped areas that can be retreated. Care must be taken at the thin tubal ostia region. Postoperative uterine cramping and serosanguineous drainage lasting for up to 3 weeks postoperatively frequently occur. In the original study, Goldrath et al reported biopsy findings of necrotic myometrium for up to 4 months postoperatively. They noted a surprising absence of inflammatory cells, except foreign body giant cells surrounding the carbon particles. One patient was found to have 2 ml of old blood; post-procedure uterine sounding was recommended to prevent hematometra. Post-ablative changes resembled third degree burns, with ridges, fibrosis, and adhesions; occasional tufts of viable endometrium were also visualized hysteroscopically.

Argon laser endometrial ablation was compared to a combined rollerball and endometrial resection procedure by McClure et al in 1992.[21] All electrocautery and most laser procedures were performed using 1.5% glycine under direct visualization. In this study, the HGM Inc Endocoagulator Model 20 (Salt Lake City, UT) was used through a Hamou operative hysteroscope. A power of 20 W was used for ablation by systematically dragging the fiber across the entire endometrial lining of the uterus. Argon lasers have lower penetration depth than Nd:YAGs (2 vs 4 mm, respectively), but the energy is selectively absorbed by red pigments. For electrocautery, the Storz resectoscope (Tuttlingen, Germany) and Valley Lab Force 2 (Denver, CO) electrosurgical generator were used. Twelve patients randomized to laser and 10 to resection were pretreated with medroxyprogesterone acetate 10 mg three times a day for 3 months prior to surgery. Women with myomas diagnosed on transvaginal ultrasound were excluded from this study. Operating time was significantly longer for the laser group compared to electrocautery (114 vs 80 min). Menstrual blood loss (MBL) was similar between groups (51.2 ml vs 30.2 ml) with a mean decrease of 68.1% vs 81% for laser and electrocautery, respectively. Two of 12 patients in the laser group and four out of 10 patients in the electrocautery group were amenorrheic at 6 months postoperatively.

A trial by Bhattacharya et al in 1997 also compared laser to TCRE in a randomized controlled trial.[22] However, this group used Nd:YAG and evaluated a large group of women enrolled during two different time periods. Results for the first group of women comparing ablation (53 in laser group and 52 in TCRE group) and hysterectomy were published first.[23] Eight months later, 267 more women were enrolled (188 patients in the laser arm and 184 in the TCRE arm). Results of the combination of these two groups were reported at 6 and 12 months following surgery. Amenorrhea, satisfaction, pain, general health, and symptoms were essentially identical between groups at 6 and 12 months. Statistically significant differences were fluid overload, fluid deficit, equipment failure, and operating time in favor of TCRE. There were, however, three uterine perforations and one hysterectomy in the TCRE group, while none occurred in the laser group. There was a trend in favor of laser for retreatment (16% for laser and 20% for TCRE).

Transcervical resection of the endometrium (or endomyoresection)

Over 4000 endometrial ablations had been performed in Great Britain before a randomized trial of these methods was performed.[24] Potential advantages of TCRE over ablative methods include histologic sampling to detect hyperplasia and carcinoma, less need for hormonal pretreatment, possible treatment of superficial adenomyosis, and simultaneous ability to resect submucous myomas without necessitating a change in equipment. TCRE was first described by DeCherney et al in 1987.[25] The procedure was adapted using a urologic cystoscope and resection performed with a wire loop at a power of 30 W of current using 32%

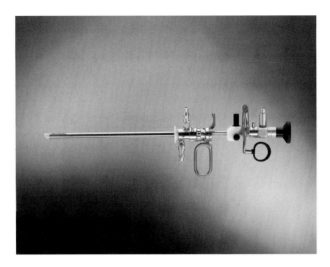

Figure 6.1 Resectoscope used for hysteroscopic trans-cervical resection of the endometrium (TCRE). Image courtesy of © Karl Storz Endoscopy America, Inc

Dextran 70 for uterine distension. A modern resecto-scope is shown in Figure 6.1.

Gannon et al in 1991[24] and Dwyer et al in 1993[26] performed the early randomized trials comparing endometrial ablation by TCRE with abdominal hys-terectomy. In Gannon's study, patients were pretreated with 150 mg of medroxyprogesterone acetate intra-muscularly 4–6 weeks prior to surgery to decrease the thickness of the endometrium. Gannon et al random-ized 51 women and Dwyer et al randomized 196 women to hysterectomy or TCRE. In the first study, no intraoperative or early postoperative complications occurred in the TCRE group, while 12 women in the hysterectomy group experienced complications (vault hemorrhage: 1, urinary retention: 4, urinary tract infection: 2, wound infection: 3, respiratory tract infec-tion: 1, granulation tissue cautery: 4). Recovery time, time off work, postoperative pain, and hospital costs were significantly less in the TCRE group. The efficacy of TCRE was not addressed in this study; authors cited the use of depot medroxyprogesterone preoperatively as a potential confounder, which may have affected vaginal bleeding for up to 1 year.

In Dwyer's study, no endometrial thinning agents were given and patients were followed for 4 months. Postoperative complications were statistically signifi-cantly higher in the hysterectomy group, and included transfusion, pyrexia, pelvic infection, hematoma, wound infection, urinary tract infection, urinary reten-tion, and anemia. Operating time, postoperative pain, time off work, return to daily activities, and return to intercourse were all significantly less in the TCRE group. However, satisfaction rates, as well as rates of improve-ment in dysmenorrhea, premenstrual bloating, and

premenstrual breast tenderness, were also lower in this group. Amenorrhea (13 of 95), hypomenorrhea (76 of 95), and no change in vaginal bleeding (nine of 95) were all significantly worse in the TCRE group com-pared to hysterectomy (presumably 100% amenor-rhea). Premenstrual mood changes were noted to improve in both groups to a similar degree.

Crosignani et al compared TCRE to vaginal hys-terectomy in a 1997 Italian study of 85 women who were followed for 2 years.[27] The only complication observed during the study (vaginal vault hematoma) occurred in the hysterectomy group. Operating time (13 vs 71 min), hospital stay (1 vs 5 days), return to normal activities (8 vs 13 days), and return to work (14 vs 30 days) were all significantly shorter for the TCRE group. Amenorrhea (22%), spotting (11%), hypomenorrhea (28.7%), and normal menstrual peri-ods (34.4%) were all significantly worse in the TCRE group compared to vaginal hysterectomy (presumably 100% amenorrhea). Although satisfaction rates and sexual function scores were not statistically different, quality of life outcomes were all in favor of vaginal hysterectomy.

In 1997, O'Connor et al published the Medical Research Council trial comparing TCRE with both abdominal and vaginal hysterectomy.[4] Two hundred and two women were randomized to TCRE or hys-terectomy in a 2:1 fashion and followed for 3 years. Fifty-seven women underwent hysterectomy; the choice of abdominal vs vaginal was decided by the sur-geon. One hundred and nineteen underwent TCRE; the use of pretreatment thinning agents was decided by the individual surgeon. Intraoperative adverse events such as hemorrhage and anesthesia complications occurred only in the hysterectomy group, while fluid overload, perforation, cervical tears, and abandonment of the surgery were observed only in the TCRE group. Blood loss and operating time were significantly less in the TCRE group. Postoperative complications during hospitalization such as sepsis, hemorrhage, and transfu-sion (13%) were found only in the hysterectomy group. After discharge, complications remained significantly more frequent in the hysterectomy group (32% vs 13% in the TCRE group) and included sepsis and hematomas. Satisfaction rates did not reach significance, but the trends were in favor of hysterectomy over TCRE. The amenorrhea rate fell from the first year (46%) to the third year (21%). Although at least 80% of patients reported improvement in menstrual symptoms, 22% required further surgery for persistent bleeding or pain during the 3-year follow-up.

In 1994, Pinion et al[23] compared abdominal hys-terectomy, Nd:YAG laser, and TCRE in a study involving

204 women followed for 1 year postoperatively. No statistically significant differences were detected between these two types of ablation procedures except for operating time (50.3 vs 39.9 min) and fluid deficit (766 vs 414 ml) for laser and TCRE, respectively. Major complications occurred more frequently in the hysterectomy group (five of 99) vs hysteroscopy (two of 103). Minor complications were also more frequent in the hysterectomy group, but overall infectious morbidity (32% lower) was the only category to reach statistical significance. Recovery time, time off work, and time to resumption of intercourse were all less with hysteroscopy. At 12 months, 22% of patients were amenorrheic and 62% were hypomenorrheic. Fourteen per cent of patients required a hysterectomy within the first 12 months.

Four-year follow-up of this same study was provided by the Aberdeen Endometrial Ablation Trials group in 1999.[28] Satisfaction rates remained high in both groups but those rating their health as 'much better' were statistically higher in the hysterectomy group (89% vs 80%). In addition, 38% of patients in the TCRE group received further surgery for menorrhagia. Amenorrhea rates were 45% for the TCRE group and 98% for hysterectomy. Two per cent of TCRE patients reported no change in their menstrual symptoms. Premenstrual breast tenderness and irritability were higher in the TCRE group.

In summary, TCRE is highly effective, permits tissue sampling, and results in high patient satisfaction rates. Compared to hysterectomy, TCRE affords patients a quicker recovery time and return to work, is associated with less perioperative morbidity, and requires shorter operating times. Complications of TCRE include uterine perforations, cervical lacerations, and fluid overload. Compared to laser ablation, TCRE appears to be faster. However, compared to subsequent ablation methods, considerable surgical skills are required and intraoperative complications occur more frequently with TCRE, which will be described in detail below.

Notably, in spite of a higher rate of complications, hysterectomy appears to result in overall better long-term patient satisfaction.

Rollerball

Rollerball endometrial ablation was first described in 1988 by Lin et al[29] and in 1989 by Vancaillie.[30] Its popularity grew because it was safer than TCRE, less expensive than laser, and easier to perform than both. Initially, these procedures were performed with a urologic resectoscope used for prostate resections. Now,

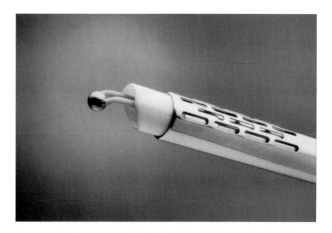

Figure 6.2 Rollerball used for endometrial ablation through an operative hysteroscope. Image courtesy of © Karl Storz Endoscopy America, Inc

dedicated operative hysteroscopes with operating channels for instruments are used routinely (Figure 6.2). The electrocautery unit is typically set at 50–120 W of coagulation current. A non-conducting medium is used for uterine distension (e.g. glycine or sorbitol–mannitol). Coagulation is performed with the rollerball in a systematic manner, usually starting at the tubal ostia, proceeding to the fundus, and then anterior, posterior, and lateral uterine walls down to the level of the internal cervical os. At times, tissue will adhere to the rollerball; if this occurs, the instrument is removed from the cavity and cleared. It is important to closely monitor fluid deficit during the procedure. If this level exceeds 1000–1500 ml, standard of care dictates stopping the procedure. Adequate coagulation results in a yellow-brown appearance with flecks of black char.

Boujida et al performed a study comparing TCRE to rollerball and reported 5-year follow-up results.[31] Operating time was significantly less in the rollerball group (13 vs 20 minutes). Thirty-six per cent of patients required a second procedure during this time (20 in the rollerball and 16 in the TCRE group), with younger patients being more likely to require a second operation. No differences were detected in bleeding rates between groups. Satisfaction rates were also equivalent. Infectious complications were significantly lower in patients who received prophylactic antibiotics.

Vaporizing electrode

Vercellini et al introduced the vaporizing electrode in 1996.[32] This device is larger than the typical rollerball and has three grooves that provide eight edges along which the energy density is greatest, to allow cell vaporization on contact. The purported advantages include faster treatment times given the larger surface area of the bar, no need to repeatedly remove endomyometrial fragments from the electrode (which can prolong surgical time), and ability to treat submucosal fibroids. In addition, a deeper penetration of thermal necrosis occurs beyond the surface ablation. This method purportedly seals myometrial vessels and thus contributes to the decreased absorption of distension medium compared to TCRE.

To perform this type of ablation, the uterine cavity is distended with a non-conductive, hypo-osmolar solution (e.g. 2.7% sorbitol and 0.54% mannitol) to 100–120 mmHg of pressure and a vacuum of 230–240 mmHg applied for suction. Pure cutting waveform current for endometrial vaporization is performed at 200 W. The endometrium is ablated in a radial fashion starting from the tubal ostia, withdrawing the electrode toward the cervix at 1–1.5 cm/second, with minimal pressure on the uterine wall. The fundus and any remaining areas are treated to the level of the isthmus.[33]

Vercellini et al conducted an Italian study directly comparing TCRE to the vaporizing electrode in 1999.[33] Ninety-one women were randomized and results were reported at 1 year of follow-up. Fluid deficit (109 vs 367 ml) and operating time (9.2 vs 10.7 min) were significantly less for vaporizing electrode compared to TCRE, respectively. Amenorrhea rates were similar in both groups.

SECOND GENERATION PROCEDURES

Hot water balloon ablation

Given the complications and technical difficulty of the early endometrial ablation methods, safer and easier systems were needed. One of the first of these next generation devices was a hot water balloon attached to a thin probe that can be inserted into the uterine cavity without an operative hysteroscope. The hot water balloon introduced in the USA by Singer et al[15] in 1994 is called ThermaChoice® (Gynecare, Ethicon, Inc, Johnson & Johnson). The ThermaChoice system consists of a uterine balloon catheter (16 cm long and 5 mm wide) with a single use latex balloon at the tip of the catheter, where the heating element is also located. The central monitor controls balloon temperature, duration, and pressure. This central unit is connected to the probe via a multilumen catheter.

Briefly, the procedure is performed as follows. First, proper function of the system is checked by inflating the balloon outside the uterine cavity. A paracervical block can be administered at this point (with or without general anesthesia), in order to lessen postoperative pain. When necessary, the cervix should be dilated to accommodate the 5-mm instrument. Often cervical dilatation is unnecessary, particularly in parous or heavily bleeding women. The early protocols first evaluating the hot water balloon included a brief suction curettage to decrease the thickness of the endometrium. Although pretreatment with GnRH analogs, progestins, or oral contraceptives to decrease endometrial thickness may improve success rates, these medications were not specifically approved for this use during the initial studies evaluating this device. However, at present, the use of these agents in lieu of suction curettage is common. The balloon catheter is then inserted into the uterine cavity through the cervix. Care should be taken not to create a false passage; excessive resistance should not be encountered under normal circumstances. The uterus can be sounded to obtain a sense of uterine size and position, which can aid when introducing the balloon catheter into the uterus. Resistance is felt when the tip of the probe reaches the fundus; insertion of the probe is performed very gently to avoid uterine perforation. Perforation or cervical lacerations are rarely reported with this device.

After satisfactory uterine placement of the device, the balloon is inflated with sterile 5% dextrose in water via the port on the probe. Depending on the size of the uterine cavity, approximately 2–30 ml is needed to reach the goal intrauterine pressure of 160–180 mmHg, which is monitored and displayed by base unit. Insufflation allows contact of the balloon with the entire surface of a regularly shaped endometrium. A minimum pressure of 150 mmHg must be achieved in order for the device to activate; an automatic shutoff feature turns off the device below this threshold. The fluid inside the balloon is heated to approximately 87°C (170°F) by the indwelling thermistor. Treatment time is preset for 8 minutes. After completion of the heat cycle, fluid is removed from the balloon via the port and the balloon catheter is removed from the uterus.

The second hot water balloon system was described in 1996 by Friberg et al; this system, called Cavaterm™ (Wallsten Medical SA, Morges, Switzerland), was initially introduced clinically in 1993.[34] Like the ThermaChoice system, the Cavaterm system also utilizes a disposable balloon that can be inflated with heated fluid to destroy the endometrial lining of the uterus. However, these systems differ in several details. The Cavaterm balloon is made of silicone and can be customized to accommodate different sizes of uterine cavities by adjusting the balloon length. Length of balloon needed is determined by sounding the uterus and subtracting the cervical length. The purported advantage is to minimize cervical damage in smaller cavities and ensure adequate ablation of the lower uterine segment in larger uteri. The central control unit contains a pump, pressure safety device, pressure monitoring device, and battery generated power source (24 V, 4 A, 100 W). The system is pretested and primed with air by attaching the supplied syringe to the three-way tap, which is held in the vertical position. Next, the cervix is dilated to Hegar 8–9 and the 8-mm diameter Cavaterm catheter is inserted until the fundus is reached. The syringe is then filled with 30 ml of 1.5% glycine. The balloon is filled until a stable pressure of 160–200 mmHg is obtained to ensure contact of the balloon with the entire endometrial surface; this represents a pressure that surpasses systolic blood pressure flowing to the uterus, but lower than intrauterine pressures measured during dysmenorrhea. This device also includes an oscillating pump in the central unit, which serves to circulate the fluid in the balloon. It also maintains a stable intrauterine pressure by adding fluid during the procedure if needed. The catheter includes an automated drain mechanism, which draws off excess fluid if the predetermined pressure threshold is overcome. The balloon houses a heating element, called Soft Heat™ (Wallsten Medical SA, Morges, Switzerland), which maintains a temperature of about 80°C. This element maximizes surface area using closely spaced, thin lamellae. The initial phase of heating utilizes full electrical power. Once the preset goal temperature is near, the central controller drops electrical power to 10–20 W. At this point, the generator is only producing enough heat to maintain the temperature. This ability to rapidly respond and accommodate allows the unit to maintain a constant temperature at a safe range. These temperatures achieve endometrial destruction to a depth of about 5 mm. The first 60 women reported were treated for 30 minutes, but since 1995 length of treatment has been 15 minutes.

Since the efficacy of first generation hysteroscopic techniques such as rollerball and transcervical resection of the endometrium (TCRE) using operative hysteroscopes had already been tested against hysterectomy, the newer second generation techniques were tested against these first generation 'gold standards'. One of the first randomized trials was by Meyer et al,[35] comparing uterine balloon therapy (UBT) ablation (ThermaChoice) with rollerball ablation, and provides one of the longest follow-up data sets available

for these newer techniques. The purpose of this study was to demonstrate that this new technique was as effective and as safe as the rollerball. The trial enrolled 275 women with menorrhagia and normal endometrial cavities at 14 centers, two in Canada and 12 in the USA. Participants were at least 30 years old, were premenopausal, and had a normal cavity, benign Pap test and endometrial biopsy (EMB), no infection or malignancy, and no desire for future fertility. No endometrial thinning agents were given preoperatively, but a 3-minute suction curettage was performed in both groups prior to ablation. Follow-up data for 1, 2, 3, and 5 years were published for this trial.

Overall, outcomes of UBT and rollerball ablation were quite similar in this study. Amenorrhea rates increased over time, and were slightly higher in the rollerball group at each analysis: 23% for UBT and 33% for rollerball after 5 years. Rates of normal bleeding or less were also non-significantly higher, but converged over time to 95.1% for UBT and 96.7% for rollerball at 5 years. Satisfaction, hysterectomy, dysmenorrhea, and overall success rates were similar after 5 years. Intraoperative complications were lower in the UBT group (0%) vs rollerball (3.2%), which included fluid overload, cervical laceration, and uterine perforation. Immediate postoperative adverse events were similar (2.9% UBT and 2.4% rollerball), and included endometritis, hematometra, urinary tract infection (UTI), and post-ablation sterilization syndrome.

In 2001, Soysal et al[36] published a small prospective randomized trial of 45 women with menorrhagia comparing rollerball endometrial ablation with the ThermaChoice system for treating small fibroids. Most previous studies excluded women with myomas. In fact, many of the treatment failures were attributed to myomatous uteri upon pathologic inspection following treatment failures requiring subsequent hysterectomy. Study design was similar to the above described study by Meyer et al. Notable differences included pretreatment with GnRH analogs and inclusion of myomatous uteri detected by ultrasound examination. Exclusion criteria were: the presence of any myoma larger than 3 cm in diameter or >50% submucous component and uterine size >12 weeks.

The results of this trial by Soysal et al were similar to those of Meyer's study. After 12 months of follow-up, bleeding was significantly lower, and similar in both groups as defined by the Pictoral Blood-loss Assessment Chart or PBAC (384 to 41.1 for UBT and 385 to 40 for rollerball). The PBAC is a validated method that uses a chart with pictures indicating the amount of staining on a pad or tampon. Mean hemoglobin levels were also similar and increased significantly in both groups (from 10 to 12.8 g/dl for UBT and from 9.8 to 12.9 for rollerball). Rates of hysterectomy and postoperative complications were comparable. ThermaChoice therapy was associated with a slightly lower amenorrhea rate at 12 months (11% vs 16% for rollerball), though this difference was not statistically significant. The two significant differences were in operating time (11.5 min for UBT vs 37 min for rollerball) and intraoperative complications (0% UBT vs 10.4% rollerball). Based on the above findings, the authors concluded that myomatous uteri less than 12 weeks in size may be treated by either method.

ThermaChoice was compared to rollerball ablation again in 2003 in a single-blinded randomized controlled trial by van Zon-Rabelink et al[37] to look specifically at technical and safety aspects. One hundred and thirty-nine premenopausal women were randomized after pretreatment with GnRH analog (goserelin 3.6 mg given subcutaneously, 2 and 6 weeks prior to surgery). In this study, UBT had a statistically significant lower rate of intraoperative complications. Impressively, no intraoperative complications occurred in the UBT group, while eight (14%) occurred in the rollerball group, including uterine perforation (3), cervical laceration (3), electrolyte imbalance (1), and suspicion of perforation requiring a diagnostic laparoscopy (1). Technical complications such as device malfunctions were similar (17% in UBT vs 16% in rollerball). Operating time was lower in the UBT group (18 min vs 35 min for rollerball). The sole benefit in the rollerball group was seen in the rate of postoperative medication prescribed.

van Zon-Rabelink et al also compared UBT (ThermaChoice) to rollerball in 2004.[38] One hundred and thirty-seven women were randomized and followed for 2 years. MBL was significantly less in the UBT group at 24 months. Success rates (menstrual score < 185) and satisfaction rates (75% for rollerball and 80% for uterine balloon) were equivalent at 12 and 24 months postoperatively.

A subsequent study by Pellicano et al in 2002[39] showed even greater benefit of Cavaterm over a first generation technique. Instead of comparing balloon therapy to rollerball, this trial evaluated Cavaterm vs TCRE. Women who were < 50 years old, had failed 3 months of medical therapy, had a uterus < 12 weeks size, and had no submucosal fibroids were enrolled in this Italian study. Ninety-six subjects were randomized and outcomes were reported at 3 months, 1 year, and 2 years. The TCRE group was treated with GnRH analog (Enantone®), but the UBT group had no pretreatment

because the drug was not approved for this use at the time of the study.

The UBT group compared favorably to TCRE significantly with respect to operating time (24 vs 37 min), intraoperative blood loss (7.2 vs 89 ml), postoperative vaginal bleeding (5.2 vs 7.8 days), immediate postoperative pain (3.2 vs 3.8 on scale from 1 = no pain to 5 = not tolerable pain), 'excellent' satisfaction assessment rates (67.5% vs 50% at 3 months, 54% vs 31.5% at 1 year, 45.7% vs 6% at 2 years), bleeding recurrence (5.4% vs 15.7% at 1 year and 8.5% vs 24.2% at 2 years), pain recurrence (2.7% vs 18.4% at 1 year and 2.7% vs 27.2%), and reoperation rates (5.4% vs 10.4% at 1 year and 5.7% vs 15.1% at 2 years). Though not statistically significant, no intraoperative complications occurred in the UBT group, while eight (five fluid overloads, one cervical tear, and two conversions to hysterectomy for severe uterine perforation) occurred in the TCRE group. Only postoperative pain at discharge (1.9 vs 1.5) was worse in patients who underwent UBT.

The following year (2003), Hawe et al[40] compared Cavaterm to Nd:YAG laser endometrial ablation by randomizing 72 women pretreated with one dose of goserelin 3.6 mg, 4–5 weeks prior to either procedure. The study was double-blind: neither patients nor researchers evaluating outcomes knew which treatment was used. There was no statistically significant difference between groups for any of the outcomes measured, except laser ablation was less painful at 4 hours postoperatively than Cavaterm. Amenorrhea rates for Cavaterm and laser ablation, respectively, were 40.5% and 29% at 6 months and 37% and 39% at 12 months. There were no major intraoperative complications in either group. At 6 and 12 months, respectively, 95% and 93% of women were satisfied or very satisfied with Cavaterm compared to 91% and 96% of those treated with laser. MBL was decreased by 80.5% and 83.5% at 12 months as measured by the visual analog scale in women who underwent Cavaterm and laser ablation, respectively. Although operating time was not reported, the authors concluded that Cavaterm demonstrated equivalent effectiveness and appeared easier to use.

Taken together, the balloon systems represent safe, effective, and minimally invasive approaches to treat menorrhagia. They are easier to learn, faster, and are associated with fewer complications compared to first generation techniques. Some studies show slightly higher amenorrhea rates with traditional methods such as rollerball than with UBT; however, satisfaction rates remain high, and similar, to those with first

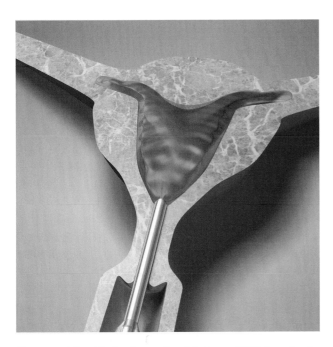

Figure 6.3 Hydrothermal ablation (HTA) of the endometrium, a second generation ablation method utilizing direct circulation of hot water through the uterine cavity. Image courtesy of Boston Scientific

generation techniques. There were a few studies that showed slightly higher rates of pain with UBT compared to the first generation methods in the immediate or intermediate postoperative period as evidenced by both pain scores and pain medications prescribed.[37,39] Hysterectomies are effectively avoided in the majority of women undergoing these procedures.

Hydrothermal ablation

Hydrothermal ablation (HTA) was first described by Goldrath et al in pigs[41] and first reported in a human trial by das Dores et al.[42] The concept was to ensure treatment of the entire endometrial surface, simplify the ablation procedure, and minimize risks of perforation. Because the water fills the entire cavity, all surfaces are treated, even in the presence of significant cavity irregularities. The procedure begins by dilating the cervix to 8 mm in diameter. The 7.8-mm insulated hysteroscope and HTA cannula are then introduced into the uterine cavity (Figure 6.3); instruments should fit snugly to prevent leaking of hot fluid into the vagina. If necessary, a tenaculum can be placed on the cervix to achieve a tight fit. A diagnostic hysteroscopy is performed to rule out unidentified pathology, followed by a flush cycle with saline after the cannula is introduced into the uterus. The cannula

is then positioned at the endocervical junction with the lower uterine segment, and 90°C saline is circulated through the cavity for 10–15 minutes at approximately 50–55 mmHg. This intrauterine pressure is chosen to be well below the minimum pressure of 70 mmHg required to open the fallopian tubes. The endometrium is flushed again with room-temperature saline to cool the instrument and cavity (for approximately 1 min), followed by removal of the HTA cannula. The procedure is performed under direct hysteroscopic visualization.

Corson published a multicenter randomized controlled trial in 2001 involving 276 women randomized in a 2:1 fashion to HTA (Hydro ThermAblator™; BEI Medical Systems, Teterboro, NJ) and rollerball.[43] Success (82% vs 77%) and amenorrhea (51% vs 40%) rates were slightly higher for rollerball than for HTA at 12-month follow-up. Improvements in quality of life (QOL) measures were similar.

Three-year follow-up results of this study were reported by Goldrath in 2003.[44] HTA, compared to rollerball ablation, was associated with higher amenorrhea (53% vs 46%), reduction of bleeding to normal level (94% vs 91%), and satisfaction (98% vs 97%) rates after 3 years. Subsequent interventions for menorrhagia were similar between groups.

Disadvantages include the risk of burns to the cervix, vagina, or peritoneal cavity due to leakage of hot water through the fallopian tubes. A safety mechanism built into this system automatically turns off the instrument if more than 10 ml of fluid is lost. Pain can be significant from both the thermal necrosis and cervical dilatation required in order to pass the 8-mm instrument, which usually requires the use of general anesthesia.

Bipolar desiccation

Another commonly performed second generation ablation method is bipolar desiccation of the endometrial lining. The product (NovaSure®) is produced by Novacept (Mountain View, CA), and utilizes bipolar radiofrequency (RF) to desiccate the endometrium and superficial myometrium (Figure 6.4). The system consists of a disposable probe connected to a portable controller and is operated using a foot pedal. The gold-plated, porous electrode array is mounted on a conformable and expandable mesh, which is housed in a protective sheath. The cervix is first dilated to approximately 8 mm diameter to accommodate the 7.2-mm probe. After transcervical introduction into the endometrial cavity, the sheath is retracted. This

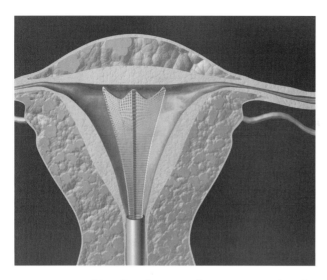

Figure 6.4 NovaSure® second generation bipolar endometrial ablation technique. Image courtesy of Cytyc Corporation and affiliates

deploys the mesh, which expands to conform to the uterine cavity. A vacuum is then created in the cavity to generate sufficient pressure to achieve contact with the entire surface of the cavity and to continuously suction steam and moisture as tissue is desiccated and resistance increases. The system is impedance controlled; it automatically detects when 50 ohms of resistance is reached. This usually takes 1–2 minutes. In addition, the device adjusts its power output based on operator and device measurements of uterine size. The average depth of ablation is 4–5 mm, but is tapered to allow for a shallower ablation at the cornua and internal cervical os. NovaSure is performed blindly: no hysteroscopic visualization is required. Because this may contribute to unrecognized perforations, a safety feature was added to the design. The device first insufflates the uterine cavity with CO_2 until a pressure of 50 mmHg is achieved and maintained for 4 seconds; this implies the uterine cavity integrity has not been compromised by perforation.

The procedure obviates the risks associated with distension media, and associated fluid overload. Notably, a fairly regular endometrial contour is required. Like other second generation methods, the procedure is fast and easy to learn.

The efficacy of NovaSure was first studied in a multicenter randomized controlled trial by Cooper et al in 2002.[17] Women were randomized in a 2:1 fashion to NovaSure and rollerball and followed for 1 year. NovaSure use was associated with significantly shorter operative times (4.2 vs 24 min) and less cervical dilatation (7.7 vs 9.6 mm). Intraoperative (0.6% vs 6.7%) and postoperative (13% vs 25.3%) complications were

less frequent with NovaSure than with rollerball. Success rates were high (88.3% for NovaSure and 81.7% for rollerball) as defined by PBAC < 75. Amenorrhea rates were similar (41% for NovaSure vs 35% for rollerball). NovaSure was significantly more likely to be used with local anesthesia (73%) vs rollerball (18%). Quality of life outcomes were similar.

The Hawe group published a report in 2003 comparing the Cavaterm balloon device to NovaSure.[45] Fifty-seven women were randomized in a 2:1 fashion (NovaSure, 38; Cavaterm, 19) in an intention to treat analysis. No medical pretreatment was used in either group, but women in the Cavaterm group underwent curettage immediately prior to surgery. Operative time was significantly shorter in the NovaSure group (4 vs 23 min). Amenorrhea (12% vs 43%) rates were lower, but hypomenorrhea rates higher (59% vs 27%) in the NovaSure group compared to the Cavaterm group. Although not statistically significant, six women in the NovaSure group underwent a second surgery (including one dilatation and curettage (D&C) for hematometra) within 12 months compared to none in the Cavaterm group. There were no major intraoperative complications, but frequent equipment problems did occur (11% in Cavaterm and 8% in NovaSure). All three of the cases associated with generator dysfunction in the NovaSure group resulted in the need for a second procedure (two repeat ablations and one hysterectomy).

In another study, ThermaChoice UBT was compared to NovaSure by Bongers et al in 2004.[46] In this Dutch trial, 126 women were randomly assigned to either group and subsequently followed for 12 months. Amenorrhea rates (43% vs 8%) and satisfaction rates (90% vs 79%) were significantly higher in the NovaSure group. Quality of life outcomes for this same study were published in 2005.[47] Interestingly, there were no significant differences between health-related quality of life parameters measured, including the medical outcomes Short-Form 36, the Self-rating Depression Scale, the Rotterdam Symptom Checklist, the State-Trait Anxiety Inventory, and structured clinical history questionnaire.

Another bipolar device, Vesta, was introduced by Soderstrom et al in 1996.[16] Vesta consists of an inflatable, inverted triangle shaped balloon with 12 individually controlled bipolar electrodes on its surface. Each electrode is connected by a separate thermistor. Only one electrode is activated at a time on a preset program by the generator. The probe is 8 mm in diameter and includes a sheath that retracts after intrauterine placement is achieved to expose the balloon. The balloon is then inflated with 12–15 ml of air to expand the balloon and ensure good contact with the endometrial surface. A central channel allows a small amount of fluid or air to be instilled, which can detect fundal perforation. The electrosurgical generator charges for 90 seconds and monitors impedance at each of the 12 electrodes independently every 0.33 seconds. High readings suggest non-contact or perforation, and the system automatically shuts down. Cornual electrodes are set at 72°C while the remaining electrodes are set at 75°C. The control box automatically initiates a 4-minute treatment cycle using 45 W undampened current.

The Vesta system was compared in a randomized controlled trial to ablation through a combined TCRE/rollerball ablation procedure, and results were reported in 1999 and 2000.[48,49] Results were similar to those of NovaSure. Procedure time was shorter with Vesta (23 vs 39 min). General anesthesia was less frequent with Vesta (16.7% vs 79.7%). Success (86.9% vs 83%) and amenorrhea (31.1% vs 34.8%) rates were similar between Vesta and TCRE/rollerball, respectively. Intraoperative (1.4% vs 3.3%) and postoperative (2.2% vs 3.5%) complications were lower with Vesta.

Microwave ablation

Microwave ablation was first described by Sharp et al in 1995.[14] It was designed to improve on the available ablative options by developing a faster, safer, and easier technique to learn. Microwave energy at 20 W generated by a frequency of 9.2 GHz was chosen to achieve tissue penetration of no more than 5–6 mm. The active tip of the device is placed in the uterine cavity via an 8-mm diameter probe (Figure 6.5). The energy is generated by a magnetron in the base unit and passes through the cable to the probe tip; the device is controlled by the operator using a footswitch. Intrauterine temperature is continuously monitored by thermocouples on the exterior surface of the waveguide, which is displayed and recorded by the central controller.

Under general or local anesthesia the cervix is dilated to 9 mm and the length of the uterine cavity is measured. The entire procedure is performed using real time temperature feedback. First the applicator is advanced to the mid-fundus and wide lateral sweeping is begun. Sweeping continues until the temperature reaches the therapeutic band of 70–80°C. At this time the applicator is pointed to each cornu, one then the other, followed by wide lateral sweeping as the applicator is slowly withdrawn to treat the corpus and lower segment. Care is taken during each step to keep

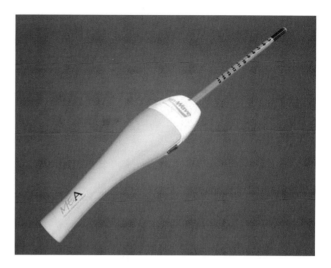

Figure 6.5 Microsulis second generation microwave endometrial ablation system for use with femWave™ single use endometrial ablation applicators. Image courtesy of Microsulis Americas, Inc

the temperature in the therapeutic band. The procedure lasts less than 5 min. Microwave ablation (Microsulis, Waterlooville, Hampshire, UK) uses a relatively cost-effective disposable probe. Initially developed in the UK, the femWAVE™ system is now approved by the Food and Drug Administration (FDA).

Cooper's group conducted a randomized controlled trial in 240 women comparing microwave ablation to TCRE after pretreatment with goserelin. Amenorrhea rates, success rates, satisfaction rates, and complications were comparable between groups. Operating time was significantly shorter in the microwave group (11.4 vs 15 min). Bain et al reported 2-year follow-up data in 2002 of this same study.[50] Amenorrhea rates were slightly better in the microwave group (47%) vs TCRE (41%), but did not reach statistical significance. Satisfaction rates did reach statistical significance in favor of microwave (79% vs 67%). Quality of life, complication, and reintervention rates were similar. At the 5-year follow-up,[51] statistical significance was achieved in favor of microwave ablation for satisfaction (86% vs 74%), acceptability, and the proportion that would recommend the treatment to a friend. Amenorrhea (65% vs 69%) rates appeared slightly higher in TCRE and subsequent surgical intervention rates were slightly lower (24% vs 28%) for microwave ablation compared to TCRE, though neither difference reached statistical significance.

Cooper et al then compared microwave ablation to rollerball in a 2004 multicenter, randomized controlled trial of 322 women randomized in a 2:1 fashion and followed for 1 year.[52] Success (87% vs 83%)

and amenorrhea (55.3% vs 45.8%) rates appeared slightly higher for microwave vs rollerball treatment, though the effects were not statistically different. Local vs general anesthesia was much more likely in the microwave (62% vs 37%) than in the rollerball group (18% vs 76%). Reintervention and postoperative complications were similar between groups. No major intraoperative complications were reported. However, vomiting and uterine cramping were statistically higher in the microwave group compared to rollerball. Despite this, satisfaction rates remained high for both microwave and rollerball groups, respectively (98.5% and 99%).

ELITT™ (endometrial laser intrauterine thermal therapy)

ELITT is a global laser technique not currently available in the USA. This device contains a 20-W, 830-nm diode laser attached to a 6-mm probe (GyneLase™; ESC/Sharplan, Needham, MA). Three laser beams are emitted simultaneously through separate channels. This system does not require direct contact with the endometrium; the lasers diffuse in irregularly shaped cavities to treat the entire endometrial surface. Unlike traditional TCRE procedures, the cornual areas do not need to be treated separately. The 830-nm wavelength is absorbed by hemoglobin and penetrates the endometrium, where it is transformed to heat energy and induces coagulation. The cervix is dilated to 7 mm in diameter to accommodate the light diffuser handpiece. The distal end is advanced to the fundus and then the side diffusers are opened to form an 'inverted triangle'. The device consists of three fibers: two lateral fibers diffuse light up to 3 cm away and the middle fiber diffuses light to 4 cm. The device is preset for 7 minutes treatment length, programmed with the following settings: 20 W during the first 90 seconds, 18 W during the next 90 seconds, and 16 W during the final 240 seconds. At the end of the procedure, the wings are collapsed and the probe is removed from the uterus. The entire procedure is performed blindly and no distension medium is used. Given the small size of the probe and lack of distension medium needed, it is a possible candidate for use in the office setting.

Perino et al conducted an Italian trial comparing ELITT to TCRE, published in 2004.[53] One hundred and eleven women were randomized, and follow-up reported for 3 years. The amenorrhea rate was markedly

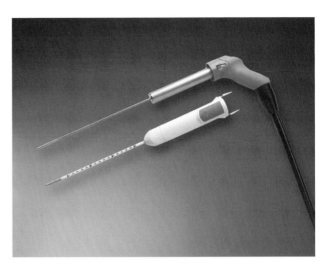

Figure 6.6 Her Option™ endometrial cryoablation technique, a second generation technique. Image courtesy of American Medical Systems, Inc

better in the ELITT group (59%) vs only 24% in the TCRE group. Complication, satisfaction, and retreatment rates were similar between the two groups. Pain scores were statistically significantly higher in the ELITT group (4.4 vs 3.7; scale from 1 to 10), but the clinical significance of this difference appears minimal. No significant complications occurred in either group and both groups were pretreated with a GnRH agonist.

Cryoablation

Cryoablation was first described by Droegemueller et al in 1971,[54] and the first randomized trial of this technique performed by Pittrof et al in 1993.[11] The device used by Pittrof et al resembled a Hegar 8 dilator with a central lumen through which 3–15 ml of saline could be instilled into the uterine cavity. The device was then activated for 5 min and the temperature decreased to −45°C. The ice mold was then allowed to melt and the tip of the device was placed into the opposite cornu. The improvement rate among 67 women in this early trial was 63% at 3–18 months' follow-up.[55]

The modern cryoablation system currently available in the USA is Her Option™ (American Medical Systems, Minnesota) shown in Figure 6.6. Cryoablation as performed at present differs from typical global ablation procedures: it is not automated and the progress of the procedure is monitored using real time ultrasound. The probe, measuring 5.5 mm in diameter, is perfused with a closed-system gas mixture that is cooled based on the Joule–Thomson principle: pressurized gas is passed through a small orifice, thereby producing a cooling effect. After the probe is inserted into the uterine cavity, the cavity is cooled to approximately −90°C, producing an elliptical ice ball. Ultrasound is used to follow the progression of the ice front. The temperature at the edge of the ice front is only −2°C, while tissue death usually occurs at approximately −20°C. This means that all of the tissue visualized on ultrasound within the ice ball is not being destroyed; the outermost 4–6 mm is usually not permanently ablated. The cooling cycle is usually terminated after 7–8 minutes, or sooner when the ice front reaches between 3 and 5 mm from the surface of the uterine serosa. The probe is then warmed (which releases it from the frozen tissue) and repositioned to the next area. Typically, two or three freezes adequately treat the entire endometrium, taking 10–20 minutes. In an average uterus (sounding less than 10 cm), usually two freezes suffice: the probe tip is placed first in the proximity of one and then the opposite cornu. Larger uteri may require additional freezes in the central fundus and/or lower uterine segment. By using a freezing technique to ablate the endometrium, the nociceptive response is decreased, resulting in less pain and cramping than with heat based therapies. Also, since the operator can directly observe the progression of the ice front using ultrasound, the risk of complications such as unrecognized uterine perforations or thermal bowel injury is minimized. Particular attention must be paid to sonographic monitoring of the expansion of the freeze zone in the lower uterine segment in patients with previous cesarean sections, as this area may be much thinner than the fundus or even the cornual area. Because this procedure is well tolerated, cryoablation can be performed in an office setting.

Her Option (Cryogen, San Diego, CA) was compared to rollerball in a randomized controlled trial by Duleba et al[56] in 2003 of 279 women randomized in a 2:1 fashion. Success rates were 77.3% for cryoablation and 83.8% for rollerball; bleeding declined by 92% and 94%, respectively, at 1 year. In the cryoablation group, the amenorrhea rate was significantly lower (27.6% vs 55.6%) and the persistent menorrhagia rate was higher (12.2% vs 6.9%). However, patients undergoing cryoablation were significantly more likely to recommend the procedure to a friend and to not require general anesthesia. Treatment effect persisted at 24–30 months.[57] Retreatment rates, as well as complication rates, were similar between groups.

Although it is usually performed on normal endometrial cavities, successful cryoablations of submucosal fibroids ≤ 3 cm have been reported.[58]

Progesterone intrauterine devices

Progesterone impregnated intrauterine devices are also a safe and minimally invasive treatment alternative for menorrhagia. When compared with the levonorgestrel IUS, endometrial ablation was found to be more effective in controlling menstrual blood loss at 1 year, but was equivalent at 2 and 3 years. Satisfaction rates and quality of life were equivalent at 1, 2, and 3 years with both treatments.[59]

CONCLUSIONS

Endometrial ablations have several advantages. They are generally outpatient procedures, have low morbidity, and are less invasive than hysterectomy. Disadvantages include risks of persistent or recurrent bleeding and possible need for repeat ablation or hysterectomy. Up to 40% of patients undergoing electrocautery, laser, or radiofrequency ablations required a second ablation or hysterectomy within 4 years compared to only 1% risk of repeat surgery for patients who were primarily managed with a hysterectomy.[60] A Cochrane review found that subsequent operative rates or need for a second procedure were not significantly different between standard and second generation techniques including balloon, Vesta, microwave, and Hydro ThermoAblator.[60] Long-term outcome studies on some of the newest ablative procedures are not yet available.

Most short-term complications are more frequent following hysterectomy when compared to endometrial ablation techniques. Hysterectomy is associated with significant risk of sepsis, blood transfusion, urinary retention, anemia, febrile illness, and vaginal cuff and wound hematoma. Hysteroscopic ablations are associated with risks related to uterine perforation and complications of distension fluid media. All ablations also carry the risk of endometritis, hematometra, and thermal injuries to surrounding structures, including bowel injury.[61]

Overall, second generation techniques appear similar in efficacy to first generation techniques but are technically easier to perform; the procedures are generally faster, more likely to be tolerated under local anesthesia, and associated with lower risk of complication.

Table 6.2 summarizes salient features of the different endometrial ablation procedures.

Table 6.2 Summary of endometrial ablation techniques

Procedure	Cervical dilatation	Anesthesia	Procedure time	Satisfaction rate	Amenorrhea rate	Advantages	Disadvantages
Standard ablation (e.g. laser, rollerball, wire loop resection)	10–12 mm	Usually general	10–40 min (varies widely with operator skill)	82–99% at 1 year	35–50% at 1 year	Irregular cavities may be treated under direct visualization; injury minimized by immediate recognition of perforations	Requires operative hysteroscope, general anesthesia, significant operator skill, close fluid monitoring
Vaporizing electrode	10–12 mm	Usually general	10 min	96% at 1 year	36% at 1 year	Fluid deficit less than first generation methods	Requires operative hysteroscope
Hot water balloon (ThermaChoice®, Cavaterm™)	5 mm	Usually general	15 min	91–96% at 1 year	8–37% at 1 year	Easy to perform, small probe diameter	Performed blindly
Hydrothermal ablation	8 mm	Usually general	15 min	98% at 3 years	40% at 1 year	Performed under direct visualization; water fills entire surface of even irregularly shaped cavities	Requires an 8-mm hysteroscope; risk of hot water leakage causing burns of cervix, vagina, or through fallopian tubes to peritoneum
Bipolar mesh dessication (NovaSure®)	8 mm	Usually general	1–2 min	91% at 1 year	41–43% at 1 year	Quick and easy to learn and perform	Requires a smooth endometrial cavity; performed blindly
Microwave (femWAVE™)	9 mm	Usually general	3–5 min	99% at 1 year	59% at 3 years	High success rate	Requires a large hysteroscope; performed blindly
Laser (ELITT)	7 mm	Usually general	7 min	95% at 1 year	55% at 1 year	Energy diffuses to treat irregularly shaped cavities; uses small hysteroscope	Is performed blindly
Cryoablation (Her Option™)	5.5 mm	Usually local	10–20 min	96% at 1 year	28% at 1 year	Can monitor progress in real time by ultrasound thereby minimizing risk for injury; less pain because cold is used instead of heat, can be performed in the office setting; possible efficacy in treating small fibroids	As with all methods, care must be exercised in the setting of previous c-section because the lower uterine segment may be much more thin, leading to thermal injury beyond the uterine serosa in this area

REFERENCES

1. Scott-Levin. Physician Drug & Diagnosis Audit, MAT. Yardley, PA: Verispan, 2002.

2. National Hospital Discharge and Ambulatory Surgery Data. Hyattsville, MD: National Center for Health Statistics, 1996.

3. Garry R, Fountain J, Mason S et al. The eVALuate study: two parallel randomised trials, one comparing laparoscopic with abdominal hysterectomy, the other comparing laparoscopic with vaginal hysterectomy. BMJ 2004; 328: 129.

4. O'Connor H, Broadbent JA, Magos AL, McPherson K. Medical Research Council randomised trial of endometrial resection versus hysterectomy in management of menorrhagia. Lancet 1997; 349: 897–901.

5. Stenchever MA, Oroegemuller W, Herbst AL, Mishell D, eds. Comprehensive Gynecology, 4th edn. Philadelphia: Harcourt Health Sciences, 2001.

6. Cole S, Billewizc W, Thomson A. Sources of variation in menstrual blood loss. J Obstet Gynaecol Br Commonw 1971; 78: 933–9.

7. Hallberg L, Hogdahel AM, Nilsson L, Rybo G. Menstrual blood loss – a population study. Variation at different ages and attempts to define normality. Acta Obstet Gynecol Scand 1966; 45: 320–51.

8. Fraser IS, McCarron G. Randomized trial of 2 hormonal and 2 prostaglandin-inhibiting agents in women with a complaint of menorrhagia. Aust NZ J Obstet Gynaecol 1991; 31: 66–70.

9. Lethaby A, Irvine G, Cameron I. Cyclical progestogens for heavy menstrual bleeding. Cochrane Database Syst Rev 2000; (2): CD001016.

10. Taylor HS. Endometrial cells derived from donor stem cells in bone marrow transplant recipients. JAMA 2004; 292: 81–5.

11. Pittrof R, Majid S, Murray A. Initial experience with transcervical cryoablation using saline as a uterine distension medium. Minim Invas Ther 1993; 2: 69–73.

12. Baggish M, Paraiso M, Breznock EM, Griffey S. A computer-controlled, continuously circulating, hot irrigating system for endometrial ablation. Am J Obstet Gynecol 1995; 173: 1842–8.

13. Donnez J, Polet R, Mathieu PE et al. Endometrial laser interstitial hyperthermy: a potential modality for endometrial ablation. Obstet Gynecol 1996; 87: 459–64.

14. Sharp NC, Cronin N, Feldberg I et al. Microwaves for menorrhagia: a new fast technique for endometrial ablation. Lancet 1995; 346: 1003–4.

15. Singer A, Almanza R, Gutierrez A et al. Preliminary clinical experience with a thermal balloon endometrial ablation method to treat menorrhagia. Obstet Gynecol 1994; 83: 732–4.

16. Soderstrom RM, Brooks PG, Corson SL et al. Endometrial ablation using a distensible multielectrode balloon. J Am Assoc Gynecol Laparosc 1996; 3: 403–7.

17. Cooper J, Gimpelson R, Laberge P et al. A randomized, multicenter trial of safety and efficacy of the NovaSure system in the treatment of menorrhagia. J Am Assoc Gynecol Laparosc 2002; 9: 418–28.

18. Fehr MK, Madsen SJ, Svaasand LO et al. Intrauterine light delivery for photodynamic therapy of the human endometrium. Hum Reprod 1995; 10: 3067–72.

19. Sowter MC, Lethaby A, Singla AA. Pre-operative endometrial thinning agents before endometrial destruction for heavy menstrual bleeding. Cochrane Database Syst Rev 2002; (3): CD001124.

20. Goldrath MH, Fuller TA, Segal S. Laser photovaporization of endometrium for the treatment of menorrhagia. Am J Obstet Gynecol 1981; 140: 14–19.

21. McClure N et al. A quantitative assessment of endometrial electrocautery in the management of menorrhagia and a comparative report on argon laser endometrial ablation. Gynaecol Endosc 1992; 1: 199–202.

22. Bhattacharya S, Cameron IM, Parkin DE et al. A pragmatic randomised comparison of transcervical resection of the endometrium with endometrial laser ablation for the treatment of menorrhagia. Br J Obstet Gynaecol 1997; 104: 601–7.

23. Pinion SB, Parkin DE, Abramovich DR et al. Randomised trial of hysterectomy, endometrial laser ablation, and transcervical endometrial resection for dysfunctional uterine bleeding. BMJ 1994: 309: 979–83.

24. Gannon MJ, Holt EM, Fairbank J et al. A randomised trial comparing endometrial resection and abdominal hysterectomy for the treatment of menorrhagia. BMJ 1991; 303: 1362–4.

25. DeCherney AH, Diamond MP, Lavy G, Polan ML. Endometrial ablation for intractable uterine bleeding: hysteroscopic resection. Obstet Gynecol 1987; 70: 668–70.

26. Dwyer N, Hutton J, Stirrat GM. Randomised controlled trial comparing endometrial resection with abdominal hysterectomy for the surgical treatment of menorrhagia. Br J Obstet Gynaecol 1993; 100: 237–43.

27. Crosignani PG, Vercellini P, Apolone G et al. Endometrial resection versus vaginal hysterectomy for menorrhagia: long-term clinical and quality-of-life outcomes. Am J Obstet Gynecol 1997; 177: 95–101.

28. A randomised trial of endometrial ablation versus hysterectomy for the treatment of dysfunctional uterine bleeding: outcome at four years. Aberdeen Endometrial Ablation Trials Group. Br J Obstet Gynaecol 1999; 106: 360–6.

29. Lin BL, Tomomatsu M, Kuribayashi Y et al. [The development of a new operating hysteroscopic fiberscope and its clinical application.] Nippon Sanka Fujinka Gakkai Zasshi 1988; 40: 1733–9. [in Japanese]

30. Vancaillie TG. Electrocoagulation of the endometrium with the ball-end resectoscope. Obstet Gynecol 1989; 74: 425–7.

31. Boujida VH, Philipsen T, Pelle J, Joergensen JC. Five-year follow-up of endometrial ablation: endometrial coagulation versus endometrial resection. Obstet Gynecol 2002; 99: 988–92.

32. Vercellini P, Oldani S, DeGiorgi O et al. Endometrial ablation with a vaporizing electrode in women with regular uterine cavity or submucous leiomyomas. J Am Assoc Gynecol Laparosc 1996; 3 (Suppl): S52.

33. Vercellini P, Oldani S, Yaylayan L et al. Randomized comparison of vaporizing electrode and cutting loop for endometrial ablation. Obstet Gynecol 1999; 94: 521–7.

34. Friberg B et al. A new, simple, safe, and efficient device for the treatment of menorrhagia. J Gynecol Tech 1996; 2: 103–8.

35. Meyer WR, Walsh BW, Grainger DA et al. Thermal balloon and rollerball ablation to treat menorrhagia: a multicenter comparison. Obstet Gynecol 1998; 92: 98–103.

36. Soysal ME, Soysal SK, Vicdan K. Thermal balloon ablation in myoma-induced menorrhagia under local anesthesia. Gynecol Obstet Invest 2001; 51: 128–33.

37. van Zon-Rabelink IA, Vleugels MP, Merkus HM, de Graaf R. Endometrial ablation by rollerball electrocoagulation compared to uterine balloon thermal ablation. Technical and safety aspects. Eur J Obstet Gynecol Reprod Biol 2003; 110: 220–3.

38. Van Zon-Rabelink IA, Vleugels MP, Merkus HM, de Graaf R. Efficacy and satisfaction rate comparing endometrial ablation by rollerball electrocoagulation to uterine balloon thermal ablation in a randomised controlled trial. Eur J Obstet Gynecol Reprod Biol 2004; 114: 97–103.

39. Pellicano M, Guida M, Acunzo G et al. Hysteroscopic transcervical endometrial resection versus thermal destruction for menorrhagia: a prospective randomized trial on satisfaction rate. Am J Obstet Gynecol 2002; 187: 545–50.

40. Hawe et al. 2003

41. Goldrath MH, Barrionuevo M, Husain M. Endometrial ablation by hysteroscopic instillation of hot saline solution. J Am Assoc Gynecol Laparosc 1997; 4: 235–40.

7 Medical treatment options for endometriosis

Neal G Mahutte and Aydin Arici

Endometriosis is found in up to 60% of women with dysmenorrhea, 40–50% of reproductive age women with pelvic pain or deep dyspareunia, and 30–40% of women with infertility.[1] Endometriosis is defined as the presence and proliferation of endometrial tissue outside the uterus. Endometriosis is most frequently found in the dependent portions of the pelvis, including the surface of the ovaries, the uterosacral ligaments, the pelvic sidewalls and the posterior cul-de-sac. Endometriosis may also form so-called chocolate cysts of the ovary (endometriomas), may invade the recto-vaginal septum, may appear at the sites of previous surgical incisions, or may even arise in distant parts of the body such as the lung or brain.

Endometriosis is typically associated with two major problems: pain and impaired fertility. Although not all women with endometriosis are symptomatic, cyclic bleeding from ectopic endometrium into surrounding tissue may result in inflammation, scarring and adhesions. In addition, endometriotic lesions may induce pain by direct neuronal invasion or via neuronal responses to inflammatory cytokines.

Endometriosis is an estrogen-dependent disorder and thus typically is found only in reproductive age women. When endometriosis is encountered in premenarchal girls or postmenopausal women, exogenous steroid administration or peripheral aromatization of androgens to estrogens is often the cause. Because of its estrogen dependence, virtually all commonly used medical treatments for endometriosis-associated pain derive their efficacy by suppressing estrogen production or opposing estrogen action. In either case, the treatment typically succeeds or fails based on the extent to which it induces hypo/amenorrhea.

The association between endometriosis and infertility is less well understood. In terms of medical treatments, it is clear that the hormonal suppressive therapies most commonly used to treat endometriosis-associated pain do not improve spontaneous fecundity rates. In contrast, there is some evidence to support surgical management, and compelling evidence to support treating women with endometriosis-associated infertility in a manner similar to that of women with unexplained infertility. Superovulation combined with intrauterine insemination or in vitro fertilization consistently provides higher per cycle pregnancy rates than surgical approaches for endometriosis-associated infertility. Thus, non-invasive and minimally invasive therapies form the foundation of treatment for both endometriosis-associated pain and endometriosis-associated infertility in the 21st century.

DIAGNOSIS OF ENDOMETRIOSIS

The gold standard diagnosis of endometriosis relies on surgery and the histologic demonstration of ectopic endometrial glands and stroma. Reliance solely on clinical symptomatology, e.g. pelvic pain, dysmenorrhea, or visual inspection at the time of laparoscopy is unreliable.[2] Although there is a role for presumptive treatment of dysmenorrhea or pelvic pain with medications, the clinical suspicion of endometriosis should always be confirmed by histologic findings before the patient is definitively labeled with this diagnosis.

Peritoneal endometriotic implants may appear bluish-black, white, red, or clear. Variability in the appearance of endometriosis corresponds with varying degrees for which lesions are confirmed histologically. For example, typical blue-black powder-burn lesions correlate with histology in 75–90% of cases,[3,4] while atypical lesions correlate less frequently with strict histologic criteria (Table 7.1).[5]

Curiously, misdiagnosis of endometriosis may also result from over-reliance on the 'gold standard' histologic criteria. For example, biopsy of visually normal-appearing peritoneum in asymptomatic, fertile women may occasionally demonstrate all the histologic elements for endometriosis.[4,6] Similarly, surgical specimens from obvious endometriotic lesions do not always meet strict histologic criteria.

Non-invasive techniques to diagnose endometriosis

Our ability to study and effectively treat endometriosis would be greatly aided by a non-invasive method to accurately diagnose it.[7] Although much effort has been made to identify substances that could be detected

Table 7.1 Frequency with which specific types of lesions meet the strict histologic criteria for endometriosis[3–5]

	Likelihood of histologic diagnosis of endometriosis (%)
• Classic blue-black lesion	75–90
• Red, flame-like lesion	60–80
• White opacified peritoneum	60–80
• Glandular lesions	60–70
• Subovarian adhesions	20–50
• Yellow-brown peritoneum	45–50
• Peritoneal windows	12–45
Completely normal peritoneum	**6–13**

with a routine blood test that would distinguish women with endometriosis from those without it, we have yet to succeed. At one time there was hope that CA125 would provide this capability.[8] Serum CA125 is elevated in 50–80% of untreated women with moderate–severe stage endometriosis and 10–30% of women with minimal–mild stage disease.[9–11] However, serum CA125 is not a reliable marker for endometriosis. CA125 varies during the menstrual cycle, and may be elevated by a variety of other gynecologic conditions including pregnancy, fibroids, infection, peritoneal inflammation, and ovarian cancer. At best, serum CA125 may have a role in monitoring response to treatment or reactivation of disease in women previously known to have endometriosis and an elevated serum CA125 pre-treatment.[11–14]

Unfortunately, diagnostic imaging with ultrasound or magnetic resonance imaging (MRI) also has a limited role.[15] Although both modalities are superb at diagnosing endometriomas, neither modality is reliable at detecting peritoneal endometriosis. On ultrasound, endometriomas typically appear as persistent, thick-walled cystic ovarian masses with fine, diffuse homogeneous echoes. Endometriomas may also be septated or fluid filled. In very large studies using transvaginal ultrasound to diagnose endometriomas, sensitivity rates approaching 90% and specificity rates approaching 99% have been reported.[16] The accuracy of MRI appears to be similar to that of ultrasound, but may also offer the ability to detect deep peritoneal implants.[17] Endometriotic lesions are typically hypointense on T2 weighted images and hyperintense on T1 weighted images. With MRI, sensitivities of 61–71% and specificities of 60–98% have been reported for the detection of endometriosis.[18–21]

In the future, the application of genomic and proteomic technology is likely to produce a variety of novel diagnostic markers for endometriosis. Undoubtedly, some small studies with carefully selected patient populations will yield startling results. However, it will be critical to ensure that these diagnostic markers perform equally well when applied to broad, diverse populations of reproductive-age women with and without endometriosis. Moreover, potential confounders such as timing within the menstrual cycle, the presence of other pelvic pathology such as fibroids, adnexal masses, or adhesions, and the influence of medications will need to be addressed before these novel markers can be relied upon to accurately diagnose endometriosis.

PATHOGENESIS OF ENDOMETRIOSIS

The pathogenesis of endometriosis is unknown. In the 1920s Sampson proposed that endometriosis results from seeding of the peritoneal cavity by refluxed endometrial tissue.[22] A variety of compelling observations support Sampson's theory of retrograde menstruation (Table 7.2). Because retrograde menstruation occurs in almost all women but only a minority develop endometriosis, genetic and immune factors have been invoked to explain differences in individual susceptibility to the disease.

Five critical steps have been postulated to explain the development of endometriosis after retrograde menstruation. The two initial steps are attachment of endometrial cells to the peritoneal surface and invasion of these cells into the mesothelium. Angiogenesis around the nascent implant, endometrial cellular proliferation, and recruitment of inflammatory cells subservient to the implant then become important. It would appear that endometriotic tissues, local immune cells, and inflammatory cytokines mediate each of these steps.

However, Sampson's theory cannot explain all cases. Rarely, endometriosis may occur in the lung or brain, and these cases are believed to result from lymphovascular spread of endometrial tissue. Coelomic metaplasia may also account for certain cases of endometriosis such as those occurring in men who receive exogenous estrogen treatment or those occurring in peri-menarchal teenage girls.[31]

STAGING OF ENDOMETRIOSIS

The purpose of staging endometriosis is to provide prognostic information for patients, to allow uniform reporting of results, and to facilitate research. The current staging system for endometriosis is the revised

Table 7.2 Evidence in favor of Sampson's theory for the pathogenesis of endometriosis

- The existence of retrograde menstruation is well documented
- Endometrial debris from menstrual effluent can grow in tissue culture[23]
- Human endometrial tissue can adhere to peritoneal tissue[24]
- In animal models, menstrual endometrium transposed to the peritoneal cavity may cause endometriosis[25]
- Endometriosis implants are most frequently found in the dependent portions of the pelvis[26,27]
- There is a very high incidence of endometriosis in women who have mullerian anomalies with outflow tract obstruction[28]
- Endometriosis is associated with increased menstrual flow, frequent menstruation and early menarche[29,30]
- Even in the presence of extensive pelvic disease the fallopian tubes often remain patent

classification of the American Society for Reproductive Medicine.[32] Endometriosis is divided into four stages (minimal, mild, moderate, and severe) based on the total cumulative score derived from a weighted point system. Points are assigned based on the size and depth of peritoneal and adnexal lesions as well as the extent of pelvic adhesions.

One of the major problems with this staging system is its reliance on arbitrary scoring assignments. Scoring itself is prone to inter- and intraobserver variation, but more important than that the actual algorithm scores are not based on empiric data.[33] For example, partial obliteration of the posterior cul-de-sac is assigned a score of 4 while complete obliteration of the posterior cul-de-sac is assigned a score of 20, even though there is no evidence that one is 5 times worse than the other in terms of pain or its effect on fertility.

Studies have consistently failed to identify a close correlation between the stage of endometriosis and the presence of pain or infertility.[34-38] In a classic study, Fedele et al demonstrated that the incidences of dysmenorrhea (70–80%), dyspareunia (30%), and pelvic pain (40%) were no different in a group of 68 women with stage I–II endometriosis compared to a group of 92 women with stage III–IV endometriosis. Better correlation may exist between pain symptomatology and the depth of endometriosis lesions.[39,40]

MEDICAL MANAGEMENT OF ENDOMETRIOSIS-ASSOCIATED PAIN

Endometriosis-associated pain is among the most challenging conditions in gynecologic practice.[41] Careful evaluation of the patient is paramount to minimize the possibility of misdiagnosis and to maximize the chance of therapeutic success. Particular attention should be given to past medical and surgical treatments in planning future management. While a variety of medical treatments can effectively suppress endometriosis, they generally have little effect on other potential causes of pelvic pain such as adhesions, adnexal cysts, interstitial cystitis, or inflammatory bowel disease. For these reasons, consideration should be given to laparoscopic evaluation if the diagnosis of endometriosis is not well established.

Once the diagnosis of endometriosis-associated pain is confirmed, a broad armamentarium of medical treatments exists. In general, the efficacy of medical treatments for endometriosis-associated pain correlates with their ability to reduce menstrual bleeding or induce amenorrhea.[42] Among the options that reliably induce hypo/amenorrhea are progestins, gonadotropin releasing hormone (GnRH) agonists, and danazol. All of these have been utilized to treat endometriosis-associated pain, and all have been shown to be equipotent.[43-45] The main problem with each of these treatments is the frequency and severity of side-effects (Table 7.3), and thus the choice of which therapy to use in a particular patient should be based primarily on the anticipated side-effects and cost.

It is incumbent on physicians who provide gynecologic services to women of reproductive age to be intimately familiar with the treatment options for endometriosis, and in particular with the nuances of medication delivery and combination therapy. Whenever possible, attempts should be made to mitigate potential treatment side-effects. For example, immediately combining add-back therapy with a GnRH agonist has been shown to significantly reduce vasomotor symptoms without compromising treatment efficacy. Similarly, use of the levonorgestrel intrauterine system (Mirena®) captures all the potential benefits of other progestins but significantly reduces unwanted systemic side-effects.

Non-steroidal anti-inflammatories

Although non-steroidal anti-inflammatory drugs (NSAIDs) do not directly treat endometriotic lesions, they have long been a mainstay in the treatment of endometriosis-associated pain. Unlike narcotics, NSAIDs are not addictive. Moreover, by inhibiting cyclooxygenase, NSAIDs reduce prostaglandin production and are particularly well suited to treat dysmenorrhea.[46]

Table 7.3   Side-effects of equipotent medical treatments for endometriosis

	Breakthrough bleeding (%)	Hot flashes (%)	Acne/oily skin (%)	Mood changes (%)	Weight gain (%)
High dose Provera®	70	—	30	20	50
Aygestin® 2.5 mg per day	30–50	—	5	7	30
Mirena®	30–50	—	5	5	10
Danazol	40	50	50	20	50
GnRH agonists	25	90	—	10	10
GnRH agonists with add-back Aygestin	25	50	10	10	30

A wide variety of NSAIDs are available. Naproxen and ibuprofen are among the most commonly used in gynecology. They are of similar efficacy in the relief of dysmenorrhea and pelvic pain, but differ slightly in cost and dosing schedule. One of the risks of frequent NSAID use is gastric irritation/ulceration. The risk of this complication can be reduced by taking NSAIDs only with meals and/or by using specific cyclooxygenase-2 (COX-2) inhibitors, e.g. celecoxib (Celebrex®) or rofecoxib (Vioxx®).[47–49] Another serious, but rare, complication of long-term NSAID use is kidney damage, including papillary necrosis and renal failure.

Oral contraceptives

Oral contraceptives are undoubtedly the most widely used hormonal therapy for endometriosis-associated pain. Oral contraceptives provide continuous progestin opposition to actions of estrogen, and reduce menstrual blood loss. Oral contraceptives are generally inexpensive and well tolerated.

Despite these attributes, there have been relatively few studies critically examining the use of oral contraceptives in women with endometriosis.[50] The first of these was a prospective, randomized trial comparing a cyclic low-dose oral contraceptive (20 μg ethinyl estradiol + 0.15 mg of desogestrel) to a GnRH agonist. Although both treatments reduced dysmenorrhea, dyspareunia, and pelvic pain, the relief of dysmenorrhea and dyspareunia after 6 months of therapy was less pronounced with the oral contraceptive than with the GnRH agonist.[51] A second randomized trial compared cyclic use of an oral contraceptive (30 μg ethinyl estradiol + 0.75 mg of gestodene) to a 4-month course of a GnRH agonist followed by 8 additional months of the same oral contraceptive used in the study group.[52] At the end of 1 year only 35% of the study participants in each group continued to have dysmenorrhea, and only about 40% reported ongoing pelvic pain.

There are now data confirming that women who do not benefit from a cyclic monophasic oral contraceptive may benefit from starting a new pill pack every 21 days, i.e. taking the pill continuously. Vercellini et al offered 50 women with recurrent dysmenorrhea following surgery and use of a cyclic oral contraceptive the opportunity to convert to a continuous regimen (20 μg ethinyl estradiol + 0.15 mg desogestrel).[53] This method provides constant progestin-mediated suppression of endometrial growth, and achieves complete amenorrhea in close to 40% of patients. After 2 years of follow-up, 80% of study participants were either satisfied (54%) or very satisfied (26%) with the treatment, and only 14% reported moderate or severe side-effects.

One of the potential pitfalls of continuous oral contraceptive use is spotting or frank breakthrough bleeding. In general, episodes of bleeding tend to be associated with exacerbation of pain. If bleeding is prolonged (> 1 week) then it is recommended to stop the oral contraceptive for 7 days to allow the endometrium to stabilize. If a 3-month trial of continuous oral contraceptives and a NSAID are ineffective, then more aggressive hormonal therapy is warranted. There is no evidence that switching from one oral contraceptive to another or one NSAID to another is beneficial in this setting.

Danazol

Danazol is a synthetic derivative of 17-ethynyltestosterone and has been used in the treatment of endometriosis since the 1970s. For much of the 1980s it was considered the gold standard for medical therapy. However, since the 1990s the use of danazol has markedly declined due to its high cost and significant side-effect profile.

Danazol derives its efficacy from its capacity to produce a high androgen/low estrogen environment.[54–57]

Danazol also suppresses the mid-cycle surge of luteinizing hormone (LH) and follicle stimulating hormone (FSH).[58] This hormone profile results in endometrial atrophy both within the uterus and at ectopic sites.[59,60] As a result, most women using high-dose danazol experience amenorrhea.

In the 1980s, two small prospective randomized trials validated the efficacy of danazol 600 mg/day compared to placebo for the treatment of endometriosis-associated pain.[61,62] These results were in keeping with earlier cohort studies reporting improvements in pain scores for 80–90% of women with endometriosis using danazol 600–800 mg/day.[63–65] As one would expect, women who develop amenorrhea on danazol have the highest response rate.[64]

Unfortunately, up to 80% of women using danazol 600–800 mg per day experience major androgenic side-effects, e.g. acne, oily skin, hirsutism, and/or irreversible deepening of the voice.[66] Other common side-effects with danazol include breakthrough bleeding, edema, and muscle cramps. Because of these problems, lower doses of danazol (in the range of 50–200 mg daily) have been investigated.[64,67–70] Although participants in these studies reported fewer side-effects, most of them continued to menstruate, and as a result clinical efficacy rates declined to levels similar to those of oral contraceptives, i.e. 60–75%. If one considers using danazol it is important to keep in mind that danazol is a potential teratogen, and thus an alternative form of contraception is indicated with this therapy.

Progestins

A number of studies have shown that progestins are as effective as danazol in the treatment of endometriosis-associated pain.[61,62,71–73] The earliest studies described the use of oral medroxyprogesterone acetate (Provera®) at doses of 50–100 mg per day. At these dosages approximately 80–90% of women with endometriosis-associated pain reported symptomatic improvement. An alternative route to oral medroxyprogesterone acetate is intramuscular or subcutaneous depot medroxyprogesterone acetate (Depo-Provera®). Depo-Provera is inexpensive, and within 6–12 months most women develop amenorrhea. In a prospective randomized trial, Depo-Provera was shown to be as effective as very low dose danazol combined with an oral contraceptive.[74] Another prospective, randomized trial compared Depo-Provera to a GnRH agonist and found no difference in clinical efficacy between the two treatments.[75] However, major disadvantages of Depo-Provera include

the inability to rapidly stop treatment if untoward side-effects occur, and the fact that there is often a significant delay in the resumption of ovulatory cycles after treatment is stopped.

A promising alternative to medroxyprogesterone acetate is norethindrone acetate (also known as norethisterone acetate, Aygestin®). A study in the 1990s suggested that dosages between 5 and 20 mg per day relieved pain in over 90% of women with endometriosis.[76] More recently, a well-designed prospective randomized trial evaluated the benefit of low dose Aygestin (2.5 mg per day) in 45 women with recurrent symptomatic rectovaginal endometriosis.[77] Although five women withdrew from the study because of medication side-effects, 85% of the women who completed the 12-month study were satisfied with the results. Moreover, pain scores showed gradual improvement from month to month throughout the 12 months in which they were measured, suggesting that patients who attempt this treatment should be encouraged to continue with it for at least 6 months (assuming it is well tolerated) before deciding whether they believe it has helped.

Progestins cause eutopic and ectopic endometrial tissue to undergo atrophic changes and pseudodecidualized reaction. In addition, progestins may have other properties that support their use for women with endometriosis. These include the observation that progestins inhibit the expression of matrix metalloproteinases and plasminogen activator, substances that play a role in tissue invasion and angiogenesis.[78,79] Progestins may also have anti-inflammatory properties that reduce peritoneal fluid leukocyte counts and cytokine production.[80,81]

An unfortunate frequent side-effect of progestins is breakthrough bleeding. As with other medical treatments, pain is often exacerbated when bleeding is present. Moreover, persistent breakthrough bleeding may limit the patient's tolerance for continued progestin use. In general, the incidence of breakthrough bleeding declines over time, but many women with endometriosis-associated pain struggle to hold on for hypo/amenorrhea to arrive. Other potential side-effects with progestins include fluid retention, weight gain, breast tenderness and mood changes.[61,71]

The levonorgestrel releasing intrauterine system (Mirena) is an effective alternative to systemic progestins for women with endometriosis-associated pain.[82] Because progestin levels are concentrated locally within the pelvis, therapeutic efficacy can be maximized while minimizing side-effects. Moreover, because treatment with Mirena requires only one medical intervention every 5 years it may become the treatment of choice for selected women with endometriosis-associated pain. Two pilot studies that investigated Mirena in women with endometriosis-associated pain reported excellent patient satisfaction rates (85–95%) and significant reductions in pain scores.[83,84] Women with endometriosis of the rectovaginal septum also appear to respond well to Mirena.[84] Finally, in a recent multicenter prospective randomized trial involving 82 women, Mirena was highly effective and equivalent to a GnRH agonist in terms of reducing pain scores.[85]

Gonadotropin releasing hormone agonists

After an initial gonadotropin flare, GnRH agonists induce pituitary downregulation and hypoestrogenism, and for this reason have proved very useful in the treatment of endometriosis-associated pain.[86] Two randomized, placebo-controlled, double blind trials have demonstrated the efficacy of GnRH agonists.[87,88] In one study 94% of the women assigned the GnRH agonist were satisfied with the treatment, while 77% of the participants assigned to placebo withdrew because of worsening pain.[87]

Numerous randomized controlled trials have compared the efficacy of GnRH agonists to danazol.[89–101] In every case, GnRH agonists and danazol were equivalent at reducing pain. There does not appear to be any therapeutic advantage of one GnRH agonist over another.[102,103] However, because of the flare effect at the initiation of treatment and the potential for the gonadotropin surge to result in a surge of estrogen and functional ovarian cyst formation, it is generally advisable to initiate GnRH agonists in the luteal phase of the menstrual cycle as opposed to the early follicular phase.

Most side-effects of GnRH agonists are related to hypoestrogenism. The vast majority (80–90%) of women using GnRH agonists alone experience hot flashes.[87,104] GnRH agonists also have adverse effects on bone density and lipid profiles. After a 6-month course of a GnRH agonist the average loss of bone density is 4–6%. Although most women regain any losses in bone density when the treatment is stopped, the use of unopposed GnRH agonists is limited to 6 months unless add-back therapy plus supplemental calcium/vitamin D is used.

Hormonal add-back therapy relies on the hierarchy of end-organ responses to estrogen. The concept is that the threshold level of estrogen required to avoid hot flashes or loss of bone density is lower than the threshold estrogen level required to stimulate ectopic endometrial tissue.[105] Thus, one may add back sufficient amounts of estrogen to alleviate vasomotor symptoms and avert losses in bone density without compromising the efficacy of the GnRH agonist. The simplest add-back regimen proven to mitigate vasomotor symptoms and preserve bone density for up to 1 year of continuous GnRH agonist use is norethindrone acetate (Aygestin) 5 mg per day combined with supplemental calcium and vitamin D.[106,107] Moreover, this regimen, unlike those utilizing conjugated equine estrogens, does not reduce the clinical efficacy of GnRH agonists compared to the use of a GnRH agonist alone.[107–111] In short, the immediate introduction of add-back Aygestin significantly reduces vasomotor symptoms and averts any loss of bone density without compromising pain relief.

Other medical treatments

The antiprogestin mifepristone (RU 486) has been studied in women with endometriosis because it inhibits ovulation and disrupts endometrial integrity. In small, open-label cohort studies, dosages between 50 and 100 mg per day have been shown to induce amenorrhea (without hypoestrogenism) and lower pain scores.[112,113] However, long-term administration of mifepristone leads to mixed proliferative/secretory endometrium and alters glucocorticoid levels. To date, mifepristone has not been widely used for the treatment of endometriosis-associated pain.

Although not available in the United States, gestrinone has been used successfully in Europe to treat women with endometriosis-associated pain. Gestrinone is derived from a 19-nortestosterone steroid nucleus and has both antiestrogen and antiprogesterone effects on the endometrium. Gestrinone bears many similarities to danazol. Like danazol, gestrinone results in endometrial atrophy and amenorrhea.[114] Like danazol, the side-effects of gestrinone include acne, hirsutism, and hot flashes. Several large randomized trials have demonstrated gestrinone (2.5 mg twice a week) to be equivalent in clinical efficacy to danazol[115,116] and GnRH agonists.[117,118]

Aromatase inhibitors may also be helpful for women with endometriosis-associated pain.[119] The enzyme aromatase converts androgens, such as testosterone, to estrogens, such as estradiol. Although normal endometrium does not express aromatase, endometriosis implants do, and thus may convert androgens derived from the blood supply into estrogens. These estrogens promote endometrial proliferation. They may also stimulate prostaglandin E2, which in turn stimulates aromatase activity, creating a positive feedback loop within the endometriotic lesions.[120] Complicating matters, deficient 17β-hydroxysteroid dehydrogenase in endometriosis implants impairs inactivation of estradiol to estrone.[121] Studies in animal models have shown promise, with near total resolution of endometriotic nodules.[122] In humans there have been case reports describing the successful use of aromatase inhibitors to treat endometriosis in postmenopausal woman.[123,124] The only prospective studies published thus far in premenopausal women have combined the aromatase inhibitor with either low dose Aygestin (2.5 mg per day)[125] or a low dose oral contraceptive.[126]

Finally, immune system modulators may provide potential treatment options for women suffering from endometriosis. Among the inflammatory cytokines amplified in women with endometriosis is tumor necrosis factor (TNF)-α. In animals, pentoxifylline (an anti-TNF therapy) has been shown to induce lesion regression.[127,128] A small pilot study in women with endometriosis-associated infertility also suggested benefit.[129] As our understanding of the immunology of endometriosis improves, one anticipates greater interest in the application of immune system modulators to treat women with endometriosis.

Longevity of medical treatments

In general, endometriosis is a chronic disease for reproductive age women. There is a widely held misconception that hormonal suppressive therapies for endometriosis result in the permanent destruction of endometriosis implants. On the contrary, quiescent implants have been demonstrated in nearly all women treated with progestins, danazol, or GnRH agonists. In one prospective study comparing danazol to GnRH agonists, more than 80% of biopsies from previously identified endometriotic lesions demonstrated typical endometrial glands and stroma at second-look laparoscopy.[89] In another study, active endometriotic implants were demonstrated in 80% of women given 6 months of progestin treatment and in almost 70% of women given 6 months of a GnRH agonist.[130] Moreover, once treatment is stopped, both eutopic and ectopic endometrial tissues resume metabolic activity.[89,131] Therefore, hormonal treatment is suppressive therapy, not extirpative therapy, and pain relapse at treatment suspension is the rule rather than the exception.[132]

The length of time to recurrence of pain after cessation of medical therapy is variable. Recurrence rates between 30 and 70% have been reported.[63,64,67,68,87,93,104,133] The mean length of time to symptom recurrence has been reported as between 6 and 18 months.[67,87,93,133,134]

Suggested approach to medical treatment

Typically, continuous low-dose oral contraceptives and NSAIDs are first-line therapy because of their mild side-effects and low cost (Table 7.4). If adequate relief is not obtained one should consider progestins (oral Aygestin 2.5 mg per day or the Mirena intrauterine system) versus a GnRH agonist with immediate add-back Aygestin. Progestins are less expensive and can be used safely for a much longer period of time, but GnRH agonists may provide more rapid relief. If none of these options proves beneficial, or if side-effects are intolerable, then surgery is indicated for analgesic value and to reconfirm the diagnosis.

The role of medical treatment after conservative surgery for endometriosis-associated pain

Several studies have shown that a 3-month postoperative course of danazol or a GnRH agonist does not delay the recurrence of endometriosis-associated pain.[135–138] However, studies have clearly demonstrated that long-term postoperative therapies, e.g. therapies continued for 6 months or more, extend pain relief and reduce the need for future surgery.[62,70,134,139] Given the risks of surgery and the frequency with which endometriosis-associated pain recurs it would seem prudent to administer medical therapy postoperatively, assuming that treatment is well tolerated and there is no immediate desire to become pregnant. One attractive option for certain women is to place a Mirena in the operating room at the end of the laparoscopy if endometriosis has been confirmed.

MEDICAL MANAGEMENT OF ENDOMETRIOSIS-ASSOCIATED INFERTILITY

The relationship between endometriosis and infertility is complex.[140] Although advanced stages of endometriosis often manifest easily recognizable infertility factors, such as tubal distortion/obstruction or

Table 7.4 Recommended approach to the treatment of endometriosis-associated pain

1st line:	Continuous low-dose monophasic oral contraceptive contraceptive with non-steroidal anti-inflammatories
2nd line:	Progestins (oral or intrauterine) vs GnRH agonist with immediate add-back therapy
3rd line:	Repeat surgery, followed by 1st or 2nd line

ovarian compromise, the mechanisms underlying reproductive dysfunction in women with minimal or mild endometriosis are less clear. Some of the difficulties in understanding the true relationship between endometriosis and infertility derive from compromised study designs, poor control groups, and failure to account for the impact of prior surgical treatments, such as cystectomy/oophorectomy, on ovarian reserve.

It was once thought that hormonal suppressive therapies for endometriosis, e.g. progestins or danazol, might have a role in the treatment of endometriosis-associated fertility. The concept was that the suppression of endometriotic lesions would improve the peritoneal environment, and that once these treatments were discontinued, folliculogenesis, fertilization, and implantation would all be enhanced. Unfortunately, numerous prospective studies all reached the same conclusion: hormonal suppressive therapies do not improve spontaneous fecundity rates.[93,95,96,99,100,141-147] For this reason, many pundits believe that the optimal approach to endometriosis-associated infertility is surgical, not medical. Although there are valid reasons for surgery in women with endometriosis-associated infertility, there is more compelling evidence to support the application of standard fertility regimens in these women.

The best study of surgical therapy for women with minimal-to-mild stage endometriosis is the ENDO-CAN (Endometriosis-Canada) trial.[148] This multicenter study randomized 241 infertile women at the time of laparoscopy to no further treatment or surgical excision/ablation of endometriosis implants. Women randomized to surgical intervention had a significantly higher pregnancy rate (30.7%) than controls (17.7%) after 36 weeks of follow-up. The mean monthly fecundity rate was also improved from 2.4 to 4.7%. Unfortunately, the study participants were not blinded to what had been done at the time of surgery, and this may explain the slight difference in cycle fecundity rates between the two groups. Moreover, even if one accepts the results of the trial at face value it is important to consider what cycle fecundity rates might have been achieved in this patient population with other types of treatment.

Three randomized controlled trials have evaluated the benefits of clomiphene citrate or gonadotropins in women with endometriosis.[149-151] Women undergoing superovulation with or without intrauterine insemination achieved monthly fecundity rates of 10–15%. In contrast, the controls in these studies attained monthly fecundity rates of only 2–5%, within range of that reported for both the treatment and control groups of the ENDO-CAN trial. Clearly, the per-cycle chance of pregnancy with superovulation is higher than that achieved with surgical interventions. However, in the same way that the possible benefits of surgery must be balanced by their risks, the improvement in cycle fecundity with fertility medications must be balanced by the risk of multiple pregnancy and ovarian hyperstimulation syndrome.

In vitro fertilization (IVF) offers an even more potent fertility option. In general, IVF is reserved for women with endometriosis who have failed less expensive, more conservative alternatives. In the United States, endometriosis accounts for approximately 15% of all women undergoing IVF treatment.

The impact of endometriosis on IVF outcomes is controversial.[152] A recent meta-analysis suggested that pregnancy rates for women with endometriosis undergoing IVF may be lower than in women undergoing IVF for tubal factor.[153] However, this finding is not supported by data from the Society for Assisted Reproductive Technology (SART). Considering virtually all the IVF cycles done in the United States from 1997 to the latest year of publication there is no clinically significant difference in the per-cycle chance of pregnancy for women undergoing IVF for endometriosis compared to any other major infertility diagnosis, with the exception of diminished ovarian reserve. Moreover, none of the four largest studies comparing IVF outcomes in women with endometriosis to women with tubal disease reported significant differences in per-cycle pregnancy rates.[154-157]

One should not underestimate the potential role of GnRH agonists in women with endometriosis undergoing IVF treatment. Numerous studies have suggested benefits for prolonged downregulation with GnRH agonists in women with endometriosis prior to beginning controlled ovarian hyperstimulation.[158-163] Recently, this benefit was confirmed in a multicenter, prospective randomized trial offering a 3-month course of GnRH agonists prior to commencing controlled ovarian hyperstimulation.[164] Whether this effect is due to better quality oocytes or an enhanced implantation milieu is unclear, but the evidence clearly supports prolonged downregulation prior to commencing an IVF cycle.

CONCLUSION

Abundant evidence supports the use of medical treatments for endometriosis. In women with endometriosis-associated pain, hormonal suppressive regimens that include oral contraceptives, progestins, danazol, and GnRH agonists have all proved to be effective and may be used in place of or as a complement to surgical interventions. In contrast, women with endometriosis-associated infertility clearly benefit from fertility medications, and may be approached with a treatment algorithm that closely resembles that used for women with unexplained infertility.

REFERENCES

1. Eskenazi B, Warner M, Bonsignore L et al. Validation study of nonsurgical diagnosis of endometriosis. Fertil Steril 2001; 76: 929–35.
2. Ballard K, Lowton K, Wright J. What's the delay? A qualitative study of women's experiences of reaching a diagnosis of endometriosis. Fertil Steril 2006; 86: 1296–301.
3. Moen MH, Halvorsen TB. Histologic confirmation of endometriosis in different peritoneal lesions. Acta Obstet Gynecol Scand 1992; 71: 337–42.
4. Nisolle M, Paindaveine B, Bourdon A et al. Histologic study of peritoneal endometriosis in infertile women. Fertil Steril 1990; 53: 984–8.
5. Jansen RP, Russell P. Nonpigmented endometriosis: clinical, laparoscopic, and pathologic definition. Am J Obstet Gynecol 1986; 155: 1154–9.
6. Balasch J, Creus M, Fabregues F et al. Visible and non-visible endometriosis at laparoscopy in fertile and infertile women and in patients with chronic pelvic pain: a prospective study. Hum Reprod 1996; 11: 387–91.
7. Gupta S, Agarwal A, Sekhon L et al. Serum and peritoneal abnormalities in endometriosis: potential use as diagnostic markers. Minerva Ginecol 2006; 58: 527–51.
8. Mol BW, Bayram N, Lijmer JG et al. The performance of CA-125 measurement in the detection of endometriosis: a meta-analysis. Fertil Steril 1998; 70: 1101–8.
9. Barbieri RL, Niloff JM, Bast RC Jr et al. Elevated serum concentrations of CA-125 in patients with advanced endometriosis. Fertil Steril 1986; 45: 630–4.
10. Colacurci N, Fortunato N, De Franciscis P et al. Relevance of CA-125 in the evaluation of endometriosis. Clin Exp Obstet Gynecol 1996; 23: 150–4.
11. Chen FP, Soong YK, Lee N et al. The use of serum CA-125 as a marker for endometriosis in patients with dysmenorrhea for monitoring therapy and for recurrence of endometriosis. Acta Obstet Gynecol Scand 1998; 77: 665–70.
12. Fraser IS, McCarron G, Markham R. Serum CA-125 levels in women with endometriosis. Aust NZ J Obstet Gynaecol 1989; 29: 416–20.
13. Takahashi K, Musa AA, Nagata H et al. Serum CA-125 and 17 beta-estradiol in patients with external endometriosis on danazol. Gynecol Obstet Invest 1990; 29: 301–4.
14. Franssen AM, van der Heijden PF, Thomas CM et al. On the origin and significance of serum CA-125 concentrations in 97 patients with endometriosis before, during, and after buserelin acetate, nafarelin, or danazol. Fertil Steril 1992; 57: 974–9.

15. Umaria N, Olliff JF. Imaging features of pelvic endometriosis. Br J Radiol 2001; 74: 556–62.
16. Dogan MM, Ugur M, Soysal SK et al. Transvaginal sonographic diagnosis of ovarian endometrioma. Int J Gynaecol Obstet 1996; 52: 145–9.
17. Kinkel K, Chapron C, Balleyguier C et al. Magnetic resonance imaging characteristics of deep endometriosis. Hum Reprod 1999; 14: 1080–6.
18. Zawin M, McCarthy S, Scoutt L et al. Endometriosis: appearance and detection at MR imaging. Radiology 1989; 171: 693–6.
19. Arrive L, Hricak H, Martin MC. Pelvic endometriosis: MR imaging. Radiology 1989; 171: 687–92.
20. Ha HK, Lim YT, Kim HS et al. Diagnosis of pelvic endometriosis: fat-suppressed T1-weighted vs conventional MR images. AJR Am J Roentgenol 1994; 163: 127–31.
21. Stratton P, Winkel C, Premkumar A et al. Diagnostic accuracy of laparoscopy, magnetic resonance imaging, and histopathologic examination for the detection of endometriosis. Fertil Steril 2003; 79: 1078–85.
22. Sampson J. Peritoneal endometriosis due to the menstrual dissemination of endometrial tissue into the peritoneal cavity. Am J Obstet Gynecol 1927; 14: 422–69.
23. Kruitwagen RF, Poels LG, Willemsen WN et al. Endometrial epithelial cells in peritoneal fluid during the early follicular phase. Fertil Steril 1991; 55: 297–303.
24. Witz CA, Dechaud H, Montoya-Rodriguez IA et al. An in vitro model to study the pathogenesis of the early endometriosis lesion. Ann NY Acad Sci 2002; 955: 296–307.
25. D'Hooghe TM, Bambra CS, Raeymaekers BM et al. Intrapelvic injection of menstrual endometrium causes endometriosis in baboons (Papio cynocephalus and Papio anubis). Am J Obstet Gynecol 1995; 173: 125–34.
26. Jenkins S, Olive DL, Haney AF. Endometriosis: pathogenetic implications of the anatomic distribution. Obstet Gynecol 1986; 67: 335–8.
27. Ishimura T, Masuzaki H. Peritoneal endometriosis: endometrial tissue implantation as its primary etiologic mechanism. Am J Obstet Gynecol 1991; 165: 210–14.
28. Olive DL, Henderson DY. Endometriosis and mullerian anomalies. Obstet Gynecol 1987; 69: 412–15.
29. Cramer DW, Wilson E, Stillman RJ et al. The relation of endometriosis to menstrual characteristics, smoking, and exercise. JAMA 1986; 255: 1904–8.
30. Darrow SL, Vena JE, Batt RE et al. Menstrual cycle characteristics and the risk of endometriosis. Epidemiology 1993; 4: 135–42.
31. Suginami H. A reappraisal of the coelomic metaplasia theory by reviewing endometriosis occurring in unusual sites and instances. Am J Obstet Gynecol 1991; 165: 214–18.
32. Revised American Society for Reproductive Medicine classification of endometriosis: 1996. Fertil Steril 1997; 67: 817–21.
33. Hornstein MD, Gleason RE, Orav J et al. The reproducibility of the revised American Fertility Society classification of endometriosis. Fertil Steril 1993; 59: 1015–21.
34. Fedele L, Parazzini F, Bianchi S et al. Stage and localization of pelvic endometriosis and pain. Fertil Steril 1990; 53: 155–8.
35. Guzick DS, Silliman NP, Adamson GD et al. Prediction of pregnancy in infertile women based on the American Society for Reproductive Medicine's revised classification of endometriosis. Fertil Steril 1997; 67: 822–9.
36. Szendei G, Hernadi Z, Devenyi N et al. Is there any correlation between stages of endometriosis and severity of chronic pelvic pain? Possibilities of treatment. Gynecol Endocrinol 2005; 21: 93–100.
37. Vercellini P, Fedele L, Aimi G et al. Reproductive performance, pain recurrence and disease relapse after conservative surgical treatment for endometriosis: the predictive value of

the current classification system. Hum Reprod 2006; 21: 2679–85.

38. Vercellini P, Fedele L, Aimi G et al. Association between endometriosis stage, lesion type, patient characteristics and severity of pelvic pain symptoms: a multivariate analysis of over 1000 patients. Hum Reprod 2007; 22: 266–71.

39. Koninckx PR, Meuleman C, Demeyere S et al. Suggestive evidence that pelvic endometriosis is a progressive disease, whereas deeply infiltrating endometriosis is associated with pelvic pain. Fertil Steril 1991; 55: 759–65.

40. Chapron C, Fauconnier A, Dubuisson JB et al. Deep infiltrating endometriosis: relation between severity of dysmenorrhoea and extent of disease. Hum Reprod 2003; 18: 760–6.

41. Sinaii N, Cleary SD, Younes N et al. Treatment utilization for endometriosis symptoms: a cross-sectional survey study of lifetime experience. Fertil Steril 2007; 87: 1277–86.

42. Mahutte NG, Arici A. Medical management of endometriosis-associated pain. Obstet Gynecol Clin North Am 2003; 30: 133–50.

43. Olive DL, Pritts EA. The treatment of endometriosis: a review of the evidence. Ann NY Acad Sci 2002; 955: 360–72; discussion 389–93, 396–406.

44. Child TJ, Tan SL. Endometriosis: aetiology, pathogenesis and treatment. Drugs 2001; 61: 1735–50.

45. Prentice A, Deary AJ, Goldbeck-Wood S et al. Gonadotrophin-releasing hormone analogues for pain associated with endometriosis. Cochrane Database Syst Rev 2000; (2): CD000346.

46. Dawood MY. Dysmenorrhea. J Reprod Med 1985; 30: 154–67.

47. Morrison BW, Daniels SE, Kotey P et al. Rofecoxib, a specific cyclooxygenase-2 inhibitor, in primary dysmenorrhea: a randomized controlled trial. Obstet Gynecol 1999; 94: 504–8.

48. Scott LJ, Lamb HM. Rofecoxib. Drugs 1999; 58: 499–505.

49. Weaver AL. Rofecoxib: clinical pharmacology and clinical experience. Clin Ther 2001; 23: 1323–38.

50. Moore J, Kennedy S, Prentice A. Modern combined oral contraceptives for pain associated with endometriosis. Cochrane Database Syst Rev 2000; (2): CD001019.

51. Vercellini P, Trespidi L, Colombo A et al. A gonadotropin-releasing hormone agonist versus a low-dose oral contraceptive for pelvic pain associated with endometriosis. Fertil Steril 1993; 60: 75–9.

52. Parazzini F, Di Cintio E, Chatenoud L et al. Estroprogestin vs gonadotrophin agonists plus estroprogestin in the treatment of endometriosis-related pelvic pain: a randomized trial. Gruppo Italiano per lo Studio dell'Endometriosi. Eur J Obstet Gynecol Reprod Biol 2000; 88: 11–14.

53. Vercellini P, Frontino G, De Giorgi O et al. Continuous use of an oral contraceptive for endometriosis-associated recurrent dysmenorrhea that does not respond to a cyclic pill regimen. Fertil Steril 2003; 80: 560–3.

54. Selak V, Farquhar C, Prentice A, Singla A. Danazol for pelvic pain associated with endometriosis. Cochrane Database Syst Rev 2001; (4): CD000068.

55. Telimaa S, Apter D, Reinila M et al. Placebo-controlled comparison of hormonal and biochemical effects of danazol and high-dose medroxyprogesterone acetate. Eur J Obstet Gynecol Reprod Biol 1990; 36: 97–105.

56. Luciano AA, Hauser KS, Chapler FK et al. Danazol: endocrine consequences in healthy women. Am J Obstet Gynecol 1981; 141: 723–7.

57. Steingold KA, Lu JK, Judd HL et al. Danazol inhibits steroidogenesis by the human ovary in vivo. Fertil Steril 1986; 45: 649–54.

58. Barbieri RL, Ryan KJ. Danazol: endocrine pharmacology and therapeutic applications. Am J Obstet Gynecol 1981; 141: 453–63.

59. Fedele L, Marchini M, Bianchi S et al. Endometrial patterns during danazol and buserelin therapy for endometriosis: comparative structural and ultrastructural study. Obstet Gynecol 1990; 76: 79–84.

60. Sakata M, Terakawa N, Mizutani T et al. Effects of danazol, gonadotropin-releasing hormone agonist, and a combination of danazol and gonadotropin-releasing hormone agonist on experimental endometriosis. Am J Obstet Gynecol 1990; 163: 1679–84.

61. Telimaa S, Puolakka J, Ronnberg L et al. Placebo-controlled comparison of danazol and high-dose medroxyprogesterone acetate in the treatment of endometriosis. Gynecol Endocrinol 1987; 1: 13–23.

62. Telimaa S, Ronnberg L, Kauppila A. Placebo-controlled comparison of danazol and high-dose medroxyprogesterone acetate in the treatment of endometriosis after conservative surgery. Gynecol Endocrinol 1987; 1: 363–71.

63. Barbieri RL, Evans S, Kistner RW. Danazol in the treatment of endometriosis: analysis of 100 cases with a 4-year follow-up. Fertil Steril 1982; 37: 737–46.

64. Moore EE, Harger JH, Rock JA et al. Management of pelvic endometriosis with low-dose danazol. Fertil Steril 1981; 36: 15–19.

65. Buttram VC Jr, Reiter RC, Ward S. Treatment of endometriosis with danazol: report of a 6-year prospective study. Fertil Steril 1985; 43: 353–60.

66. Selak V, Farquhar C, Prentice A, Singla A. Danazol for pelvic pain associated with endometriosis. Cochrane Database Syst Rev 2000; (2): CD000068.

67. Biberoglu KO, Behrman SJ. Dosage aspects of danazol therapy in endometriosis: short-term and long-term effectiveness. Am J Obstet Gynecol 1981; 139: 645–54.

68. Dmowski WP, Kapetanakis E, Scommegna A. Variable effects of danazol on endometriosis at 4 low-dose levels. Obstet Gynecol 1982; 59: 408–15.

69. Vercellini P, Trespidi L, Panazza S et al. Very low dose danazol for relief of endometriosis-associated pelvic pain: a pilot study. Fertil Steril 1994; 62: 1136–42.

70. Morgante G, Ditto A, La Marca A et al. Low-dose danazol after combined surgical and medical therapy reduces the incidence of pelvic pain in women with moderate and severe endometriosis. Hum Reprod 1999; 14: 2371–4.

71. Vercellini P, Cortesi I, Crosignani PG. Progestins for symptomatic endometriosis: a critical analysis of the evidence. Fertil Steril 1997; 68: 393–401.

72. Luciano AA, Turksoy RN, Carleo J. Evaluation of oral medroxyprogesterone acetate in the treatment of endometriosis. Obstet Gynecol 1988; 72: 323–7.

73. Prentice A, Deary AJ, Bland E. Progestagens and antiprogestagens for pain associated with endometriosis. Cochrane Database Syst Rev 2000; (2): CD002122.

74. Vercellini P, De Giorgi O, Oldani S et al. Depot medroxyprogesterone acetate versus an oral contraceptive combined with very-low-dose danazol for long-term treatment of pelvic pain associated with endometriosis. Am J Obstet Gynecol 1996; 175: 396–401.

75. Schlaff WD, Carson SA, Luciano A et al. Subcutaneous injection of depot medroxyprogesterone acetate compared with leuprolide acetate in the treatment of endometriosis-associated pain. Fertil Steril 2006; 85: 314–25.

76. Muneyyirci-Delale O, Karacan M. Effect of norethindrone acetate in the treatment of symptomatic endometriosis. Int J Fertil Womens Med 1998; 43: 24–7.

77. Vercellini P, Pietropaolo G, De Giorgi O et al. Treatment of symptomatic rectovaginal endometriosis with an estrogen-progestogen combination versus low-dose norethindrone acetate. Fertil Steril 2005; 84: 1375–87.

78. Huang HF, Hong LH, Tan Y et al. Matrix metalloproteinase 2 is associated with changes in steroid hormones in the sera and peritoneal fluid of patients with endometriosis. Fertil Steril 2004; 81: 1235–9.

79. Osteen KG, Bruner-Tran KL, Keller NR et al. Progesterone-mediated endometrial maturation limits matrix metalloproteinase (MMP) expression in an inflammatory-like environment: a regulatory system altered in endometriosis. Ann NY Acad Sci 2002; 955: 37–47; discussion 86–8, 396–406.

80. Haney AF, Weinberg JB. Reduction of the intraperitoneal inflammation associated with endometriosis by treatment with medroxyprogesterone acetate. Am J Obstet Gynecol 1988; 159: 450–4.

81. Zhao D, Lebovic DI, Taylor RN. Long-term progestin treatment inhibits RANTES (regulated on activation, normal T cell expressed and secreted) gene expression in human endometrial stromal cells. J Clin Endocrinol Metab 2002; 87: 2514–19.

82. Vercellini P, Vigano P, Somigliana E. The role of the levonorgestrel-releasing intrauterine device in the management of symptomatic endometriosis. Curr Opin Obstet Gynecol 2005; 17: 359–65.

83. Vercellini P, Aimi G, Panazza S et al. A levonorgestrel-releasing intrauterine system for the treatment of dysmenorrhea associated with endometriosis: a pilot study. Fertil Steril 1999; 72: 505–8.

84. Fedele L, Bianchi S, Zanconato G et al. Use of a levonorgestrel-releasing intrauterine device in the treatment of rectovaginal endometriosis. Fertil Steril 2001; 75: 485–8.

85. Petta CA, Ferriani RA, Abrao MS et al. Randomized clinical trial of a levonorgestrel-releasing intrauterine system and a depot GnRH analogue for the treatment of chronic pelvic pain in women with endometriosis. Hum Reprod 2005; 20: 1993–8.

86. Belchetz PE, Plant TM, Nakai Y et al. Hypophysial responses to continuous and intermittent delivery of hypopthalamic gonadotropin-releasing hormone. Science 1978; 202: 631–3.

87. Dlugi AM, Miller JD, Knittle J. Lupron depot (leuprolide acetate for depot suspension) in the treatment of endometriosis: a randomized, placebo-controlled, double-blind study. Lupron Study Group. Fertil Steril 1990; 54: 419–27.

88. Bergqvist A, Bergh T, Hogstrom L et al. Effects of triptorelin versus placebo on the symptoms of endometriosis. Fertil Steril 1998; 69: 702–8.

89. Bulletti C, Flamigni C, Polli V et al. The efficacy of drugs in the management of endometriosis. J Am Assoc Gynecol Laparosc 1996; 3: 495–501.

90. Cirkel U, Ochs H, Schneider HP. A randomized, comparative trial of triptorelin depot (D-Trp6-LHRH) and danazol in the treatment of endometriosis. Eur J Obstet Gynecol Reprod Biol 1995; 59: 61–9.

91. Adamson GD, Kwei L, Edgren RA. Pain of endometriosis: effects of nafarelin and danazol therapy. Int J Fertil Menopausal Stud 1994; 39: 215–17.

92. Rock JA, Truglia JA, Caplan RJ. Zoladex (goserelin acetate implant) in the treatment of endometriosis: a randomized comparison with danazol. The Zoladex Endometriosis Study Group. Obstet Gynecol 1993; 82: 198–205.

93. Nafarelin for endometriosis: a large-scale, danazol-controlled trial of efficacy and safety, with 1-year follow-up. The Nafarelin European Endometriosis Trial Group (NEET). Fertil Steril 1992; 57: 514–22.

94. Wheeler JM, Knittle JD, Miller JD. Depot leuprolide versus danazol in treatment of women with symptomatic endometriosis. I. Efficacy results. Am J Obstet Gynecol 1992; 167: 1367–71.

95. Shaw RW. An open randomized comparative study of the effect of goserelin depot and danazol in the treatment of endometriosis. Zoladex Endometriosis Study Team. Fertil Steril 1992; 58: 265–72.

96. Fraser IS, Shearman RP, Jansen RP et al. A comparative treatment trial of endometriosis using the gonadotrophin-releasing hormone agonist, nafarelin, and the synthetic steroid, danazol. Aust NZ J Obstet Gynaecol 1991; 31: 158–63.

97. Shaw RW. Nafarelin in the treatment of pelvic pain caused by endometriosis. Am J Obstet Gynecol 1990; 162: 574–6.

98. Trabant H, Widdra W, de Looze S. Efficacy and safety of intranasal buserelin acetate in the treatment of endometriosis: a review of six clinical trials and comparison with danazol. Prog Clin Biol Res 1990; 323: 357–82.

99. Fedele L, Bianchi S, Arcaini L et al. Buserelin versus danazol in the treatment of endometriosis-associated infertility. Am J Obstet Gynecol 1989; 161: 871–6.

100. Henzl MR, Corson SL, Moghissi K et al. Administration of nasal nafarelin as compared with oral danazol for endometriosis. A multicenter double-blind comparative clinical trial. N Engl J Med 1988; 318: 485–9.

101. Cheng MH, Yu BK, Chang SP et al. A randomized, parallel, comparative study of the efficacy and safety of nafarelin versus danazol in the treatment of endometriosis in Taiwan. J Chin Med Assoc 2005; 68: 307–14.

102. Agarwal SK, Hamrang C, Henzl MR et al. Nafarelin vs leuprolide acetate depot for endometriosis. Changes in bone mineral density and vasomotor symptoms. Nafarelin Study Group. J Reprod Med 1997; 42: 413–23.

103. Bergqvist A. A comparative study of the acceptability and effect of goserelin and nafarelin on endometriosis. Gynecol Endocrinol 2000; 14: 425–32.

104. Fedele L, Bianchi S, Bocciolone L et al. Buserelin acetate in the treatment of pelvic pain associated with minimal and mild endometriosis: a controlled study. Fertil Steril 1993; 59: 516–21.

105. Barbieri RL. Hormone treatment of endometriosis: the estrogen threshold hypothesis. Am J Obstet Gynecol 1992; 166: 740–5.

106. Surrey ES, Hornstein MD. Prolonged GnRH agonist and add-back therapy for symptomatic endometriosis: long-term follow-up. Obstet Gynecol 2002; 99: 709–19.

107. Hornstein MD, Surrey ES, Weisberg GW et al. Leuprolide acetate depot and hormonal add-back in endometriosis: a 12-month study. Lupron Add-Back Study Group. Obstet Gynecol 1998; 91: 16–24.

108. Franke HR, van de Weijer PH, Pennings TM et al. Gonadotropin-releasing hormone agonist plus 'add-back' hormone replacement therapy for treatment of endometriosis: a prospective, randomized, placebo-controlled, double-blind trial. Fertil Steril 2000; 74: 534–9.

109. Gregoriou O, Konidaris S, Vitoratos N et al. Gonadotropin-releasing hormone analogue plus hormone replacement therapy for the treatment of endometriosis: a randomized controlled trial. Int J Fertil Womens Med 1997; 42: 406–11.

110. Kiilholma P, Tuimala R, Kivinen S et al. Comparison of the gonadotropin-releasing hormone agonist goserelin acetate alone versus goserelin combined with estrogen-progestogen add-back therapy in the treatment of endometriosis. Fertil Steril 1995; 64: 903–8.

111. Kiesel L, Schweppe KW, Sillem M et al. Should add-back therapy for endometriosis be deferred for optimal results? Br J Obstet Gynaecol 1996; 103: 15–17.

112. Kettel LM, Murphy AA, Morales AJ et al. Treatment of endometriosis with the antiprogesterone mifepristone (RU486). Fertil Steril 1996; 65: 23–8.

113. Kettel LM, Murphy AA, Morales AJ et al. Clinical efficacy of the antiprogesterone RU486 in the treatment of endometriosis and uterine fibroids. Hum Reprod 1994; 9: 116–20.

114. Marchini M, Fedele L, Bianchi S et al. Endometrial patterns during therapy with danazol or gestrinone for endometriosis: structural and ultrastructural study. Hum Pathol 1992; 23: 51–6.

115. Halbe HW, Nakamura MS, Da Silveira GP et al. Updating the clinical experience in endometriosis–the Brazilian perspective. Br J Obstet Gynaecol 1995; 102: 17–21.

116. Bromham DR, Booker MW, Rose GL et al. Updating the clinical experience in endometriosis–the European perspective. Br J Obstet Gynaecol 1995; 102: 12–16.

117. Gestrinone versus a gonadotropin-releasing hormone agonist for the treatment of pelvic pain associated with endometriosis: a multicenter, randomized, double-blind study. Gestrinone Italian Study Group. Fertil Steril 1996; 66: 911–19.

118. Nieto A, Tacuri C, Serra M et al. Long-term follow-up of endometriosis after two different therapies (Gestrinone and Buserelin). Clin Exp Obstet Gynecol 1996; 23: 198–204.

119. Attar E, Bulun SE. Aromatase inhibitors: the next generation of therapeutics for endometriosis? Fertil Steril 2006; 85: 1307–18.

120. Bulun SE, Zeitoun KM, Takayama K et al. Molecular basis for treating endometriosis with aromatase inhibitors. Hum Reprod Update 2000; 6: 413–18.

121. Bulun SE, Zeitoun KM, Takayama K et al. Estrogen biosynthesis in endometriosis: molecular basis and clinical relevance. J Mol Endocrinol 2000; 25: 35–42.

122. Fang Z, Yang S, Gurates B et al. Genetic or enzymatic disruption of aromatase inhibits the growth of ectopic uterine tissue. J Clin Endocrinol Metab 2002; 87: 3460–6.

123. Takayama K, Zeitoun K, Gunby RT et al. Treatment of severe postmenopausal endometriosis with an aromatase inhibitor. Fertil Steril 1998; 69: 709–13.

124. Fatemi HM, Al-Turki HA, Papanikolaou EG et al. Successful treatment of an aggressive recurrent post-menopausal endometriosis with an aromatase inhibitor. Reprod Biomed Online 2005; 11: 455–7.

125. Ailawadi RK, Jobanputra S, Kataria M et al. Treatment of endometriosis and chronic pelvic pain with letrozole and norethindrone acetate: a pilot study. Fertil Steril 2004; 81: 290–6.

126. Amsterdam LL, Gentry W, Jobanputra S et al. Anastrazole and oral contraceptives: a novel treatment for endometriosis. Fertil Steril 2005; 84: 300–4.

127. Steinleitner A, Lambert H, Suarez M et al. Immunomodulation in the treatment of endometriosis-associated subfertility: use of pentoxifylline to reverse the inhibition of fertilization by surgically induced endometriosis in a rodent model. Fertil Steril 1991; 56: 975–9.

128. Nothnick WB, Curry TE, Vernon MW. Immunomodulation of rat endometriotic implant growth and protein production. Am J Reprod Immunol 1994; 31: 151–62.

129. Balasch J, Creus M, Fabregues F et al. Pentoxifylline versus placebo in the treatment of infertility associated with minimal or mild endometriosis: a pilot randomized clinical trial. Hum Reprod 1997; 12: 2046–50.

130. Nisolle-Pochet M, Casanas-Roux F, Donnez J. Histologic study of ovarian endometriosis after hormonal therapy. Fertil Steril 1988; 49: 423–6.

131. Revelli A, Modotti M, Ansaldi C et al. Recurrent endometriosis: a review of biological and clinical aspects. Obstet Gynecol Surv 1995; 50: 747–54.

132. Brosens IA, Verleyen A, Cornillie F. The morphologic effect of short-term medical therapy of endometriosis. Am J Obstet Gynecol 1987; 157: 1215–21.

133. Miller JD, Shaw RW, Casper RF et al. Historical prospective cohort study of the recurrence of pain after discontinuation of treatment with danazol or a gonadotropin-releasing hormone agonist. Fertil Steril 1998; 70: 293–6.

134. Hornstein MD, Hemmings R, Yuzpe AA et al. Use of nafarelin versus placebo after reductive laparoscopic surgery for endometriosis. Fertil Steril 1997; 68: 860–4.

135. Parazzini F, Fedele L, Busacca M et al. Postsurgical medical treatment of advanced endometriosis: results of a randomized clinical trial. Am J Obstet Gynecol 1994; 171: 1205–7.

136. Bianchi S, Busacca M, Agnoli B et al. Effects of 3 month therapy with danazol after laparoscopic surgery for stage III/IV endometriosis: a randomized study. Hum Reprod 1999; 14: 1335–7.

137. Busacca M, Somigliana E, Bianchi S et al. Post-operative GnRH analogue treatment after conservative surgery for symptomatic endometriosis stage III–IV: a randomized controlled trial. Hum Reprod 2001; 16: 2399–402.

138. Loverro G, Carriero C, Rossi AC et al. A randomized study comparing triptorelin or expectant management following conservative laparoscopic surgery for symptomatic stage III–IV endometriosis. Eur J Obstet Gynecol Reprod Biol 2006 Dec 16; [Epub ahead of print].

139. Vercellini P, Crosignani PG, Fadini R et al. A gonadotrophin-releasing hormone agonist compared with expectant management after conservative surgery for symptomatic endometriosis. Br J Obstet Gynaecol 1999; 106: 672–7.

140. Mahutte NG, Arici A. New advances in the understanding of endometriosis related infertility. J Reprod Immunol 2002; 55: 73–83.

141. Noble AD, Letchworth AT. Medical treatment of endometriosis: a comparative trial. Postgrad Med J 1979; 55: 37–9.

142. Fedele L, Bianchi S, Viezzoli T et al. Gestrinone versus danazol in the treatment of endometriosis. Fertil Steril 1989; 51: 781–5.

143. Dmowski WP, Radwanska E, Binor Z et al. Ovarian suppression induced with Buserelin or danazol in the management of endometriosis: a randomized, comparative study. Fertil Steril 1989; 51: 395–400.

144. Thomas EJ, Cooke ID. Successful treatment of asymptomatic endometriosis: does it benefit infertile women? Br Med J 1987; 294: 1117–19.

145. Telimaa S. Danazol and medroxyprogesterone acetate inefficacious in the treatment of infertility in endometriosis. Fertil Steril 1988; 50: 872–5.

146. Bayer SR, Seibel MM, Saffan DS et al. Efficacy of danazol treatment for minimal endometriosis in infertile women. A prospective, randomized study. J Reprod Med 1988; 33: 179–83.

147. Fedele L, Parazzini F, Radici E et al. Buserelin acetate versus expectant management in the treatment of infertility associated with minimal or mild endometriosis: a randomized clinical trial. Am J Obstet Gynecol 1992; 166: 1345–50.

148. Marcoux S, Maheux R, Berube S. Laparoscopic surgery in infertile women with minimal or mild endometriosis. Canadian Collaborative Group on Endometriosis. N Engl J Med 1997; 337: 217–22.

149. Deaton JL, Gibson M, Blackmer KM et al. A randomized, controlled trial of clomiphene citrate and intrauterine insemination in couples with unexplained infertility or surgically corrected endometriosis. Fertil Steril 1990; 54: 1083–8.

150. Fedele L, Bianchi S, Marchini M et al. Superovulation with human menopausal gonadotropins in the treatment of infertility associated with minimal or mild endometriosis: a controlled randomized study. Fertil Steril 1992; 58: 28–31.

151. Tummon IS, Asher LJ, Martin JS et al. Randomized controlled trial of superovulation and insemination for infertility associated with minimal or mild endometriosis. Fertil Steril 1997; 68: 8–12.

152. Mahutte NG, Arici A. Endometriosis and assisted reproductive technologies: are outcomes affected? Curr Opin Obstet Gynecol 2001; 13: 275–9.

153. Barnhart K, Dunsmoor-Su R, Coutifaris C. Effect of endometriosis on in vitro fertilization. Fertil Steril 2002; 77: 1148–55.

154. Olivennes F, Feldberg D, Liu HC et al. Endometriosis: a stage by stage analysis–the role of in vitro fertilization. Fertil Steril 1995; 64: 392–8.

155. Tanbo T, Omland A, Dale PO et al. In vitro fertilization/embryo transfer in unexplained infertility and minimal peritoneal endometriosis. Acta Obstet Gynecol Scand 1995; 74: 539–43.

156. Geber S, Paraschos T, Atkinson G et al. Results of IVF in patients with endometriosis: the severity of the disease does not affect outcome, or the incidence of miscarriage. Hum Reprod 1995; 10: 1507–11.

157. Hull MG, Williams JA, Ray B et al. The contribution of subtle oocyte or sperm dysfunction affecting fertilization in endometriosis-associated or unexplained infertility: a controlled comparison with tubal infertility and use of donor spermatozoa. Hum Reprod 1998; 13: 1825–30.

158. Dicker D, Goldman GA, Ashkenazi J et al. The value of pretreatment with gonadotrophin releasing hormone (GnRH) analogue in IVF-ET therapy of severe endometriosis. Hum Reprod 1990; 5: 418–20.

159. Nakamura K, Oosawa M, Kondou I et al. Menotropin stimulation after prolonged gonadotropin releasing hormone agonist pretreatment for in vitro fertilization in patients with endometriosis. J Assist Reprod Genet 1992; 9: 113–17.

160. Marcus SF, Edwards RG. High rates of pregnancy after long-term down-regulation of women with severe endometriosis. Am J Obstet Gynecol 1994; 171: 812–17.

161. Kim CH, Cho YK, Mok JE. Simplified ultralong protocol of gonadotrophin-releasing hormone agonist for ovulation induction with intrauterine insemination in patients with endometriosis. Hum Reprod 1996; 11: 398–402.

162. Damario MA, Moomjy M, Tortoriello D et al. Delay of gonadotropin stimulation in patients receiving gonadotropin-releasing hormone agonist (GnRH-a) therapy permits increased clinic efficiency and may enhance in vitro fertilization (IVF) pregnancy rates. Fertil Steril 1997; 68: 1004–10.

163. Rickes D, Nickel I, Kropf S et al. Increased pregnancy rates after ultralong postoperative therapy with gonadotropin-releasing hormone analogs in patients with endometriosis. Fertil Steril 2002; 78: 757–62.

164. Surrey ES, Silverberg KM, Surrey MW et al. Effect of prolonged gonadotropin-releasing hormone agonist therapy on the outcome of in vitro fertilization-embryo transfer in patients with endometriosis. Fertil Steril 2002; 78: 699–704.

8 Medical treatment options for leiomyomas

Jason G Bromer and Aydin Arici

INTRODUCTION

Uterine leiomyomas are the most common benign tumors of reproductive age women, affecting between 20 and 50% of these women. Thus, it is not surprising that leiomyomas are among the most commonly encountered clinical entities by gynecologists in practice.[1-5] They increase in prevalence with age, and they are more common in certain ethnic populations. For example, African-American women have a threefold greater frequency of myomas than Caucasian women. Other risk factors for leiomyomas include obesity, early age of menarche, race, and nulliparity, whereas protective factors include smoking and parity.[1,6]

While at least 50% of women with leiomyomas are asymptomatic, uterine myomas are responsible for a large diversity of symptoms. Menstrual abnormalities occur in 30% of women with uterine myomas.[7] Other symptoms include pelvic pain or pressure, menometrorrhagia, dysmenorrhea, urinary retention, bowel dysfunction, and reproductive problems ranging from infertility to preterm labor.[1,2,6,8,9] An estimated 3-5 billion dollars is spent annually in the United States for the diagnosis and management of myomas,[10] making them also an important public health problem. A diagnosis of uterine myomas accounts for 35% of the approximately 600 000 hysterectomies performed yearly in the United States, contributing significantly to the cost associated with this common disorder.[2,11-13] While surgery is indicated in a subgroup of women with uterine myomas (Table 8.1),[2] given the associated cost and morbidity, conservative management has become the preferred first line of treatment for the majority of cases (Table 8.2).

The goal of medical therapy for uterine myomas is symptomatic relief. Hormonal therapies can act both to shrink large myomas and to regulate the menstrual cycle, thus improving symptomatic bleeding. Pressure related symptoms may be alleviated by medical therapies that decrease myoma volume. Medical therapy has the advantages of uterine conservation and an avoidance of surgical complications. A trial of medical therapy before surgical intervention is often reasonable and may be especially useful in women with concomitant issues, such as oligo-ovulation, which may be contributing to abnormal uterine bleeding or infertility.[14]

Table 8.1 Indications for surgical intervention in the management of uterine myomas

Abnormal uterine bleeding not responsive to conservative treatment
Anemia secondary to chronic blood loss
Growth after menopause
High level of suspicion for malignancy
Infertility with distortion of the endometrial cavity
Pain or pressure symptoms interfering with quality of life
Recurrent pregnancy loss with distortion of the endometrial cavity
Urinary tract symptoms

Table 8.2 Currently available conservative therapies for management of symptomatic uterine myomas

Medical	Non-medical
NSAIDs	Image-guided surgical therapy
Estrogen and progestin therapy	Percutaenous laser ablation
Inhibitors of steroid synthesis	Cryomyolysis
GnRH agonists and	MRI-guided ultrasound
antagonists aromatase	Uterine artery embolization
inhibitors	
Steroid receptor modulators	
SERMs	
SPRMs	
Androgen therapy	
danazol	
gestrinone	
Progestin-containing IUD	

It should be noted that one area of myoma symptoms that is not amenable to medical therapy is infertility. Both fibroid size and location are known to influence outcomes for in vitro fertilization and embryo transfer. Specifically, for submucosal myomas or intramural or subserosal myomas with a diameter greater than 4 cm, myomectomy has been shown to have benefit in fertility outcomes (Table 8.3).[15-17] Furthermore, most hormonal regimens available are incompatible with pregnancy or attempting pregnancy.

PATHOGENESIS OF UTERINE MYOMAS

Fibroids are benign tumors composed of smooth muscle cells and an overly abundant extracellular matrix,

Table 8.3 Indications for myomectomy in the setting of infertility

Submucosal or intracavitary component
Intramural fibroid >4 cm
Subserosal fibroid >4 cm that may deform the tubo-ovarian
   relationship
Myoma leading to tubal obstruction

Table 8.4 Hormonally responsive growth factors implicated in myoma pathogenesis

Growth factor	Affect of steroid hormone	Action on leiomyoma
TGF-β3	Induced by estrogen	Induces formation of ECM products, and inhibits their degradation
EGF	Induced by progesterone	Implicated in myoma growth
Bcl-2	Induced by progesterone	Inhibits apoptosis
TNF-α	Suppressed by progesterone	Induces apoptosis
IGF-I	Suppressed by progesterone	Promotes mitotic activity, upregulates Bcl-2 expression

with increased amounts of fibronectin, elastin, and type I and type III collagen. The pathophysiology of uterine myomas is not very well understood; however, it has been established that fibroids are monoclonal tumors, which appear to be the result of at least two distinct events: (1) the transformation of a normal myocyte to an abnormal one, and (2) clonal expansion of the myocyte leading to tumor growth.[18]

Myomas are hormonally responsive, specifically to estrogen and progesterone. Estrogen and progesterone receptors are present within uterine myomas in higher concentrations than in the surrounding myometrium.[19] Furthermore, aromatase activity is found in uterine myomas in higher concentration than in the surrounding myometrium, suggesting that leiomyoma smooth muscle cells synthesize estrogen in situ.[20] Supporting the theory that endocrine factors play an important role in their pathogenesis, myomas do not typically occur prior to the onset of puberty; they tend to grow during periods of increasing hormone levels such as pregnancy, and regress after menopause.[21] However, pregnancy and oral contraceptive use are also claimed to be protective against the development of uterine myomas, suggesting that additional non-hormonal factors must also play a role in myoma growth and development.[3]

While the initiating factors in the development of fibroids are unknown, there is a large body of evidence showing that estrogen and progesterone are necessary, but not sufficient, for leiomyoma growth.[19,21–24] Furthermore, the effects of these ovarian sex steroids are likely mediated through the local production and action of growth factors originating in the extracellular matrix (ECM)[25–28] (Table 8.4). For instance, one growth factor that is known both to be estrogen responsive and overexpressed in leiomyomas is transforming growth factor β3 (TGF-β3).[28–32] Progesterone acts to regulate local factors on uterine myomas as well, by upregulating the expression of epidermal growth factor and Bcl-2, and downregulating tumor necrosis factor α (TNF-α) and insulin like growth factor I (IGF-I) expression.[28,33]

As it is clearly evident that myoma growth is regulated by complex biochemical interactions, and that steroid hormones have a significant impact on these processes, almost all current medical therapies for myomas involve attempting to manipulate the hormonal milieu of the myoma in order to achieve symptomatic relief. This chapter will cover the available medical therapies for symptomatic relief of uterine myomas (Table 8.2). Likely future management options which act to take advantage of the local environment of growth factors will also be discussed.

NON-STEROIDAL ANTI-INFLAMMATORY DRUGS

Non-steroidal anti-inflammatory drugs (NSAIDs), while useful in the management of other types of menorrhagia, have not been extensively studied in the management of uterine myomas. In one trial, ibuprofen at a daily dose of 1200 mg reduced median blood loss by approximately 25% in primary menorrhagia but had no effect on blood loss in women with uterine fibroids.[34] A second study showed a similar (35.7%) decrease in blood loss in women with primary menorrhagia with the use of 500–1000 mg of naproxen daily, but no consistent effect on menorrhagia secondary to myomas.[35] Therefore, although they may be useful in the management of myoma associated pain, the current literature does not support the use of NSAIDs alone for the management of myoma related menorrhagia.

ESTROGEN AND PROGESTIN THERAPY

The first-line treatment option for uterine myomas is frequently progestin-only or combined estrogen and progestin therapy, due to their high tolerability, low cost, and their usefulness in patients with other concomitant gynecologic problems.[14] They likely act by managing the abnormal uterine bleeding caused by myomas by producing endometrial stabilization and, eventually, atrophy. However, estrogen and progestin therapy has not been shown to reduce the size of uterine myomas;[36] thus, it will have limited efficacy in treating mechanical or anatomical symptoms of large myomas (e.g. urinary retention).

Few studies have addressed the effects of oral estrogens or progestins alone on myoma symptoms. Instead, most studies have explored the efficacy of these medications when combined with gonadotropin releasing hormone (GnRH) agonists.[1,37,38] Furthermore, given that estrogens and progestins are known to act as stimulants for myoma growth, treatment of myomas with oral contraceptives or progestin-only therapy must be addressed with caution.[1,39] Nonetheless, Friedman and Thomas[40] addressed the question of whether treatment with low-dose oral contraceptives could affect uterine size or menstrual flow in premenopausal women with symptomatic uterine fibroids. The study was nonrandomized, with women electing to either take a low dose, monophasic oral contraceptive or go without therapy. They noted that after 12 months, the women who had taken the oral contraceptive had significantly increased hematocrits, decreased duration of menstrual flow, and no change in uterine size as assessed by ultrasound and bimanual examination. Despite the lack of randomization, this study suggests that there may be a role for oral contraceptive therapy in the management of symptomatic myoma-related bleeding.

There is conflicting evidence regarding the effects of progestins on uterine myomas. Some authors have reported a decrease in myoma size with progestin therapy,[41,42] whereas other studies using progestins in conjunction with GnRH agonists have shown a significant increase in myoma sizes.[37,43,44] Nonetheless, a positive effect has been noted in at least one study of progestin-only hormone therapy. Venkatachalam et al[7] administered depot medroxyprogesterone acetate 150 mg/month for 6 months to 20 women. They reported that 30% of the women became amenorrheic, 70% had improvement in their bleeding, and 15% had increased hemoglobin levels. They also reported a mean decrease in uterine and myoma volumes. This study is compelling as it again suggests that an inexpensive, well-tolerated medication may provide significant relief from symptomatic myomas.

Lastly, there is some evidence to support that combined estrogen/progestin or progestin-only therapy may have benefit in the prevention of uterine fibroids.

This protective benefit has been shown for combined oral contraceptive pills (OCPs) as well as for depot progestin-only injectable therapy,[45,46] but only if the use of therapy was initiated after the age of 16.[14]

INHIBITORS OF OVARIAN STEROID HORMONE SYNTHESIS

Gonadotropin releasing hormone agonists

GnRH agonists are the most widely recognized, most often used, and most successful management option for the treatment of uterine myomas. While many different formulations are available, the general premise in the creation of a GnRH agonist involves two key structural modifications at the 6th and 10th amino acid locations of the GnRH molecule (Table 8.5). These changes result in a more stable compound with a much higher receptor affinity than the native molecule.[47] GnRH agonists act both by directly binding to and by downregulating GnRH receptors in the pituitary, thus causing a profound decrease in the production of follicle stimulating hormone (FSH) and luteinizing hormone (LH). These decreases, in turn, lead to a drastic decrease in ovarian steroidogenesis and, thus, the production of a hypoestrogenic environment. Another mechanism by which GnRH agonists act is through suppression of aromatase within the leiomyoma, which decreases endogenous estrogen production.[48]

It should be noted that there is a transient (usually 1 week or less) 'flare-up' phase at the beginning of GnRH agonist therapy.[6] While this period is typically not noticeable clinically, patients with concomitant diagnoses such as endometriosis may notice a transient worsening of symptoms at the beginning of this therapy.

GnRH agonists and antagonists are available in a wide variety of formulations. They can be delivered nasally or subcutaneously in rapid fashion; however, the most common formulation for management of uterine myomas is the long acting depot injection, which is typically administered intramuscularly. These forms are typically administered monthly for a period of 3–6 months. Longer treatment times than these regimens are associated with profound side-effects secondary to hypoestrogenism; therefore, their usage is typically limited to the perioperative time period in the premenopausal patient or in the perimenopause.[1,2,9] Along these lines, the United States Food and Drug Administration has approved use of leuprolide acetate (the most commonly used GnRH agonist in

Table 8.5   GnRH agonists and antagonists and their amino acid substitutions

	pGlu	His	Trp	Ser	Tyr	Gly	Leu	Arg	Pro	Gly-NH$_2$
GnRH agonist										
Buserelin						D-Ser				NH-Eth
Deslorelin						D-Trp				NH-Eth
Goserelin						D-Ser				Aza-Gly
Histrelin						D-His				NH-Eth
Leuprolide						D-Leu				NH-Eth
Nafarelin						D-Nap				
Tryptorelin						D-Trp				
GnRH antagonist										
Abarelix	D-Ala	D-Phe	D-Ala			D-Asp		Lys(iPr)		D-Ala
Cetrorelix	D-Nal	D-Phe	D-Pal			D-Cit				D-Ala
Ganirelix	D-Nal	D-Phe	D-Pal			D-hArg		hArg		D-Ala

D-Nap, D-naphthylalanine; NH-Eth, NH-ethylamide

the United States) for the preoperative time period in women with myomas, but not for solitary medical management.[14]

Treatment with GnRH agonists leads to amenorrhea in most women, and, within 3 months of initiating treatment, a significant reduction of uterine volume. With this shrinkage, many of the symptoms of uterine myomas are alleviated as well. Stewart recently reviewed a series of studies looking at changes in myoma volume after beginning leuprolide acetate GnRH agonist therapy.[14] These studies showed an initial decrease in volume of 51–100%. Other clinical trials have shown an initial reduction in volume of 35–65% after the first 3 months of treatment.[49–52] However, the final change in volume at the maximal time of therapy recorded in all trials varied from 0 to 95%. This significant variation in response is likely due to the heterogeneous nature of individual myomas.[53] All studies of GnRH agonists have shown a rapid return to menses and pretreatment myoma volume after discontinuation of treatment.

The limiting factor in the use of GnRH agonist therapy is the significant side-effects encountered secondary to hypoestrogenism. These effects can vary from bothersome (headaches, insomnia, hot flashes, vaginal dryness) to serious medical comorbidities (depression, bone mineral loss, osteoporosis).[1,2,9,14,21,54] Bone loss is the most clinically relevant longer-term toxicity of these medications; a bone loss of about 3% occurs after 3 months of treatment.[6] These side-effects can be largely ameliorated by the administration of 'add-back' therapy using estrogen, a progestin, or a combination; however, this addition can lead to a decrease in efficacy in reducing myoma volume[37,43,44] This is especially true for progestin-only add-back therapy, which can completely abolish the clinical efficacy of GnRH agonists at reducing uterine volume. Friedman et al compared GnRH agonist with or without the addition of medroxyprogesterone acetate for 24 weeks in a randomized double blinded trial. While both groups showed statistically significant increases in serum hematocrits and serum iron levels after 24 weeks of therapy, only the patients without the added progestin showed a significant reduction in uterine volume.[38]

The addition of low doses of estrogen alone or combination low dose estrogen and progestin may, however, be sufficient to prevent the hypoestrogenic side-effects of GnRH agonists while maintaining amenorrhea and without stimulating the growth of myomas.[55] Friedman et al demonstrated that estrogen induced proliferative effects on uterine myomas only when plasma concentrations exceeded 50 pg/ml.[56] This finding is also supported by another study by Friedman et al, which showed greater reduction in pretreatment uterine volume (75% on initial volume) after 1 year of GnRH agonist with estrogen and progestin add-back than with progestin-only add-back (92% of initial volume).[43]

Overall, existing data support the use of GnRH agonists for reduction of myoma volume and improvement of bleeding, and they should be considered a first-line treatment therapy for preoperative or perimenopausal women with symptomatic myomas and anemia.

Gonadotropin releasing hormone antagonists

GnRH antagonists have also been used to treat uterine myomas, often prior to surgery.[1] Unlike GnRH agonists, the antagonists differ significantly in structure from the endogenous molecule (Table 8.5), and they bind the GnRH receptor with nine times the affinity.[57] Their onset of action is immediate, causing a decrease in concentrations of FSH and LH within hours of administration. Maximum reduction in endogenous steroid hormone production is seen within 14 days, which is a shorter time than with GnRH agonists. In addition, there is no 'flare-up' initial response as with GnRH agonists. Therefore, GnRH antagonists may be a preferable agent when a shorter duration of both treatment and hypoestrogenic side-effects is preferred.[6]

Several recent studies have also looked at the clinical efficacy of GnRH antagonists on symptomatic uterine myomas.[58–60] Two trials have evaluated the use of cetrorelix in premenopausal women who were candidates for hysterectomy or myomectomy. Gonzalez-Barcena et al showed a reduction of uterine volume to 56% of pretreatment volume after 3 months of daily administration.[60] Similarly, Felberbaum et al used a depot form of cetrorelix and showed a 33% reduction in largest myoma volume after 6 or 8 weeks of treatment.[59] A more recent clinical trial examined the other available formulation of GnRH antagonist, ganirelix. Using magnetic resonance imaging (MRI) and ultrasound to compare myoma volume, Flierman et al showed a 25–40% regression in myoma volume after a mean of 19 days of therapy.[58] In all of these studies, side-effects were similar to those seen with GnRH agonists, and these effects resolved after discontinuation of therapy.

Overall, while they have been less extensively studied for myoma therapy than the agonists, GnRH antagonists are likely to also be clinically useful. While they may provide a faster onset of action and more rapid effect on myoma volume, there is no additional benefit conferred by choosing an antagonist over an agonist.

Aromatase inhibitors

Aromatase inhibitors are a class of compounds which bind to the heme-containing enzyme aromatase-P450, which is responsible for the conversion of androgens to estrogens. While two classes of aromatase inhibitors have been developed,[61] only the type II non-steroidal triazoles such as anastrozole and letrozole have been studied in myoma management. When used, aromatase inhibitors directly inhibit estrogen synthesis, leading to a rapid state of hypoestrogenism.[62,63] As uterine myomas are known to directly overexpress aromatase,[62,63] aromatase inhibitors pose a compelling possibility for myoma management.

There have only been two reports of the usage of aromatase inhibitors in the treatment of uterine myomas. In one case, a 53-year-old woman who was suffering from urinary retention secondary to a uterine leiomyoma was treated with fadrozole. Her urinary retention resolved after 2 weeks of treatment, and the myoma volume decreased by 71% after 8 weeks of treatment.[63] A second case report involved a 93-year-old woman who had been using tamoxifen therapy for 5 years as a treatment for breast cancer. She presented acutely with a 24-week pregnancy size myomatous uterus and urinary symptoms. Treatment with anastrozole led to a reduction to an 18-week pregnancy size after 5 weeks of treatment, and a 12–14-week pregnancy size after 9 weeks of treatment, with complete resolution of her symptoms.[64]

While there have been no large scale clinical trials performed with aromatase inhibitors for the management of uterine myomas, these case reports are compelling. Furthermore, the rapid onset of hypoestrogenism makes them a promising therapeutic option. Lastly, the fact that aromatase is specifically overexpressed in leiomyomas relative to the ovaries could provide a key therapeutic benefit. Specifically, it may be possible to formulate a concentration of aromatase inhibitor that could have a suppressive effect on leiomyomas without significantly affecting ovarian hormone production.[62]

STEROID RECEPTOR MODULATORS

Selective estrogen receptor modulators

Selective estrogen receptor modulators (SERMs) are a relatively new class of non-steroidal medications that were developed for and shown to be efficacious in the treatment of estrogen responsive breast cancers. They act by directly binding to the estrogen receptor; however, they show tissue specific responses, acting as agonists in some tissues and antagonists in others.[65] The two major SERMs that have been studied for uterine myoma therapy are tamoxifen and raloxifene.

Tamoxifen is a SERM that acts as an antagonist in the breast, therefore acting as a potent antiestrogen in the treatment of breast cancer. However, it has agonist action in bone, cardiovascular tissue, and the endometrium.[65] Thus, the gynecologist must be wary of the increased risks for endometrial hyperplasia and cancer in patients using this medication. Only one prospective study has investigated the use of tamoxifen in the treatment of uterine fibroids. Sadan et al[66] reported on a group of 20 women of reproductive age complaining of abdominal pain and bleeding secondary to uterine fibroids. Ten women received daily tamoxifen and 10 received placebo for a period of 6 months. The patients were then reinterviewed after 5 years. While there was no reported decrease in uterine size, the patients using tamoxifen did report a subjective decrease of bleeding by 40–50% while the placebo group reported a slight increase over the same time period. Hemoglobin levels remained unchanged in both groups. The patients taking tamoxifen also reported a substantial decrease in pain by 4 months of therapy. However, the tamoxifen group had a significant amount of side-effects with therapy, including ovarian cyst formation in 70%, hot flashes and dizziness in 80%, and endometrial thickening (without evidence of neoplasia). The authors concluded that treatment of uterine myomas with tamoxifen added only marginal benefit while causing unacceptable side-effects, and its use for myoma management should be discouraged.

Raloxifene is a newer SERM that has been more widely studied in the management of leiomyomas. Unlike tamoxifen, raloxifene has no agonist effect on the endometrium. Palomba et al[67] first studied raloxifene in the management of fibroids in postmenopausal women. These women were treated for 12 months with 60 mg/day of raloxifene or placebo. Uterine and myoma size were evaluated by ultrasound at entry and every 3 months. They showed a statistically significant decrease in both uterine and myoma size at 6, 9, and 12 months of therapy, but no change in bleeding profiles in the women.

The same group also looked at the effects of raloxifene on uterine and myoma size in premenopausal women. They compared raloxifene at 60 or 180 mg/day and placebo. After 12 months of therapy, there was no change in uterine size, myoma size, or bleeding in any of the groups. The authors concluded that raloxifene had no significant effect on uterine and leiomyoma size or on menstrual bleeding in premenopausal women.[68] However, a different group of authors compared 3 months of treatment with raloxifene 180 mg/day versus no treatment.[69] They found that raloxifene was very well tolerated and resulted in a decrease in myoma size. Furthermore, while there was progression of uterine myomas in the control group, raloxifene appeared to inhibit myoma growth in the treatment group.

Palomba et al have also explored the effects of combining raloxifene with a GnRH agonist, in a study of 100 women randomized to receive either leuprolide acetate depot plus raloxifene 60 mg/day or leuprolide plus placebo tablet for 6 months.[70] A significant decrease in uterine, leiomyoma, and non-leiomyoma sizes was detected in both groups after 6 months compared to baseline; however, only leiomyoma sizes were decreased in the patients taking raloxifene compared to placebo at the end of the study. There was also no difference in myoma related symptoms between the two groups. More important, they also showed that treatment could be extended to 18 months with stable myoma sizes, without any reduction in bone mineral density.[71] An additional study also showed that while treatment of women with GnRH agonist caused alterations in serum lipoprotein levels, homocysteine levels, and increased insulin resistance, these metabolic changes could be prevented or reduced by coincident treatment with raloxifene.[72]

While the data on the use of raloxifene alone for the management of myomas may be conflicting, it appears that it may be a useful as an adjunct to GnRH agonist treatment. Its benefits may be twofold: increasing the efficacy of the GnRH agonist, while at the same time providing a protective effect against the side-effects of the GnRH agonist.

Selective progesterone receptor modulators

Although estrogen has been classically described as the key steroidogenic hormone in myoma growth and development, there is increasing belief that progesterone also plays a crucial role in these processes. Furthermore, progesterone receptors have been found in higher concentrations in uterine myomas than in surrounding myometrium.[19] Therefore, a novel treatment strategy for leiomyomas has involved the use of molecules that modulate activity at the progesterone receptor. In addition to synthetic progestins, the class of compounds known to be progesterone receptor modulators includes progesterone antagonists and selective progesterone receptor modulators (SPRMs). Collectively, these compounds show a wide spectrum of activity at the reproductive tissues (Table 8.6).

SPRMs represent a new class of progesterone receptor ligands that effect partial agonist and antagonist activities in vivo. They demonstrate a high degree of receptor and tissue selectivity, with a high binding affinity for the progesterone receptor. At the same time, they demonstrate only moderate affinity for the glucocorticoid receptor, low affinity for the androgen receptor, and no binding affinity for the estrogen or mineralocorticoid receptors.[73] SPRMs have specific application to gynecology, as they appear to target the endometrium directly and produce amenorrhea, without much effect on ovulation, and without any

Table 8.6 Spectrum of activity for different progesterone receptor modulators used in the treatment of uterine fibroids

	Progestins	Selective progesterone receptor modulators	Progesterone antagonists
Ovary			
ovulation	↓	↓ or ↔	↓
estrogen	↓	↔	↔
progesterone	↓	↓ or ↔	↓
Endometrium			
bleeding	Breakthrough	Amenorrhea	Amenorrhea
Leiomyoma			
size	↑ / ↓	↓	↓
Examples	Medroxyprogesterone acetate, norethindrone, combined OCP	Asoprisnil (J 867) CDB-2914 Org 33628	Mifepristone (RU 486)

↓=suppressed or inhibited; ↑=promoted or enhanced; ↔=no change
OCP, oral contraceptive pill

significant breakthrough bleeding. Furthermore, treatment with these compounds is not associated with hypoestrogenism and bone loss.[21,74]

Asoprisnil is the first SPRM to reach an advanced stage of clinical development to be studied for the treatment of symptomatic uterine myomas.[75] There has been one large phase II trial completed with asoprisnil.[76] In this double blinded, placebo-controlled study of women with symptomatic fibroids, asoprisnil was used in three dosages (5, 10, or 25 mg/day) for 12 weeks. Asoprisnil was shown to suppress both the duration and intensity of bleeding in a dose-dependent fashion, without any breakthrough bleeding. Hemoglobin concentrations were significantly increased compared with placebo. With the highest dosage, there was an 80% amenorrhea rate. The two higher dosages were also successful at shrinking myoma size, as shown by ultrasound measurement of the largest uterine fibroid in each patient.

Recent in vitro studies have attempted to address the mechanism of action of asoprisnil on uterine fibroids. Chen et al recently showed that treatment of in vitro cultured leiomyoma cells with asoprisnil both inhibited proliferation as shown by the proliferating cell nuclear antigen (PCNA)-positive rate, and induced apoptosis, as shown by the terminal deoxynucleotide transferase-mediated dUTP nick-end labeling (TUNEL)-positive rate.[77] Wang et al have also shown recently that asoprisnil inhibits the expression of epidermal growth factor (EGF), IGF-I, TGF-β3 and their receptors in cultured leiomyoma cells.[78] Most interesting, in both of these studies, the effects were limited to the cultured leiomyoma cells, and there were no significant effects on matched normal myometrial cells. These results provide more compelling evidence that

SPRMs may have true selective efficacy in the management of uterine myomas and that additional large scale trials are warranted.

Antiprogestins, such as mifepristone (RU 486), are another subset of progesterone receptor modulators with an essentially pure antagonist action.[79] The mechanism of action was recently shown to be by reducing the number of progesterone receptors found in uterine fibroids.[80] This direct antiprogestin effect is believed to result in suppression of myomas as well as impacting their vascular supply. In addition, amenorrhea results as acyclicity is achieved, with maintenance of a hormonal state consistent with the early follicular phase.[79–81] Interestingly, there does appear to be a mild hypoestrogenic state induced by mifepristone, suggesting that it may also act as non-competitive antagonist at the estrogen receptor. Nonetheless, there does not appear to be any significant effect on bone density with mifepristone use, in doses up to 50 mg/day.[6]

Steinaur et al recently performed a systematic review of six small clinical trials involving the treatment of symptomatic fibroids with mifepristone. The studies involved a total of 166 women receiving between 5 and 50 mg/day of mifepristone for a total of 3–6 months. While none of the trials were blinded or placebo-controlled, the results were compelling. The trials showed reductions in leiomyoma volumes ranging from 26 to 74%. Mifepristone treatment also reduced dysmenorrhea, menorrhagia, and pelvic pressure. Amenorrhea rates ranged from 63 to 100%. Toxicities were limited and involved hot flashes in 38%, and transient elevations in transaminases in 4%. Endometrial hyperplasia was detected in 28% of women who were biopsied.[79]

Mifepristone may prove to be a useful treatment modality for symptomatic myomas, but the risk of endometrial hyperplasia may limit its efficacy. Nonetheless, a recent study was undertaken to assess the long-term effects of lower dose therapy mifepristone on myoma regression, symptoms, and endometrial pathology. This study followed 40 women with symptomatic myomas who received mifepristone at doses of 5 or 10 mg/day for 1 year. These doses resulted in similar reductions of myoma volume and amenorrhea rates to those in previous studies. Endometrial hyperplasia was identified in 13.9% of the women at 6 months but only in 4.8% at 12 months. All cases of hyperplasia occurred in the 10-mg group and all cases were simple hyperplasia without atypia. The authors concluded that low-dose mifepristone was effective in management of symptomatic myomas and resulted in modest rates of low-grade endometrial hyperplasia, without evidence of malignant potential.[82]

ANDROGEN THERAPY

With the advent of newer therapies such as GnRH agonists, androgen therapy is now rarely employed in the management of symptomatic myomas. Its use is discussed here for historical purposes and perspective.

Danazol

Danazol is a synthetic steroid derivative of 19-nortestosterone. It has antigonadotropic properties, including amenorrhea, blockage of ovarian steroid production, and blockage of gonadotropin release from the pituitary.[83] It also appears to have a significant suppressive effect on sex hormone binding globulin.[6] Therefore, the effects of danazol work through decreased GnRH, FSH, and LH release from the pituitary, changes in the growth of ovarian follicles, and direct suppression of growth on the endometrium. These effects are mainly androgenic, but danazol also has lesser progestogenic, antiprogestogenic, and anti-estrogenic activity.[83]

Danazol has been studied in the treatment of uterine fibroids. De Leo et al treated 20 women with symptomatic fibroids with danazol 400 mg/day for 4 months.[83] These women had an average 23.6% reduction in fibroid volume at the end of therapy. All women in the study reported improvement or complete relief of symptoms while taking the therapy. Six months after completing treatment, there was some increase in fibroid volume, but not to the pretreatment volumes. A second study by the same group of

researchers used danazol at 100 mg/day for 6 months. They showed similar effects on myoma volume after 6 months of therapy (37.6%), but in addition they showed a significant increase in uterine artery pulsatility index, suggestive of increased resistance to flow.[84] These results suggest that the impact of danazol on uterine fibroids may be related to vascular effects as well as hormonal ones. Lastly, a third study evaluated the use of danazol 100 mg/day for 6 months following 3 months of GnRH agonist administration.[85] The women who received danazol had a 30% reduced rebound uterine volume after discontinuation of GnRH agonist compared to controls. Furthermore, bone mineral density, which had decreased during GnRH administration, improved significantly with danazol administration.

Severe androgenic side-effects are the limiting factors in danazol therapy. These include weight gain, edema, decreased breast size, acne, oily skin, hirsutism, voice deepening, headache, hot flashes, changes in libido, and muscle cramps. One or more of these side-effects occur in more than 75% of patients using danazol,[6] and may lead to discontinuation of therapy.

Gestrinone

Gestrinone is a trienic steroid, and it is a synthetic derivative of ethinyl nortestosterone. It has antiestrogenic and antiprogestogenic properties.[6] Like danazol, it has been shown to decrease myoma volume and to improve myoma related bleeding. In two studies by Coutinho et al, gestrinone was given either orally or vaginally, at doses of 2.5 or 5 mg 2–3 times/week, for 4–24 months.[86–89] The dose and regimen were tailored to fibroid size. Amenorrhea resulted in 95% of patients. Abdominal pain, dyspareunia, and dysuria were progressively alleviated during treatment. Uterine volume was reduced in all patients, with an average reduction of 40–50%. More important, 89% of women who were treated for 6 months maintained a uterine volume smaller than pretreatment volume for 18 months.[89] There were no adverse effects on bone mineral density. Most patients experienced side-effects associated with androgenicity. These included weight gain, seborrhea, acne, nervousness, myalgias, and arthralgias. Hirsutism, hoarseness, and increase in libido were less common, and all side-effects were reversible upon discontinuation of treatment.

As gestrinone has a similar side-effect profile to danazol, it has no additional advantage when compared to danazol. It is not currently available in the United States.

PROGESTIN-CONTAINING INTRAUTERINE DEVICES

Progestin-containing intrauterine devices (IUDs) have been extensively evaluated for the treatment of menorrhagia. They have been shown to decrease blood loss and relieve dysmenorrhea,[90] and have been shown to be equally effective in the treatment of menorrhagia as endometrial ablation.[91] Therefore, these devices have been long considered a safe, reversible form of management for menorrhagia. The mechanism of action is believed to be through the induction of endometrial decidualization and glandular atrophy.[92–94]

Despite these successes, there have been no randomized studies evaluating use of the two commercially available progestin-containing IUDs for treatment of menorrhagia related to uterine leiomyoma. Large or distorted uterine cavities or the presence of submucosal fibroids are contraindications to these devices, so their use may be limited in the management of symptomatic myomas.[14] Nonetheless, several small case series and non-randomized trials have been reported, which have shown significant reductions in menorrhagia as well as a decrease in myoma size.[95,96] In the largest study to date, Grigorieva et al followed prospectively 67 women with myomatous uteri who had chosen the levonorgestrel-containing IUD for contraception. They showed significant reductions in menstrual blood flow as well as increased hemoglobin and ferritin levels over 1 year of use.[97] A second observational study by Mercorio et al followed 19 patients with recurrent menorrhagia and uterine fibroids who were treated for 12 months with a levonorgestrel-containing IUD. The women were followed subjectively using a pictorial blood loss assessment chart score (PBAC). The median score before treatment was 310, and the PBAC score gradually decreased from 186 at 3 months to a value of 155, 108, and 96 at 6, 9, and 12 months of treatment, respectively. Despite the statistically significant change in PBAC score, persistent menorrhagia, defined as a monthly PBAC score of 100 or higher, was observed at 12 months in nearly 75% of the patients, with only one woman becoming amenorrheic. They concluded that the levonorgestrel-containing IUD showed reduced clinical effectiveness in the treatment of myoma-related menorrhagia.[98] Most recently, Soysal et al compared a series of women with menorrhagia and at least one uterine myoma using the levonorgestrel-containing IUD to historical controls who had undergone thermal balloon endometrial ablation. Throughout the 12-month study, they found statistically significant decreases in menstrual blood flow and increases in hemoglobin values. Furthermore, the IUD was found to be as effective as thermal balloon ablation.[99]

Inki et al studied the levonorgestrel-containing IUD in the treatment of menorrhagia versus hysterectomy. They noted that an IUD was associated with the development of asymptomatic ovarian cysts. While IUD use decreased endometrial thickness, it did not affect the size of the uterus or the size of uterine fibroids.[100] These data, which conflict with some of the previous studies, was suggested to be possibly due to a dual action of progestin on uterine fibroids. As discussed earlier, progesterone acts by upregulating the expression of EGF and Bcl-2, and downregulating TNF-α and IGF-I expression, suggesting that the local growth factor environment may determine the ultimate effects of progestins.[33] The conflicting results with the use of progestin-containing IUDs may suggest that certain patients are better candidates for such therapy than others. Further studies are warranted for this type of therapy.

POTENTIAL FUTURE THERAPIES

No medication currently available has been approved for the long-term management of myomas, and it is still unclear how long-term medical therapy may impact on future fertility. Furthermore, with medical therapy, complete regression of the myoma is not realized, and thus definitive treatment is not achieved. For these reasons, surgery remains the treatment standard of care for large symptomatic myomas in patients who desire future fertility.[1]

As we look to the future on strategies for medical management for leiomyomas, one important area will be optimizing the current therapies available for long-term use and minimization of toxicity. GnRH agonists are currently considered the gold standard therapy; however, they have significant side-effects. Studies are needed not only to compare GnRH agonists with the other newer, effective therapies discussed in this chapter, but also to evaluate the utility of these medications as add-back therapy. The data on raloxifene to date are promising, and more long-term, prospective studies are warranted.

Another important area to consider as we look to the future is the explosion of research into the molecular pathophysiology of uterine fibroids. Most current medical therapies for myomas involve attempts to manipulate steroid hormones. While these therapies are effective on the myomas, they also affect other steroid-responsive tissues, causing toxicities and unwanted side-effects such as mastalgia, bone loss, and menopausal symptoms.[101] By trying to more selectively target the localized growth factors responsible for myoma growth and development, a less toxic therapy might be developed.

Somatostatin analogs

One potential group of medications that has received some attention has been the somatostatin analogs. These medications are believed to have an antiproliferative effect on target tissues by inhibiting growth factors and decreasing IGF-I and -II production.[10] Over 40 years ago, it was demonstrated that estrogen and growth hormone (GH) acted synergistically to increase uterine size in adult rats.[102] More recently, it was demonstrated that patients who have acromegaly (a disorder characterized by high levels of GH and IGF) have a prevalence of 81% for uterine myomas.[103] Furthermore, recent studies have shown that IGF-I and -II mRNA are present in uterine tissue, and that estrogen stimulation increases their expression. In addition, fibroids contain more binding sites for IGF-I than do normal myometrial tissues.[104,105]

De Leo et al recently studied the administration of the somatostatin analog lanreotide in fertile women with symptomatic fibroids. Using a depot formulation of lanreotide, the mean reduction in total uterine volume was 24% and the mean reduction in myoma volume was 41.6%.[106] These data suggest that the GH–IGF system may play an important role in the growth and development of uterine fibroids, and that somatostatin analogs may be an important future treatment option.

A role for antifibrotic agents

Another important area for consideration in the search for agents of leiomyoma inhibition is in the molecular pathways for fibrosis. Fibroids express increased amounts of extracellular matrix, and, as discussed earlier, TGF-β3 has been convincingly demonstrated to be overexpressed in uterine myomas.[28-32] Other members of the TGF-β signaling family, including its receptor TGF-β RII, have also been recently suggested to be overexpressed in fibroids,[107] indicating that the entire TGF-β signaling pathway emanating from the ECM may be overexpressed in fibroids. As TGF-β is known to affect the transcription of genes encoding collagen chains, Leppert et al recently examined the expression of collagen genes in uterine fibroids. Consistent with the activation of

TGF-β signaling in leiomyoma cells, they noted that many genes encoding collagen chains showed increased expression.[108] The group further examined the ultrastructural organization of ECM in fibroids and noted that, unlike the ECM of myometrium, collagen fibrils were randomly oriented in fibroids. Noting that fibroids seem to have many similarities to keloids both in molecular expression and in molecular arrangement, they hypothesized that fibroid formation may be more due to an abnormal healing process than an oncogenic one. Finally, they suggested that if fibroid formation more closely resembled a disorder of healing than of oncogenesis, one could envision management strategies that interfere with collagen formation.[108]

Pirfenidone is an antifibrotic agent that has been investigated in patients with pulmonary fibrosis. It has been shown to produce antifibrotic effects and to inhibit fibroblast proliferation in vitro.[6] In studies of bleomycin-induced pulmonary fibrosis in the rat lung, it has been shown to inhibit the production of TGF-β and collagen.[108-110] Lee et al demonstrated that pirfenidone inhibited leiomyoma proliferation and collagen production in cultured leiomyoma cells in vitro.[110] There has also been one small pilot study of eight women who received pirfenidone 400 mg/kg twice daily for 3 months. In this study, the authors reported ultrasound-determined reductions in fibroid volume from 32 to 56%.[108]

CONCLUSIONS

It is clear that there is a wide range of hormonal treatment options for the medical management of uterine myomas. Real reductions in both myoma size and symptoms can be achieved in short periods of time without the associated morbidities of surgery. However, the use of these therapies must be weighed against the possible toxicities and long-term effects on the patient, as well as the patient's reproductive goals. Newer non-hormonal medical options may prove to be exciting additions to the current arsenal of medical therapies, and as the molecular pathophysiology of uterine fibroids is further explored, even more medical options for therapy may be discovered.

REFERENCES

1. Rackow BW, Arici A. Options for medical treatment of myomas. Obstet Gynecol Clin North Am 2006; 33: 97–113.
2. Wallach EE, Vlahos NF. Uterine myomas: an overview of development, clinical features, and management. Obstet Gynecol 2004; 104: 393–406.
3. Stewart EA. Uterine fibroids. Lancet 2001; 357: 293–8.

4. Manyonda I, Sinthamoney E, Belli AM. Controversies and challenges in the modern management of uterine fibroids. BJOG 2004; 111: 95–102.

5. Vollenhoven BJ, Lawrence AS, Healy DL. Uterine fibroids: a clinical review. Br J Obstet Gynaecol 1990; 97: 285–98.

6. De Leo V, Morgante G, La Marca A et al. A benefit-risk assessment of medical treatment for uterine leiomyomas. Drug Saf 2002; 25: 759–79.

7. Venkatachalam S, Bagratee JS, Moodley J. Medical management of uterine fibroids with medroxyprogesterone acetate (Depo Provera): a pilot study. J Obstet Gynaecol 2004; 24: 798–800.

8. Practice Committee of the American Society for Reproductive Medicine. Myomas and reproductive function. Fertil Steril 2004; 82 (Suppl 1): S111–16.

9. Olive DL, Lindheim SR, Pritts EA. Non-surgical management of leiomyoma: impact on fertility. Curr Opin Obstet Gynecol 2004; 16: 239–43.

10. Brahma PK, Martel KM, Christman GM. Future directions in myoma research. Obstet Gynecol Clin North Am 2006; 33: 199–224, xiii.

11. Calson K, Nichols D, Schiff I. Indications for hysterectomy. N Engl J Med 1993; 328: 856–60.

12. Cramer SF, Patel A. The frequency of uterine leiomyomas. Am J Clin Pathol 1990; 94: 435–8.

13. Wilcox LS, Koonin LM, Pokras R et al. Hysterectomy in the United States, 1988–1990. Obstet Gynecol 1994; 83: 549–55.

14. Treatment of uterine leiomyomas. 2005. Accessed at http://www.uptodate.com.

15. Rackow BW, Arici A. Fibroids and in-vitro fertilization: which comes first? Curr Opin Obstet Gynecol 2005; 17: 225–31.

16. Pritts EA. Fibroids and infertility: a systematic review of the evidence. Obstet Gynecol Surv 2001; 56: 483–91.

17. Oliveira FG, Abdelmassih VG, Diamond MP et al. Impact of subserosal and intramural uterine fibroids that do not distort the endometrial cavity on the outcome of in vitro fertilization-intracytoplasmic sperm injection. Fertil Steril 2004; 81: 582–7.

18. Epidemiology, pathogenesis, diagnosis, and natural history of uterine leiomyomas. 2006. Accessed at http://www.uptodate.com.

19. Nisolle M, Gillerot S, Casanas-Roux F et al. Immunohistochemical study of the proliferation index, oestrogen receptors and progesterone receptors A and B in leiomyomata and normal myometrium during the menstrual cycle and under gonadotrophin-releasing hormone agonist therapy. Hum Reprod 1999; 14: 2844–50.

20. Folkerd EJ, Newton CJ, Davidson K, Anderson MC, James VH. Aromatase activity in uterine leiomyomata. J Steroid Biochem 1984; 20: 1195–200.

21. Chwalisz K, DeManno D, Garg R et al. Therapeutic potential for the selective progesterone receptor modulator asoprisnil in the treatment of leiomyomata. Semin Reprod Med 2004; 22: 113–19.

22. Flake GP, Andersen J, Dixon D. Etiology and pathogenesis of uterine leiomyomas: a review. Environ Health Perspect 2003; 111: 1037–54.

23. Kawaguchi K, Fujii S, Konishi I et al. Mitotic activity in uterine leiomyomas during the menstrual cycle. Am J Obstet Gynecol 1989; 160: 637–41.

24. Rein MS, Barbieri RL, Friedman AJ. Progesterone: a critical role in the pathogenesis of uterine myomas. Am J Obstet Gynecol 1995; 172: 14–18.

25. Barbarisi A, Petillo O, Di Lieto A et al. 17-beta estradiol elicits an autocrine leiomyoma cell proliferation: evidence for a stimulation of protein kinase-dependent pathway. J Cell Physiol 2001; 186: 414–24.

26. Lippman ME, Dickson RB, Kasid A et al. Autocrine and paracrine growth regulation of human breast cancer. J Steroid Biochem 1986; 24: 147–54.

27. Sozen I, Arici A. Interactions of cytokines, growth factors, and the extracellular matrix in the cellular biology of uterine leiomyomata. Fertil Steril 2002; 78: 1–12.

28. Sozen I, Arici A. Cellular biology of myomas: interaction of sex steroids with cytokines and growth factors. Obstet Gynecol Clin North Am 2006; 33: 41–58.

29. Arici A, Sozen I. Transforming growth factor-beta3 is expressed at high levels in leiomyoma where it stimulates fibronectin expression and cell proliferation. Fertil Steril 2000; 73: 1006–11.

30. Lee BS, Nowak RA. Human leiomyoma smooth muscle cells show increased expression of transforming growth factor-beta 3 (TGF beta 3) and altered responses to the antiproliferative effects of TGF beta. J Clin Endocrinol Metab 2001; 86: 913–20.

31. Catherino WH, Prupas C, Tsibris JC et al. Strategy for elucidating differentially expressed genes in leiomyomata identified by microarray technology. Fertil Steril 2003; 80: 282–90.

32. Tsibris JC, Segars J, Coppola D et al. Insights from gene arrays on the development and growth regulation of uterine leiomyomata. Fertil Steril 2002; 78: 114–21.

33. Maruo T, Matsuo H, Shimomura Y et al. Effects of progesterone on growth factor expression in human uterine leiomyoma. Steroids 2003; 68: 817–24.

34. Makarainen L, Ylikorkala O. Primary and myoma-associated menorrhagia: role of prostaglandins and effects of ibuprofen. Br J Obstet Gynaecol 1986; 93: 974–8.

35. Ylikorkala O, Pekonen F. Naproxen reduces idiopathic but not fibromyoma-induced menorrhagia. Obstet Gynecol 1986; 68: 10–12.

36. Stewart EA, Nowak RA. Leiomyoma-related bleeding: a classic hypothesis updated for the molecular era. Hum Reprod Update 1996; 2: 295–306.

37. Carr BR, Marshburn PB, Weatherall PT et al. An evaluation of the effect of gonadotropin-releasing hormone analogs and medroxyprogesterone acetate on uterine leiomyomata volume by magnetic resonance imaging: a prospective, randomized, double blind, placebo-controlled, crossover trial. J Clin Endocrinol Metab 1993; 76: 1217–23.

38. Friedman AJ, Barbieri RL, Doubilet PM, Fine C, Schiff I. A randomized, double-blind trial of a gonadotropin releasing-hormone agonist (leuprolide) with or without medroxyprogesterone acetate in the treatment of leiomyomata uteri. Fertil Steril 1988; 49: 404–9.

39. Harrison-Woolrych M, Robinson R. Fibroid growth in response to high-dose progestogen. Fertil Steril 1995; 64: 191–2.

40. Friedman AJ, Thomas PP. Does low-dose combination oral contraceptive use affect uterine size or menstrual flow in premenopausal women with leiomyomas? Obstet Gynecol 1995; 85: 631–5.

41. Vikhliaeva EM. [Conservative treatment of patients with uterine myoma]. Akush Ginekol (Mosk) 1987; 11: 63–7. [in Russian]

42. Tiltman AJ. The effect of progestins on the mitotic activity of uterine fibromyomas. Int J Gynecol Pathol 1985; 4: 89–96.

43. Friedman AJ, Daly M, Juneau-Norcross M et al. A prospective, randomized trial of gonadotropin-releasing hormone agonist plus estrogen-progestin or progestin 'add-back' regimens for women with leiomyomata uteri. J Clin Endocrinol Metab 1993; 76: 1439–45.

44. Friedman AJ, Daly M, Juneau-Norcross M et al. Long-term medical therapy for leiomyomata uteri: a prospective, randomized study of leuprolide acetate depot plus either oestrogen-progestin or progestin 'add-back' for 2 years. Hum Reprod 1994; 9: 1618–25.

45. Lumbiganon P, Rugpao S, Phandhu-fung S et al. Protective effect of depot-medroxyprogesterone acetate on surgically

treated uterine leiomyomas: a multicentre case – control study. Br J Obstet Gynaecol 1996; 103: 909–14.

46. Wise LA, Palmer JR, Harlow BL et al. Reproductive factors, hormonal contraception, and risk of uterine leiomyomata in African-American women: a prospective study. Am J Epidemiol 2004; 159: 113–23.

47. Nestor JJ Jr, Ho TL, Simpson RA et al. Synthesis and biological activity of some very hydrophobic superagonist analogues of luteinizing hormone-releasing hormone. J Med Chem 1982; 25: 795–801.

48. Shozu M, Sumitani H, Segawa T et al. Inhibition of in situ expression of aromatase P450 in leiomyoma of the uterus by leuprorelin acetate. J Clin Endocrinol Metab 2001; 86: 5405–11.

49. Coddington CC, Collins RL, Shawker TH et al. Long-acting gonadotropin hormone-releasing hormone analog used to treat uteri. Fertil Steril 1986; 45: 624–9.

50. Lumsden MA, West CP, Baird DT. Goserelin therapy before surgery for uterine fibroids. Lancet 1987; 1: 36–7.

51. Matta WH, Shaw RW, Nye M. Long-term follow-up of patients with uterine fibroids after treatment with the LHRH agonist buserelin. Br J Obstet Gynaecol 1989; 96: 200–6.

52. Maheux R, Samson Y, Farid NR, Parent JG, Jean C. Utilization of luteinizing hormone-releasing hormone agonist in pulmonary leiomyomatosis. Fertil Steril 1987; 48: 315–17.

53. Nowak RA. Fibroids: pathophysiology and current medical treatment. Baillieres Best Pract Res Clin Obstet Gynaecol 1999; 13: 223–38.

54. Maheux R, Lemay A, Blanchet P, Friede J, Pratt X. Maintained reduction of uterine leiomyoma following addition of hormonal replacement therapy to a monthly luteinizing hormone-releasing hormone agonist implant: a pilot study. Hum Reprod 1991; 6: 500–5.

55. Thomas EJ. Add-back therapy for long-term use in dysfunctional uterine bleeding and uterine fibroids. Br J Obstet Gynaecol 1996; 103 (Suppl 14): 18–21.

56. Friedman AJ, Lobel SM, Rein MS, Barbieri RL. Efficacy and safety considerations in women with uterine leiomyomas treated with gonadotropin-releasing hormone agonists: the estrogen threshold hypothesis. Am J Obstet Gynecol 1990; 163: 1114–19.

57. Rabinovici J, Rothman P, Monroe SE, Nerenberg C, Jaffe RB. Endocrine effects and pharmacokinetic characteristics of a potent new gonadotropin-releasing hormone antagonist (Ganirelix) with minimal histamine-releasing properties: studies in postmenopausal women. J Clin Endocrinol Metab 1992; 75: 1220–5.

58. Flierman PA, Oberye JJ, van der Hulst VP, de Blok S. Rapid reduction of leiomyoma volume during treatment with the GnRH antagonist ganirelix. BJOG 2005; 112: 638–42.

59. Felberbaum RE, Germer U, Ludwig M et al. Treatment of uterine fibroids with a slow-release formulation of the gonadotrophin releasing hormone antagonist Cetrorelix. Hum Reprod 1998; 13: 1660–8.

60. Gonzalez-Barcena D, Alvarez RB, Ochoa EP et al. Treatment of uterine leiomyomas with luteinizing hormone-releasing hormone antagonist Cetrorelix. Hum Reprod 1997; 12: 2028–35.

61. Miller WR. Aromatase inhibitors: mechanism of action and role in the treatment of breast cancer. Semin Oncol 2003; 30 (Suppl 14): 3–11.

62. Shozu M, Murakami K, Inoue M. Aromatase and leiomyoma of the uterus. Semin Reprod Med 2004; 22: 51–60.

63. Shozu M, Murakami K, Segawa T, Kasai T, Inoue M. Successful treatment of a symptomatic uterine leiomyoma in a perimenopausal woman with a nonsteroidal aromatase inhibitor. Fertil Steril 2003; 79: 628–31.

64. Attilakos G, Fox R. Regression of tamoxifen-stimulated massive uterine fibroid after conversion to anastrozole. J Obstet Gynaecol 2005; 25: 609–10.

65. Cook JD, Walker CL. Treatment strategies for uterine leiomyoma: the role of hormonal modulation. Semin Reprod Med 2004; 22: 105–11.

66. Sadan O, Ginath S, Sofer D et al. The role of tamoxifen in the treatment of symptomatic uterine leiomyomata – a pilot study. Eur J Obstet Gynecol Reprod Biol 2001; 96: 183–6.

67. Palomba S, Sammartino A, Di Carlo C et al. Effects of raloxifene treatment on uterine leiomyomas in postmenopausal women. Fertil Steril 2001; 76: 38–43.

68. Palomba S, Orio F Jr, Morelli M et al. Raloxifene administration in premenopausal women with uterine leiomyomas: a pilot study. J Clin Endocrinol Metab 2002; 87: 3603–8.

69. Jirecek S, Lee A, Pavo I et al. Raloxifene prevents the growth of uterine leiomyomas in premenopausal women. Fertil Steril 2004; 81: 132–6.

70. Palomba S, Russo T, Orio F Jr et al. Effectiveness of combined GnRH analogue plus raloxifene administration in the treatment of uterine leiomyomas: a prospective, randomized, single-blind, placebo-controlled clinical trial. Hum Reprod 2002; 17: 3213–19.

71. Palomba S, Orio F Jr, Russo T et al. Long-term effectiveness and safety of GnRH agonist plus raloxifene administration in women with uterine leiomyomas. Hum Reprod 2004; 19: 1308–14.

72. Palomba S, Russo T, Orio F Jr et al. Lipid, glucose and homocysteine metabolism in women treated with a GnRH agonist with or without raloxifene. Hum Reprod 2004; 19: 415–21.

73. DeManno D, Elger W, Garg R et al. Asoprisnil (J867): a selective progesterone receptor modulator for gynecological therapy. Steroids 2003; 68: 1019–32.

74. Chabbert-Buffet N, Meduri G, Bouchard P, Spitz IM. Selective progesterone receptor modulators and progesterone antagonists: mechanisms of action and clinical applications. Hum Reprod Update 2005; 11: 293–307.

75. Chwalisz K, Perez MC, Demanno D et al. Selective progesterone receptor modulator development and use in the treatment of leiomyomata and endometriosis. Endocr Rev 2005; 26: 423–38.

76. Chwalisz K, Parker L, Williamson S. Treatment of uterine leiomyomas with the novel selective progesterone receptor modulator [SPRM] [Abstract]. J Soc Gynecol Investig 2003; 10: 301a.

77. Chen W, Ohara N, Wang J et al. A novel selective progesterone receptor modulator asoprisnil (J867) inhibits proliferation and induces apoptosis in cultured human uterine leiomyoma cells in the absence of comparable effects on myometrial cells. J Clin Endocrinol Metab 2006; 91: 1296–304.

78. Wang J, Ohara N, Wang Z et al. A novel selective progesterone receptor modulator asoprisnil (J867) down-regulates the expression of EGF, IGF-I, TGFbeta3 and their receptors in cultured uterine leiomyoma cells. Hum Reprod 2006; 21: 1869–77.

79. Steinauer J, Pritts EA, Jackson R, Jacoby AF. Systematic review of mifepristone for the treatment of uterine leiomyomata. Obstet Gynecol 2004; 103: 1331–6.

80. Murphy AA, Kettel LM, Morales AJ, Roberts VJ, Yen SS. Regression of uterine leiomyomata in response to the antiprogesterone RU 486. J Clin Endocrinol Metab 1993; 76: 513–17.

81. Murphy AA, Morales AJ, Kettel LM, Yen SS. Regression of uterine leiomyomata to the antiprogesterone RU486: dose-response effect. Fertil Steril 1995; 64: 187–90.

82. Eisinger SH, Bonfiglio T, Fiscella K, Meldrum S, Guzick DS. Twelve-month safety and efficacy of low-dose mifepristone for uterine myomas. J Minim Invasive Gynecol 2005; 12: 227–33.

83. De Leo V, la Marca A, Morgante G. Short-term treatment of uterine fibromyomas with danazol. Gynecol Obstet Invest 1999; 47: 258–62.

84. La Marca A, Musacchio MC, Morgante G, Petraglia F, De Leo V. Hemodynamic effect of danazol therapy in women with uterine leiomyomata. Fertil Steril 2003; 79: 1240–2.

85. De Leo V, Morgante G, Lanzetta D, D'Antona D, Bertieri RS. Danazol administration after gonadotrophin-releasing hormone analogue reduces rebound of uterine myomas. Hum Reprod 1997; 12: 357–60.

86. Coutinho EM. Treatment of large fibroids with high doses of gestrinone. Gynecol Obstet Invest 1990; 30: 44–7.

87. Coutinho EM, Boulanger GA, Goncalves MT. Regression of uterine leiomyomas after treatment with gestrinone, an antiestrogen, antiprogesterone. Am J Obstet Gynecol 1986; 155: 761–7.

88. Coutinho EM. Gestrinone in the treatment of myomas. Acta Obstet Gynecol Scand Suppl 1989; 150: 39–46.

89. Coutinho EM, Goncalves MT. Long-term treatment of leiomyomas with gestrinone. Fertil Steril 1989; 51: 939–46.

90. Sivin I, Stern J. Health during prolonged use of levonorgestrel 20 micrograms/d and the copper TCu 380Ag intrauterine contraceptive devices: a multicenter study. International Committee for Contraception Research (ICCR). Fertil Steril 1994; 61: 70–7.

91. Crosignani PG, Vercellini P, Mosconi P et al. Levonorgestrel-releasing intrauterine device versus hysteroscopic endometrial resection in the treatment of dysfunctional uterine bleeding. Obstet Gynecol 1997; 90: 257–63.

92. Stewart A, Cummins C, Gold L, Jordan R, Phillips W. The effectiveness of the levonorgestrel-releasing intrauterine system in menorrhagia: a systematic review. BJOG 2001; 108: 74–86.

93. Scommegna A, Pandya GN, Christ M, Lee AW, Cohen MR. Intrauterine administration of progesterone by a slow releasing device. Fertil Steril 1970; 21: 201–10.

94. Hurskainen R, Paavonen J. Levonorgestrel-releasing intrauterine system in the treatment of heavy menstrual bleeding. Curr Opin Obstet Gynecol 2004; 16: 487–90.

95. Starczewski A, Iwanicki M. [Intrauterine therapy with levonorgestrel releasing IUD of women with hypermenorrhea secondary to uterine fibroids]. Ginekol Pol 2000; 71: 1221–5. [in Polish]

96. Fong YF, Singh K. Effect of the levonorgestrel-releasing intrauterine system on uterine myomas in a renal transplant patient. Contraception 1999; 60: 51–3.

97. Grigorieva V, Chen-Mok M, Tarasova M, Mikhailov A. Use of a levonorgestrel-releasing intrauterine system to treat bleeding related to uterine leiomyomas. Fertil Steril 2003; 79: 1194–8.

98. Mercorio F, De Simone R, Di Spiezio Sardo A et al. The effect of a levonorgestrel-releasing intrauterine device in the treatment of myoma-related menorrhagia. Contraception 2003; 67: 277–80.

99. Soysal S, Soysal ME. The efficacy of levonorgestrel-releasing intrauterine device in selected cases of myoma-related menorrhagia: a prospective controlled trial. Gynecol Obstet Invest 2005; 59: 29–35.

100. Inki P, Hurskainen R, Palo P et al. Comparison of ovarian cyst formation in women using the levonorgestrel-releasing intrauterine system vs. hysterectomy. Ultrasound Obstet Gynecol 2002; 20: 381–5.

101. Stewart EA, Nowak RA. New concepts in the treatment of uterine leiomyomas. Obstet Gynecol 1998; 92: 624–7.

102. Grattarola R, Li CH. Effect of growth hormone and its combination with estradiol-17 beta on the uterus of hypophysectomized and hypophysectomized-ovariectomized rats. Endocrinology 1959; 65: 802–10.

103. Cohen O, Schindel B, Homburg R. Uterine leiomyomata–a feature of acromegaly. Hum Reprod 1998; 13: 1945–6.

104. Boehm KD, Daimon M, Gorodeski IG et al. Expression of the insulin-like and platelet-derived growth factor genes in human uterine tissues. Mol Reprod Dev 1990; 27: 93–101.

105. Hoppener JW, Mosselman S, Roholl PJ et al. Expression of insulin-like growth factor-I and -II genes in human smooth muscle tumours. EMBO J 1988; 7: 1379–85.

106. De Leo V, la Marca A, Morgante G, Severi FM, Petraglia F. Administration of somatostatin analogue reduces uterine and myoma volume in women with uterine leiomyomata. Fertil Steril 2001; 75: 632–3.

107. Bromer JG, Parker CY, Mayers CM, Segars JH, Catherino WH. TGF-beta receptor II is overexpressed in human leiomyomata [Abstract]. J Soc Gynecol Investig 2005; 12 (2): 93A.

108. Leppert PC, Catherino WH, Segars JH. A new hypothesis about the origin of uterine fibroids based on gene expression profiling with microarrays. Am J Obstet Gynecol 2006; 195: 415–20.

109. Young SL, Al-Hendy A, Copland JA. Potential nonhormonal therapeutics for medical treatment of leiomyomas. Semin Reprod Med 2004; 22: 121–30.

110. Lee BS, Margolin SB, Nowak RA. Pirfenidone: a novel pharmacological agent that inhibits leiomyoma cell proliferation and collagen production. J Clin Endocrinol Metab 1998; 83: 219–23.

9 Uterine artery embolization: a minimally invasive approach for symptomatic uterine myomas

Paul B Marshburn, Michelle L Matthews, Rebecca S Usadi, and Bradley S Hurst

Uterine artery embolization (UAE) has been successfully utilized for refractory postpartum hemorrhage, bleeding after gynecologic surgery or pelvic trauma, and the treatment of pelvic arteriovenous malformation.[1,2] These initial uses of UAE were performed under emergent conditions, and offered life-saving therapy when patients could not await or withstand surgery. The desire for minimally invasive alternatives for the management of symptomatic uterine myomas prompted Ravina et al to propose UAE as an alternative to surgical treatment of uterine fibroids in 1995.[3] The demand for UAE subsequently accelerated following other reports that symptoms of uterine bleeding and pelvic discomfort were improved without the need for surgery.[4-9] The growing public demand for UAE in treating symptomatic uterine fibroids promoted use of this technique before clinical trials confirmed the relative safety, effectiveness, and indications for UAE compared with conventional surgical and medical options.

Results from clinical series indicate that UAE will help problematic pelvic symptoms and excessive bleeding from uterine leiomyomas. These observational reports, however, provide little comparative data to suggest the long-term advantages of UAE over conventional surgical options. Current randomized controlled trials of UAE versus surgery for symptomatic uterine myomas are producing critical information to help clinicians counsel patients on the risks and benefits of these options. Collaborative efforts between gynecologists and interventional radiologists are necessary to provide guidelines for selecting UAE or alternative therapies for patients to optimize safety and efficacy while minimizing cost and morbidity.

TECHNICAL OVERVIEW OF UTERINE ARTERY EMBOLIZATION

The gynecologist must partner with the interventional radiologist to establish optimal clinical guidelines for patient care. The preoperative consultation, diagnostic testing, and post-procedural follow-up are typically performed by the gynecologist. The patient should have consultations with both the referring gynecologist and the interventional radiologist for informed consent, documentation of necessary pre-procedural diagnostic testing, and to confirm the timing of the UAE procedure.

Selective occlusion of the arterial supply to myomas exclusively cannot be accomplished with UAE. Rather, the technical goal of UAE is to deliver particulate material into both uterine arteries to produce ischemic regression of myomas without causing permanent damage to other uterine tissues.[10,11] Typically, polyvinyl alcohol (PVA) particles, PVA microspheres, or gelatin-coated tris-acryl polymer microspheres are the most common embolic agents used for UAE. Investigators have examined the type, size, shape, and amount of the embolic particles that would limit normal myometrial damage while maintaining clinical efficacy. Ultimately, a comparative randomized trial failed to find any significant difference in outcome or complications between embolization with PVA microspheres and tris-acryl gelatin microspheres.[12]

After intravenous analgesia or epidural anesthesia, a single femoral artery is typically catheterized and pelvic arteriography performed to define the vascular tree (Figures 9.1 and 9.2). A bilateral femoral approach is more cumbersome, but preferred at some centers to reduce radiation exposure and procedural time. When both uterine arteries have been identified using subtraction angiography, arteriography is performed to confirm that no vascular anomalies are present. Initially, complete occlusion of both uterine arteries was the goal of UAE. Recent data with PVA or gelatin-coated tris-acryl polymer microspheres suggest that incomplete embolization of both arteries may produce effective infarction of myomas with less severe pain.[14] Technical difficulties in cannulating the uterine arteries may occur as a result of anatomical variation, arterial spasm, or prior use of gonadotropin releasing hormone analogs. Procedural failure or complications may occur due to uterine perfusion from collateral ovarian vasculature.[15] A more detailed technical

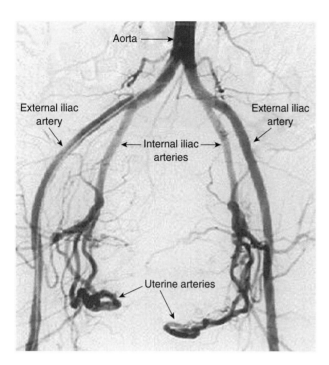

Figure 9.1 Digital subtraction flush pelvic arteriogram. A 5-French flush catheter is placed from a right common femoral approach through the right external iliac artery and positioned with the sideholes just above the aortic bifurcation. Normal pelvic vasculature with hypertrophy of the uterine arteries is seen. Reproduced with permission from reference 13

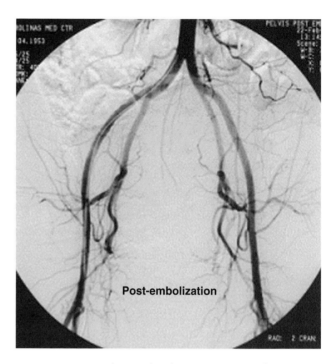

Figure 9.2 Unsubtracted pelvic arteriogram after uterine artery embolization. Reproduced with permission from reference 13

description of the UAE procedure has been summarized previously.[13]

The procedure requires approximately 1 hour to perform, and radiation exposure is comparable to that received during one or two barium enemas. Uterine cramping may be severe, but is usually reduced by non-steroidal anti-inflammatory drugs. Most patients are admitted overnight for pain control, and patient controlled analgesia provides satisfactory and timely analgesia for ischemic pain. In some circumstances, however, hospitalization may be extended for 2–4 days to provide parenteral narcotics when pain is severe or protracted.

Quality improvement guidelines and credentialing standards have recently been published to ensure safe technical practices, identify the elements of appropriate patient selection, anticipate expected outcomes, and recognize complications in a timely manner following UAE.[16]

PATIENT EVALUATION AND SELECTION FOR UTERINE ARTERY EMBOLIZATION

The counseling of patients prior to UAE or alternative treatments is based upon determination of the patient's goal of therapy, medical status, and desire for future reproduction. The referring gynecologist must know the indications and contraindications to UAE and have access to an experienced interventional radiology staff with knowledge of their center's outcomes data and procedural risks. The cost of uterine artery embolization varies by region, but is comparable to the charges for hysterectomy and is typically less than abdominal myomectomy.

The evaluation of candidates for UAE should follow a clear clinical indication for treatment. These indications are most often excessive menstrual blood loss that produces anemia and/or fibroid-related pelvic discomfort or organ dysfunction that impairs normal daily activities. All patients should have a current normal cervical cytology. An endometrial biopsy is recommended if endometrial neoplasia is suspected. UAE is typically reserved for premenopausal patients; the presence of uterine bleeding or a symptomatic pelvic mass in a postmenopausal woman should raise the specter of malignancy or a condition requiring further diagnostic evaluation. Rapid growth of a uterine mass is an exclusion criterion for UAE until the possibility of uterine sarcoma is further evaluated. Appropriate pre-procedural laboratory testing may include evaluation for concurrent blood coagulopathy, renal dysfunction, infection, or anemia. There is no evidence that pretreatment of patients with gonadotropin releasing hormone analogs improves the results of UAE.[17]

Fibroid size, location, and number should be confirmed with pelvic ultrasound. Magnetic resonance imaging (MRI) of the uterus is more sensitive than ultrasound in this regard, and can provide better determination of myoma size reduction after UAE. The extent of myoma blood flow has been correlated with UAE treatment efficacy, and this measure can be determined with contrast enhancement during MRI or Doppler flow ultrasound.[18] MRI is also very helpful to suggest the presence of coexistent adenomyosis or adenomyomas that can masquerade as myomas. Pelvic ultrasound may suggest adenomyosis, but MRI is superior to ultrasound in signifying the presence of adenomyosis with a sensitivity of more than 80%.[19] As will be discussed, the presence of adenomyosis should prompt counseling that UAE may be less effective in relieving symptoms.

The set of absolute and relative contraindications for UAE are continuing to be defined with increasing clinical experience. Pregnancy, active infection, and suspicion of uterine or ovarian cancer are absolute contraindications for UAE.[20] Relative contraindications include coagulopathy, immunocompromise, prior pelvic irradiation, a desire to maintain childbearing potential, contrast allergy, and large, pedunculated, subserosal, myomas. UAE may be the best treatment option for women with symptomatic fibroids who are not candidates for surgery or who do not wish to accept the risks of an operative procedure.

CLINICAL OUTCOMES FOR UTERINE ARTERY EMBOLIZATION

An ideal conservative treatment for leiomyomas would eliminate symptoms, markedly reduce the size of myomas, limit recurrence of future myomas, and preserve fertility. UAE has been shown to accomplish some, if not all, of these goals. Within 2–4 months after embolization, a 30–60% reduction of uterine volume may be expected. One study demonstrated that the uterine volume continues to shrink with time; however, symptomatic improvement may be achieved without remarkable change in myoma size.[9]

In reviews of published data, the symptomatic improvement rate for menorrhagia was approximately 85%.[13] Most studies reporting relief from menorrhagia after UAE have relied upon interviews or questionnaires from patients without additional objective measures such as post-treatment hemoglobin levels or

control groups. Investigators who have published case series since the year 2000 have reported reductions in menorrhagia between 84 and 93% at 1 year based upon patient impressions from interviews and questionnaires. An outline of treatment outcomes, lengths of post-procedural observation, and comments on complications for the major studies of UAE for uterine fibroids are summarized in Table 9.1.

The location of the myoma, not the size, is the most important factor that contributes to myoma-induced menorrhagia. Symptoms of pelvic discomfort, and impairment of normal bowel and urinary function, however, are related to the bulk effect of myoma size. Some experts have questioned whether there is an upper limit for uterine size beyond which UAE should not be recommended. Potentially, UAE for symptoms of the massively enlarged uterus could be less effective or could increase necrosis-related complications. Results from UAE, however, indicate little correlation between initial uterine volume and treatment outcome.[6] Failure was more likely when patients had undergone prior pelvic surgery. Poorer results following UAE have also been reported when myoma blood flow has lower peak systolic velocity determined by Doppler flow measurement.[18]

No studies have determined the efficacy of UAE specifically for submucous myomas. Transcervical leiomyoma expulsion after UAE most commonly originates from detachment of submucosal myomas, and is often associated with painful uterine contractions, fever, nausea, vomiting, and vaginal bleeding. Some treatment failures with continued abnormal uterine bleeding are due to submucous myomas.[7] Until studies establish the safety, efficacy, and cost-effectiveness of UAE for this indication, hysteroscopic resection of isolated submucosal myomas should be considered the preferred approach if feasible.

Pedunculated, subserosal myomas have generally been considered a relative contraindication for UAE, mainly because of the risk of detachment from the uterus after embolization.[38] If the stalk of a pedunculated, subserosal myoma is less than 3 cm and the myoma is solitary, surgical candidates are often best served by outpatient laparoscopic myomectomy. Nonetheless, relief of bulk-related symptoms was achieved following UAE without complication in 12 patients with pedunculated, subserosal myomas having a mean diameter of 8 cm and mean stalk diameter of 3 cm at 2 years' follow-up.[39]

Adenomyosis is characterized by the presence of endometrial glands and stroma within the myometrium, and may be associated with uterine enlargement,

Table 9.1   Outcome of uterine artery embolization for symptomatic leiomyomas

Authors	Number of patients	Decrease in uterine volume (%)	Decrease in menorrhaghia (%)	Follow-up interval (months)	Complications and comments
Ravina et al, 1997[21]	88	69	89	2–6	8 hysterectomy or myomectomy 2 D&C required
Goodwin et al, 1997[5]	11	40	20	6	1 hysterectomy
Worthington-Kirsch et al, 1998[8]	53	53	46	3	1 hysterectomy 1 upper GI bleed
Bradley et al, 1998[22]	8	51	80	3	1 ovarian failure 1 myoma expulsion
Goodwin et al, 1999[6]	60	43	81	10	6 hysterectomies 4 myoma expulsion 1 ovarian failure
Spies et al, 1999[23]	169	35	88	12	1 myoma expulsion 1 hysteroscopic resection 1 D&C required 2 hysterectomy 2 ovarian failure
Hutchins et al, 1999[24]	305	48	86%, 3 months 85%, 6 months 92%, 12 months	12	1 hysterectomy 4 puncture site hematoma 2 pain readmission
Ravina et al, 1999[25]	184	87% of patients, 6 months	90	29	1 hysterectomy with bowel obstruction 6 myoma expulsion
Siskin et al, 2000[26]	49	47.5%, 6 months	88.5	—	1 hysterectomy 1 prolonged fever
Pelage et al, 2000[27]	80	20%, 2 months 52%, 6 months	94	—	1 hysterectomy 4 amenorrhea 4 myoma expulsion
Brunereau et al, 2000[28]	58	23%, 3 months 43%, 6 months 51%, 1 year	90%, 3 months 92%, 6 months 93%, 1 year	12	1 external iliac artery dissection
McLucas et al, 2001[29]	167	49%, 6 months 52%, 12 months	82%, 6 months	6	1 hysterectomy 8 myoma expulsion
Anderson et al, 2001[30]	62	68%, 6 months	96	6	1 endometritis 2 myoma expulsion
Spies et al, 2001[31]	200	42%, 3 months 60%, 1 year	86%, 3 months 88%, 6 months 90%, 1 year	21	2 endometritis 1 myoma expulsion 2 thromboembolism
Katsumori et al, 2002[32]	60	55%, 4 months 70%, 12 months	98%, 4 months 100%, 12 months	—	2 myoma expulsion 1 amenorrhea
Walker and Pelage, 2002[33]	400	64% by MRI 73% by US	84	17	3 hysterectomy 26 amenorrhea 9 myoma expulsion 13 chronic vaginal discharge
Pron et al, 2003[34]	538	42	83	3	21 amenorrhea
Pinto et al, 2003[35]	36	46	86	24	UAE: shorter hospital stay and fewer complications than hysterectomy
Hehenkamp et al, 2005[36]	88	—	—	1.5	UAE: shorter hospital stay, but higher complications than hysterectomy

(Continued)

Table 9.1   Continued

Authors	Number of patients	Decrease in uterine volume (%)	Decrease in menorrhaghia (%)	Follow-up interval (months)	Complications and comments
Mara et al, 2005[37]	30	30	—	17	UAE: shorter hospital stay, but higher reintervention rate than myomectomy

D&C, dilatation and curettage; GI, gastrointestinal

abnormal uterine bleeding, and dysmenorrhea.[40] Some women with adenomyosis, however, will undergo UAE for coexistent uterine fibroids. In fact, preliminary reports have shown a relatively high incidence of adenomyosis in the uterus of UAE treatment failures who ultimately require hysterectomy.[6] Nonetheless, successful outcomes have been reported in women with adenomyosis following UAE. In 43 women with MRI-documented adenomyosis, significant improvement of dysmenorrhea and menorrhagia was achieved and a reduction in adenomyotic volume was detected at 3.5 months' follow-up.[41] Experienced interventional radiologists have recommended that if adenomyosis is identified before UAE, then a lower expectation for clinical success should be related to patients.[29] On the basis of these limited reports, the risk of treatment failure is probably increased, but adenomyosis should not be considered a contraindication for UAE.

Currently, four prospective randomized controlled trials have compared the clinical outcomes of UAE to hysterectomy and myomectomy.[35–37,42] In these studies, the clinical success rate of UAE for fibroid-related menstrual blood loss was 85%, with a mean dominant fibroid volume reduction by 30–46%. Compared to either hysterectomy or myomectomy, women receiving UAE had a shorter hospital stay and resumed normal activities sooner. Minor post-procedural complications such as vaginal discharge, venipuncture hematomas, and symptoms of post-embolization syndrome (pain, fever, nausea, and vomiting) were higher in patients receiving UAE. No differences in major complications were detected between surgery (myomectomy or hysterectomy) and UAE. Currently, only short-term clinical results are available. The Randomized trial of Embolization versus Surgical Treatment (REST) for Fibroids trial has provided 1-year follow-up quality of life data on patients randomized to surgery (hysterectomy or myomectomy) or UAE.[42] The REST trial investigators concluded that the faster recovery and decreased short-term morbidity following UAE should be balanced against the greater need for further

treatment by 1 year after UAE compared to surgery. The ongoing long-term results from the EMbolization versus hysterectoMY (EMMY) study will provide much needed prospective data for the clinical outcomes of UAE compared to conventional surgical option.[36]

UAE was initially used as a surgical adjuvant to reduce bleeding for women who were scheduled for abdominal myomectomy. This use of UAE quickly became secondary, as embolization was shown to improve fibroid-related symptoms. As UAE became a primary treatment for uterine fibroids, the role of UAE as a surgical adjuvant has remained largely unexplored.

In theory, UAE could be used as a surgical adjuvant in several clinical situations. Since UAE reduces uterine bleeding, its preoperative use may correct anemia and shrink the uterus before hysterectomy or myomectomy. Intraoperatively, embolization could be used during myomectomy if hemorrhage cannot be controlled surgically. Further, combined UAE plus hysteroscopic myomectomy would be expected to reduce bulk symptoms, limit menorrhagia, and prevent extrusion of submucous myomas (Figure 9.3). Embolization may be the most suitable option when multiple small fibroids remain following myomectomy, especially for those with 'innumerable' fibroids. Finally, if pregnancy outcomes after UAE are compromised because of the remaining myomas and not because of uterine vascular compromise, outcomes might be improved if UAE and myomectomy are combined, compared with UAE alone.

Few researchers, however, have explored the potential application of UAE as a surgical adjuvant, but studies have not shown the combined approach to be beneficial. The complication rate and long-term outcomes are not improved when UAE is performed before abdominal myomectomy. In a prospective observational study of 42 women scheduled for myomectomy, 20 received pre-surgical embolization.[43] Preoperative UAE did not reduce the mean intraoperative blood loss, although four required transfusion in the non-UAE group. Furthermore, if uterine healing is compromised after combined embolization and

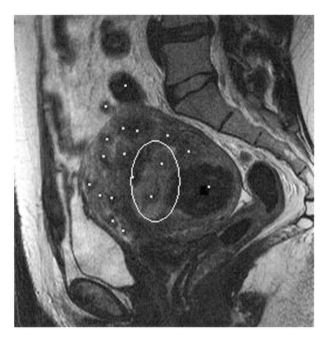

Figure 9.3 Magnetic resonance image of 'innumerable' fibroids, including two submucous myomas (circled) in a 42-year-old with severe menorrhagia and a desire for uterine preservation. Individual fibroids in this plane are indicated by white dots. In this clinical setting, combined uterine artery embolization and hysteroscopic myomectomy may be more beneficial than either approach alone

myomectomy, the risk for uterine rupture during pregnancy may increase. Finally, any marginal clinical benefit of UAE to reduce uterine size prior to hysterectomy would be offset by the increased treatment cost. In conclusion, no studies support the usefulness of UAE as a surgical adjuvant, and it cannot be recommended for routine clinical settings.

RISKS OF UTERINE ARTERY EMBOLIZATION FOR UTERINE MYOMAS

A recent Cochrane review reports the overall complication rate of UAE to be 10.5%, with a 1.5% major complication rate.[44] The most common minor complications following UAE included hot flashes (20%) and vaginal passage of fibroid tissue (15%).[36] Inguinal hematomas were experienced by about 20% of patients in this study, which was a higher rate of groin hematoma than reported by others (less than 4%).[6]

Fetid vaginal discharge occurred after UAE in 4–7% of patients, but the discharge resolved spontaneously in 90% of these cases.[33] The persistent vaginal discharge in these patients appears secondary to fluid accumulation within infarcted myomas that drains into the endometrial cavity. Fibroid extrusion occurs in

10% of patients following UAE, and can occur up to a year following the procedure.[6] Hysteroscopic resection of necrotic submucosal myomas after UAE usually cures persistent vaginal discharge and bleeding from degenerating myomas.[9] Resection of an unattached intracavitary myoma, however, may prove more difficult than resection of an attached submucous myoma.

Transient or permanent ovarian failure has been reported in up to 15% of cases following UAE.[45] The etiology of the ovarian failure is, in some cases, secondary to embolic material gaining access to ovarian vasculature, but also may be simply coincident with natural menopause. After UAE, the acute onset of ovarian failure occurs in approximately 15% of patients over age 45. Several observational studies have examined the effect of UAE on ovarian reserve testing in women of different ages. The largest study involved 73 women who were followed for 6 months with basal follicle stimulating hormone (FSH) testing. The majority of patients did not have any short-term change in basal FSH level; however, about 15% of women over age 45 had a significant elevation in FSH levels compared to their pre-UAE testing.[46] Taken together, these studies suggest that the ovarian effects of UAE may be age-dependent. Therefore, discussing the possibility of diminished ovarian reserve after UAE is prudent, especially when counseling women of advanced reproductive age.

The rate of major complications after UAE appears to compare favorably with the rate following myomectomy or hysterectomy.[44] Major complications following UAE for uterine fibroids are estimated to occur in 1–5% of patients based on either the American College of Obstetricians and Gynecologists (ACOG) or the Society of Cardiovascular and Interventional Radiology (SCVIR) classifications of adverse events. The most common major adverse event following UAE was hospital readmission for inadequate pain relief (2–4%). A need to evaluate fever was the second reason for readmission (0.5%) in these studies. Approximately a third of all patients develop post-embolization fever. Fever and leukocytosis are likely the result of myoma infarction and necrosis and may be associated with nausea, vomiting, malaise, and anorexia. This 'post-embolization syndrome' may occur in as many as 15% of patients, and may require readmission for the evaluation of pelvic or systemic infection. Serious infectious complications, however, occur in 1–2% of patients, and are more frequently encountered following embolization of larger fibroids.[47]

The FIBROID (Fibroid Registry for Outcomes Data) study reported that 1% of patients required a surgical intervention within 30 days following UAE.[48] In the

1-year follow-up of this study, 3% required hysterectomy and 10% required other interventions such as repeat embolization, myomectomy, dilatation and curettage, or bilateral oophorectomy. A prospective study with a 5-year follow-up reported that 20% of 200 patients had procedural failures or recurrent symptoms after UAE.[49] About 14% of these women underwent subsequent hysterectomy, 4% had myomectomy, and 2% required repeat embolization for continued symptoms relating to degenerating or persistent myomas.

Major complications from ischemic injury to nontarget tissues have been reported. Case reports have described labial, vaginal, cervical, buttock, or bladder necrosis, vesicouterine fistula, uterine wall defects, and abscess formation.[50] Ischemic rupture of the uterus after UAE has also been reported. Leiomyosarcoma was diagnosed in a patient who underwent UAE and subsequently exhibited an enlarging uterine mass.

At least three deaths have been reported following UAE relating to either sepsis or pulmonary embolism. The evidence is not currently available to sufficiently compare mortality rates following UAE versus major operative interventions. Procedure related death following UAE, however, is unlikely to exceed that following hysterectomy.

PREGNANCY OUTCOME AFTER UTERINE ARTERY EMBOLIZATION

Successful pregnancy outcome has been reported following UAE; however, there are insufficient data to conclude that UAE be recommended for women interested in future fertility. The FIBROID study has collected prospective data on over 3000 women undergoing UAE, and more than 700 of them reported that they are considering future pregnancy.[48] Only short-term outcomes have been reported thus far, but a goal of the registry is to collect data on fertility rates, miscarriage rates, and pregnancy outcome after UAE for the purpose of counseling women who wish to become pregnant after this procedure.

Normal pregnancy and delivery can be achieved following UAE for uterine leiomyomas. The first report of pregnancy after UAE occurred in 1995.[3] Approximately 136 pregnancies have been reported after UAE for leiomyomas, and delivery outcome is provided for 76 of those pregnancies (Table 9.2). Most pregnancies were delivered at term without complications. Despite these encouraging results, no randomized, controlled trials have evaluated the effect of UAE versus surgery on fertility or pregnancy outcome.

Unfortunately, the majority of retrospective studies have not documented the number of women who attempted pregnancy following embolization, and thus, cycle conception and fecundity rates cannot be calculated. One study evaluating fertility after UAE reported conception in 31% of patients.[62] The mean age at the completion of pregnancy was 37 years, and, of the 60 documented pregnancies, 19 patients experienced a delay to conception ranging from 18 months to 8 years.

Prospective trials that compare fertility rates after UAE to untreated control patients are unlikely to be completed. Such studies would be complicated by confounding factors including age, fibroid size and location, and the theoretical effect of UAE on the uterine vasculature. Both submucosal myomas and intramural leiomyomas (greater than 4 cm) reduce fertility.[63] Therefore, residual submucosal and/or intramural fibroids after UAE may adversely affect embryo implantation and pregnancy continuation. In addition, fertility may be diminished if ovarian function is compromised following UAE. Dissemination of embolization material may also impact on myometrial and endometrial vasculature, affecting embryo implantation. In fact, embolization particles have been identified after UAE in structures adjacent to leiomyomas such as the myometrium, parametrium, and mesoovarium. Myometritis, endomyometritis, and/or acute endometritis after UAE have also been reported.[64] Fortunately, in most cases, there generally does not appear to be any significant histologic impact on the endometrium, presumably because myometrial vessels trap particles before arrival in the endometrium. However, decreased vascularity and inflammation of the uterine myometrium and endometrium could affect embryo implantation and fertility rates.

The dissemination of embolization materials within the uterus could result in a deleterious effect on maintenance of pregnancy, and complications during labor and delivery. Theoretically, a uterus with areas of devascularized leiomyomata would likely be structurally weaker or exhibit contractile dysfunction during labor, resulting in an increased risk of cesarean section or uterine rupture. However, we could find no documented report of uterine rupture during labor following UAE only. However, the rate of cesarean section after UAE appears higher than in the general population. Of the 60 patients with term deliveries reporting mode of delivery, 40 were delivered by cesarean section (67%). Walker and McDowell reported that of 23 term cesarean sections, 13 were elective for prior cesearean section or fibroids.[62] Other

Table 9.2 Pregnancy outcome after uterine artery embolization

Authors	Number of UAE subjects	Number of pregnancies (with outcome information)	Number of deliveries	Comments
Bradley et al, 1998[22]	8	1	NS	1st trimester viability
Pron et al, 1999[51]	77	1	NS	1st trimester viability
Nicholson and Ettles, 1999[52]	24	1	1	1 term CS
Forman et al, 1999[53]	1000	14	NS	
Ravina et al, 2002[54]	184	12	7	2 term SVD
				2 term CS
				3 preterm (septicemia, twins + preeclampsia)
				5 SAB
Vashist et al, 2001[55]	NS	1	1	1 term CS
Ciraru-Vigneron and Ravina, 2001[56]	NS	5	3	2 term SVD
				1 term CS
				1 SAB
				1 EAB
McLucas et al, 2001[57]	400	15	10	2 term SVD
				7 term CS (2 breech)
				1 preterm (previa, abruption)
				5 SAB
Goldberg et al, 2002[58]	NS	2	2	1 term CS (twins)
				1 preterm CS (PROM, abruption)
Kovacs et al, 2002[59]	NS	1	NS	2nd trimester viability
D'Angelo et al, 2003[60]	NS	1	1	1 preterm CS (34-week twins)
Pron et al, 2005[61]	555	24	18	9 term SVD; 5 term CS:
				3 small for gestational age
				2 previa + hemorrhage
				4 preterm (htn, prior preterm delivery, previa + hemorrhage)
				4 SAB
				2 EAB
Walker and McDowell, 2006[62]	1200	56	33	4 term SVD; 23 term CS
				6 preterm (SROM, HELLP, pre-eclampsia, abruption)
				17 SAB
				3 EAB
				2 stillbirth
				1 ectopic
Total		134	76	60 term, 16 preterm

NS, not stated; CS, cesarean section; SVD, vaginal delivery; SAB, spontaneous abortion; EAB, elective abortion; PROM, premature rupture of the membranes; htn, hypertension; SROM, spontaneous rupture of the membranes; HELLP, hemolysis, elevated liver enzymes, low platelets

indications included breech presentation, placenta previa, preeclampsia, cephalopelvic disproportion, and chorioamnionitis. Based on limited data, there is insufficient evidence to conclude that UAE increases the rate of dysfunctional labor resulting in cesarean section.

It is unclear whether UAE by itself increases the risk of preterm delivery. These patients commonly possess established risk factors for preterm delivery, and often include women with advanced age and residual fibroids.[65] Of 76 patients with delivery information, 16 preterm deliveries were reported (21%), which is higher than the expected rate for the general population. The causes for

preterm labor in these cases included septicemia, preeclampsia, multiple pregnancy, prior preterm delivery, abruption, and hemorrhage secondary to placenta previa.

Theoretically, UAE could contribute to abnormal placentation over areas of devascularized endometrium and myometrium, which could increase the risk of placental abruption. The 20% incidence of preterm delivery due to placental abruption appears higher than the expected incidence of 1%. Pron et al reported a possible correlation between UAE and abnormal placentation contributing to hemorrhage.[51] In their series of 18 deliveries, three cases of abnormal placentation with placenta previa and/or accreta and subsequent antepartum or postpartum hemorrhage were reported. Postpartum hemorrhage occurred in approximately 20% of patients in the largest follow-up study of pregnancy after UAE.[62] Until further outcome information is available, patients should be advised of a potential increased risk of antepartum and postpartum hemorrhage following UAE.

No controlled trials are available to assess whether UAE may be associated with an increased risk of miscarriage. Of the 136 pregnancies summarized in Table 9.2, several were electively terminated or outcome information was not available, leaving a total of 117 pregnancies for consideration. Thirty-two pregnancies were reported as spontaneous losses, for a spontaneous abortion rate of 27%. This miscarriage rate is similar to that in the largest study, which reported miscarriage rates of 30% after UAE.[62] This incidence of pregnancy loss following UAE is higher than the accepted overall 15% clinical miscarriage rate in the general population. In a different UAE study, however, the miscarriage rate was similar to this overall early pregnancy loss rate. Pron et al reported a spontaneous abortion rate of 16.7% in women who delivered after UAE, with an average age of 36 years for these women.[61] Further study will be required to assess the impact of the UAE procedure on the risk of miscarriage.

In conclusion, fertility may be affected by residual fibroids or the effect of UAE on ovarian and uterine vasculature. Uncomplicated pregnancy and delivery can be expected for most patients after UAE based on small studies. However, there may be an increased risk of miscarriage, preterm delivery, and placental abnormalities, contributing to an increased risk of abruption and postpartum hemorrhage. Spies and colleagues reserve UAE for women who do not desire future fertility, but will consider UAE for women wishing to maintain reproductive capability if hysterectomy or repeat extensive myomectomy are the only other options.[9] Other groups have taken a more open approach, and now offer UAE to patients who desire future fertility.[3,66] Patients should be advised that there may be a detrimental effect on future fertility and pregnancy outcome if embolization is performed for those interested in future childbearing.

ALTERNATIVES TO UTERINE ARTERY EMBOLIZATION

While UAE provides a new alternative to hysterectomy and myomectomy for many women with symptomatic uterine fibroids, it may not be the most appropriate choice. The challenge is to choose the most suitable approach among the many available treatments. There are several options for treating symptomatic fibroids, and the choice depends on three major considerations: (1) uterine preservation, (2) desire for fertility, and (3) the extent of endometrial distortion caused by fibroids. Treatment should be chosen to provide maximal efficacy with the lowest risk, least expense, and fastest recovery. According to ACOG guidelines, observation without intervention is most appropriate for asymptomatic women with uterine fibroids, regardless of the size, number, or growth rate. UAE is not appropriate for these women.

Because pregnancy outcomes may be compromised with UAE, surgery is a better option for women who wish to preserve fertility. Surgery may include hysteroscopic resection of submucosal myomas and abdominal or laparoscopic myomectomy for intramural and subserosal lesions, depending on the skill of the surgeon and the location and number of fibroids.[67]

Hysteroscopic myomectomy for submucous myomas is an accepted therapy for women who desire fertility preservation, and conception occurs in nearly 50% of patients after surgery.[68] For intramural or submucous myomas, hospitalization is shorter with laparoscopic myomectomy, recovery is faster, there is less postoperative morbidity, and pregnancy and recurrence rates are equivalent, compared to abdominal myomectomy.[67] In contrast to UAE, pregnancies after laparoscopic myomectomy have lower rates of preterm delivery and malpresentation.[69] When needed, laparoscopic and hysteroscopic myomectomy can be combined during a single anesthesia to complete resection of multiple fibroids. Overall, 40–50% of infertile women conceive after myomectomy, and miscarriage rates are reduced following abdominal myomectomy.

Hysteroscopic myomectomy is reserved for patients with submucosal myomas. UAE and hysteroscopic myomectomy both control excessive uterine bleeding in 85–90%, and hysteroscopic myomectomy can be combined with endometrial ablation.[70] Hysteroscopic myomectomy, however, often does not result in an appreciable reduction in uterine size, a disadvantage compared to UAE.

The long-term outcomes of myomectomy and UAE are similar.[71] UAE requires more invasive treatments for myomas than myomectomy in the 3–5-year interval after the initial therapy. Patient satisfaction is high with both procedures (94% UAE, 79% abdominal myomectomy), and resolution of menorrhagia and anemia is similar. Less is known about leiomyoma recurrence following UAE than following myomectomy.

Table 9.3 Indications for ablative therapy for uterine leiomyomas: abdominal myomectomy versus uterine artery embolization. From reference 13

Condition	Myomectomy	UAE
Multiple symptomatic subserosal, intramural, and submucous myomas	+	+
Rapidly enlarging myoma	+	0
Infertility	+	0
Desire to retain fertility	+	?
Does not desire future fertility, but wishes to retain uterus	?	+
Poor surgical risk	0	+
Hemodynamic instability due to hemorrhage	0	+
Diffuse multiple uterine leiomyomas	0	+
Hydrosalpinx	+	0
Adnexal mass	+	0

Patient age and the number and location of the myomas affect recurrence rates. The recurrence rate requiring further surgery after myomectomy is estimated to be 15–20%. However, new myomas are found by ultrasound in over 50% of patients 5 years after myomectomy.[72] These rates compare to a symptom recurrence rate of 10% at 2 years after UAE.[73]

Myomectomy is almost exclusively reserved for women desiring future pregnancy. Myomectomy and UAE, however, may be offered to those who desire preservation of the uterus, but do not desire conception, if they are willing to accept the potential for recurrence of myoma related symptoms. For these individuals there are several additional options, including medical therapies, endometrial ablation, myolysis, uterine artery ligation, and MRI-directed high-intensity ultrasound myoma focused ablation.

Medical therapies (gonadotropin releasing analogs, the progestin intrauterine system, aromatase inhibitors, progesterone receptor antagonists, selective progesterone receptor antagonists, and antifibrotic agents) have not been compared to UAE in clinical trials. In some cases, medical therapies might temporize symptoms in perimenopausal women in an attempt to avoid surgery or UAE.[67]

Several new minimally invasive approaches are under development for uterine fibroids, but no clinical studies have directly compared these modalities to UAE. Promising interventions include ultrasound-directed transvaginal myolysis, ultrasound- or MRI-directed high-intensity focused ultrasound myoma ablation, and vaginal uterine artery ligation.[74–76]

Finally, hysterectomy is the only proven definitive treatment for symptomatic fibroids, and therefore remains an appealing approach for many women.

Compared to UAE, hospitalization and recovery time is longer for hysterectomy, but no comparative studies have assessed these outcomes for vaginal, laparoscopy-assisted vaginal, and laparoscopic hysterectomy.[35,36,42]

COLLABORATIVE MANAGEMENT OF SYMPTOMATIC LEIOMYOMAS

Collaboration between the gynecologist and the interventional radiologist is necessary to optimize the safety and efficacy of UAE. The primary candidates for this procedure include those with symptomatic uterine fibroids who no longer desire fertility, but wish to avoid surgery or are poor surgical risks (Table 9.3). The gynecologist is likely to be the primary initial consultant for patients presenting with complaints of symptomatic myomas, and therefore must be familiar with the indications, exclusions, outcome expectations, and complications of UAE in their particular center. Appropriate diagnostic testing should aid in the exclusion of most but not all gynecologic cancers and pregnancy.

Any center that offers UAE should adhere to published clinical guidelines, maintain ongoing assessment of quality improvement measures, and observe strict criteria for obtaining procedural privileges.[20] The complexity of pelvic arterial anatomy, the skill required to master modern coaxial microcatheters, and the hazards of significant patient radiation exposure are cited as reasons that sound training and demonstration of expertise be obtained prior to the credentialing of clinicians for the performance of UAE.

Uterine artery embolization is a unique new treatment for uterine myomas and is no longer considered investigational for symptomatic uterine fibroids. Current efforts to provide prospective objective assessment of treatment outcomes and complications after UAE will help to optimize patient selection and clinical guidelines. The Fibroid Registry for Outcomes Data (FIBROID) should provide critical information for the assessment of safety and outcomes measures in women receiving UAE for symptomatic uterine myomas. Continued results from prospective trials that are newly completed or ongoing will provide valuable long-term data.

REFERENCES

1. Heaston DK, Mineau DE, Brown BJ, Miller FJ. Transcatheter arterial embolization for control of persistent massive puerperal hemorrhage after bilateral surgical hypogastric artery ligation. AJR Am J Roentgenol 1979; 133: 152–4.

2. Oliver JA, Lance JS. Selective embolization to control massive hemorrhage following pelvic surgery. Am J Obstet Gynecol 1979; 135: 431–2.

3. Ravina JH, Herbreteau D, Ciraru-Vigneron N et al. Arterial embolization to treat uterine myomata. Lancet 1995; 346: 671–2.

4. McLucas B, Goodwin S, Vedantham S. Embolic therapy for myomata. Minim Invasive Ther Allied Technol 1996; 5: 336–8.

5. Goodwin SC, Vedantham S, McLucas B, Forno AE, Perrella R. Preliminary experience with uterine artery embolization for uterine fibroids. J Vasc Interv Radiol 1997; 8: 517–26.

6. Goodwin SC, McLucas B, Lee M et al. Uterine artery embolization for the treatment of uterine leiomyomata midterm results. J Vasc Intervent Radiol 1999; 10: 1159–65.

7. Goodwin SC, Walker WJ. Uterine artery embolization for the treatment of uterine fibroids. Curr Opin Obstet Gynecol 1998; 10: 315–20.

8. Worthington-Kirsch RL, Popky GL, Hutchins FL Jr. Uterine arterial embolization for the management of leiomyomas: quality-of-life assessment and clinical response. Radiology 1998; 208: 625–9.

9. Spies JB, Scialli AR, Jha RC et al. Initial results from uterine fibroid embolization for symptomatic leiomyomata. J Vasc Interv Radiol 1999; 10: 1149–57.

10. Pelage JP, Soyer P, LeDref O et al. Uterine arteries: bilateral catheterization with a single femoral approach and a single 5-F catheter-technical note. Radiology 1999; 210: 573–5.

11. Joffre F, Tubina JM, Pelage JP; Group FEMIC. FEMIC (Fibromes Embolisés aux MICrosphères calibrées): uterine fibroid embolization using tris-acryl microspheres. A French multicenter study. Cardiovasc Intervent Radiol 2004; 27: 600–6.

12. Spies JB, Allison S, Flick P et al. Polyvinyl alchohol particles and tris-acyl gelatin microspheres for uterine artery embolization for leiomyomas: results of a randomized comparative study. J Vasc Interv Radiol 2004; 15: 793–800.

13. Hurst BS, Stackhouse DJ, Matthews ML, Marshburn PB. Uterine artery embolization for symptomatic uterine myomas. Fertil Steril 2000; 74: 855–69.

14. Spies JB. Recovery after uterine artery embolization: understanding and managing short-term outcomes. J Vasc Interv Radiol 2003; 14: 1219–22.

15. Nikolic B, Spies JB, Abbara S, Goodwin SC. Ovarian artery supply of uterine fibroids as a cause of treatment of failure after uterine artery embolization: a case report. J Vasc Interv Radiol 1999; 10: 1167–70.

16. Spies JB, Sacks D. Credentials for uterine artery embolization. J Vasc Interv Radiol 2004; 15: 111–13.

17. Vilos GA, Vilos AG, Abu-Rafea B et al. Administration of goserelin acetate after uterine artery embolization does not change the reduction rate and volume of uterine myomas, Fertil Steril 2006; 85: 1478–83.

18. McLucas B, Pevella R, Goodwin S et al. Role of uterine artery Doppler flow in fibroid embolization. J Ultrasound Med 2002; 21: 113–20.

19. Ascher SM, Arnold LL, Patt RH et al. Adenomyosis: prospective comparison of MR imaging and transvaginal sonography, 1994; 190: 803–6.

20. Hovsepian DM, Siskin GP, Bonn J et al. Quality improvement guidelines for uterine artery embolization for symptomatic leiomyomata. Cardiovasc Intervent Radiol 2004; 27: 307–13.

21. Ravina JH, Bouret JM, Ciraru-Vigneron N et al. Application of particulate arterial embolization in the treatment of uterine fibromyomata. Bull Acad Natl Med 1997; 181: 233–43.

22. Bradley EA, Reidy JF, Forman RG, Jarosz J, Braude PR. Transcatheter uterine artery embolization to treat large uterine fibroids. Br J Obstet Gynaecol 1998; 105: 235–40.

23. Spies JB, Levy EB, Gomez-Jorge J et al. Uterine fibroid embolization: midterm results. Abstract presented at 25th Annual Scientific Meeting of the Society of Cardiovascular and Interventional Radiology, March, 1999, San Diego.

24. Hutchins FL Jr, Worthington-Kirsch R, Berkowitz RP. Selective uterine artery embolization as primary treatment for symptomatic leiomyomata uteri. J Am Assoc Gynecol Laparosc 1999; 6: 279–84.

25. Ravina J, Cirau-Vigneron N, Aymard A et al. Uterine artery embolisation for fibroid disease: results of a 6 year study. Minim Invasive Ther Allied Technol 1999; 8: 441–7.

26. Siskin GP, Stainken BF, Dowling K et al. Outpatient uterine artery embolization for symptomatic uterine fibroids: experience in 49 patients. J Vasc Interv Radiol 2000; 11: 305–11.

27. Pelage JP, Le Dref O, Soyer P et al. Fibroid-related menorrhagia: treatment with superselective embolization of the uterine arteries and midterm follow-up. Radiology 2000; 215: 428–31.

28. Brunereau L, Herbreteau D, Gallas S et al. Uterine artery embolization in the primary treatment of uterine leiomyomas: technical features and prospective follow-up with clinical and sonographic examinations in 58 patients. AJR Am J Roentgenol 2000; 175: 1267–72.

29. McLucas B, Adler L, Perrella R. Uterine fibroid embolization: nonsurgical treatment for symptomatic fibroids. J Am Coll Surg 2001; 192: 95–105.

30. Anderson PE, Lund N, Justesen P et al. Uterine artery embolization of symptomatic uterine fibroids: initial success and short-term results. Acta Radiol 2001; 42: 234–8.

31. Spies JB, Ascher SA, Roth AR et al. Uterine artery embolization for leiomyomata, 2001; 98: 29–34.

32. Katsumori T, Nakajima K, Mihara T, Tokuhiro M. Uterine artery embolization using gelatin sponge particles alone for symptomatic uterine fibroids: midterm results. AJR Am J Roentgenol 2002; 178: 135–9.

33. Walker WJ, Pelage JP. Uterine artery embolisation for symptomatic fibroids: clinical results in 400 women with imaging follow-up. Br J Obstet Gynaecol 2002; 109: 1262–72.

34. Pron G, Bennett J, Common A et al. The Ontario Uterine Fibroid Embolization Trial. Part 2: uterine fibroid reduction and symptom relief after uterine artery embolization for fibroids. Fertil Steril 2003; 79: 120–7.

35. Pinto I, Chimeno P, Romo A et al. Uterine fibroids: uterine artery embolization versus abdominal hysterectomy for treatment – a prospective, randomized, and controlled clinical trial. Radiology 2003; 226: 425–31.

36. Hehenkamp WJK, Volkers NA, Donderwinkel PFJ et al. Uterine artery embolization versus hysteresctomy in the treatment of symptomatic uterine fibroids (EMMY trial): peri- and

postprocedural results from a randomized trial. Am J Obstet Gynecol 2005; 193: 1618–29.

37. Mara M, Fucikova Z, Maskova J, Kuzel D, Haakova L. Uterine fibroid embolization versus myomectomy in women wishing to preserve fertility: preliminary results of a randomized controlled trial. Eur J Obstet Gynecol 2006; 126: 226–33.

38. Braude P, Reidy J, Nott V, Taylor A, Forman R. Embolization of uterine leiomyomata: current concepts in management. Hum Reprod Update 2000; 6: 603–8.

39. Katsumori T, Akazawa K, Mihara T. Uterine artery embolization for pedunculated subserosal fibroids. Am J Radiol 2005; 184: 399–402.

40. Vavilis D, Agorastos T, Tzafetas J et al. Adenomyosis at hysterectomy: prevalence and relationship to operative findings and reproductive and menstrual factors. Clin Exp Obstet Gynecol 1997; 24: 36–8.

41. Kim MD, Won JW, Lee DY, Ahn C-S. Uterine artery embolization for adenomyosis without fibroids. Clin Radiol 2004; 59: 520–6.

42. Edwards RD, Moss JG, Lumsden MA et al. Committee of the Randomized Trial of Embolization versus Surgical Treatment for Fibroids. Uterine-artery embolization versus surgery for symptomatic uterine fibroids. N Engl J Med 2007; 356: 360–70.

43. Djabbari M, Denys AL, Anquetil C, Levardon M, Menu YM. Preoperative bilateral uterine arterial embolization before multiple myomectomies: is it useful to reduce preoperative bleeding? Abstract presented at Radiological Society of North American Scientific Assembly and Annual Meeting, November, 1999, Chicago.

44. Gupta JK, Sinha AS, Lumsden MA, Hickey M. Uterine artery embolization for symptomatic uterine fibroids. Cochrane Database Syst Rev 2006; (4): 1–28.

45. Chrisman HB, Saker MB, Ryu RK et al. The impact of uterine fibroid embolization on resumption of menses and ovarian function. J Vasc Interv Radiol 2000; 11: 699–703.

46. Spies JB, Roth AR, Gonsalves SM, Murphy-Skrzyniarz KM. Ovarian function after uterine artery embolization for leiomyomata: assessment with use of serum follicle stimulating hormone assay. J Vasc Interv Radiol 2001; 12: 437–42.

47. Rajan DK, Beecroft JR, Clark TWI et al. Risk of intrauterine infectious complications after uterine artery embolization. J Vasc Interv Radiol 2004; 15: 1415–21.

48. Worthington-Kirsch R, Spies JB, Myers ER et al. FIBROID Investigators. The Fibroid Registry for outcomes data (FIBROID) for uterine embolization: short-term outcomes. Obstet Gynecol 2005; 106: 52–9.

49. Spies JB, Bruno J, Czeyda-Pommersheim F et al. Long-term outcome of uterine artery embolization of leiomyomata. Obstet Gynecol 2005; 106: 933–9.

50. American College of Obstetricians and Gynecologists Committee on Gynecologic Practice. Uterine Artery Embolization. ACOG Committee Opinion 2004, No 293. Compendium of Selected Publications. Washington, DC: American College of Obstetricians and Gynecologists, 2006: 262–3.

51. Pron G, Simons M, Common A et al. Uterine artery embolization for symptomatic fibroids: sarcoma, pregnancy and other reasons for treatment relapse or failure. Abstract presented at SMIT/CIMIT 11th Annual Scientific meeting, September, 1999, Boston.

52. Nicholson A, Ettles D. Fibroid embolization: observations in 24 patients. Abstract presented at SMIT/CIMIT 11th Annual Scientific meeting, September, 1999, Boston.

53. Forman RG, Reidy J, Nott V, Braude P. Fibroids and fertility. Minim Invasive Ther Allied Technol 1999; 8: 415–19.

54. Ravina JH, Ciraru-Vigneron N, Aymard A, LeDrref O, Merland JJ. Pregnancy after embolization of uterine myoma: report of 12 cases. Fertil Steril 2002; 73: 1241–3.

55. Vashist A, Smith JR, Thorpe-Beeston G, McCall J. Pregnancy subsequent to uterine artery embolization. Fertil Steril 2001; 75: 1246–8.

56. Ciraru-Vigneron N, Ravina JH. Pregnancy subsequent to uterine artery embolization. Fertil Steril 2001; 75: 1247–8.

57. McLucas B, Goodwin S, Adler L et al. Pregnancy following uterine fibroid embolization. Int J Gynaecol Obstet 2001; 74: 1–7.

58. Goldberg J, Periera L, Berghella V. Pregnancy after uterine artery embolization, Obstet Gynecol 2002; 100: 869–72.

59. Kovacs P, Stangel JJ, Santoro NF, Leiman H. Successful pregnancy after transient ovarian failure following treatment of symptomatic leiomyoma. Fertil Steril 2002; 77: 1292–5.

60. D'Angelo AD, Amso NN, Wood A. Spontaneous multiple pregnancy after uterine artery embolization for uterine fibroid: a case report. Eur J Obstet Gynecol Reprod Biol 2003; 110: 245–6.

61. Pron G, Mocarski E, Bennett J, Vilos G, Common A. Pregnancy after uterine artery embolization for leiomyomata: the Ontario multicenter trial. Obstet Gynecol 2005; 105: 67–76.

62. Walker J, McDowell S. Pregnancy after uterine artery embolization for leiomyomata: a series of 56 completed pregnancies. Am J Obstet Gynecol 2006; 106: 52–9.

63. Eldar-Geva T, Meagher S, Healy DL et al. Effect of intramural, subserosal, and submucosal uterine fibroids on the outcome of assisted reproductive technology treatment. Fertil Steril 1998; 70: 687–91.

64. Colgan TJ, Pron G, Mocarski EJM et al. Pathologic features of uteri and leiomyomas following uterine artery embolization for leiomyomas. Am J Surg Pathol 2003; 27: 167–77.

65. Committee on Technical Bulletins of the American College of Obstetricians and Gynecologists. Assessment of Risk Factors for Preterm Birth. ACOG Technical Bulletin 2001, No 31. Compendium of Selected Publications. Washington, DC: American College of Obstetricians and Gynecologists, 2005: 303–10.

66. Vedantham S, Goodwin SC, McLucas B et al. Uterine artery embolization for fibroids: considerations in patient selection and clinical follow-up. Medscape Women's Health 1999; 4: 2.

67. Hurst BS, Matthews ML, Marshburn, PB. Laparoscopic myomectomy for symptomatic uterine myomas. Fertil Steril 2005; 83: 1–23.

68. Candiani GB, Fedele L, Parazzini F, Villa L. Risk of recurrence after myomectomy. Br J Obstet Gynaecol 1991; 98: 385–9.

69. Goldberg J, Pereira L, Berghella V et al. Pregnancy outcomes after treatment for fibromyomata: uterine artery embolization versus laparoscopic myomectomy. Am J Obstet Gynecol 2004; 191: 18–21.

70. Vercellini P, Zaina B, Yaylayan L et al. Hysteroscopic myomectomy: long-term effects on menstrual pattern and fertility. Obstet Gynecol 1999; 94: 341–7.

71. Broder MS, Goodwin S, Chen G et al. Comparison of long-term outcomes of myomectomy and uterine artery embolization. Obstet Gynecol 2002; 100: 864–8.

72. Fedele L, Parazzini F, Luchini L et al. Recurrence of fibroids after myomectomy: a transvaginal ultrasonographic study. Hum Reprod 1995; 10: 1795–6.

73. Marret H, Alonso AM, Cottier JP et al. Leiomyoma recurrence after uterine artery embolization. J Vasc Interv Radiol 2003; 14: 1395–9.

74. Hurst S, Marshburn PB, Elliot M, Matthews MM. New minimally invasive treatment of uterine fibroids: transvaginal ultrasound-directed myolysis. Preclinical study to determine optimal use of prototype. Fertil Steril 2004; 82: S10–11.

75. Smart OC, Hindley JT, Regan L, Gedroyc WG. Gonadotropin-releasing hormone and magnetic-resonance-guided ultrasound surgery for uterine leiomyomata. Obstet Gynecol 2006; 108: 49–54.

76. Akinola OI, Fabamwo AO, Ottun AT, Akinniyi OA. Uterine artery ligation for management of uterine fibroids. Int J Gynaecol Obstet 2005; 91: 137–40.

10 Infertility

Beth W Rackow and Emre Seli

The involvement of a couple, not just an individual, makes infertility a unique medical condition encountered in the outpatient practice of an obstetrician–gynecologist. *Fertility* is defined as the ability of a couple to conceive and bear offspring. Approximately 80–90% of couples will conceive within 12 months of attempting pregnancy; the failure of a couple to conceive after 12 months of unprotected frequent intercourse defines *infertility*. *Fecundability* is the probability of achieving a pregnancy in one menstrual cycle, and is estimated at 20–25% in healthy young couples.[1] *Fecundity* is the probability of achieving a live birth in one menstrual cycle. Both fecundability and fecundity decrease over time, and after 6–12 months without conception, it is reasonable for couples to seek evaluation and treatment. Infertility is not an all-or-none situation, but encompasses a wide spectrum of reversible and irreversible disorders, and a multitude of successful treatments are available.

The clinical definition of infertility is based on several large retrospective studies. In 1956, Guttmacher[2] studied 5574 English and American women who engaged in unprotected intercourse and ultimately conceived between 1946 and 1956. In this cohort, 50% of women conceived within 3 months, 72% within 6 months, and 85% within 12 months. Another study from 1950 demonstrated that in normal healthy couples, conception occurred in 25% within 1 month, 70% within 6 months, and 90% within 12 months.[3] Furthermore, the probability of conception was related to the age of the couple and the frequency of coitus. Although the majority of couples conceive within 12 months, most pregnancies occur in the first 6 months. After 12 months without success, approximately 50% of couples will conceive spontaneously within the next 36 months.[4] If a couple do not conceive after 3 years, infertility will likely persist without medical intervention.

Based on data from the 1995 National Survey of Family Growth, the prevalence of infertility among reproductive aged nulliparous women has remained stable: 13.3% in 1965, 13.9% in 1982, 13.7% in 1988, and 13.5% in 1995.[5,6] However, the total number of women aged 15–44 seeking infertility care increased from 6.6 million women (12%) in 1982 to 9.3 million

(15%) in 1995.[7] Women seeking infertility services, compared with the general population, were more likely older (age 35–44 years), nulliparous, married, and relatively affluent, and had healthcare insurance.[7] Greater numbers of women seeking infertility treatment are attributed to significant improvements in the array and availability of infertility services, improvements in physicians' ability to evaluate and diagnose infertility, increased public awareness of infertility and available treatments, and improved social acceptance of infertility, which increases the seeking of care and self-reporting.

ETIOLOGY OF INFERTILITY

Successful conception requires the orchestration of a series of specific events: ovulation of a competent oocyte, production of competent sperm, juxtaposition of oocyte and sperm in the reproductive tract and subsequent fertilization, generation of a viable embryo, transport of the embryo to the uterine cavity, and implantation of the embryo into the endometrium. Defects in any of these necessary steps can result in diminished fertility. Furthermore, a combination of factors may contribute to a couple's infertility. Overall, there are four major categories of conditions affecting fecundability:

- abnormalities in oocyte production and ovulation
- abnormalities of female reproductive tract transport: cervical, uterine, tubal, and peritoneal factors
- abnormalities in sperm production
- unexplained or other conditions.

Male and female partners contribute similarly to a couple's infertility; some degree of male infertility is implicated in up to 40% of couples.[8] A review of over 14 000 infertile couples from 21 published reports identified the distribution of primary clinical diagnoses to be 27% ovulatory factor, 25% male factor, 22% tubal factor, 17% unexplained, and 9% other diagnoses (Figure 10.1).[9] The rate of unexplained infertility depends on the level of evaluation prior to making this diagnosis.

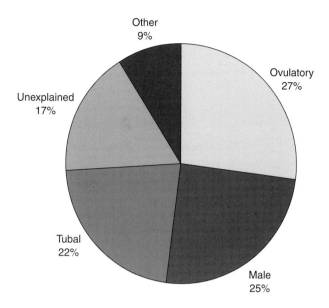

Figure 10.1   Prevalence of etiologies of infertility[9]

EVALUATION OF INFERTILITY

The evaluation of infertility investigates the most common causes of male and female reproductive dysfunction. Despite the widespread use of certain tests, there are few data regarding their predictive value; an abnormal test does not necessarily determine the cause of infertility in a particular couple.[10] Furthermore, there may be more than one factor involved in a couple's infertility, including mild abnormalities that tests do not routinely discover. In the following discussion we will review the initial and supplemental tests to evaluate infertility, and the data supporting current use or abandonment of each test (Table 10.1).

The timing of the infertility evaluation depends on the age of the female partner and the couple's risk factors for infertility. In the United States, maternal age-specific birth rates for 2004 highlight the decrease in fecundity with increasing maternal age (Figure 10.2).[11] Due to this decline in fecundity with maternal age, a marker of ovarian aging, it is recommended that women over age 35 undergo an evaluation of infertility prior to 12 months of attempted conception.[12] Furthermore, women with a history of oligomenorrhea or amenorrhea, endometriosis, known or suspected uterine or tubal disease, chemotherapy or radiation exposure, or subfertility, or with a subfertile partner, warrant expedited evaluation and treatment.[12]

History and physical examination

A detailed history and physical examination are invaluable for identifying symptoms or signs that suggest potential etiologies for infertility, and guide the subsequent diagnostic evaluation. Both female and male partners should be questioned about their duration of infertility and any previous evaluation or treatment; fertility in previous relationships; medical history including previous hospitalizations and serious illnesses or injuries; surgical history; current medications and allergies; use of tobacco, alcohol, and other drugs; lifestyle issues such as exercise, dieting, and stress; occupational and environmental exposures; and family history of birth defects, mental retardation, or reproductive failure. Relevant history for the female partner includes a thorough gynecologic history including pubertal course, menstrual history and occurrence of dysmenorrhea, sexually transmitted diseases or pelvic inflammatory disease, abnormal Pap tests and subsequent treatment, contraceptive use, coital frequency, and a detailed obstetric history. The male partner may be questioned about his developmental and pubertal history, previous genital trauma or surgery, sexual history including sexually transmitted diseases, and sexual function. The review of systems should include symptoms of thyroid disease, galactorrhea, hirsutism or changes in hair growth patterns, changes in weight, acne, headaches or vision changes, pelvic or abdominal pain, and dyspareunia.

Physical examination of the female should identify the following: weight and body mass index; thyroid enlargement, nodularity, or tenderness; breast mass or nipple discharge; signs of androgen excess including abnormalities of the skin or hair growth; pelvic or abdominal tenderness, mass, or organomegaly; vaginal or cervical abnormality or discharge; uterine size, shape, position, and mobility; adnexal mass or tenderness; and cul-de-sac mass, tenderness, or nodularity.

Assessment of ovulation

A woman's menstrual history helps to determine whether she has ovulatory menstrual cycles. Predictable, cyclic menses every 25–35 days with moliminal symptoms (breast tenderness, dysmenorrhea, bloating) almost always signify regular ovulation, and are likely associated with a normal hormone profile including follicle stimulating hormone (FSH), luteinizing hormone (LH), estradiol (E2), prolactin (PRL), and androgens. Laboratory documentation of ovulation may not be necessary in these women. In contrast, oligomenorrhea implies infrequent ovulation and thus irregular menses; assessment of ovulation may be helpful, and evaluation of the cause of ovulatory dysfunction is warranted.

Several tests provide indirect evidence of ovulation. The basal body temperature chart reveals a biphasic

Table 10.1 Tests that aid in evaluation of the infertile couple

Etiology of infertility	Initial evaluation	Further testing	Not indicated
Ovulatory dysfunction	History Basal body temperature charting Ovulation predictor kit	Mid-luteal phase progesterone Ultrasonography	Endometrial biopsy
Cervix	None	None	Postcoital test
Uterus	Ultrasonography	Sonohysterography Hysterosalpingography Hysteroscopy MRI	
Fallopian tubes and peritoneum	Hysterosalpingography	Laparoscopy with chromopertubation Chlamydia antibody testing Air-contrast sonohysterography	
Diminishing ovarian reserve	Cycle day-3 FSH and estradiol Antral follicle count	Clomiphene citrate challenge test	
Male	Semen analysis with migration	Genetic evaluation FSH, LH, testosterone Prolactin Scrotal or rectal ultrasonography	

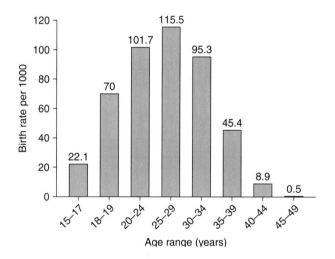

Figure 10.2 Maternal age-specific birth rates for 2004[11]

curve during most ovulatory cycles. An elevation of early morning core temperature by 0.5–1.0°F is associated with progesterone production by the corpus luteum, and retrospectively identifies the occurrence of an LH surge 1–2 days prior to the change in temperature. This inexpensive but cumbersome method can be difficult to interpret, and may not reliably identify ovulation. Over-the-counter urinary LH kits prospectively identify the presence and timing of ovulation; ovulation occurs the day after evidence of an LH surge. Due to variability in timing of the LH surge and renal clearance of LH, the once-daily test may only identify 85% of LH surges.[10] Another test used to retrospectively confirm ovulation is the mid-luteal phase serum progesterone. The progesterone level is obtained 18–24 days after menses; a value greater than 3 ng/ml is diagnostic of ovulation, although levels of

6–25 ng/ml are preferred. Due to the variability of pulsatile LH release, a single low progesterone value should be repeated. For women with severe oligomenorrhea (cycle lengths greater than 45 days), LH or progesterone measurements have little utility, and evaluation of the cause of oligo-ovulation is paramount.

The luteal phase endometrial biopsy has been used to assess ovulation. The presence of secretory endometrium requires progesterone, and hence ovulation is implied. Normal histologic development of the secretory phase endometrium has been described.[13] Therefore, adequate steroid hormone levels and an appropriate endometrial response are presumed when the assigned histologic date is within 2 days of the cycle day calculated from the LH surge (day 14). Two 'out-of-phase' biopsies (defined as histologic dating more than 2 days delayed) have been used to diagnose a luteal phase defect, believed to be associated with defective corpus luteum production of progesterone or poor endometrial response to progesterone. However, fertile women can also have out-of-phase luteal phase biopsies.[12,14] Moreover, the ability of an endometrial biopsy to accurately identify abnormalities in the endometrium is questioned, since histologic studies of secretory phase endometrium do not reliably discriminate fertile from infertile women.[15–17] Therefore, luteal phase endometrial biopsies should not be routinely performed.

Once the presence of anovulation is established, further testing is necessary to identify the underlying cause (Table 10.2). Common causes of anovulation include thyroid disorders and hyperprolactinemia, and therefore serum thyroid stimulating hormone (TSH) and prolactin levels should be assessed. Evaluation

Table 10.2 Tests to evaluate the etiology of anovulation or oligo-ovulation

Test	Comments
TSH	Evaluate for thyroid disease
Prolactin	Evaluate for hyperprolactinemia
FSH, LH, estradiol	Assessment for hypogonadotropic hypogonadism or premature ovarian failure
Free and total testosterone	Evaluate for hyperandrogenism
Fasting glucose and insulin	Evaluate for impaired glucose tolerance and insulin resistance
17-hydroxyprogesterone	Evaluate for congenital adrenal hyperplasia
DHEAS	If hyperandrogenism is present, evaluate for adrenal etiology
Free cortisol, 24-hour urine collection	To rule out Cushing's syndrome

of the thyroid is also important, because abnormalities are implicated in reproductive disorders such as ovulatory subfertility and pregnancy loss. An elevated serum prolactin warrants a repeat morning fasting level, and if persistently elevated then head magnetic resonance imaging (MRI) is indicated to investigate whether a pituitary adenoma is present. Oligomenorrheic women with signs of hyperandrogenism should be evaluated for polycystic ovarian syndrome as well as adrenal disorders such as adult-onset congenital adrenal hyperplasia and androgen-producing tumors. Important laboratory tests include total testosterone, 17-hydroxyprogesterone, and dehydroepiandrosterone sulfate (DHEAS) levels. Treatment of the cause of ovulatory dysfunction may result in resumption of ovulation, and hence improved fertility.

Amenorrhea may signify anovulation, but requires a different approach. First, pregnancy should be excluded. A progestin challenge test (such as medroxyprogesterone acetate 10 mg/day for 10 days) should result in bleeding within 1 week after the course of medication; this identifies the presence of adequate estrogen levels to stimulate endometrial growth and a patent outflow tract. Absence of a progesterone withdrawal bleed may result from hypothalamic dysfunction, ovarian failure, or an outflow tract abnormality such as cervical stenosis or intrauterine synechiae. Pelvic imaging and further hormonal evaluation (FSH, LH, estradiol) are indicated.

Assessment of cervical factor

In reproduction, normal midcycle cervical mucus facilitates the transport of sperm into the uterus. The history and physical examination may elicit potential problems with the cervix, including prior infection, cytologic abnormality, surgery, or a congenital malformation that may impair cervical function. Documentation of a recent normal Pap smear and cervical cultures is reasonable.

The postcoital test has been used to evaluate the adequacy of cervical mucus and its interaction with sperm. This test requires obtaining a sample of cervical mucus 2–12 hours after intercourse that occurs 1–3 days prior to ovulation. Standard criteria include the presence of cervical mucus ferning, more than 5 cm of spinnbarkeit (the distance the mucus can be stretched before breaking), and at least five motile sperm per high-powered field.[10] The utility and validity of the postcoital test have been questioned. Routine use of this test leads to additional tests and treatment, but similar pregnancy rates when compared with infertility evaluations that did not use the test.[18] Furthermore, there is no consensus on test technique and interpretation, and the reproducibility of the test is poor.[12] Contemporary fertility treatment with intrauterine insemination or in vitro fertilization bypasses any abnormality of the cervix or cervical mucus. Due to limited diagnostic utility, routine use of the postcoital test is not indicated.[12,19]

Assessment of uterine factor

Uterine abnormalities sufficient to cause infertility are uncommon, but must be investigated. Details in a woman's medical history such as abnormal uterine bleeding, miscarriage, prior uterine surgery, or diethylstilbestrol exposure may heighten suspicion of a significant uterine abnormality such as leiomyomas, endometrial polyps, intrauterine adhesions, or Mullerian anomalies. Overall, uterine pathology is present in up to 10% of infertile women, and in 15–55% of women with recurrent pregnancy loss.[20] Acquired uterine abnormalities may impair embryo implantation; congenital anomalies are associated with difficulty maintaining a pregnancy, not an impaired ability to conceive.[20–22] The septate uterus is the most common Mullerian anomaly; it has a prevalence of 1% in infertile women and 3.3% in women with recurrent pregnancy loss.[23]

Assessment of the uterus and endometrial cavity is accomplished with transvaginal ultrasonography, hysterosalpingography (HSG), or saline-infusion sonohysterography (SHG); hysteroscopy is usually reserved for evaluation and treatment of abnormalities identified by less invasive methods. Each test has inherent strengths and weaknesses, and therefore a combination of modalities may be reasonable: transvaginal ultrasonography assesses the uterus and adnexa but may not recognize an abnormal uterine cavity; HSG evaluates the fallopian tubes and provides a limited-to-adequate view of the uterine cavity; SHG assesses the uterus, endometrial cavity, and adnexa, and can be used to evaluate the fallopian tubes. Furthermore, magnetic resonance imaging provides excellent delineation of pelvic structures and is considered the gold standard for the evaluation of Mullerian anomalies.[24]

A comparison of methods to evaluate submucosal myomas determined that SHG was the most accurate for detecting size, location, and intracavitary growth; transvaginal ultrasonography was less accurate in determining the intracavitary involvement; and hysteroscopy was the least accurate for predicting size, but precisely diagnosed the type of mass and its location.[25] When hysteroscopy was performed after HSG, 43% of subjects with normal HSG results had abnormal surgical findings.[26] For evaluation of the uterus, SHG is comparable to hysteroscopy, and superior to HSG or transvaginal ultrasonography.[27]

Assessment of tubal and peritoneal factors

Abnormalities of the fallopian tubes and pelvic peritoneum may impair transport of the oocyte, sperm, and embryo. A history of pelvic inflammatory disease or other pelvic infection, endometriosis, abdominal or pelvic surgery, or pelvic pain may be associated with tubal or peritoneal pathology. Evaluation of the fallopian tubes and pelvis may be achieved with hysterosalpingography, air-contrast sonohysterography, or diagnostic laparoscopy, and chlamydia antibody testing is an effective screening test.

Hysterosalpingography documents patency of the fallopian tubes or the location of tubal obstruction; it has less utility for evaluation of the uterine cavity. This test is commonly performed between the end of menses and ovulation. Pre-procedure administration of a non-steroidal anti-inflammatory medication such as ibuprofen may decrease patient discomfort during the test, and a short course of antibiotics (e.g. doxycycline 100 mg orally twice daily for 3 days) may be prescribed as prophylaxis against infection. Compared with laparoscopy with chromopertubation, HSG has lower sensitivity (54–65%) and specificity (83%) for tubal disease.[28,29] It is reliable for detecting significant tubal pathology and obstruction, but misses 20–30% of tubal abnormalities such as subtle peritubal or peritoneal

adhesions or partial tubal obstruction.[30] Furthermore, proximal tubal obstruction on HSG may be a false-positive finding 50% of the time.[31] Rotation of the patient so that the obstructed tube is inferior may resolve this finding in 50% of cases.[32] HSG has several advantages: it is minimally invasive, it is relatively quick to perform, and no anesthesia is needed.[33,34] In addition, tubal flushing during HSG with oil-soluble contrast medium is associated with a significant increase in the likelihood of pregnancy compared with no intervention; water-soluble contrast medium appears to be similarly effective, although the data on this contrast medium are less clear.[35]

Air-contrast SHG involves the injection of saline solution into the uterine cavity followed with a small amount of air, and passage of bubbles through the cornua and fallopian tubes is assessed.[36] Findings in this procedure are 79.4% concordant with laparoscopic chromopertubation.[36] Beyond assessing tubal patency, this method provides evaluation of the uterus and ovaries.[37] Furthermore, this method is inexpensive and better tolerated by patients than HSG, and provides rapid results.[38,39]

Laparoscopy with chromopertubation is considered the gold standard for evaluating tubal patency and function. Furthermore, laparoscopy enables the diagnosis and treatment of pelvic abnormalities such as partial tubal obstruction, peritubal adhesions, hydrosalpinges, and endometriosis. Endometriosis occurs with higher frequency among infertile women compared with fertile women.[40] It is reasonable to consider laparoscopy in infertile women with pelvic pain or other symptoms of endometriosis, a history of infection or surgery, an abnormal HSG, or unexplained infertility, especially when a period of treatment has not led to conception.

Lastly, chlamydia antibody testing (CAT) is a cost-effective and non-invasive approach for assessing a previous infection with *Chlamydia trachomatis*, and hence indirectly evaluates the fallopian tubes.[41] Several serologic techniques are available. A meta-analysis determined that CAT can be used instead of HSG as an initial screen for tubal disease since the discriminative ability of the two tests is comparable.[41] However, this test does not provide information about the pelvic anatomy, and has no potentially therapeutic effect.

Assessment of ovarian reserve

Increasing maternal age is associated with a predictable decrease in fecundability due to a decline in oocyte quantity and quality (Figure 10.2). Aging oocytes have chromosomal, morphologic, and functional abnormalities, ovaries with fewer oocytes exhibit decreased ovarian reserve, and ovulatory dysfunction can result from an altered hormonal environment.[42–45] Furthermore, older women have had more time to develop conditions associated with infertility such as endometriosis, uterine myomas, and pelvic infections, as well as more time for exposure to environmental insults such as tobacco smoke, radiation, or occupational exposures.

The probability of clinical pregnancy in fertile women with similarly aged partners after intercourse on the most fertile day of the cycle is 50% at 19–26 years, 40% at 27–34 years, and 30% at 35–39 years.[46] Similarly, age is the most important predictor of pregnancy rates for women undergoing in vitro fertilization (IVF).[45] Ovarian reserve should be assessed in women aged 35 and older, and in women with other risk factors for ovarian dysfunction or premature ovarian failure such as previous ovarian surgery or oophorectomy, poor response to fertility treatment, exposure to chemotherapy or radiation therapy, tobacco use, and unexplained infertility.[12]

The evaluation of ovarian reserve to predict the quality and quantity of remaining oocytes, and hence to assess the chance of pregnancy, is imperfect; many infertile women have normal tests, and women with abnormal testing still conceive. Along with maternal age, early follicular phase serum FSH and estradiol levels are the most commonly used tests to assess ovarian reserve.[47] An elevated cycle day-3 serum FSH level indicates a depleted follicular pool and decreased fecundability, and a high cycle day-3 estradiol level suggests fewer available oocytes and rapid follicular recruitment. However, prediction of pregnancy rates based on an elevated basal FSH is limited in women with ovulatory menstrual cycles.[48] A basal FSH level of 15–20 mIU/ml or a basal estradiol level exceeding 100 pg/ml is concerning for diminished ovarian reserve and thus a lower chance of conception (these values depend on a given laboratory's threshold for normal values). Overall, basal FSH as a marker of ovarian reserve may be better predictive of oocyte production capacity, and maternal age may be more indicative of oocyte quality.[49,50] With fertility treatment, approximately 5% of women with diminished ovarian reserve will achieve pregnancy.[51]

The limited predictive value of age and cycle day-3 serum FSH has led to the use of the clomiphene citrate challenge test (CCCT), a more dynamic assessment of ovarian reserve.[52] In the CCCT, clomiphene citrate (100 mg) is administered daily on cycle days 5–9, and the serum FSH level is measured on cycle days 3 and 10. An abnormal elevation of serum FSH on either day indicates decreased ovarian reserve. Women with a normal CCCT respond better to controlled ovarian hyperstimulation, and this test has been shown to be more sensitive than basal FSH alone.[53] As for the ability of the CCCT to predict fertility treatment outcome, a normal result has low utility, since many infertile women have normal testing.[54] Although an abnormal CCCT strongly suggests that treatment will not result in pregnancy, one study of women less than 40 years old undergoing IVF determined that there was no CCCT FSH threshold value above which conception did not occur.[54,55]

Ovarian characteristics on transvaginal ultrasonography have been used to further assess ovarian potential during hormone stimulation.[56–59] Among the ultrasonography markers, a decreased basal antral follicle count has been shown to be a predictor of poor ovarian response to controlled ovarian stimulation.[60] In a prospective study of 120 women undergoing their first IVF cycle, the antral follicle count was the best single predictor of poor ovarian response compared with total ovarian volume, basal FSH, estradiol, and inhibin-B levels to determine ovarian reserve.[47] Furthermore, the antral follicle count (AFC) has been shown to correlate with maternal age, and may reflect the size of the available primordial follicle pool.[61] Currently, the antral follicle count seems to promise better prognostic information about ovarian response during hormone stimulation for IVF than does the patient's chronologic age and available endocrine markers.[62–64]

Assessment of male factor

During evaluation of an infertile couple, an appropriate history should be obtained from the male partner as detailed above. The male partner should undergo semen analysis. Physical examination of the male partner may not be necessary unless the history or semen analysis indicates a potential abnormality.

Etiologies of male infertility include hypothalamic–pituitary disease (1–2%; congenital, acquired, or systemic disorders causing gonadal dysfunction), testicular disease (30–40%; congenital, acquired, or systemic disorders causing testicular abnormalities), post-testicular defects (10–20%; disorders of sperm transport or ejaculation), and unexplained infertility (40–50%; abnormal semen analysis with unidentifiable cause; inability to achieve pregnancy with a seemingly normal female partner). Occasionally, male infertility may be the presenting sign of a serious underlying medical condition

Table 10.3   Reference values for semen analysis

Parameter	Normal values
Ejaculate volume	1.5–5.0 ml
pH	>7.2
Sperm concentration	>20 million/ml
Total sperm number	>40 million/ejaculate
Percentage motility	>50%
Forward progression	>2 (scale 0–4)
Normal morphology	>50% normal (WHO, 1987[66])
	>30% normal (WHO, 1992[67])
	>14% normal (Kruger Strict Criteria, WHO, 1999[68])
Sperm agglutination	<2 (scale 0–3)
Viscosity	<3 (scale 0–4)

such as testicular cancer or a pituitary tumor, and thus an appropriate evaluation is essential.[65]

Semen analysis

The semen sample should be obtained after 2–3 days of abstinence. Although a masturbated sample collected in the physician's office is preferred, other options include a specimen collected at home or in condoms without chemical additives, provided that the laboratory receives the specimen within 1 hour. The standard semen analysis measures seminal volume, pH, liquefaction time, sperm concentration, sperm motility and morphology, and microscopic debris and agglutination.

The World Health Organization (WHO) established normal semen measurements based on a study from 1951[66–68] (Table 10.3). Although these standards are widely used, significant overlap exists between semen parameters of fertile and infertile men. Recently, sperm concentration, motility, and morphology of fertile and infertile men were compared, and fertile and subfertile cut-off values were identified with a sizable 'indeterminate' range between the two values.[69] No single parameter is able to predict fertility; however, the percentage of sperm with normal morphology appears to be the best discriminator.[70] An abnormal semen analysis should prompt a repeat test with emphasis on abstinence and specimen collection and transport. Due to the inherent variability of semen samples, some authorities recommend routine collection of two semen samples 1–2 weeks apart. A persistently abnormal semen analysis should instigate further evaluation and referral to a urologist or reproductive endocrinologist specializing in male infertility.

Certain abnormalities identified by semen analysis may point toward an etiology of male infertility. Sperm concentration is usually 20 million/ml or greater,

although lower counts do not preclude fertility.[68] Azoospermia (no sperm present) or severe oligospermia (fewer than 5 million/ml) may be associated with problems such as defective testicular sperm production, genital tract obstruction, retrograde ejaculation, a varicocele, a genetic or endocrine disorder, toxin exposure, infection, or a medication effect. Low semen volume with severe oligospermia or azoospermia is characteristic of genital tract obstruction (such as congenital absence of the vas deferens and ejaculatory duct obstruction). An absent vas deferens on physical examination and a low semen pH diagnose congenital absence of the vas deferens; transrectal ultrasonographic identification of dilated seminal vesicles diagnoses ejaculatory duct obstruction. Asthenospermia (low sperm motility) is concerning for antisperm antibodies, partial obstruction, infection, or sperm structural defects. Teratospermia (abnormal morphology) suggests a genetic disorder, varicocele, infection, medication effect, or toxin exposure. Identification of white blood cells in semen suggests the presence of infection or inflammation. Abnormalities in sperm concentration, motility, and morphology may also be idiopathic. Further testing of sperm function with specialized diagnostic tests is seldom performed, and rarely warranted in the routine evaluation of infertile men.[71]

Sperm agglutination (sperm clumping visualized on microscopy) suggests autoimmunity; sperm autoantibodies are present in approximately 4–8% of subfertile men.[72] These antibodies are also implicated in abnormal postcoital tests.[72] The occurrence of these antibodies may be due to a disruption of the blood–testis barrier such as with trauma, testicular torsion, vasectomy reversal, obstruction of the vas deferens, and genital tract infection. Antibodies are considered clinically significant when they coat more than 50% of spermatozoa and when the spermatozoa fail to penetrate preovulatory cervical mucus or achieve fertilization.[72]

A varicocele can be found in men with normal semen parameters and normal fertility; however, it is more common in men with abnormal semen.[73] In appropriate candidates, varicocele repair has been shown to improve semen parameters, and this low-risk procedure may improve fertility.[74] However, two meta-analyses reported no fertility benefit of varicocele repair,[75,76] and therefore the procedure is not routinely recommended.

Genetic testing

Genetic testing is appropriate for men with severe oligospermia and azoospermia (Table 10.4); genetic

Table 10.4   Recommended testing for severe male factor infertility

Test	Indication
Repeat semen analysis	Recommended if first analysis is abnormal
Post-ejaculatory urinalysis	Low volume (< 1.0 ml) or absent ejaculate concerning for retrograde ejaculation
Transrectal ultrasonography	Low volume, oligoasthenospermic, or azoospermic ejaculate concerning for complete or partial ejaculatory duct obstruction
Scrotal ultrasonography	May identify non-palpable scrotal abnormalities, can clarify ambiguous examintion findings
Endocrine evaluation	Abnormal semen analysis (especially with concentration < 10 million/ml), impaired sexual function, concern for an endocrinopathy
• Initial: FSH, total testosterone	
• If low testosterone: check total and free testosterone, LH, prolactin	
Cystic fibrosis gene mutations	Obstructive azoospermia, physical examination reveals absent vas deferens
Karyotype Y-chromosome microdeletions	Non-obstructive azoospermia or severe oligospermia

abnormalities may affect sperm production or transport. Assisted reproductive technologies (ART) give these men a chance to father a child; however, the risk of transmitting a genetic disorder must be addressed. The cystic fibrosis transmembrane conductase regulator (CFTR) gene mutations, somatic and sex chromosome abnormalities, and microdeletions of the Y chromosome are the most common abnormalities identified. As with any identified genetic condition, genetic counseling is recommended prior to fertility treatment.

Mutations in one or both copies of the CFTR gene are associated with congenital bilateral absence of the vas deferens (CBAVD);[77] however, many of these men have no pulmonary symptoms. Approximately two-thirds of men with CBAVD have a CFTR gene mutation, while the majority of men with clinical cystic fibrosis have CBAVD.[71] Other findings associated with CFTR gene abnormalities include congenital bilateral obstruction of the epididymides or unilateral agenesis of the vas deferens.[71] If a man has any of these abnormalities and a CFTR gene mutation is not identified, it should be assumed that he carries an abnormality that is currently unidentifiable.[71] Furthermore, the female partner must also undergo CFTR gene testing.

The prevalence of karyotype abnormalities is inversely related to the sperm concentration; karyotype abnormalities are identified in 10–15% of azoospermic men, 5% of oligospermic men, and less than 1% of men with normal sperm counts.[71] Klinefelter's syndrome (47,XXY) accounts for approximately two-thirds of the chromosomal abnormalities identified in infertile men.[78] Abnormalities of autosomal chromosomes, such as inversions and translocations, are identified more frequently in infertile compared with fertile men.[71] These chromosomal defects are associated with miscarriage,

and offspring with chromosomal and congenital abnormalities. Therefore, a karyotype is indicated in men with severe oligospermia or non-obstructive azoospermia prior to attempting conception with ART.

Microdeletions in the Y chromosome have been identified in 10–15% of men with severe oligospermia or azoospermia;[79] these deletions are rarely found in men with sperm concentrations greater than 5 million/ml.[80] The microdeletions are found along the long arm of the Y chromosome in three main loci of the azoospermic factor (AZF) region (AZFa, AZFb, AZFc),[80,81] and are not detected by routine karyotype analysis. If conception occurs with ART then Y chromosome microdeletions, and hence altered testicular development and spermatogenesis, can be transmitted from father to son.[82]

Endocrine testing

Endocrine evaluation is appropriate for infertile men with abnormal sperm concentrations or signs of androgen deficiency (Table 10.4). Serum total testosterone is utilized as the initial screening test; a borderline value can be further assessed by checking the serum free testosterone level. Low testosterone levels require evaluation of FSH and LH levels. Primary hypogonadism is suggested by low total testosterone, and elevated LH and FSH levels. Low levels of total testosterone, LH, and FSH indicate secondary hypogonadism. A low LH level in the setting of oligospermia and a well-androgenized man is suspicious for exogenous steroid use (steroids suppress LH secretion); total testosterone levels can be variable. Serum prolactin testing is indicated to rule out a pituitary adenoma in men with low serum testosterone and normal to low serum LH levels.

Diagnosis of unexplained infertility

Unexplained infertility is diagnosed when a comprehensive evaluation does not reveal an identifiable etiology of the couple's infertility. This diagnosis implies a normal semen analysis, evidence of ovulation, adequate ovarian reserve, a normal uterine cavity, and bilateral tubal patency; approximately 10–15% of infertile couples meet these criteria. The diagnosis of unexplained infertility likely signifies the presence of one or more mild abnormalities in follicular development, ovulation, oocyte or sperm function, fertilization, implantation, or early embryo development that may not be detected by current tests. The presence of several borderline factors can be additive, causing a decrease in fertility. With expectant management, 1–3% of couples with unexplained infertility conceive each month;[12,83,84] however, this rate is influenced by the age of the female partner and duration of infertility.[9]

The use of diagnostic laparoscopy to evaluate a woman with unexplained infertility remains controversial. Despite a normal pelvic examination and HSG, laparoscopy may identify abnormal fallopian tubes, pelvic adhesions, endometriosis, or other pelvic pathology in a number of women. These findings can be treated at the time of diagnosis, and may improve fertility in a subset of patients.[85,86] Furthermore, surgical findings may encourage more aggressive medical treatment of fertility such as controlled ovarian hyperstimulation (COH) or IVF. However, it is also reasonable to proceed with medical treatment options for infertility without laparoscopy.[86]

Assessment of lifestyle factors affecting fertility

Certain lifestyle factors may impact on fertility, and attention should be paid to those over which one has some control: weight, cigarette smoking, alcohol consumption, marijuana use, caffeine consumption, and stress. There are no prospective randomized controlled trials to support certain recommendations, and most studies investigating the effect of these exposures on fertility are observational, and thus subject to bias and confounding factors. Although most of these lifestyle factors do not cause sterility, they may impair fecundability, lengthen the time to conception, or result in a cumulative negative effect.[87]

Extremes of body mass index (BMI) are associated with health risks and reproductive dysfunction.

Underweight (BMI $<17\,\text{kg/m}^2$), overweight (BMI $25–29.9\,\text{kg/m}^2$), and obese (BMI $>30\,\text{kg/m}^2$) women have an increased rate of anovulatory infertility.[88] Abnormalities of gonadotropin releasing hormone (GnRH) and pituitary gonadotropin secretion are common in underweight, overweight, and obese women.[88] Weight reduction in obese infertile women is associated with increased frequency of ovulation and likelihood of pregnancy.[89] For optimal health and fertility potential, a BMI of $20–25\,\text{kg/m}^2$ is recommended.

Up to 13% of infertility may be attributable to cigarette smoking.[90,91] Smoking more than 10 cigarettes a day has been associated with decreased fertility in females due to tubal abnormalities, cervical abnormalities, premature ovarian aging and depletion of oocytes, spontaneous abortion, and ectopic pregnancy.[90,92] A meta-analysis of reproductive-aged women including 11 000 smokers and 20 000 non-smokers identified an association between cigarette smoking and an increase in infertility and time to conception.[91] In contrast, smoking has not been shown to affect male fertility, despite modest reductions in semen quality and altered hormone levels.[93]

Other types of substance abuse can adversely affect fertility. Moderate alcohol consumption in women has been shown to increase the risk of anovulatory infertility and endometriosis-associated infertility,[94,95] and to delay time to conception.[96] Heavy alcohol consumption in men is associated with reduced testosterone production, decreased semen quality, and impotence.[95] Marijuana inhibits the secretion of GnRH and thus can suppress reproductive function in either partner,[97] and can impair ovulatory function in women.[98] Caffeine consumption of more than 250 mg daily (approximately 2–3 cups of coffee daily) is associated with a delay in time to conception,[99] and greater consumption may increase the risk of spontaneous abortion.[100]

Based on reasonable evidence, several recommendations can be made for couples attempting to conceive. Maintenance of a BMI of $20–25\,\text{kg/m}^2$ is ideal for long-term and reproductive health. Both partners should be encouraged to quit smoking due to adverse effects on health, fertility, and pregnancy outcome. Much of the subfertility attributed to smoking may be reversed within 1 year.[90] Due to the association between moderate alcohol consumption and subfertility as well as the negative effects of alcohol on a developing fetus, consumption should be limited to four drinks per week when attempting to conceive, and abstinence should be maintained during pregnancy. Caffeine intake should be less than 250 mg daily. It is noteworthy that although sensible, these lifestyle modifications have not yet been proven to benefit fertility.

APPROACHES TO INFERTILITY TREATMENT

A couple's infertility may be due to a single identified abnormality, or may be multifactorial. Numerous medical, surgical, and assisted reproductive technology treatments are available to help a couple conceive. This section will review the most common therapies for fertility treatment. Common disorders and the therapies recommended to maximize the chance of conception will follow.

Ovulation induction

The goal of ovulation induction is monofollicular development in women with ovulatory disorders. The most commonly used medication is *clomiphene citrate*, a selective estrogen receptor modulator (SERM) that competitively inhibits estrogen binding to the estrogen receptor and has both estrogen agonist and antagonist effects depending on the target tissue. Antiestrogen effects of clomiphene promote gonadotropin release from the pituitary while they may cause thinning of the endometrium and decreased cervical mucus.[101] This medication is most effective in oligo-ovulatory women with normal gonadotropin and estrogen levels (WHO class 2), and is often ineffective in hypoestrogenic women with low or high gonadotropin levels (WHO classes 1 and 3). Clomiphene is started between cycle days 3 and 5 at a dose of 50 mg daily for 5 days. The LH surge can occur from 5 to 12 days after the last pill, or human chorionic gonadotropin (hCG) may be used to trigger ovulation in a timed manner. Regular midcycle intercourse, intercourse timed to the urinary LH kit or ultrasonographic evidence of a mature follicle, or intrauterine inseminations timed similarly may be done. A mid-luteal phase progesterone level can also be used to confirm ovulation. If ovulation does not occur, the dose is increased by 50 mg. The maximum clomiphene dose recommended is 150 mg, although dosages up to 250 mg can be used.[102]

A maximum of six ovulatory clomiphene cycles without conception is recommended prior to more aggressive treatment. Clomiphene therapy is associated with an ovulation rate of 73%, a pregnancy rate of 36%, and a multiple pregnancy rate of approximately 10%, the majority of which are twin gestations.[103] The discrepancy between the ovulation and pregnancy rates is attributed

to the antiestrogen effects of clomiphene which may impair fertilization and implantation.[103] Uncomplicated ovarian enlargement may occur, but ovarian hyperstimulation syndrome is rare. If conception is not achieved after six cycles, re-evaluation is recommended.

Tamoxifen is another SERM that can induce ovulation. At the endometrial level, this medication has less antiestrogenic effect compared to clomiphene. Similar to the clomiphene protocol, 20 mg of tamoxifen is given for 5 days starting between cycle days 3 and 5. Tamoxifen has a similar ovulation and pregnancy rate compared with clomiphene.[104]

Aromatase inhibitors such as letrozole and anastrozole block the conversion of testosterone to estradiol, and androstenedione to estrone. Markedly decreased systemic estrogen levels reduce the negative feedback of estrogen on the pituitary. Studies have shown that aromatase inhibitors are effective for ovulation induction; however, this is not an approved indication. Although a potential risk of fetal teratogenicity has been reported, findings from a recent large study support the safety and efficacy of letrozole for ovulation induction.[105] Due to fewer antiestrogenic effects on the endometrium and cervical mucus, aromatase inhibitors may be a reasonable alternative for women who have a suboptimal response to clomiphene. Other advantages with this therapy include the production of fewer follicles, lower estrogen levels, and a lower risk of multiple gestation.[106]

Controlled ovarian hyperstimulation

Gonadotropin therapy can be used to achieve monofollicular ovulation in anovulatory women, and for COH in women where the goal is several mature follicles. Available preparations include human menopausal gonadotropins (hMG: LH and FSH extracted from the urine of postmenopausal women) and recombinant human FSH. Various low-dose medication protocols are effective for ovulation induction, including those in which the dose of FSH is raised (step-up protocol) or lowered (step-down protocol) during stimulation. Based on body weight, age, infertility diagnosis, and response to previous fertility therapy, a higher dose of gonadotropins may be used for COH. Due to the potency of gonadotropin preparations, follicular growth should be monitored with transvaginal ultrasonography and serial serum estradiol measurements. A dose of hCG is administered when at least one follicle appears to be mature: follicle diameter of 18 mm or serum estradiol concentration of 200 pg/ml per dominant follicle. Intrauterine inseminations are commonly performed within 12–36 hours from hCG administration to optimally time the placement of semen in the uterus.

Risks of COH include ovarian hyperstimulation syndrome (OHSS), multiple gestations, and an increased rate of ectopic pregnancy. OHSS is a potentially life-threatening complication of ovarian stimulation. Mild forms of OHSS involve marked ovarian enlargement with multiple cysts, abdominal distension, and discomfort; severe OHSS is associated with hemoconcentration, third-spacing of fluid, and possibly thromboembolism, stroke, and death. Mild OHSS can occur in up to 25% of women undergoing ovarian stimulation; severe OHSS occurs in 1–2% of COH patients and 0.2% of IVF patients.[107] The risk of multiple gestations depends on the number of mature follicles at the end of ovarian stimulation,[108] and is greater with gonadotropin therapy than with other ovulation induction agents (25% vs 10% of those who conceive).

Intrauterine insemination

The process of intrauterine insemination involves washing an ejaculated semen specimen to remove prostaglandins, bacteria, and proteins, suspending the sperm in a small volume of culture media, and placing a thin catheter through the cervix into the endometrial cavity where the sperm suspension is released. In men with retrograde ejaculation, intrauterine insemination (IUI) can be performed after sperm are retrieved from a urine sample and washed. Using ovulation predictor kits or an hCG injection, IUI is timed to coincide with ovulation. Abstinence from ejaculation for 48–72 hours prior to IUI is associated with higher pregnancy rates.[109] A total motile sperm count of at least one million must be inseminated; pregnancy is rarely achieved with lower counts.[110] In couples with male infertility, pregnancy rates are significantly increased with IUI.[111] One trial compared IUI with intracervical insemination in couples with the majority having unexplained infertility; a significant increase in pregnancy rates was noted with IUI cycles (4.9% vs 2.0%).[112] Furthermore, the addition of IUI to clomiphene or gonadotropin therapy in couples with unexplained infertility or endometriosis in the female partner increases the pregnancy rate.[112]

Assisted reproductive technologies

Assisted reproductive technologies (ART) include all procedures that involve manipulation of gametes,

zygotes, or embryos to achieve pregnancy. IVF accounts for more than 99% of all ART procedures in the United States.[113] In general, the IVF procedure involves retrieval of oocytes from a woman's ovaries, oocyte fertilization *in vitro* in the laboratory, and transfer of the resulting embryo(s) into a woman's uterus through the cervix. For some IVF procedures, fertilization involves intracytoplasmic sperm injection (ICSI) in which a single sperm is injected directly into the oocyte. In addition, ART are often categorized according to whether the procedure used a woman's own oocytes (non-donor) or oocytes from another woman (donor), and according to whether the embryos were newly fertilized (fresh) or previously fertilized, cryopreserved, and then thawed (frozen).

Indications for IVF include absent or blocked fallopian tubes, failed tuboplasty, severe pelvic disease, severe endometriosis, diminished ovarian reserve, oligo-ovulation, severe male factor infertility, unexplained infertility, or failed treatment with less invasive therapies. IVF involves exogenous gonadotropin administration (usually recombinant FSH) to achieve the development of multiple follicles, a GnRH agonist or antagonist to prevent the endogenous LH surge and ovulation, and administration of hCG to initiate the ovulation of mature follicles.

IVF medication protocols vary based on preparation, dose, and timing of gonadotropins and GnRH analogs used. During COH, close monitoring with transvaginal ultrasonography and serum estradiol levels is necessary to maximize adequate response and safety, and enable medication adjustments. When follicles are determined to be mature, ovulation is triggered with hCG, and 36 hours later, oocyte retrieval is performed by transvaginal ultrasonography-guided follicle aspiration. After retrieval, oocytes are inseminated (mixed with spermatozoa in a small amount of culture medium) or undergo ICSI as indicated, and the woman begins progesterone supplementation. Fertilization is evident approximately 18 hours after exposure of the oocyte to sperm. Embryos are maintained in culture for several days, during which development is carefully monitored. The number and quality of embryos determines the timing of embryo transfer, between 3 and 5 days after oocyte retrieval. If preimplantation genetic diagnosis (PGD) is required, a post-fertilization polar body or an 8-cell embryo is biopsied, and, depending on the test results, the embryo is transferred on day 5. Transcervical embryo transfer is commonly performed with transabdominal ultrasonographic guidance. If viable embryos remain after transfer, embryo cryopreservation may be considered. If conception occurs, intramuscular or vaginal progesterone supplementation continues until 10–12 weeks gestational age; progesterone supplementation in ART is associated with increased pregnancy rates.[114]

The Society of Assisted Reproductive Technology reported that more than 122 000 IVF cycles were performed in 2005 (Figure 10.3).[113] In IVF cycles for women less than 35 years of age using fresh non-donor oocytes, a mean number of 2.4 embryos were transferred, achieving a 42.9% pregnancy rate and a 37.1% live birth rate. However, IVF pregnancy and live birth rates are age dependent (Figure 10.4). Of those cycles that resulted in live births, approximately 30% resulted in twins and 2–3% resulted in triplets or greater. When fresh donor oocytes were used, transfer of a mean number of 2.3 embryos resulted in a 52.2% live birth rate, including a 40% multiple live birth rate. The multiple pregnancy rate is determined by the patient's age, embryo quality, and number of embryos transferred into the uterus: the more embryos transferred, the greater the chance of pregnancy and the greater chance of a multiple gestation. With IVF, the spontaneous abortion rate is approximately 15%, and depends on the woman's age and the number of gestations present.

TREATMENT OPTIONS FOR SPECIFIC ETIOLOGIES OF INFERTILITY

Ovulation disorders

Ovulatory disorders have been classified by the WHO, and the etiology of ovulatory dysfunction determines the treatment options for achieving pregnancy. WHO class 1 anovulation is hypogonadotropic hypogonadism (i.e. hypothalamic amenorrhea, Kallman's syndrome) and accounts for 5–10% of anovulation. These women have low levels of FSH and estradiol due to decreased GnRH secretion from the hypothalamus or abnormal pituitary response to GnRH, and many are amenorrheic. Reversible etiologies of hypothalamic amenorrhea include high levels of stress, intense exercise, and low body weight. It is recommended that attempts be made to reverse these lifestyle factors before considering treatment with medications. Due to low levels of endogenous gonadotropins in this situation, the most effective treatment is ovulation induction with gonadotropins.

Normogonadotropic normoestrogenic anovulation comprises the WHO class 2 category, and represents 70–85% of anovulatory women. The most common disorder is polycystic ovarian syndrome (PCOS). This

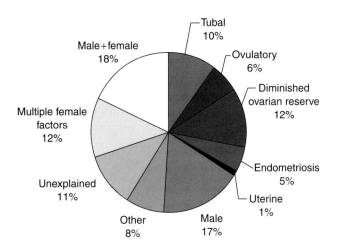

Figure 10.3 Etiologies of infertility in women undergoing IVF. Data from the Society for Assisted Reproductive Technology, 2005[113]

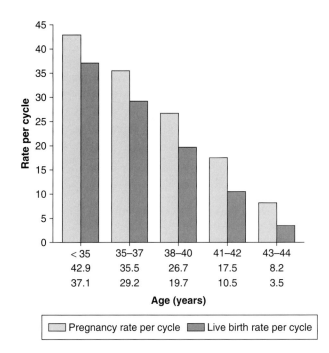

Figure 10.4 Pregnancy rate and live birth rate per IVF cycle based on the woman's age. Data from the Society for Assisted Reproductive Technology, 2005[113]

condition is often associated with increased body mass index, and loss of 5–10% of body weight can restore ovulation in at least 50% of overweight women with PCOS within 6 months.[115] In women who demonstrate insulin resistance, insulin-sensitizing agents are used to normalize insulin and glucose levels and may restore ovulation. Metformin, an oral biguanide, is commonly used in this situation; it acts to improve peripheral sensitivity to insulin and to decrease hepatic glucose production. Treatment of PCOS, including the use of metformin, is discussed in detail in Chapter 12. Ovulation may be restored with metformin or induced with clomiphene citrate, or a combination of the two therapies can be used.[116–118] A recent study determined that clomiphene alone is superior to metformin for achieving live birth in infertile women with PCOS.[119] If conception is not achieved with metformin and/or ovulation induction with clomiphene, other options include gonadotropin stimulation alone or combined with intrauterine insemination, in vitro fertilization, or surgery. Laparoscopic ovarian wedge resection and ovarian drilling are surgical treatments for PCOS. These procedures decrease the androgen-producing ovarian stroma which may induce ovulation, but do not affect serum insulin levels.[120] After this procedure, the pregnancy rate at 6–12 months is similar to that achieved with 3–6 months of ovulation induction with gonadotropins, and the multiple pregnancy rate is lower;[121] this must be weighed against surgical risks including pelvic adhesions and ovarian damage.

WHO class 3 anovulation is defined by hypergonadotropic hypogonadism (i.e. premature ovarian failure, gonadal dysgenesis), and occurs in 10–30% of anovulatory women. Common etiologies include premature ovarian failure and ovarian resistance, and most of these women are amenorrheic. A large majority of these women do not respond to ovarian stimulation with gonadotropin therapy and hence require oocyte donation to conceive.

Hyperprolactinemic anovulation (5–10%) constitutes WHO class 4 anovulation. Elevated serum prolactin levels inhibit gonadotropin secretion, and hence estrogen secretion is decreased and anovulation occurs. These women may experience oligomenorrhea or amenorrhea. Head MRI can determine the presence of a pituitary microadenoma (< 1 cm) or macroadenoma (> 1 cm). Hyperprolactinemia with or without a pituitary adenoma is initially treated with dopamine agonist therapy; bromocriptine or cabergoline effectively normalize the serum prolactin level in more than 90% of patients. Ovulation usually returns with treatment of hyperprolactinemia, and if the woman remains anovulatory then ovulation induction methods can be utilized. Pituitary adenomas that are symptomatic or persist require evaluation by a neurosurgeon.

Uterine infertility

Uterine abnormalities that affect the endometrial cavity can be associated with poor reproductive outcomes: infertility and recurrent pregnancy loss (RPL).

Therefore, surgical correction is recommended for submucosal leiomyomas, endometrial polyps, and intrauterine adhesions; operative hysteroscopy is the preferred approach for isolated intrauterine pathology. Surgical repair of Mullerian anomalies is indicated in women with pelvic pain, endometriosis, an obstructive anomaly, recurrent pregnancy loss, and preterm delivery.[122] Uterine septa are also commonly resected in women with infertility.

Uterine leiomyomas with a submucosal component and intramural myomas that distort the endometrial cavity are associated with lower pregnancy and implantation rates with IVF, and outcomes improve after myomectomy.[123–125] The impact of intramural myomas without cavity distortion on fertility and reproductive outcomes remains unclear;[126] multiple studies demonstrate no effect of intramural myomas on IVF outcomes;[125,127,128] however, other studies identify lower IVF pregnancy rates with intramural myomas present,[129–131] especially when myomas measure 4 cm or greater.[132] Subserosal myomas do not affect reproductive outcomes.[124]

The surgical approach for uterine myomas is dictated by the location, number, and size of the myomas. Hysteroscopic myomectomy is preferred if more than 50% of the myoma is submucosal in location. If a transmural myoma with a submucosal component is present, or if the uterine cavity is distorted by multiple intramural and submucosal myomas, then an abdominal myomectomy may be the most effective procedure to correct uterine anatomy. The laparoscopic approach is feasible; however, a skilled laparoscopic surgeon is necessary, and this technique is associated with a higher risk of uterine rupture during a subsequent pregnancy.[133,134] Hysteroscopic or abdominal myomectomy does not appear to negatively impact on implantation or clinical pregnancy rates in subsequent IVF cycles.[135]

Endometrial polyps are commonly found in reproductive age women, and have been associated with spontaneous abortion after IVF[58] and lower pregnancy rates with IUI; pregnancy rates with IUI were markedly improved after hysteroscopic polypectomy.[136] When hysteroscopy is performed to evaluate an intrauterine lesion, and since data support that uterine cavity distortion with myomas adversely affects reproductive outcome, it is recommended that endometrial polyps, even if asymptomatic, be removed in infertile women.

Intrauterine adhesions (Asherman's syndrome) may develop as a result of intrauterine trauma, usually due to surgery or infection. Common sequelae of intrauterine adhesions are infertility (43%) and menstrual irregularity (62%).[137] Hysteroscopic lysis of adhesions in infertile women is associated with a live birth rate of up to 47%.[138,139] Overall, reproductive outcomes correlate best with the initial severity of intrauterine adhesions and the clinical presentation; women with recurrent pregnancy loss fare better than women with infertility.[138]

Unicornuate, didelphic, bicornuate, septate, arcuate, and diethylstilbestrol-exposed uteri are associated with adverse reproductive outcomes such as RPL and preterm delivery, but not infertility. Surgical repair of a didelphic or bicornuate uterus requires a major abdominal procedure such as the Strassman metroplasty, and should be considered in select women with poor reproductive outcomes.[140,141] In contrast, the septate uterus is associated with the poorest reproductive outcomes.[23] Although a uterine septum is not considered a cause of infertility, the association with RPL, the ease and low morbidity of hysteroscopic metroplasty, and the documented improvement in obstetrical outcomes after septum resection makes this a reasonable procedure to perform in women with infertility, RPL, and prior to undergoing ART.[22,142,143]

Tubal infertility

Management of tubal infertility depends on the location and degree of tubal impairment, the age and ovarian reserve of the woman, and the presence of other causes of infertility.[37] Overall, the most effective and successful management of all types of tubal infertility is to bypass the fallopian tubes with IVF. IVF is appropriate for women who decline surgery, who have other concomitant causes of infertility, or who have diminished ovarian reserve. Surgery is a reasonable initial option for mild to moderate tubal disease and for women who cannot afford IVF; women at advanced reproductive age and those with severe tubal disease should proceed directly to IVF.[144,145]

Proximal tubal occlusion diagnosed by HSG may be a false-positive result, and thus laparoscopy should be considered to better evaluate tubal patency and treat any other pelvic pathology. Proximal tubal occlusion can be treated with transcervical tubal cannulation. Hysteroscopic and fluoroscopic approaches are most commonly used, and have ongoing pregnancy rates of approximately 50% and 25%, respectively.[146] Although many proximal occlusions can be treated with cannulation, there is a risk of tubal perforation and further tubal damage, ectopic pregnancy, and reocclusion.[146] Another strategy for proximal occlusion is to excise

the occluded isthmic portion of tube and perform microsurgical tubocornual anastamosis; the ongoing pregnancy rate is 47%.[146]

Tubal surgery is most successful for distal occlusions, either with fimbrioplasty (lysis of fimbrial adhesions or dilatation of strictures) or neosalpingostomy (creation of a new distal tubal opening). Although laparotomy with microsurgical salpingostomy is associated with the highest ongoing pregnancy rates, the laparoscopic approach is less invasive and a reasonable option.[145] Pregnancy rates after salpingostomy for mild, moderate, and severe distal tubal disease are 81, 31, and 16%, respectively.[147] Distal tubal occlusion with hydrosalpinges can occur from pelvic infection or endometriosis. Management options for hydrosalpinx include needle drainage, salpingostomy, proximal tubal ligation, and salpingectomy.[148] The tubal fluid has been shown to have a direct toxic effect on embryos and a negative effect on the endometrium.[149–151] Data support that laparoscopic salpingectomy for hydrosalpinges prior to IVF improves implantation and pregnancy rates.[152–154]

Tubal occlusion due to prior sterilization may be amenable to surgical treatment depending on the method and location of sterilization, the degree of tubal damage, and the length of residual tube. Compared with electrocautery, sterilization with rings or clips is associated with more successful tubal anastamosis.[155] Isthmus–isthmus anastamoses are the most successful, and have a pregnancy rate of 81%.[156] The length of the longest anastamosed tube (in centimeters) multiplied by 10 reasonably approximates the subsequent term delivery rate.[156] Sterilization reversal in younger women with no other causes of infertility has a high success rate, and provides the opportunity for multiple subsequent pregnancies.

Endometriosis

Endometriosis is more commonly seen among infertile women compared with fertile women.[40] The association between endometriosis and infertility is attributed to distorted pelvic anatomy, altered peritoneal function, altered hormonal and cell-mediated function, endocrine and ovulatory abnormalities, and abnormal endometrial function and impaired implantation.[157] Medical management of any stage of endometriosis precludes pregnancy and does not improve fecundity,[86,157] and thus is not a reasonable option in women who wish to conceive.

Laparoscopy may be indicated in infertile women with pelvic pain or with known endometriosis, especially without another etiology of infertility. Two randomized trials explored rates of spontaneous conception in women with minimal-to-mild endometriosis after laparoscopy (diagnostic or for treatment of endometriosis);[158,159] results were conflicting, but a meta-analysis revealed that surgical treatment appears to improve fertility.[85] Although ablation of endometriosis and adhesiolysis for minimal-to-mild endometriosis may improve fecundity, women with endometriosis demonstrate reduced fecundity compared with normal fertile women.[85,86,157] There is no evidence that postoperative medical treatment enhances fertility, and it unnecessarily delays fertility treatment and the time to conception.[157]

No randomized prospective trials have investigated fecundity after conservative surgical treatment for moderate-to-severe endometriosis, but some data suggest that surgery may improve fecundity.[86,157,160] However, more than one surgery for advanced-stage endometriosis is not effective in improving fertility.[161] Although controversial, laparoscopic cystectomy for ovarian endometriomas greater than 4 cm may improve fertility in women with endometriosis who are attempting to conceive, particularly if undergoing IVF.[86] Cystectomy is preferable to and more effective than endometrioma drainage and coagulation.[86] Women with endometriomas should be counseled about the risk of decreased ovarian function after ovarian cystectomy, and the risk of oophorectomy.

Provided that the fallopian tubes are patent, ovulation stimulation with clomiphene or gonadotropins plus IUI is a reasonable initial therapy in infertile women with early-stage or advanced-stage endometriosis. It is appropriate to proceed with IVF for endometriosis-associated infertility if fallopian tubes are compromised, if other causes of infertility are present, or if prior therapies including surgery have failed.[86] However, women with endometriosis demonstrate lower IVF pregnancy rates than women with tubal infertility.[86,162] Prolonged GnRH agonist therapy for 3–6 months prior to IVF in women with endometriosis should be considered; this treatment has been shown to improve pregnancy rates.[163]

Male infertility

Treatment of male infertility includes endocrine therapies, intrauterine insemination (IUI), assisted reproductive technologies (ART), and use of donor sperm. Many of these therapies are best managed by a urologist or reproductive endocrinologist specializing in male fertility. Only men with infertility due to hypogonadotropic hypogonadism are candidates for specific medical treatments. Hyperprolactinemia (from a lactotroph adenoma) should be treated with a dopamine agonist such as bromocriptine or cabergoline.

Hypothalamic disease can be treated with gonadotropin-releasing hormone, and both hypothalamic and pituitary disease can be treated with gonadotropin therapy (using hCG). The process of normal spermatogenesis takes 3 months; thus, hormonal therapy to restore a normal sperm count can take at least 3–6 months after prolactin and testosterone levels are normalized. Empiric treatment of idiopathic male infertility with clomiphene citrate, other hormones, or vitamins has not been shown to be clinically effective.[164] As previously discussed, IUI with or without ovulation stimulation significantly increases pregnancy rates in couples with male infertility, female infertility, or both, by approximately 50%.

ART are utilized for severe male infertility, or if significant female infertility is also a factor. If the sperm concentration is below 5 million/ml with poor sperm motility, oocyte fertilization rates and pregnancy rates are much lower than with a normal sperm count.[165] Intracytoplasmic sperm injection (ICSI) involves the injection of a spermatozoan into the cytoplasm of an oocyte, and has markedly improved oocyte fertilization rates in men with a low sperm count (oligospermia), low motility (asthenospermia), a high proportion of abnormal sperm morphology (teratospermia), or no sperm in the ejaculate (azoospermia). Sperm for IVF–ICSI can be obtained through percutaneous epididymal sperm aspiration (PESA) or microsurgical epididymal sperm aspiration (MESA) from men with obstructive azoospermia (normal testicular size and histology, normal serum FSH), and through testicular sperm extraction (TESE) from men with non-obstructive azoospermia. ICSI achieves a fertilization rate of approximately 50–60%, and results are not affected by the etiology of the sperm abnormality or the origin of the spermatozoa.[165] Surgical anastamosis for epididymal lesions or prior vasectomy may be feasible, but is most successful for prior vasectomy.[166] In the absence of male infertility, the use of ICSI offers no identified advantage compared with conventional IVF.[167] For couples who fail to conceive with ART or who are unable to undergo ART, insemination with donor sperm is a reasonable option with high pregnancy rates depending on the fertility status of the female partner.

Unexplained infertility

Treatment strategies for unexplained infertility are empiric, and may counter the effects of one or several mild abnormalities. Clomiphene therapy, with or without inseminations, is a reasonable initial treatment for unexplained infertility, and is superior to no treatment or to placebo.[168] If conception does not occur, a 3-month trial of COH with gonadotropin injections plus inseminations is recommended; the majority of conceptions occur within the first three cycles.[169,170] For couples with unexplained infertility, IVF offers the highest pregnancy rate per cycle but is a more intense and costly therapy.

CONCLUSIONS

Although the prevalence of infertility is stable, the number of infertile couples presenting for evaluation and treatment is increasing due to delayed childbearing, increased public knowledge about infertility, and a greater range of available therapies. A thorough history and evidence-based evaluation of each partner is essential, since one or more causes of infertility may affect a couple. Consultation with an infertility specialist is recommended for women over age 35, women with endometriosis or a prior history of pelvic surgery, women with a history of radiation or chemotherapy, for men with an abnormal semen analysis, and after 6–12 months of fertility treatment without conception. As each couple's situation is assessed, the risks, benefits, and alternatives to fertility treatment must be addressed, and realistic expectations should be set. Couples need to be aware of all options, including availability of donor sperm, oocyte donation, gestational surrogacy, adoption, and childlessness.

REFERENCES

1. Cramer DW, Walker AM, Schiff I. Statistical methods in evaluating the outcome of infertility therapy. Fertil Steril 1979; 32: 80–6.
2. Guttmacher AF. Factors affecting normal expectancy of conception. J Am Med Assoc 1956; 161: 855–60.
3. Tietze C, Guttmacher AF, Rubin S. Time required for conception in 1727 planned pregnancies. Fertil Steril 1950; 1: 338–46.
4. Gnoth C, Godehardt E, Frank-Herrmann P et al. Definition and prevalence of subfertility and infertility. Hum Reprod 2005; 20: 1144–7.
5. Abma JC, Chandra A, Mosher WD et al. Fertility, family planning, and women's health: new data from the 1995 National Survey of Family Growth. Vital Health Stat 23 1997 May; (19): 1–114.
6. Chandra A, Stephen EH. Impaired fecundity in the United States: 1982–1995. Fam Plann Perspect 1998; 30: 34–42.
7. Stephen EH, Chandra A. Use of infertility services in the United States: 1995. Fam Plann Perspect 2000; 32: 132–7.
8. Mosher WD, Pratt WF. Fecundity and infertility in the United States: incidence and trends. Fertil Steril 1991; 56: 192–3.
9. Collins JA, So Y, Wilson EH et al. Clinical factors affecting pregnancy rates among infertile couples. Can Med Assoc J 1984; 130: 269–73.
10. Guzick DS. Evaluation of the infertile couple. In: Rose BD, ed. UpToDate. Waltham, MA: UpToDate, 2007.
11. Martin JA, Hamilton BE, Sutton PD et al. Births: final data for 2004. Natl Vital Stat Rep 2006; 55: 1–101.
12. Practice Committee of the American Society for Reproductive Medicine. Optimal evaluation of the infertile female. Fertil Steril 2006; 86: S264–7.
13. Noyes RW, Hertig AF, Rock J. Dating the endometrial biopsy. Fertil Steril 1950; 1: 3–25.
14. Li TC, Dockery P, Cooke ID. Endometrial development in the luteal phase of women with various types of infertility: comparison with women of normal fertility. Hum Reprod 1991; 6: 325–30.
15. Coutifaris C, Myers ER, Guzick DS et al. Histological dating of timed endometrial biopsy tissue is not related to fertility status. Fertil Steril 2004; 82: 1264–72.
16. Davis OK, Berkeley AS, Naus GJ et al. The incidence of luteal phase defect in normal, fertile women, determined by serial endometrial biopsies. Fertil Steril 1989; 51: 582–6.
17. Batista MC, Cartledge TP, Merino MJ et al. Midluteal phase endometrial biopsy does not accurately predict luteal function. Fertil Steril 1993; 59: 294–300.
18. Oei SG, Helmerhorst FM, Bloemenkamp KW et al. Effectiveness of the postcoital test: randomised controlled trial. BMJ 1998; 317: 502–5.
19. Griffith CS, Grimes DA. The validity of the postcoital test. Am J Obstet Gynecol 1990; 162: 615–20.
20. Lindheim SR, Adsuar N, Kushner DM et al. Sonohysterography: a valuable tool in evaluating the female pelvis. Obstet Gynecol Surv 2003; 58: 770–84.
21. Grimbizis GF, Camus M, Tarlatzis BC et al. Clinical implications of uterine malformations and hysteroscopic treatment results. Hum Reprod Update 2001; 7: 161–74.
22. Lin PC, Bhatnagar KP, Nettleton GS, Nakajima ST. Female genital anomalies affecting reproduction. Fertil Steril 2002; 78: 899–915.
23. Homer HA, Li TC, Cooke ID. The septate uterus: a review of management and reproductive outcome. Fertil Steril 2000; 73: 1–14.
24. Troiano RN, McCarthy SM. Mullerian duct anomalies: imaging and clinical issues. Radiology 2004; 233: 19–34.
25. Cicinelli E, Romano F, Anastasio PS et al. Transabdominal sonohysterography, transvaginal sonography, and hysteroscopy in the evaluation of submucous myomas. Obstet Gynecol 1995; 85: 42–7.
26. Shamma FN, Lee G, Gutmann JN, Lavy G. The role of office hysteroscopy in in vitro fertilization. Fertil Steril 1992; 58: 1237–9.
27. Soares SR, Barbosa dos Reis MM, Camargos AF. Diagnostic accuracy of sonohysterography, transvaginal sonography, and hysterosalpingography in patients with uterine cavity diseases. Fertil Steril 2000; 73: 406–11.
28. Swart P, Mol BW, van der Veen F et al. The accuracy of hysterosalpingography in the diagnosis of tubal pathology: a meta-analysis. Fertil Steril 1995; 64: 486–91.
29. Swolin K, Rosencrantz M. Laparoscopy vs. hysterosalpingography in sterility investigations. A comparative study. Fertil Steril 1972; 23: 270–3.
30. Chen YM, Ott DJ, Pittaway DE et al. Efficacy of hysterosalpingography in evaluating tubal and peritubal disease in 200 patients with infertility. Rays 1988; 13: 27–32.
31. Novy MJ, Thurmond AS, Patton P et al. Diagnosis of cornual obstruction by transcervical fallopian tube cannulation. Fertil Steril 1988; 50: 434–40.
32. Hurd WW, Wyckoff ET, Reynolds DB et al. Patient rotation and resolution of unilateral cornual obstruction during hysterosalpingography. Obstet Gynecol 2003; 101: 1275–8.

33. Nugent D, Watson AJ, Killick SR et al. A randomized controlled trial of tubal flushing with lipiodol for unexplained infertility. Fertil Steril 2002; 77: 173–5.

34. Watson A, Vandekerckhove P, Lilford R et al. A meta-analysis of the therapeutic role of oil soluble contrast media at hysterosalpingography: a surprising result? Fertil Steril 1994; 61: 470–7.

35. Johnson N, Vandekerckhove P, Watson A et al. Tubal flushing for subfertility. Cochrane Database Syst Rev 2005; (2): CD003718.

36. Jeanty P, Besnard S, Arnold A et al. Air-contrast sonohysterography as a first step assessment of tubal patency. J Ultrasound Med 2000; 19: 519–27.

37. Kodaman PH, Arici A, Seli E. Evidence-based diagnosis and management of tubal factor infertility. Curr Opin Obstet Gynecol 2004; 16: 221–9.

38. Exacoustos C, Zupi E, Carusotti C et al. Hysterosalpingo-contrast sonography compared with hysterosalpingography and laparoscopic dye pertubation to evaluate tubal patency. J Am Assoc Gynecol Laparosc 2003; 10: 367–72.

39. Korell M, Seehaus D, Strowitzki T, Hepp H. [Radiologic versus ultrasound fallopian tube imaging. Painfulness of the examination and diagnostic reliability of hysterosalpingography and hysterosalpingo-contrast-ultrasonography with echovist 200]. Ultraschall Med 1997; 18: 3–7. [in German]

40. Mahmood TA, Templeton A. Prevalence and genesis of endometriosis. Hum Reprod 1991; 6: 544–9.

41. Mol BW, Dijkman B, Wertheim P et al. The accuracy of serum chlamydial antibodies in the diagnosis of tubal pathology: a meta-analysis. Fertil Steril 1997; 67: 1031–7.

42. Angell RR. Aneuploidy in older women. Higher rates of aneuploidy in oocytes from older women. Hum Reprod 1994; 9: 1199–200.

43. Battaglia DE, Goodwin P, Klein NA, Soules MR. Influence of maternal age on meiotic spindle assembly in oocytes from naturally cycling women. Hum Reprod 1996; 11: 2217–22.

44. Rowe T. Fertility and a woman's age. J Reprod Med 2006; 51: 157–63.

45. van Rooij IA, Bancsi LF, Broekmans FJ et al. Women older than 40 years of age and those with elevated follicle-stimulating hormone levels differ in poor response rate and embryo quality in in vitro fertilization. Fertil Steril 2003; 79: 482–8.

46. Dunson DB, Colombo B, Baird DD. Changes with age in the level and duration of fertility in the menstrual cycle. Hum Reprod 2002; 17: 1399–403.

47. Tarlatzis BC, Zepiridis L, Grimbizis G, Bontis J. Clinical management of low ovarian response to stimulation for IVF: a systematic review. Hum Reprod Update 2003; 9: 61–76.

48. van Montfrans JM, Hoek A, van Hooff MH et al. Predictive value of basal follicle-stimulating hormone concentrations in a general subfertility population. Fertil Steril 2000; 74: 97–103.

49. Bukulmez O, Arici A. Assessment of ovarian reserve. Curr Opin Obstet Gynecol 2004; 16: 231–7.

50. Creus M, Penarrubia J, Fabregues F et al. Day 3 serum inhibin B and FSH and age as predictors of assisted reproduction treatment outcome. Hum Reprod 2000; 15: 2341–6.

51. Scott RT, Opsahl MS, Leonardi MR et al. Life table analysis of pregnancy rates in a general infertility population relative to ovarian reserve and patient age. Hum Reprod 1995; 10: 1706–10.

52. Navot D, Rosenwaks Z, Margalioth EJ. Prognostic assessment of female fecundity. Lancet 1987; 2: 645–7.

53. Scott RT, Toner JP, Muasher SJ et al. Follicle-stimulating hormone levels on cycle day 3 are predictive of in vitro fertilization outcome. Fertil Steril 1989; 51: 651–4.

54. Jain T, Soules MR, Collins JA. Comparison of basal follicle-stimulating hormone versus the clomiphene citrate challenge test for ovarian reserve screening. Fertil Steril 2004; 82: 180–5.

55. Yanushpolsky EH, Hurwitz S, Tikh E, Racowsky C. Predictive usefulness of cycle day 10 follicle-stimulating hormone level in a clomiphene citrate challenge test for in vitro fertilization outcome in women younger than 40 years of age. Fertil Steril 2003; 80: 111–15.

56. Chang MY, Chiang CH, Hsieh TT et al. Use of the antral follicle count to predict the outcome of assisted reproductive technologies. Fertil Steril 1998; 69: 505–10.

57. Engmann L, Sladkevicius P, Agrawal R et al. Value of ovarian stromal blood flow velocity measurement after pituitary suppression in the prediction of ovarian responsiveness and outcome of in vitro fertilization treatment. Fertil Steril 1999; 71: 22–9.

58. Lass A, Skull J, McVeigh E et al. Measurement of ovarian volume by transvaginal sonography before ovulation induction with human menopausal gonadotrophin for in-vitro fertilization can predict poor response. Hum Reprod 1997; 12: 294–7.

59. Tomas C, Nuojua-Huttunen S, Martikainen H. Pretreatment transvaginal ultrasound examination predicts ovarian responsiveness to gonadotrophins in in-vitro fertilization. Hum Reprod 1997; 12: 220–3.

60. Bancsi LF, Broekmans FJ, Eijkemans MJ et al. Predictors of poor ovarian response in in vitro fertilization: a prospective study comparing basal markers of ovarian reserve. Fertil Steril 2002; 77: 328–36.

61. Scheffer GJ, Broekmans FJ, Dorland M et al. Antral follicle counts by transvaginal ultrasonography are related to age in women with proven natural fertility. Fertil Steril 1999; 72: 845–51.

62. Hendriks DJ, Mol BW, Bancsi LF et al. Antral follicle count in the prediction of poor ovarian response and pregnancy after in vitro fertilization: a meta-analysis and comparison with basal follicle-stimulating hormone level. Fertil Steril 2005; 83: 291–301.

63. Klinkert ER, Broekmans FJ, Looman CW et al. The antral follicle count is a better marker than basal follicle-stimulating hormone for the selection of older patients with acceptable pregnancy prospects after in vitro fertilization. Fertil Steril 2005; 83: 811–14.

64. Ng EH, Chan CC, Tang OS, Ho PC. Antral follicle count and FSH concentration after clomiphene citrate challenge test in the prediction of ovarian response during IVF treatment. Hum Reprod 2005; 20: 1647–54.

65. Honig SC, Lipshultz LI, Jarow J. Significant medical pathology uncovered by a comprehensive male infertility evaluation. Fertil Steril 1994; 62: 1028–34.

66. World Health Organization. WHO Laboratory Manual for the Examination of Human Semen and Sperm–Cervical Mucus Interaction, 2nd edn. New York: Cambridge University Press, 1987.

67. World Health Organization. WHO Laboratory Manual for the Examination of Human Semen and Sperm–Cervical Mucus Interaction, 3rd edn. New York: Cambridge University Press, 1992.

68. World Health Organization. WHO Laboratory Manual for the Examination of Human Semen and Sperm–Cervical Mucus Interaction, 4th edn. New York: Cambridge University Press, 1999.

69. Guzick DS, Overstreet JW, Factor-Litvak P et al. Sperm morphology, motility, and concentration in fertile and infertile men. N Engl J Med 2001; 345: 1388–93.

70. Bonde JP, Ernst E, Jensen TK et al. Relation between semen quality and fertility: a population-based study of 430 first-pregnancy planners. Lancet 1998; 352: 1172–7.

71. Male Infertility Best Practice Policy Committee of the American Urological Association; Practice Committee of the

American Society for Reproductive Medicine. Report on optimal evaluation of the infertile male. Fertil Steril 2006; 86: S202–9.

72. Swerdloff RS, Wang C. Evaluation of male infertility. In: Rose BD, ed. UpToDate. Waltham, MA: UpToDate, 2007.

73. The influence of varicocele on parameters of fertility in a large group of men presenting to infertility clinics. World Health Organization. Fertil Steril 1992; 57: 1289–93.

74. Practice Committee of the American Society for Reproductive Medicine. Report on varicocele and infertility. Fertil Steril 2006; 86: S93–5.

75. Evers JL, Collins JA. Assessment of efficacy of varicocele repair for male subfertility: a systematic review. Lancet 2003; 361: 1849–52.

76. Evers JL, Collins JA. Surgery or embolisation for varicocele in subfertile men. Cochrane Database Syst Rev 2004; (3): CD000479.

77. Chillon M, Casals T, Mercier B et al. Mutations in the cystic fibrosis gene in patients with congenital absence of the vas deferens. N Engl J Med 1995; 332: 1475–80.

78. De Braekeleer M, Dao TN. Cytogenetic studies in male infertility: a review. Hum Reprod 1991; 6: 245–50.

79. Pryor JL, Kent-First M, Muallem A et al. Microdeletions in the Y chromosome of infertile men. N Engl J Med 1997; 336: 534–9.

80. De Kretser DM, Baker HW. Infertility in men: recent advances and continuing controversies. J Clin Endocrinol Metab 1999; 84: 3443–50.

81. Seli E, Sakkas D. Spermatozoal nuclear determinants of reproductive outcome: implications for ART. Hum Reprod Update 2005; 11: 337–49.

82. Page DC, Silber S, Brown LG. Men with infertility caused by AZFc deletion can produce sons by intracytoplasmic sperm injection, but are likely to transmit the deletion and infertility. Hum Reprod 1999; 14: 1722–6.

83. Evers JL. Female subfertility. Lancet 2002; 360: 151–9.

84. Guzick DS, Sullivan MW, Adamson GD et al. Efficacy of treatment for unexplained infertility. Fertil Steril 1998; 70: 207–13.

85. Jacobson TZ, Barlow DH, Koninckx PR et al. Laparoscopic surgery for subfertility associated with endometriosis. Cochrane Database Syst Rev 2002; (4): CD001398.

86. Kennedy S, Bergqvist A, Chapron C et al. ESHRE guideline for the diagnosis and treatment of endometriosis. Hum Reprod 2005; 20: 2698–704.

87. Hassan MA, Killick SR. Negative lifestyle is associated with a significant reduction in fecundity. Fertil Steril 2004; 81: 384–92.

88. Grodstein F, Goldman MB, Cramer DW. Body mass index and ovulatory infertility. Epidemiology 1994; 5: 247–50.

89. Clark AM, Ledger W, Galletly C et al. Weight loss results in significant improvement in pregnancy and ovulation rates in anovulatory obese women. Hum Reprod 1995; 10: 2705–12.

90. Practice Committee of the American Society for Reproductive Medicine. Smoking and infertility. Fertil Steril 2006; 86: S172–7.

91. Augood C, Duckitt K, Templeton AA. Smoking and female infertility: a systematic review and meta-analysis. Hum Reprod 1998; 13: 1532–9.

92. Phipps WR, Cramer DW, Schiff I et al. The association between smoking and female infertility as influenced by cause of the infertility. Fertil Steril 1987; 48: 377–82.

93. Vine MF. Smoking and male reproduction: a review. Int J Androl 1996; 19: 323–37.

94. Grodstein F, Goldman MB, Cramer DW. Infertility in women and moderate alcohol use. Am J Public Health 1994; 84: 1429–32.

95. Nagy F, Pendergrass PB, Bowen DC, Yeager JC. A comparative study of cytological and physiological parameters of semen obtained from alcoholics and non-alcoholics. Alcohol Alcohol 1986; 21: 17–23.

96. Olsen J, Bolumar F, Boldsen J, Bisanti L. Does moderate alcohol intake reduce fecundability? A European multicenter study on infertility and subfecundity. European Study Group on Infertility and Subfecundity. Alcohol Clin Exp Res 1997; 21: 206–12.

97. Smith CG, Asch RH. Drug abuse and reproduction. Fertil Steril 1987; 48: 355–73.

98. Mueller BA, Daling JR, Weiss NS, Moore DE. Recreational drug use and the risk of primary infertility. Epidemiology 1990; 1: 195–200.

99. Bolumar F, Olsen J, Rebagliato M, Bisanti L. Caffeine intake and delayed conception: a European multicenter study on infertility and subfecundity. European Study Group on Infertility Subfecundity. Am J Epidemiol 1997; 145: 324–34.

100. Cnattingius S, Signorello LB, Anneren G et al. Caffeine intake and the risk of first-trimester spontaneous abortion. N Engl J Med 2000; 343: 1839–45.

101. Seli E, Arici A. Ovulation induction with clomiphene citrate. In: Rose BD, ed. UpToDate. Waltham, MA: UpToDate, 2007.

102. ACOG Committee on Practice Bulletins-Gynecology. ACOG Practice Bulletin. Clinical management guidelines for obstetrician-gynecologists number 34, February 2002. Management of infertility caused by ovulatory dysfunction. American College of Obstetricians and Gynecologists. Obstet Gynecol 2002; 99: 347–58.

103. Homburg R. Clomiphene citrate – end of an era? A mini-review. Hum Reprod 2005; 20: 2043–51.

104. Boostanfar R, Jain JK, Mishell DR Jr, Paulson RJ. A prospective randomized trial comparing clomiphene citrate with tamoxifen citrate for ovulation induction. Fertil Steril 2001; 75: 1024–6.

105. Tulandi T, Martin J, Al-Fadhli R et al. Congenital malformations among 911 newborns conceived after infertility treatment with letrozole or clomiphene citrate. Fertil Steril 2006; 85: 1761–5.

106. Casper RF, Mitwally MF. Review: aromatase inhibitors for ovulation induction. J Clin Endocrinol Metab 2006; 91: 760–71.

107. Delvigne A, Rozenberg S. Epidemiology and prevention of ovarian hyperstimulation syndrome (OHSS): a review. Hum Reprod Update 2002; 8: 559–77.

108. Dickey RP, Taylor SN, Lu PY et al. Risk factors for high-order multiple pregnancy and multiple birth after controlled ovarian hyperstimulation: results of 4,062 intrauterine insemination cycles. Fertil Steril 2005; 83: 671–83.

109. Jurema MW, Vieira AD, Bankowski B et al. Effect of ejaculatory abstinence period on the pregnancy rate after intrauterine insemination. Fertil Steril 2005; 84: 678–81.

110. Nulsen JC, Walsh S, Dumez S, Metzger DA. A randomized and longitudinal study of human menopausal gonadotropin with intrauterine insemination in the treatment of infertility. Obstet Gynecol 1993; 82: 780–6.

111. Cohlen BJ, Vandekerckhove P, te Velde ER, Habbema JD. Timed intercourse versus intra-uterine insemination with or without ovarian hyperstimulation for subfertility in men. Cochrane Database Syst Rev 2000; (2): CD000360.

112. Guzick DS, Carson SA, Coutifaris C et al. Efficacy of super-ovulation and intrauterine insemination in the treatment of infertility. National Cooperative Reproductive Medicine Network. N Engl J Med 1999; 340: 177–83.

113. SART National Summary 2005. Birmingham, AL: Society for Assisted Reproductive Technology, 2005.

114. Pabuccu R, Akar ME. Luteal phase support in assisted reproductive technology. Curr Opin Obstet Gynecol 2005; 17: 277–81.

115. Guzick DS, Wing R, Smith D et al. Endocrine consequences of weight loss in obese, hyperandrogenic, anovulatory women. Fertil Steril 1994; 61: 598–604.

116. Nestler JE, Jakubowicz DJ, Evans WS, Pasquali R. Effects of metformin on spontaneous and clomiphene-induced ovulation in the polycystic ovary syndrome. N Engl J Med 1998; 338: 1876–80.

117. Seli E, Duleba AJ. Should patients with polycystic ovarian syndrome be treated with metformin? Hum Reprod 2002; 17: 2230–6.

118. Seli E, Duleba AJ. Optimizing ovulation induction in women with polycystic ovary syndrome. Curr Opin Obstet Gynecol 2002; 14: 245–54.

119. Legro RS, Barnhart HX, Schlaff WD et al. Clomiphene, metformin, or both for infertility in the polycystic ovary syndrome. N Engl J Med 2007; 356: 551–66.

120. Lemieux S, Lewis GF, Ben-Chetrit A et al. Correction of hyperandrogenemia by laparoscopic ovarian cautery in women with polycystic ovarian syndrome is not accompanied by improved insulin sensitivity or lipid-lipoprotein levels. J Clin Endocrinol Metab 1999; 84: 4278–82.

121. Farquhar C, Vandekerckhove P, Lilford R. Laparoscopic 'drilling' by diathermy or laser for ovulation induction in anovulatory polycystic ovary syndrome. Cochrane Database Syst Rev 2001; (4): CD001122.

122. Rackow BW, Arici A. Reproductive performance of women with Mullerian anomalies. Curr Opin Obstet Gynecol 2007; 19: 229–37.

123. Donnez J, Jadoul P. What are the implications of myomas on fertility? A need for a debate? Hum Reprod 2002; 17: 1424–30.

124. Pritts EA. Fibroids and infertility: a systematic review of the evidence. Obstet Gynecol Surv 2001; 56: 483–91.

125. Surrey ES, Lietz AK, Schoolcraft WB. Impact of intramural leiomyomata in patients with a normal endometrial cavity on in vitro fertilization-embryo transfer cycle outcome. Fertil Steril 2001; 75: 405–10.

126. Rackow BW, Arici A. Fibroids and in-vitro fertilization: which comes first? Curr Opin Obstet Gynecol 2005; 17: 225–31.

127. Jun SH, Ginsburg ES, Racowsky C et al. Uterine leiomyomas and their effect on in vitro fertilization outcome: a retrospective study. J Assist Reprod Genet 2001; 18: 139–43.

128. Yarali H, Bukulmez O. The effect of intramural and subserous uterine fibroids on implantation and clinical pregnancy rates in patients having intracytoplasmic sperm injection. Arch Gynecol Obstet 2002; 266: 30–3.

129. Check JH, Choe JK, Lee G, Dietterich C. The effect on IVF outcome of small intramural fibroids not compressing the uterine cavity as determined by a prospective matched control study. Hum Reprod 2002; 17: 1244–8.

130. Eldar-Geva T, Meagher S, Healy DL et al. Effect of intramural, subserosal, and submucosal uterine fibroids on the outcome of assisted reproductive technology treatment. Fertil Steril 1998; 70: 687–91.

131. Hart R, Khalaf Y, Yeong CT et al. A prospective controlled study of the effect of intramural uterine fibroids on the outcome of assisted conception. Hum Reprod 2001; 16: 2411–17.

132. Oliveira FG, Abdelmassih VG, Diamond MP et al. Impact of subserosal and intramural uterine fibroids that do not distort the endometrial cavity on the outcome of in vitro fertilization-intracytoplasmic sperm injection. Fertil Steril 2004; 81: 582–7.

133. Advincula AP, Song A. Endoscopic management of leiomyomata. Semin Reprod Med 2004; 22: 149–55.

134. Dubuisson JB, Fauconnier A, Deffarges JV et al. Pregnancy outcome and deliveries following laparoscopic myomectomy. Hum Reprod 2000; 15: 869–73.

135. Surrey ES, Minjarez DA, Stevens JM, Schoolcraft WB. Effect of myomectomy on the outcome of assisted reproductive technologies. Fertil Steril 2005; 83: 1473–9.

136. Perez-Medina T, Bajo-Arenas J, Salazar F et al. Endometrial polyps and their implication in the pregnancy rates of patients undergoing intrauterine insemination: a prospective, randomized study. Hum Reprod 2005; 20: 1632–5.

137. Schenker JG. Etiology of and therapeutic approach to synechia uteri. Eur J Obstet Gynecol Reprod Biol 1996; 65: 109–13.

138. Pabuccu R, Atay V, Orhon E et al. Hysteroscopic treatment of intrauterine adhesions is safe and effective in the restoration of normal menstruation and fertility. Fertil Steril 1997; 68: 1141–3.

139. Zikopoulos KA, Kolibianakis EM, Platteau P et al. Live delivery rates in subfertile women with Asherman's syndrome after hysteroscopic adhesiolysis using the resectoscope or the Versapoint system. Reprod Biomed Online 2004; 8: 720–5.

140. Propst AM, Hill JA 3rd. Anatomic factors associated with recurrent pregnancy loss. Semin Reprod Med 2000; 18: 341–50.

141. Strassmann EO. Fertility and unification of double uterus. Fertil Steril 1966; 17: 165–76.

142. Fedele L, Bianchi S. Hysteroscopic metroplasty for septate uterus. Obstet Gynecol Clin North Am 1995; 22: 473–89.

143. Raga F, Bauset C, Remohi J et al. Reproductive impact of congenital Mullerian anomalies. Hum Reprod 1997; 12: 2277–81.

144. Benadiva CA, Kligman I, Davis O, Rosenwaks Z. In vitro fertilization versus tubal surgery: is pelvic reconstructive surgery obsolete? Fertil Steril 1995; 64: 1051–61.

145. Watson A, Vandekerckhove P, Lilford R. Techniques for pelvic surgery in subfertility. Cochrane Database Syst Rev 2000; (2): CD000221.

146. Honore GM, Holden AE, Schenken RS. Pathophysiology and management of proximal tubal blockage. Fertil Steril 1999; 71: 785–95.

147. Schlaff WD, Hassiakos DK, Damewood MD, Rock JA. Neosalpingostomy for distal tubal obstruction: prognostic factors and impact of surgical technique. Fertil Steril 1990; 54: 984–90.

148. Zeyneloglu HB. Hydrosalpinx and assisted reproduction: options and rationale for treatment. Curr Opin Obstet Gynecol 2001; 13: 281–6.

149. Daftary GS, Taylor HS. Hydrosalpinx fluid diminishes endometrial cell HOXA10 expression. Fertil Steril 2002; 78: 577–80.

150. Meyer WR, Castelbaum AJ, Somkuti S et al. Hydrosalpinges adversely affect markers of endometrial receptivity. Hum Reprod 1997; 12: 1393–8.

151. Seli E, Kayisli UA, Cakmak H et al. Removal of hydrosalpinges increases endometrial leukaemia inhibitory factor (LIF) expression at the time of the implantation window. Hum Reprod 2005; 20: 3012–17.

152. Dechaud H, Daures JP, Arnal F et al. Does previous salpingectomy improve implantation and pregnancy rates in patients with severe tubal factor infertility who are undergoing in vitro fertilization? A pilot prospective randomized study. Fertil Steril 1998; 69: 1020–5.

153. Johnson NP, Mak W, Sowter MC. Laparoscopic salpingectomy for women with hydrosalpinges enhances the success of IVF: a Cochrane review. Hum Reprod 2002; 17: 543–8.

154. Strandell A, Lindhard A, Waldenstrom U et al. Hydrosalpinx and IVF outcome: a prospective, randomized multicentre trial in Scandinavia on salpingectomy prior to IVF. Hum Reprod 1999; 14: 2762–9.

155. Rock JA, Guzick DS, Katz E et al. Tubal anastomosis: pregnancy success following reversal of Falope ring or monopolar cautery sterilization. Fertil Steril 1987; 48: 13–17.

156. Henderson SR. The reversibility of female sterilization with the use of microsurgery: a report on 102 patients with more than one year of follow-up. Am J Obstet Gynecol 1984; 149: 57–65.

157. Practice Committee of the American Society for Reproductive Medicine. Endometriosis and infertility. Fertil Steril 2006; 86: S156–60.

158. Marcoux S, Maheux R, Berube S. Laparoscopic surgery in infertile women with minimal or mild endometriosis. Canadian Collaborative Group on Endometriosis. N Engl J Med 1997; 337: 217–22.

159. Parazzini F. Ablation of lesions or no treatment in minimal-mild endometriosis in infertile women: a randomized trial. Gruppo Italiano per lo Studio dell'Endometriosi. Hum Reprod 1999; 14: 1332–4.

160. Schenken RS. Modern concepts of endometriosis. Classification and its consequences for therapy. J Reprod Med 1998; 43: 269–75.

161. Pagidas K, Falcone T, Hemmings R, Miron P. Comparison of reoperation for moderate (stage III) and severe (stage IV) endometriosis-related infertility with in vitro fertilization-embryo transfer. Fertil Steril 1996; 65: 791–5.

162. Barnhart K, Dunsmoor-Su R, Coutifaris C. Effect of endometriosis on in vitro fertilization. Fertil Steril 2002; 77: 1148–55.

163. Sallam HN, Garcia-Velasco JA, Dias S, Arici A. Long-term pituitary down-regulation before in vitro fertilization (IVF) for women with endometriosis. Cochrane Database Syst Rev 2006; (1): CD004635.

164. Schill WB. Survey of medical therapy in andrology. Int J Androl 1995; 18 (Suppl 2): 56–62.

165. Wang C, Swerdloff RS. Treatment of male infertility. In: Rose BD, ed. UpToDate. Waltham, MA: UpToDate, 2007.

166. Southwick GJ, Temple-Smith PD. Epididymal microsurgery: current techniques and new horizons. Microsurgery 1988; 9: 266–77.

167. Bhattacharya S, Hamilton MP, Shaaban M et al. Conventional in-vitro fertilisation versus intracytoplasmic sperm injection for the treatment of non-male-factor infertility: a randomised controlled trial. Lancet 2001; 357: 2075–9.

168. Hughes E, Collins J, Vandekerckhove P. Clomiphene citrate for unexplained subfertility in women. Cochrane Database Syst Rev 2000; (3): CD000057.

169. Aboulghar M, Mansour R, Serour G et al. Controlled ovarian hyperstimulation and intrauterine insemination for treatment of unexplained infertility should be limited to a maximum of three trials. Fertil Steril 2001; 75: 88–91.

170. Aboulghar MA, Mansour RT, Serour GI et al. Management of long-standing unexplained infertility: a prospective study. Am J Obstet Gynecol 1999; 181: 371–5.

11 Fertility preservation in women

Veronica Bianchi, Joshua Johnson, and Emre Seli

INTRODUCTION

Cancer is not uncommon among younger women. In the United States, approximately 600 000 women are diagnosed with cancer every year, and one-tenth of these women are under the age of 40.[1] Ninety per cent of teenage girls and young women diagnosed with cancer will survive,[2] and it is estimated that by 2010, one in 250 adults will be a cancer survivor.[3]

The treatment required for most of the common cancer types occurring in younger women may involve removal of the reproductive organs, and/or cytotoxic treatment that could partially or definitively affect reproductive function. Therefore, women diagnosed with cancer prior to or during their reproductive period often have to deal not only with the uncertainty of long-term survival, but also with the partial or total loss of fertility as a result of cancer treatment.

In addition, women in the Western hemisphere have been delaying initiation of childbearing. In the USA, between 1990 and 2002, the birth rate in women 35–39 years of age increased by 31%, and for women aged 40–45 increased by 51%. Furthermore, in 2002, first birth rate increased by 28% for women 35–39 years of age and 44% for women 40–45 when compared to 1990.[4] In other words, more women in their late 30s to early 40s are seeking their first pregnancy than ever before. Since the incidence of most cancers increases with age, delayed childbearing results in more female cancer survivors who may be interested in fertility preservation.

In this chapter, we will describe established and experimental strategies for fertility preservation in women with malignancies. Most available options may also be applicable to women who face gonadotoxic treatment due to non-malignant disorders (such as systemic lupus erythematosus (SLE)), or those who plan to delay fertility (until an advanced reproductive age) for personal reasons.

We will first discuss non-surgical options for fertility preservation, beginning with emerging ovarian stimulation strategies that aim to limit the increase in serum estrogen concentrations in women with estrogen-sensitive malignancies. Discussion of embryo and oocyte cryopreservation follows, and, finally, results from the use of gonadotropin releasing hormone (GnRH) agonists for the protection of the ovarian reserve from chemotherapeutic insult are considered. Surgical approaches to fertility preservation, including ovarian transposition and cryopreservation of ovarian tissue, will be summarized in the latter half of the chapter. Special considerations regarding the treatment of gynecologic malignancies are reviewed in detail in Chapters 18–20.

NON-SURGICAL APPROACHES TO FERTILITY PRESERVATION

Alternative strategies for ovarian stimulation in women with estrogen sensitive malignancies

The first consideration for a newly diagnosed cancer patient seeking fertility preservation is the preservation of mature eggs and if possible embryos, to be protected from the looming effects of treatment. Protection of the ovarian reserve and physiological ovarian function is a separate concern, and will be discussed at the end of this section.

Ovarian stimulation protocols lead to an expansion of the pool of growing follicles and thus an increase in serum estrogen. Recently, new strategies for ovarian stimulation prior to in vitro fertilization (IVF) have been investigated for women with breast cancer, with the aim of retrieving more oocytes than would be available in a natural cycle, without causing a significant increase in serum estrogen. Women with breast cancer constitute a special group due to the presence of a 6-week hiatus between surgery and chemotherapy in most treatment protocols. Oktay et al first used tamoxifen to stimulate follicle growth for IVF in 12 women with breast cancer.[5] Using a dose of 40–60 mg daily for a mean duration of 6.9 days beginning on day 2 or 3 of the menstrual cycle, they obtained a higher number of oocytes (1.6 vs 0.7, $p < 0.05$) and embryos (1.6 vs 0.6, $p < 0.05$) per cycle compared to a retrospective control group consisting of breast cancer patients attempting natural cycle IVF.[5] However, mean peak estradiol level in the tamoxifen group was significantly higher than in natural cycle IVF patients

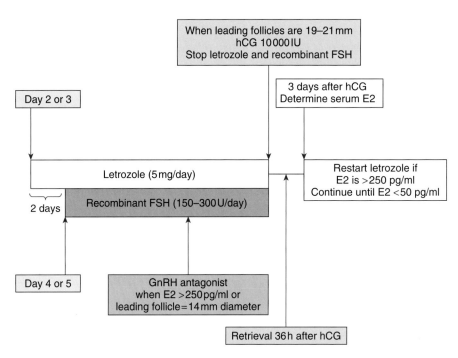

Figure 11.1   An alternative controlled ovarian stimulation protocol for women with estrogen sensitive cancer proposed by Oktay et al.[7] E2, estradiol

(442.4 vs 278 pg/ml). Following this initial study, Oktay et al reported better stimulation and embryo development using a combination of follicle stimulating hormone (FSH) with tamoxifen or letrozole (aromatase inhibitor).[6] They obtained a mean number of 5.1 mature oocytes and 3.8 embryos per cycle, with a mean peak estradiol of 1182 pg/ml using a combination of FSH and tamoxifen.[6] When they used letrozole instead of tamoxifen, in combination with FSH, they obtained a mean number of 8.5 mature oocytes and 5.3 embryos per cycle, with a mean peak estradiol of only 380 pg/ml.[6] They also reported the first pregnancy from cryopreserved embryos generated after tamoxifen stimulation.[6]

More recently, Oktay et al studied whether the combination of an aromatase inhibitor with gonadotropin treatment in breast cancer patients produces comparable results to standard IVF, without a significant increase in estradiol levels and delay in the initiation of chemotherapy.[7] They treated 47 breast cancer patients (stages I–IIIA) with 5 mg letrozole daily and 150–300 IU FSH to cryopreserve embryos or oocytes (Figure 11.1). Age-matched retrospective controls ($n=56$) were selected from women who underwent IVF for tubal disease. Stimulation with letrozole and FSH resulted in significantly lower peak estradiol levels (483 vs 1465 pg/ml) compared with controls, while the length of stimulation, number of embryos obtained, and fertilization rates were not affected. The human chorionic gonadotropin

administration criteria had to be adjusted to 20 mm follicle diameter after letrozole stimulation, compared with 17–18 mm in the controls. The mean delay from surgery to cryopreservation was 38.6 days, with 81% of all patients completing their IVF cycles within 8 weeks of surgery. These findings, although preliminary, are very encouraging for women diagnosed with breast cancer and suggest that letrozole and FSH may be a cost-effective alternative for fertility preservation in breast cancer patients that results in reduced estrogen exposure compared with standard IVF.[7] Interestingly, the combination of anastrozole with FSH does not seem to prevent the rise in serum estradiol.[8] Taking these issues into account where ovarian stimulation is indicated is leading to a successful starting point in fertility preservation for these patients. We now turn to the preservation of embryos and oocytes, until their use is possible in the assisted reproductive technologies (ART) setting.

Embryo cryopreservation

Currently, the most widely available option for fertility preservation in female patients who need chemo- and/or radiotherapy is the cryopreservation of fertilized oocytes and embryos. Cryopreservation of embryos (as well as oocytes – see below) involves an initial exposure to cryoprotectants, cooling to subzero temperatures, and storage. Upon demand, thawing occurs, and finally, a return to physiological conditions.

The methods involved in embryo cryopreservation are well-established and their risks and success rates have been investigated. Reported survival rates per thawed embryo range between 35 and 90%, and implantation rates between 8 and 30%.[9–14] In the United States, approximately 16 000 ART cycles using frozen non-donor embryos are performed yearly, with a pregnancy rate of 25% per transfer, compared to 35% pregnancy rate in cycles using fresh non-donor embryos.[15] It is noteworthy that the effects of different types of malignancies upon reproductive potential are not yet known, and these statistics may not predict the outcome in women undergoing embryo cryopreservation for fertility preservation due to malignancy.

Despite well-defined success rates, embryo cryopreservation has a few critical pitfalls. First, it requires that the patient has a male partner or uses donor sperm to fertilize retrieved eggs. Second, ovarian stimulation precedes oocyte retrieval for IVF, necessitating a delay in the initiation of chemo- or radiotherapy that may not be acceptable. Third, the high serum estrogen concentrations associated with ovarian stimulation may be contraindicated in women with estrogen sensitive malignancies. However, given the success of ovarian stimulation protocols including letrozole in leading to successful term birth,[16,17] their combination with embryo cryopreservation is also likely to be successful. Indeed, Oktay et al reported live births from cryopreserved embryos generated after ovarian stimulation using a regimen that included the combination of FSH and letrozole mentioned in the previous section.[7] Therefore, clinical progress is being made towards this last concern, and will also apply to the next technique under consideration, oocyte cryopreservation.

Oocyte cryopreservation

The cryopreservation of oocytes avoids the need for sperm, and thus is applicable to a larger group of patients compared to embryo cryopreservation. In addition, oocyte cryopreservation may circumvent ethical or legal considerations associated with embryo freezing. Moreover, it also has considerable advantages compared to ovarian tissue cryopreservation (Table 11.1), at least in the short term. However, although the first human live birth from cryopreserved oocytes was reported more than 20 years ago,[18] success rates in ART using frozen oocytes have lagged behind those using frozen embryos, most likely as a result of the biochemical and physical properties of the oocyte.

Table 11.1 Oocyte and ovarian tissue cryopreservation: differences and indications

Characteristics	Oocyte cryopreservation	Ovarian tissue cryopreservation
Requires ovarian stimulation	Yes	No
Requires delay in chemotherapy	Yes	No
Requires surgery	No	Yes
Risk of reseeding cancer	No	Yes
Appropriate in pre-puberty	No	Yes
Resumption of endocrine function	No	Yes
Human live birth	>200	2 cases

Table 11.2 Cryoprotectants: types and roles

Role	Types
Intracellular (penetrating)	
Prevention of intracellular damage	Dimethyl sulfoxide (DMSO) Ethylene glycol 1,2-propanediol (PROH) Glycerol
Extracellular (non-penetrating)	
Dehydration and rehydration	Sucrose Ficoll® Raffinose

Cell survival after freezing is intimately associated with the composition and permeability characteristics of the cell membrane, the surface to volume ratio of the cell, and the difference in osmotic pressure between the two sides of the membrane.[19,20] Additional factors associated with oocyte survival and developmental competence after freezing include developmental stage at freezing (isolation at the germinal vesicle (GV), meiotic metaphase I (MI) versus meiotic metaphase II (MII) stages of development), cryoprotectant type and concentration (Table 11.2), and the method or 'protocol' of cryopreservation. Interestingly, oocyte survival with a specific protocol can also vary according to species. This is largely believed to be related to oocyte size, but other biochemical properties may contribute to such an outcome.

Mostly due to a low efficiency of oocyte maturation in vitro, mature MII oocytes are most commonly used for cryopreservation. MII oocytes are among the

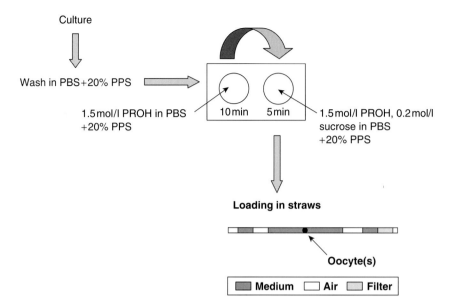

Figure 11.2 Slow freezing: equilibration and loading. PBS, phosphate buffered saline; PPS, plasma protein supplement; PROH, 1,2 propanediol

largest cells in the human body and contain the delicate meiotic spindle. As their cytoplasm contains a high proportion of water in comparison to other cells, damage due to ice crystal formation was an initial hurdle to oocyte viability after frozen storage. Protocols that include dehydration of oocytes before and/or during the cooling procedure reduced ice crystal formation and led to much improved clinical outcomes.

Cryopreservation of mature oocytes has also been shown to cause hardening of the zona pellucida, resulting in adverse effects upon fertilization.[21] Significant improvements in the fertilization of cryopreserved oocytes was achieved with the use of intracytoplasmic sperm injection (ICSI),[22,23] undoubtedly at least in part due to avoiding the effects of zona hardening.

The two most common freezing protocols used are referred to as slow cooling and vitrification. In the last 2 years, each protocol has shown increasing promise, indicating that oocyte cryopreservation is becoming more routine and less experimental.

Slow cooling procedure

The first protocol used to freeze oocytes was based on a slow cooling/rapid thawing method that had already been applied successfully for the cryopreservation and subsequent survival of embryos. In 1986, Chen[18] used this protocol to achieve the first pregnancy with frozen/thawed oocytes. Since then, much progress has been made, most of all in the optimization of cryoprotectant concentration and exposure time(s). The so-called 'curve', or temperature versus time protocol used for

slow freezing, has remained essentially unchanged from that used by Lassalle et al[24] in the first embryo freezing protocol.

As implied by the procedure's name, slow cooling makes use of a very slow rate of decreasing temperature (< 1°C/min) over time (Figures 11.2 and 11.3). These 'curves' of specimen temperature were formulated using mathematical models based on observations of the survival of different types of cells when frozen and thawed under different thermal conditions.[25,26] A modern curve is achieved using an automated chilling system capable of tightly controlled changes in temperature as follows. Freezing solutions are cooled from 20°C to –8°C at a rate of 2°C/min. Manual seeding of oocytes (Figure 11.4) within plastic straws is performed at near –8°C, and this temperature is maintained for 10 minutes in order to allow uniform ice propagation. The temperature is then decreased to –30°C at a rate of 0.3°C/min and then (relatively rapidly) brought to –150°C at a rate of 50°C/min. Straws are then plunged directly into liquid nitrogen at –196°C and stored. Thawing consists of rapid re-warming and the subsequent stepwise dilution of the cryoprotectants, and finally the return of oocytes to supportive culture media at 37°C (Table 11.3).

Several studies using slow freezing protocols have been conducted in order to analyze possible damage to subcellular structures such as the meiotic spindle and mitochondria. Rienzi et al[27] showed that the meiotic spindle is able to reform after disappearing temporarily during the freeze/thaw procedure, but not in all the oocytes analyzed;[28] further, sucrose concentrations in

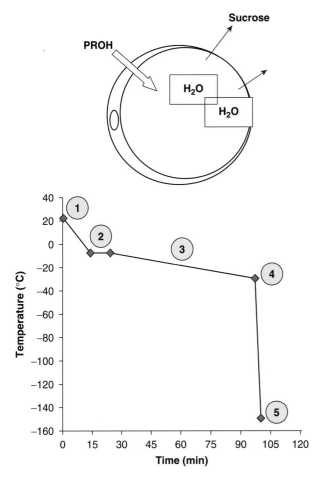

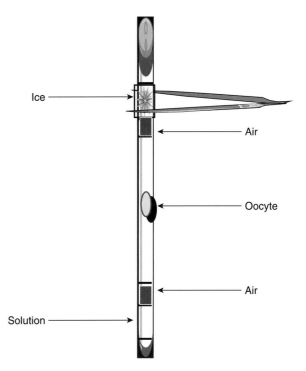

Figure 11.3 Slow freezing: curve for temperature lowering. (1) Room temperature to −8°C, −2°C/min; (2) seeding at −8°C (hold, 10 min); (3) −8°C to −30°C, −0.3°C/min; (4) −30°C to −150°C, −50°C/min; (5) plunge into liquid nitrogen

Figure 11.4 Seeding. For most slow cooling protocols for embryos and oocytes it is necessary to induce ice formation in the external solution manually; this prevents supercooling and starts the dehydration process. This procedure is called seeding, and ice formation is induced manually at temperatures ranging from −5 to −8°C. The usual procedure is to make a small portion of the solution very cold, for example by touching the wall of the container with an object cooled to −196°C

solution have been shown to affect the rate of normal spindle recovery after thawing.[29]

Clinical outcomes   Clinical outcomes after oocyte cryopreservation have been determined for different protocols. The first protocol used was exactly the same as formulated for embryo freezing.[24,30] Equilibration in the freezing mixtures 1.5 mol/l 1,2 propanediol (PROH) in phosphate buffered saline (PBS), followed by 1.5 mol/l PROH with 0.1 mol/l sucrose in PBS, preceded freezing. A stepwise dilution of PROH (1.0–0.5 mol/l) with an unvaried 0.2 mol/l sucrose concentration in PBS was used for thawing solutions. While this protocol resulted in sporadic pregnancies, results were not consistent within a large cohort of patients.[31] In 2001, Fabbri et al[32] reported significantly improved post-thaw survival rates when the concentration of sucrose was increased from 0.1 mol/l (34%) to 0.2 mol/l (60%) or 0.3 mol/l (82%) in both freezing and thawing solutions. This change resulted in improved oocyte dehydration, which correlated with higher post-thaw survival rates.

Table 11.3 Rapid thawing protocol: the thawing solutions contain a gradually decreasing concentration of 1,2-propanediol (PROH) and a constant 0.3 mol/l sucrose concentration

Rapid thawing program	
Room temperature (RT)	30 s
Waterbath at 30°C	40 s
Cryoprotectant removal	
• 1.0 mol/l PROH + 0.3 mol/l sucrose + 20% PPS	5 min
• 0.5 mol/l PROH + 0.3 mol/l sucrose + 20% PPS	5 min
• 0.3 mol/l sucrose + 20% PPS	5 min
• PBS + 20% PPS (RT)	10 min
• PBS + 20% PPS (37°C)	10 min
• Culture in medium (37°C and 5% CO$_2$)	

PPS, plasma protein supplement; PBS, phosphate buffered saline

However, those promising results did not lead to improvements in pregnancy rates. Protocols including solutions with high sucrose concentrations have been successful in terms of post-thaw survival, fertilization, and cleavage rates, but have resulted in conflicting and usually unsatisfying clinical outcomes.[33] Clinical studies using 0.3 mol/l sucrose[34,35] reported low implantation and pregnancy rates compared to fresh cycles, despite an improvement in post-thaw viability and fertilization rates of eggs.

The recent meta-analysis of Oktay et al[36] calculated the combined outcome(s) of a total of 26 reports using slow freezing, mature oocytes, and ICSI, published prior to June 2005. In these studies, the outcomes of a total of approximately 4000 thawed oocytes were reported. Clinical pregnancy per thawed oocyte was 2.4%, and a 13.1% implantation rate per transferred embryo was found. When separate analysis of seven studies using slow freezing published between June 2005 and March 2006 was done, clinical pregnancy per thawed oocyte ($n = 2409$) was 2.2%, while the implantation rate per transferred embryo was down to 6.5%. The majority (approximately 85%) of oocytes in this second group were derived from the two studies by Levi Setti and Borini,[34,35] and reflected the results of protocols using 0.3 mol/l sucrose. These clinical pregnancy rates are especially low when compared to embryo cryopreservation, where a 4–5% live birth rate per oocyte used to generate the cryopreserved embryos has been calculated.

A report by Paynter et al[37] suggested that the increased rate and extent of oocyte shrinkage that result from the high sucrose concentration during freezing might be related to this outcome. On the basis of that study, Bianchi et al[38] established a modified cryopreservation protocol in which the freezing solution contains 1.5 mol/l PROH and 0.2 mol/l sucrose in order to reduce the impact of shrinkage during cooling procedures. The higher sucrose concentration (0.3 mol/l) was used during thawing, after Fabbri et al,[32] in keeping with the original idea of Lassalle[24] who used a thawing solution in which the sucrose concentration was higher than that employed in the freezing solution.

Using this protocol, Bianchi et al thawed 403 oocytes of which 306 survived (76.0%).[38] Two hundred and fifty-two oocytes (a maximum of three oocytes per patient according to Italian law) were inseminated by ICSI and 192 fertilized normally, for a rate of 76.2%. One hundred and eighty of the 192 zygotes cleaved (93.7%), and 178 were transferred. In the end, 17 pregnancies were confirmed by ultrasound assessment, with 24 gestational sacs and 19 fetuses with heartbeats. Pregnancy rates were 21.2%, 18.9%, and 21.8% per embryo transfer, thaw cycle, and patient, respectively, and the implantation rate was 13.4%. Pregnancy rate per cryopreserved/thawed oocyte was 4.9% and the implantation rate per oocyte was 6.9%. The multiple pregnancy rate was 29.4%

(5/17), with three twin and two triplet gestations. Two patients miscarried, resulting in a miscarriage rate of 11.8%. When results were analyzed by taking into consideration only patients aged ≤38 years, 325 oocytes were thawed with a survival rate of 75.1%. Two hundred and three oocytes were microinjected and 157 (77.3%) fertilized normally. The cleavage rate was 93.0%. In this group of younger patients, 72 thawing cycles were performed, with 144 embryos transferred in 65 transfers. Pregnancy rates were 26.1%, 23.6%, and 27.4% per transfer, thaw cycle, and patient, respectively; the implantation rate was 16.6%.

These results demonstrate a significant improvement in the outcome of oocyte cryopreservation in terms of pregnancy and implantation rates. Most likely, the 0.2 mol/l sucrose concentration used during freezing provides a more optimal dehydration compared to previous protocols that used 0.1 mol/l sucrose (which may not be sufficient for adequate oocyte dehydration prior to lowering of the temperature), or 0.3 mol/l sucrose (that leads to more rapid dehydration, and possible damage to the oocyte). Moreover, the higher (0.3 mol/l) sucrose concentration used during thawing may provide a more controlled water exchange between the oocytes and the thawing solutions by slowing the entry of water. Confirmation of these results and their biological underpinnings is awaited.

Vitrification

Vitrification may be defined as a physical process by which a highly concentrated solution of cryoprotectants solidifies during cooling without the formation of ice crystals. The solid, called a glass, retains the normal molecular and ionic distribution of the liquid state and can be considered to be an extremely viscous supercooled liquid.[39] Vitrification has certain advantages over freezing because it avoids the damage caused by intracellular ice formation and the osmotic effects caused by extracellular ice formation. Further, it is a faster procedure than conventional slow cooling as it does not require seeding or a controlled freezing rate that necessitates a machine. Several reviews have been offered that describe the theory behind vitrification.[39–41]

A vitrification solution usually consists of one or more cryoprotectants in excess of 40% (v/v). There is, however, a possible toxicity to cells at 20°C, so exposure to the final concentrated solution is usually performed at low temperatures (0–4°C).[42] During vitrification, oocytes are incubated in the equilibration solution (7.5% ethylene glycol, 7.5% dimethyl sulfoxide (DMSO),

20% plasma protein supplement (PPS), each in M199 H medium) for around 8 minutes and then transferred to vitrification drop solutions (15% ethylene glycol, 15% DMSO, 0.5 mol/l sucrose, 20% PPS, each in M199 H) where the passages are very quick (5 s, 5 s, and 10 s, respectively, per drop). Samples are then plunged into liquid nitrogen. The thawing solutions are based on a series of solutions containing decreasing sucrose concentrations (1.0 mol/l, 0.5 mol/l, and 0 mol/l) with 20% PPS in M199 H.

Kuleshova et al[43] reported the first human live birth after oocyte vitrification, using open-pulled straws to load oocytes and high concentrations of ethylene glycol and sucrose. Shortly afterwards, Yoon et al[44] reported a pregnancy and the delivery of healthy infants developed from vitrified oocytes using a vitrification method based on ethylene glycol and sucrose as cryoprotectants and an electron microscope copper grid as oocyte vehicle. Since then, vitrification has been used sporadically in multiple centers with success.

The meta-analysis by Oktay et al[36] included only four reports of vitrification published prior to June 2005. These studies reported the outcome of 503 thawed oocytes, with a 2.0% live birth rate per thawed oocyte and a total of 10 live births. However, the five more recent reports discussed separately, published between June 2005 and March 2006, showed significant improvement. These latter reports included 636 oocytes, with 6% clinical pregnancy and 4.6% live birth rates per thawed oocyte. In these studies, the live birth rate per transfer was 39%, and the impantation rate was 20.5%. More recently Antinori et al[45] found similar results using the Cryotop vitrification method previously reported by Kuwayama et al.[46] In this study, 330 oocytes were thawed with a survival rate of 99.4%. The fertilization, pregnancy, and implantation rates were 92.9, 32.5, and 13.2%, respectively. It seems that very rapid improvements in the efficiency of vitrification leading to live births are under way.

Overall, slow freezing and vitrification have been shown to be increasingly mature clinical techniques. The use of oocyte cryopreservation is likely to become more prevalent in the near future.

Gonadotropin releasing hormone agonist cotreatment

Based on the postulated role of gonadal suppression in the preservation of testicular function in men receiving chemotherapy, and the belief that the fertility of pre-pubertal girls is not affected by gonadotoxic treatment,

the effect of gonadotropin releasing hormone agonist (GnRHa) treatment in preserving fertility by creating a pre-pubertal hormonal milieu has been investigated.[14]

Animal studies have shown a protective role for GnRHa treatment against chemotherapy-induced gonadal damage.[47,48] Ataya et al demonstrated that loss of primordial follicles in response to cyclophosphamide chemotherapy was significantly less in rhesus monkeys receiving GnRHa cotreatment compared to those receiving chemotherapy alone (65% vs 29%, respectively).[49] Interestingly, using the same model, they did not find GnRHa cotreatment to be effective in protecting against radiotherapy-induced gonadal damage.[50]

Following encouraging findings in animal models, non-randomized studies with short-term follow-up suggested a protective role for GnRHa cotreatment.[51-55] These studies were criticized for their lack of randomization, different follow-up periods for treatment and control groups, and the use of ovarian failure as endpoint, which may not reflect the decrease in primordial follicle count in response to chemotherapy in young women.[14]

The mechanism by which GnRHa cotreatment may protect against chemotherapy-induced gonadal damage is still debated, as is the presence of FSH receptors in primordial follicles.[14,56-58] Moreover, GnRH antagonists (unlike GnRHa) do not seem to be protective against cyclophosphamide-induced primordial follicle loss in mice.[59]

At present, despite encouraging reports, the benefits and long-term effects of GnRHa cotreatment are unclear, and a consensus regarding the effectiveness of ovarian suppression is lacking.

Currently, there are a multitude of ongoing prospective randomized trials investigating the role of GnRH agonists in the prevention of chemotherapy-induced gonadotoxicity. Among these, the Prevention of Chemotherapy Induced Ovarian Failure With Goserelin in BC Patients (ZORO) study is being conducted by the German breast group. It is a prospective randomized multicenter study that investigates whether GnRHa goserelin prevents chemotherapy-induced ovarian failure in young, hormone-insensitive breast cancer patients receiving anthracycline-containing neoadjuvant chemotherapy. In this study, all patients will receive an anthracycline-containing polychemotherapy. Patients randomized to goserelin will receive their first injection of 3.6 mg at least 2 weeks before the start of chemotherapy. Goserelin will be given as a subcutaneous injection in the abdominal wall every 4 weeks (28±3 days) until the end of the last chemotherapy cycle. The primary objective is to increase the percentage of patients with normal ovarian function at 6 months after the application of (neo)adjuvant, anthracycline-containing polychemotherapy in parallel with goserelin, compared to chemotherapy alone. Another study, very similar in design and using goserelin with a longer (5 years) follow-up, is the ovarian protection in premenopausal breast cancer patients or 'OPTION' study, conducted by the Anglo-Celtic cooperative oncology group. Other studies by the Italian breast cancer group, the German Hodgkin's lymphoma group, the Spanish lymphoma group, and the German SLE group are ongoing. Until the results of these studies become available, GnRHa cotreatment for the prevention of chemotherapy-induced gonadotoxicity should be offered to patients only with appropriate informed consent in an investigational protocol.

SURGICAL OPTIONS FOR FERTILITY PRESERVATION

Ovarian transposition

Transposition of the ovaries (oophoropexy) outside the pelvis to protect them from pelvic radiation was initially described in 1958.[60] The procedure is indicated in patients diagnosed with malignancies that require pelvic radiation, but not removal of the ovaries, as part of their treatment. The most common indications are Hodgkin's disease, cervical and vaginal cancer, and pelvic sarcomas.

Initially, the procedure was performed through a laparotomy incision. More recently, oophoropexy has been described laparoscopically.[61] There are several descriptions of laparoscopic oophoropexy with small variations. In the most commonly described method, the ovaries are completely separated from the uterus and fallopian tubes by dividing the utero-ovarian ligament and incising the mesovarium. The peritoneum along the infundibulopelvic ligament is also incised, and the ovaries are transposed laterally to the paracolic gutters and sutured. The left ovary is placed at the level of the aortic bifurcation and the right ovary is placed above the pelvic brim, between the level of the aortic bifurcation and the lower pole of the right kidney.[61] Alternative approaches advocate less mobilization of the ovary. The utero-ovarian ligament is transected, but the ovary is not separated from the fallopian tube and the infundibulopelvic ligament is not completely dissected. The ovaries are then sutured anteriorly and laterally at the level of the anterosuperior iliac spines.[62]

During the last four decades, several reports have documented different degrees of ovarian function preservation and ability to conceive a pregnancy after radiation treatment. The procedure has been successful in 16–90% of reported cases.[14,62,63] The variation is due to the inability to calculate and prevent scatter radiation, concomitant use of chemotherapy, and different doses of radiation utilized.[14] In summary, laparoscopic ovarian transposition is a relatively simple, minimally invasive, and effective procedure that may be offered to reproductive-age patients who need pelvic radiation.

Ovarian tissue cryopreservation

Cryopreservation of primordial follicles within ovarian tissue has potential advantages over both embryo and oocyte freezing. Hundreds of primordial follicles containing immature oocytes may be cryopreserved without the necessity of ovarian stimulation and delay in initiating cancer treatment. Moreover, primordial follicles are significantly less susceptible to cryoinjury compared to both mature and immature oocytes due to their smaller size, slower metabolic rate, and absence of zona pellucida. Two alternative approaches are being investigated: cryopreservation of ovarian cortical strips or whole ovaries.

Cryopreservation of ovarian cortical tissue

The outer cortical layer of the ovary contains most of the primordial follicles. Therefore, it is conceivable to cryopreserve pieces of ovarian cortical tissue. The ovarian cortex is removed via laparoscopy or laparatomy and cut into strips of tissue around 1–3 mm in thickness and less than or equal to $1\,cm^2$ in total area, in order to ensure adequate penetration of cryoprotectants.[64] A slow-cooling technique has traditionally been applied[65] (Figure 11.5). It is advisable to analyze a piece of the cortical tissue to confirm the presence of follicles and the absence of malignant metastasis.[14,56] Once the ovarian tissue is cryopreserved, future options include transplantation of the tissue back to the donor (autotransplantation) or to nude mice (xenotransplantation), or to culture the follicles in vitro.

Autotransplantation   At the present time, the most promising approach seems to be transplantation of the ovarian tissue back to the donor. Autotransplantation studies using animal models have resulted in the return of ovarian function as well as pregnancies and live births with this approach.[65–67] Two different surgical

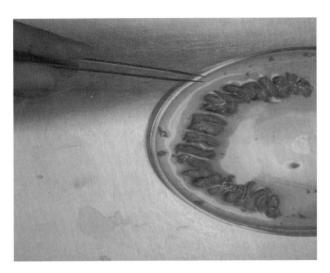

Figure 11.5 Slow freeze protocol for ovarian tissue cryopreservation. (1) Equilibrate cortical slices in cryoprotectant for 30 min at 0°C; (2) cool at 2°C/min to −9°C; (3) soak for 10 min and seed; (4) cool at 0.3°C/min to −40°C; (5) cool at 10°C/min to −140°C; (6) transfer to liquid nitrogen (−196°C)

approaches have been used in humans for transplantation: orthotopic (pelvic) or heterotopic.

Orthotopic (pelvic) transplantation places ovarian tissue in close proximity to the infundibulopelvic ligament with the hope that natural pregnancy may occur. Until recently, there has been only a single case report of this technique in which ovarian endocrine function resumed; even so, ovulation did not occur in that patient.[68] In 2004, Donnez et al reported the return of ovarian endocrine function and a spontaneous live birth following the orthotopic transplantation of cryopreserved ovarian tissue in a woman treated for Hodgkin's lymphoma.[69] This study has been criticized for not providing definitive evidence of a pregnancy resulting from cryopreserved and transplanted ovarian tissue, as the patient had not undergone oophorectomy, and ovarian failure prior to transplantation was found to be questionable.[70] More recently, Meirow et al reported a live birth after IVF following the transplantation of thawed cryopreserved ovarian cortical tissue into the ovaries of a 28-year-old woman who had ovarian failure after high-dose chemotherapy for non-Hodgkin's lymphoma.[71] However, although spontaneous menstruation resumed after delivery, her endocrine profile 22 months after transplantation indicated low ovarian reserve.[72]

Heterotopic transplantation is an alternative approach in which cryopreserved ovarian tissue is transplanted to a site outside the pelvis. Transplantation to a heterotopic site such as the forearm[64,73] or abdomen[74] is both technically easier and imposes fewer surgery-associated risks, compared to orthotopic transplantation. It also allows easier monitoring of follicle growth. Even so, it is clear that IVF–embryo transfer is absolutely necessary to achieve pregnancy. In 2001, Oktay et al were first to report the return of ovarian endocrine function with the development of a dominant follicle and resumption of menstrual cycles in two women using this approach.[73] In one case, after blocking the patient's pituitary function with gonadotropin releasing hormone antagonist, and stimulating her with human menopausal gonadotropins for 11 days, they performed percutaneous oocyte retrieval from the forearm. Unfortunately, fertilization could not be achieved with ICSI.[73] More recently, Oktay et al, by transplanting the cryopreserved ovarian tissue beneath the abdominal skin, were able to restore ovarian function in a woman previously treated for breast cancer. They performed eight cycles of controlled ovarian stimulation using GnRH antagonist or agonist for suppression and a combination of recombinant FSH and human menopausal gonadotropins for stimulation. In eight cycles, a total of 20 oocytes were retrieved. Of the eight oocytes suitable for IVF, one fertilized normally and developed into a 4-cell embryo that was transferred to the patient, but pregnancy did not occur.[74]

A significant source of concern associated with autotransplantation is the risk of transmission of metastatic cancer cells. This risk has been estimated to be highest for blood-borne cancers such as leukemia and lymphoma.[75] Histological evaluation of ovarian samples has been suggested in order to prevent cancer transmission, although it is not possible to completely eliminate the risk of transmission in hematologic or disseminated malignancies.

Xenotransplantation Mice with severe combined immunodeficiency (SCID) can accommodate tissues from foreign species without host-versus-graft response due to a deficiency in both T and B cell-mediated immunity.[76] Xenotransplantation of cryopreserved ovarian tissue into SCID mice has also shown success, with healthy follicles present in the graft when removed 22 weeks after the initial transplantation.[77] Using this option, the possibility of cancer cell transmission and relapse is eliminated, as individual oocytes are retrieved from the host animal. Another advantage is the possible application in women in whom hormonal stimulation is contraindicated. Indeed, following subcutaneous placement of human ovarian cortical tissue into mice, follicular growth in response to exogenous gonadotropin stimulation, follicle maturation, and corpus luteum formation have been observed.[78,79] Additional advantages of xenotransplantation include convenient monitoring of follicular development, and easy access to follicle aspiration. However, possible transmission of zoonoses to humans is a serious concern, and this method is unlikely to be clinically available in the near future.

In vitro maturation   In vitro maturation of follicles from cryopreserved ovarian tissue is of significant interest as it may eliminate the risk of transmission of metastatic cancer cells. However, only in the mouse has the production of live young from cultured primordial follicles been successful.[80,81] Eppig and O'Brien developed a two-stage culture system: primordial follicles were grown in organ culture to secondary follicles, and the secondary follicles were then isolated enzymatically and cultured further to mature oocytes, followed by routine IVF and embryo transfer. The first mouse born was extremely obese, and postmortem examination revealed multiple malformations,[80] and to date, only 59 live offspring (5.7% of embryos transferred) have been obtained.[81]

Preantral follicles have also been grown to the antral phase in vitro[82,83] using the mouse model. Here, oocytes were matured to metaphase II after human chorionic gonadotropin (hCG) stimulation[84] and were fertilized. Subsequently, development into blastocysts[85] and the production of live births after embryo transfer[86] were achieved.

Newton and Illingworth[87] reported the survival and in vitro growth of murine follicles after isolation from ovarian tissues cryopreserved by a slow freezing method. They indicated that follicles isolated from frozen/thawed tissue were able to give rise to mature oocytes, but at the end of the culture period, the diameter of the frozen/thawed follicles was smaller than that of fresh ones. More recently, Segino et al demonstrated that cryopreservation of mouse ovarian tissues by rapid freezing is successful in allowing the oocytes to maintain their ability to complete meiosis and participate in preimplantation development in vitro.[88] Isolation of oocytes from antral follicles of cryopreserved mouse ovaries, and their competence to undergo maturation, fertilization, embryogenesis, and development to term, have also been demonstrated.[89]

Human data on in vitro maturation of follicles from ovarian tissue are scarce. Competence to complete nuclear and cytoplasmic maturation is acquired only during the final stages of antral follicle development, a time when the large size of human antral follicles may be prohibitive to successful cryopreservation. However, eventually it may be possible to grow human oocytes from the much smaller primordial, primary, or even secondary follicle stages in vitro, as reported for the mouse, after cryopreservation. It will be important to establish whether this success can be achieved with cryopreserved material, although ultimate success seems likely.

Cryopreservation of whole ovaries

Animal studies suggest that fresh whole ovaries can be successfully transplanted. Although the duration of subsequent ovarian function has initially been limited, mostly due to ischemia resulting from thrombosis,[90] the use of microsurgical techniques has led to improvements in graft survival.[90-94] In addition, careful dissection of ovarian vessels during ovariectomy and perfusion of the ovary with cryoprotectants through these vessels improved tissue survival and led to similar rates of follicular viability and apoptosis, compared to ovarian cortical strips.[92] Recently, a successful pregnancy was achieved following transplantation of frozen/thawed rat ovaries.[94] More recently, Arav et al reported oocyte recovery, embryo development, and ovarian function maintained for 36 months after transplantation of cryopreserved whole ovary in sheep.[95]

In the human, Bedaiwy and colleagues[96] investigated the immediate post-thawing injury to the ovary that was cryopreserved as a whole with its vascular pedicle or as cortical strips. Bilateral oophorectomy was performed in two women (46 and 44 years old) undergoing hysterectomy. In both patients, one of the harvested ovaries was sectioned and cryopreserved as ovarian cortical strips. The other ovary was cryopreserved intact with its vascular pedicle. After thawing 7 days later, the overall viability of the primordial follicles was 75–78% in intact cryopreserved/thawed ovaries and 81–83% in ovarian cortical strips. Comparable primordial follicle counts, and absence of features of necrosis or apoptotic markers, led them to conclude that cryopreservation injury is not associated with significant follicular damage. Martinez-Madrid et al reported similar findings.[97]

While these results are encouraging, definitive restoration of fertility resulting from the transplantation of a cryopreserved/thawed whole human ovary remains to be demonstrated. This technique does carry potentially increased risk of returning metastatic disease to the patient, compared to the handling of oocytes or even cortical strips.

SUMMARY AND FUTURE CONSIDERATIONS

Fertility preservation in females diagnosed with cancer has become an important area of investigation due to increasing cancer survival rates combined with delayed childbearing. Alternative treatment strategies for early stage gynecologic cancers have recently been studied with promising results for both survival and fertility preservation. In addition to embryo cryopreservation, encouraging findings have recently been reported using oocyte cryopreservation, ovarian cryopreservation, and GnRHa cotreatment with chemotherapy. Improvement of these techniques as well as better characterization of their success rates and risks awaits further investigation.

REFERENCES

1. American Cancer Society. Cancer Facts & Figures 2001. Atlanta, GA: ACS, 2001.
2. Ries LAG, Percy CL, Bunin GR. Introduction. In: Ries LAG, Smith MA, Gurney JG, eds. Cancer Incidence and Survival among Children and Adolescents: United States SEER Program 1975–1995. Bethesda, MD: National Cancer Institute, 1999.
3. Bleyer WA. The impact of childhood cancer on the United States and the world. Cancer 1990; 40: 355–67.
4. Martin J, Hamilton B, Sutton P et al. Births: final data for 2002. Natl Vital Stat Rep December 2003; 52(10).
5. Oktay K, Buyuk E, Davis O et al. Fertility preservation in breast cancer patients: IVF and embryo cryopreservation after ovarian stimulation with tamoxifen. Hum Reprod 2003; 18: 90–5.
6. Oktay K, Buyuk E, Libertella N et al. Fertility preservation in breast cancer patients: a prospective controlled comparison of ovarian stimulation with tamoxifen and letrozole for embryo cryopreservation. J Clin Oncol 2005; 23: 4347–53.
7. Oktay K, Hourvitz A, Sahin G et al. Letrozole reduces estrogen and gonadotropin exposure in women with breast cancer undergoing ovarian stimulation before chemotherapy. J Clin Endocrinol Metab 2006; 91: 3885–90.
8. Azim AA, Costantini-Ferrando M, Lostritto K, Oktay K. Relative potencies of anastrozole and letrozole to suppress estradiol in breast cancer patients undergoing ovarian stimulation before in vitro fertilization. J Clin Endocrinol Metab 2007; 92: 2197–200.
9. Son WY, Yoon SH, Yoon HJ, Lee SM, Lim JH. Pregnancy outcome following transfer of human blastocysts vitrified on electron microscopy grids after induced collapse of the blastocoele. Hum Reprod 2003; 18: 137–9.
10. Wang JX, Yap YY, Matthews CD. Frozen-thawed embryo transfer: influence of clinical factors on implantation rate and risk of multiple conception. Hum Reprod 2001; 16: 2316–19.
11. Senn A, Vozzi C, Chanson A, De Grandi P, Germond M. Prospective randomized study of two cryopreservation policies avoiding embryo selection: the pronucleate stage leads to a higher cumulative delivery rate than the early cleavage stage. Fertil Steril 2000; 74: 946–52.
12. Frederick JL, Ord T, Kettel LM et al. Successful pregnancy outcome after cryopreservation of all fresh embryos with subsequent transfer into an unstimulated cycle. Fertil Steril 1995; 64: 987–90.
13. Selick CE, Hofmann GE, Albano C et al. Embryo quality and pregnancy potential of fresh compared with frozen embryos – is freezing detrimental to high quality embryos? Hum Reprod 1995; 10: 392–5.
14. Sonmezer M, Oktay K. Fertility preservation in female patients. Hum Reprod Update 2004; 10: 251–66.
15. Centers for Disease Control. Assisted reproductive technology success rates. In: National Summary and Fertility Clinic Reports. Atlanta, GA: US Department of Health and Human Services, 2002.
16. Baysoy A, Serdaroglu H, Jamal H et al. Letrozole versus human menopausal gonadotrophin in women undergoing intrauterine insemination. Reprod Biomed Online 2006; 13: 208–12.
17. Bedaiwy MA, Forman R, Mousa NA, Al Inany HG, Casper RF. Cost-effectiveness of aromatase inhibitor cotreatment for controlled ovarian stimulation. Hum Reprod 2006; 21: 2838–44.
18. Chen C. Pregnancy after human oocyte cryopreservation. Lancet 1986; 1: 884–6.
19. Jackowski S, Leibo SP, Maxur P. Glycerol permeabilities of fertilized and infertilized mouse ova. J Exp Zool 1980; 212: 329–41.
20. Leibo SP. Water permeability and its activation energy of fertilized and unfertilized mouse ova. J Membr Biol 1980; 53: 179–88.
21. Matson PL, Graefling J, Junk SM, Yovich JL, Edirisinghe WR. Cryopreservation of oocytes and embryos: use of a mouse model to investigate effects upon zona hardness and formulate treatment strategies in an in-vitro fertilization programme. Hum Reprod 1997; 12: 1550–3.
22. Porcu E, Fabbri R, Seracchioli R et al. Birth of a healthy female after intracytoplasmic sperm injection of cryopreserved human oocytes. Fertil Steril 1997; 68: 724–6.
23. Polak de Fried E, Notrica J, Rubinstein M, Marazzi A, Gomez Gonzalez M. Pregnancy after human donor oocyte cryopreservation and thawing in association with intracytoplasmic sperm injection in a patient with ovarian failure. Fertil Steril 1998; 69: 555–7.
24. Lassalle B, Testart J, Renard JP. Human embryo features that influence the success of cryopreservation with the use of 1,2 propanediol. Fertil Steril 1985; 44: 645–51.
25. Leibo SP. Fundamental cryobiology of mouse ova and embryos. Ciba Found Symp 1977; 52: 69–96.
26. Mazur P. Freezing of living cells: mechanisms and implications. Am J Physiol 1984; 247: 125–42.
27. Rienzi L, Martinez F, Ubaldi F et al. Polscope analysis of meiotic spindle changes in living metaphase II human oocytes during the freezing and thawing procedures. Hum Reprod 2004; 19: 655–9.
28. Bianchi V, Coticchio G, Fava L, Flamigni C, Borini A. Meiotic spindle imaging in human oocytes frozen with a slow freezing procedure involving high sucrose concentration. Hum Reprod 2005; 20: 1078–83.
29. Coticchio G, De Santis L, Rossi G et al. Sucrose concentration influences the rate of human oocytes with normal spindle and chromosome configurations after slow-cooling cryopreservation. Hum Reprod 2006; 21: 1771–6.
30. Gook DA, Osborn SM, Johnston WI. Cryopreservation of mouse and human oocytes using 1,2-propanediol and the configuration of the meiotic spindle. Hum Reprod 1993; 8: 1101–9.
31. Borini A, Coticchio G, Flamigni C. Oocyte freezing: a positive comment based on our experience. Reprod Biomed Online 2003; 7: 120.
32. Fabbri R, Porcu E, Marsella T et al. Human oocyte cryopreservation: new perspectives regarding oocyte survival. Hum Reprod 2001; 16: 411–16.
33. Huang J, Tan SL, Chian RC. Fertility preservation for female. J Reprod Contracept 2006; 17: 1–20.

34. Borini A, Sciajno R, Bianchi V et al. Clinical outcome of oocyte cryopreservation after slow cooling with a protocol utilizing a high sucrose concentration. Hum Reprod 2006; 21: 512–17.

35. Levi Setti PE, Albani E, Novara PV, Cesana A, Morreale G. Cryopreservation of supernumerary oocytes in IVF/ICSI cycles. Hum Reprod 2006; 21: 370–5.

36. Oktay K, Cil PA, Bang H. Efficiency of oocyte cryopreservation: a meta-analysis. Fertil Steril 2006; 86: 70–80.

37. Paynter SJ, Borini A, Bianchi V et al. Volume changes of mature human oocytes on exposure to cryoprotectant solutions used in slow cooling procedures. Hum Reprod 2005; 20: 1194–9.

38. Bianchi V, Coticchio G, Distratis V et al. Differential sucrose concentration during dehydration (0.2 mol/l) and rehydration (0.3 mol/l) increases the implantation rate of frozen human oocytes. Reprod Biomed Online 2007; 14: 64–71.

39. Mazur P. Equilibrium, quasi-equilibrium, and nonequilibrium freezing of mammalian embryos. Cell Biophys 1990; 17: 53–92.

40. Rall WF. Factors affecting the survival of mouse embryos cryopreserved by vitrification. Cryobiology 1987; 24: 387–402.

41. Fahy GM. Vitrification. In: McGrath JJ, Diller KR, eds. Low Temperature Biotechnology: Emerging Applications and Engineering Contributions. New York: ASME, 1988.

42. Kasai M, Korni JH, Takakarmo A et al. A simple method for mouse embryo cryopreservation in a low toxicity vitrification solution, without appreciable loss of viability. J Reprod Fertil 1990; 89: 91–7.

43. Kuleshova L, Gianaroli L, Magli C, Ferraretti A, Trounson A. Birth following vitrification of a small number of human oocytes: case report. Hum Reprod 1999; 14: 3077–9.

44. Yoon TK, Chung HM, Lim JM et al. Pregnancy and delivery of healthy infants developed from vitrified oocytes in a stimulated in vitro fertilization-embryo transfer program. Fertil Steril 2000; 74: 180–1.

45. Antinori M, Licata E, Dani G et al. Cryotop vitrification of human oocytes results in high survival rate and healthy deliveries. Reprod Biomed Online 2007; 14: 72–9.

46. Kuwayama M, Vajta G, Kato O, Leibo S. Highly efficient vitrification method for cryopreservation of human oocytes. Reprod Biomed Online 2005; 11: 300–8.

47. Glode LM, Robinson J, Gould SF. Protection from cyclophosphamide-induced testicular damage with an analogue of gonadotropin-releasing hormone. Lancet 1981; 1: 1132–4.

48. Ataya K, Moghissi K. Chemotherapy-induced premature ovarian failure: mechanisms and prevention. Steroids 1989; 54: 607–26.

49. Ataya K, Rao LV, Lawrence E, Kimmel R. Luteinizing hormone-releasing hormone agonist inhibits cyclophosphamide-induced ovarian follicular depletion in rhesus monkeys. Biol Reprod 1995; 52: 365–72.

50. Ataya K, Pydyn E, Ramahi-Ataya A, Orton CG. Is radiation-induced ovarian failure in rhesus monkeys preventable by luteinizing hormone-releasing hormone agonists?: Preliminary observations. J Clin Endocrinol Metab 1995; 80: 790–5.

51. Blumenfeld Z, Avivi I, Linn S et al. Prevention of irreversible chemotherapy-induced ovarian damage in young women with lymphoma by a gonadotrophin-releasing hormone agonist in parallel to chemotherapy. Hum Reprod 1996; 11: 1620–6.

52. Blumenfeld Z, Avivi I, Ritter M, Rowe JM. Preservation of fertility and ovarian function and minimizing chemotherapy-induced gonadotoxicity in young women. J Soc Gynecol Invest 1999; 6: 229–39.

53. Blumenfeld Z, Shapiro D, Shteinberg M, Avivi I, Nahir M. Preservation of fertility and ovarian function and minimizing gonadotoxicity in young women with systemic lupus erythematosus treated by chemotherapy. Lupus 2000; 9: 401–5.

54. Blumenfeld Z, Dann E, Avivi I, Epelbaum R, Rowe JM. Fertility after treatment for Hodgkin's disease [see Comment]. Ann Oncol 2002; 13 (Suppl 1): 138–47.

55. Recchia F, Sica G, De Filippi S et al. Goserelin as ovarian protection in the adjuvant treatment of premenopausal breast cancer: a phase II pilot study. Anticancer Drugs 2002; 13: 417–24.

56. Blumenfeld Z. Gynaecologic concerns for young women exposed to gonadotoxic chemotherapy. Curr Opin Obstet Gynecol 2003; 15: 359–70.

57. Blumenfeld Z. Ovarian cryopreservation versus ovarian suppression by GnRH analogues: primum non nocere. Hum Reprod 2004; 19: 1924–5.

58. Oktay K, Sonmezer M, Oktem O. 'Ovarian cryopreservation versus ovarian suppression by GnRH analogues: primum non nocere': Reply. Hum Reprod 2004; 19: 1681–3.

59. Danforth DR, Roberts A, Arbogast LK, Friedman CL. Follicular preservation during cyclophosphamide treatment: GnRH agonist vs antagonist. J Soc Gynecol Investig 2003; 10: 135A.

60. McCall ML, Keaty EC, Thompson JD. Conservation of ovarian tissue in the treatment of carcinoma of the cervix with radical surgery. Am J Obstet Gynecol 1958; 75: 590–600.

61. Morice P, Castaigne D, Haie-Meder C et al. Laparoscopic ovarian transposition for pelvic malignancies: indications and functional outcomes. Fertil Steril 1998; 70: 956–60.

62. Bisharah M, Tulandi T. Laparoscopic preservation of ovarian function: an underused procedure. Am J Obstet Gynecol 2003; 188: 367–70.

63. Morice P, Thiam-Ba R, Castaigne D et al. Fertility results after ovarian transposition for pelvic malignancies treated by external irradiation or brachytherapy. Hum Reprod 1998; 13: 660–3.

64. Oktay K, Buyuk E, Rosenwaks Z, Rucinski J. A technique for transplantation of ovarian cortical strips to the forearm. Fertil Steril 2003; 80: 193–8.

65. Gosden RG, Baird DT, Wade JC, Webb R. Restoration of fertility to oophorectomised sheep by ovarian autografts stored at –196°C. Hum Reprod 1994; 9: 597–603.

66. Salle B, Demirci B, Franck M et al. Normal pregnancies and live births after autograft of frozen-thawed hemi-ovaries into ewes. Fertil Steril 2002; 77: 403–8.

67. Sztein J, Sweet H, Farley J, Mobraaten L. Cryopreservation and orthotopic transplantation of mouse ovaries: new approach in gamete banking. Biol Reprod 1998; 58: 1071–4.

68. Radford JA, Lieberman BA, Brison DR et al. Orthotopic reimplantation of cryopreserved ovarian cortical strips after high-dose chemotherapy for Hodgkin's lymphoma. Lancet 2001; 357: 1172–5.

69. Donnez J, Dolmans MM, Demylle D et al. Livebirth after orthotopic transplantation of cryopreserved ovarian tissue. Lancet 2004; 364: 1405–10.

70. Oktay K, Tilly J. Livebirth after cryopreserved ovarian tissue autotransplantation. Lancet 2004; 364: 2091–2.

71. Meirow D, Levron J, Eldar-Geva T et al. Pregnancy after transplantation of cryopreserved ovarian tissue in a patient with ovarian failure after chemotherapy. N Engl J Med 2005; 353: 318–21.

72. Meirow D, Levron J, Eldar-Geva T et al. Monitoring the ovaries after autotransplantation of cryopreserved ovarian tissue: endocrine studies, in vitro fertilization cycles, and live birth. Fertil Steril 2007; 87: 418.e7–e15.

73. Oktay K, Economos K, Kan M et al. Endocrine function and oocyte retrieval after autologous transplantation of ovarian cortical strips to the forearm [see Comment]. JAMA 2001; 286: 1490–3.

74. Oktay K, Buyuk E, Veeck L et al. Embryo development after heterotopic transplantation of cryopreserved ovarian tissue [see Comment]. Lancet 2004; 363: 837–40.

75. Shaw JM, Bowles J, Koopman P, Wood EC, Trounson AO. Fresh and cryopreserved ovarian tissue samples from donors with lymphoma transmit the cancer to graft recipients. Hum Reprod 1996; 11: 1668–73.

76. Bosma GC, Custer RP, Bosma MJ. A severe combined immunodeficiency mutation in the mouse. Nature 1983; 301: 527–30.

77. Oktay K, Newton H, Gosden R. Transplantation of cryopreserved human ovarian tissue results in follicle growth initiation in SCID mice. Fertil Steril 2000; 73: 599–603.

78. Weissman A, Gotlieb L, Colgan T et al. Preliminary experience with subcutaneous human ovarian cortex transplantation in the NOD-SCID mouse. Biol Reprod 1999; 60: 1462–7.

79. Revel A, Davis VJ, Casper RF. Ovarian cortex cryopreservation in pediatric and adolescent medicine. J Pediatr Adolesc Gynecol 2000; 13: 95.

80. Eppig JJ, O'Brien MJ. Development in vitro of mouse oocytes from primordial follicles. Biol Reprod 1996; 54: 197–207.

81. O'Brien MJ, Pendola JK, Eppig JJ. A revised protocol for in vitro development of mouse oocytes from primordial follicles dramatically improves their development competence. Biol Reprod 2003; 68: 1682–6.

82. Qvist R, Blackwell LF, Bourne H, Brown JB. Development of mouse ovarian follicles from primary to preovulatory stages in vitro. J Reprod Fertil 1990; 89: 169–80.

83. Nayudu PL, Osborn SM. Factors influencing the rate of preantral and antral growth of mouse ovarian follicles in vitro. J Reprod Fertil 1992; 95: 349–62.

84. Cortvrindt R, Smitz J. Early preantral mouse follicle in vitro maturation: oocyte growth, meiotic maturation and granulosa-cell proliferation. Theriogenology 1998; 49: 845–59.

85. Cortvrindt R, Smitz J, Van Steirteghem AC. In vitro maturation, fertilization and embryo development of immature oocytes from early preantral follicles from prepubertal mice in a simplified culture system. Hum Reprod 1996; 11: 2656–66.

86. Spears N, Boland NI, Murray AA, Gosden RG. Mouse oocytes derived from in vitro grown primary ovarian follicles are fertile. Hum Reprod 1994; 9: 527–32.

87. Newton H, Illingworth P. In vitro growth of murine pre-antral follicles after isolation from cryopreserved ovarian tissue. Hum Reprod 2001; 16: 423–9.

88. Segino M, Ikeda M, Hirahara F, Sato K. In vitro follicular development of cryopreserved mouse ovarian tissue. Reproduction 2005; 130: 187–92.

89. Sztein JM, O'Brien MJ, Farley JS, Mobraaten LE, Eppig JJ. Rescue of oocytes from antral follicles of cryopreserved mouse ovaries: competence to undergo maturation, embryogenesis, and development to term. Hum Reprod 2000; 15: 567–71.

90. Yin H, Wang X, Kim SS et al. Transplantation of intact rat gonads using vascular anastomosis: effects of cryopreservation, ischaemia and genotype. Hum Reprod 2003; 18: 1165–72.

91. Jeremias E, Bedaiwy MA, Nelson D, Biscotti CV, Falcone T. Assessment of tissue injury in cryopreserved ovarian tissue. Fertil Steril 2003; 79: 651–3.

92. Bedaiwy MA, Jeremias E, Gurunluoglu R et al. Restoration of ovarian function after autotransplantation of intact frozen-thawed sheep ovaries with microvascular anastomosis. Fertil Steril 2003; 79: 594–602.

93. Jeremias E, Bedaiwy MA, Gurunluoglu R et al. Heterotopic autotransplantation of the ovary with microvascular anastomosis: a novel surgical technique. Fertil Steril 2002; 77: 1278–82.

94. Wang X, Chen H, Yin H et al. Fertility after intact ovary transplantation. Nature 2002; 415: 385.

95. Arav A, Revel A, Nathan Y et al. Oocyte recovery, embryo development and ovarian function after cryopreservation and transplantation of whole sheep ovary. Hum Reprod 2005; 20: 3545–59.

96. Bedaiwy MA, Hussein MR, Biscotti C, Falcone T. Cryopreservation of intact human ovary with its vascular pedicle. Hum Reprod 2006; 21: 3258–69.

97. Martinez-Madrid B, Camboni A, Dolmans MM et al. Apoptosis and ultrastructural assessment after cryopreservation of whole human ovaries with their vascular pedicle. Fertil Steril 2007; 87: 1153–65.

12 Medical management of polycystic ovarian syndrome and its sequelae

Pinar H Kodaman and Antoni J Duleba

INTRODUCTION

Polycystic ovarian syndrome (PCOS) is a heterogeneous endocrine disorder that affects 6–8% of reproductive aged women.[1] Despite the prevalence of this disorder, its definition remains controversial. The 2003 joint meeting of the European Society for Human Reproduction and Embryology and the American Society for Reproductive Medicine (ESHRE/ASRM) defined PCOS as having at least two of the following three criteria: (1) chronic oligo- or anovulation, (2) hyperandrogenemia or clinical evidence of androgen excess, and (3) polycystic ovaries.[2] Furthermore, other etiologies of hyperandrogenism or anovulation, such as congenital adrenal hyperplasia, androgen secreting tumors, or Cushing's syndrome, must be excluded prior to making the diagnosis of PCOS (Table 12.1).

Recently, these diagnostic criteria for PCOS have come into question in favor of the 1990 National Institutes of Health (NIH) definition of PCOS, which comprises women who have: (1) oligo-ovulation, (2) hyperandrogenism and/or hyperandrogenemia, and (3) the exclusion of other disorders.[3] This definition narrows the spectrum of women affected by PCOS in that it excludes ovulatory women with hyperandrogenism and polycystic ovaries and anovulatory women with polycystic ovaries, but no hyperandrogenism. It is argued that the inclusion of these two phenotypes as a part of PCOS is premature, because there is insufficient evidence to show that they lead to the metabolic complications and ovulatory dysfunction associated with classical PCOS.[3] Whether the presence of polycystic ovaries will ultimately be considered in the diagnosis of PCOS is unclear, and further studies are warranted.

Women with PCOS present with a variety of clinical signs and symptoms, including those related to menstrual dysfunction, androgen excess, and infertility. Poor reproductive function is due to anovulation as well as a high rate of early pregnancy loss.[4,5] In the long term, women with PCOS are at increased risk for dyslipidemia, hypertension, and related cardiovascular morbidity and mortality.[6–9] Insulin resistance is also

Table 12.1 Current consensus definitions of polycystic ovarian syndrome (PCOS). To fulfill the criteria for both definitions, other etiologies of androgen excess and/or ovulatory dysfunction must be excluded

1990 NIH criteria	2003 ESHRE/ASRM criteria (at least 2 of 3)
Oligo-ovulation	Oligo- or anovulation
Hyperandrogenism or hyperandrogenemia	Hyperandrogenism or hyperandrogenemia
	Polycystic ovaries

prevalent among both lean and obese women with PCOS, and, not surprisingly, women with PCOS have an increased risk of developing type II diabetes mellitus compared to controls (15% vs 2.3%, respectively).[8]

Given the significant sequelae of PCOS, prompt diagnosis and effective treatment are warranted. The recommended laboratory tests for the diagnosis and evaluation of PCOS are illustrated in Table 12.2 and will be further alluded to below. As the presentation of this syndrome can be variable, and because it affects women who may or may not be interested in conceiving, treatment must be tailored to the individual. This chapter will address the various approaches to the treatment of PCOS, focusing on medical management. Symptomatic treatment of PCOS will be addressed first followed by a review of other therapeutic options that target the underlying pathophysiology of this common endocrinopathy. Figure 12.1 represents graphically a paradigm of PCOS, its sequelae, and proposed treatments to be discussed below.

SYMPTOMATIC TREATMENT OF POLYCYSTIC OVARIAN SYNDROME

Anovulation

The etiology of anovulation in PCOS is multifactorial, and includes alterations in gonadotropin secretion such that most women with PCOS have elevated plasma concentrations of luteinizing hormone (LH)

Table 12.2 Laboratory tests aiding in the diagnosis and evaluation of PCOS. Blood may be drawn in the fasting state on days 3–7 of a spontaneous or progestin-induced cycle

Test	Comments
TSH	To rule out thyroid disease
Prolactin	To rule out hyperprolactinemia
FSH	Assessment for hypogonadotropic
LH	hypogonadism; LH to FSH ratio
17-hydroxyprogesterone	To rule out congenital adrenal hyperplasia
Free and total testosterone SHBG	Indirect assessment of hyperinsulinemia; facilitates calculation of free testosterone[a] and free testosterone index
DHEAS	Assessment for adrenal etiology of hyperandrogenism
Lipid panel Lipoprotein(a) hs-CRP (high sensitivity C-reactive protein assay)	Assessment of cardiovascular risk factors
2-hour GTT (75 g); determinations of glucose and insulin at 0, 30, 60, 90, and 120 min	Assessment for impaired glucose tolerance and hyperinsulinemia/insulin resistance
Free cortisol 24-hour urine collection	To rule out Cushing's syndrome
Test for microalbuminuria	Assessment of renal function/endothelial function

[a]Free testosterone calculation according to Vermeulen et al[10]
TSH, thyroid stimulating hormone; GTT, glucose tolerance test

and normal or decreased serum levels of follicle stimulating hormone (FSH).[11] The LH-enriched milieu promotes thecal steroidogenesis and thus contributes to the hyperandrogenism typically seen with this disorder.

At the level of the ovary, there are increased numbers of small, antral follicles, which appear to be developmentally arrested at approximately 5–8 mm in diameter and are located under a thickened ovarian capsule. This polycystic ovarian appearance can be appreciated sonographically as 12 or more follicles measuring less than 10 mm in diameter.[2] The granulosa cells within these follicles have decreased aromatase activity, and produce minimal estrogen despite the ample amounts of androgen substrate and normal FSH concentration within the follicular fluid.[12] Furthermore, these granulosa cells express LH receptors and undergo premature luteinization.[13] Thus, in PCOS, normal follicular development is altered in such a way that a dominant follicle is not selected, while most antral follicles persist and do not exhibit markers of atresia, but rather evidence of early luteinization.[13]

For those women with PCOS who suffer from anovulation and wish to become pregnant, it is imperative as always to first complete a basic infertility evaluation of

the couple, including a semen analysis, before medical treatment of anovulation is pursued. Clomiphene citrate is a first-line approach for anovulation related infertility among women with PCOS. A typical initial regimen is 25–50 mg a day for 5 days starting on day 3–5 of the menstrual cycle. If ovulation does not occur, the dose can be increased, usually in 50-mg increments and up to the maximum dose of 150 or 200 mg a day. Higher doses may be used; however, the antiestrogenic effects of clomiphene citrate may prevail, particularly with respect to the cervical mucus. Intrauterine inseminations are often recommended to overcome this barrier.

Approximately 60–85% of women with PCOS will ovulate in response to clomiphene citrate, and up to 50% will become pregnant.[14] Women who do not ovulate in response to a 150-mg dose of clomiphene citrate are usually considered resistant to this medication; such resistance affects 15–40% of women with PCOS.[15,16] Options for this subset of women with PCOS include the addition of metformin, a biguanide that improves insulin sensitivity and/or laparoscopic ovarian drilling, both of which will be discussed subsequently, as these treatments address underlying etiologies of anovulation in PCOS, namely, insulin resistance with resultant hyperinsulinemia and hyperandrogenemia, respectively.

Aromatase inhibitors and gonadotropins represent alternative options for women with PCOS who do not respond to clomiphene citrate. The use of these medications avoids some of the negative antiestrogenic effects of clomiphene, including those on the endometrium and cervical mucus. Letrozole, a selective aromatase inhibitor, can successfully induce ovulation in women with PCOS, resulting in a 20% pregnancy rate.[17,18] A dose of 2.5 mg a day is typically given on cycle days 3–7, and as with clomiphene, the mechanism of action of this drug involves negative feedback on the hypothalamus and pituitary, resulting in increased gonadotropin secretion. A recent randomized trial of ovulation induction with letrozole and clomiphene citrate among women with PCOS demonstrated that these two medications are comparable with respect to pregnancy rates.[19] Despite a report of potential teratogenic effects of letrozole,[20] which led to a warning from the manufacturer regarding its off-label use, this medication has a short half-life and appears to be safe for use in ovulation induction.[21-23]

Ovulation induction with exogenous gonadotropins leads to ovulation and pregnancy rates of 72 and 45%, respectively.[24] Risks of ovulation induction with gonadotropins, particularly among women with PCOS, include the ovarian hyperstimulation syndrome (OHSS)

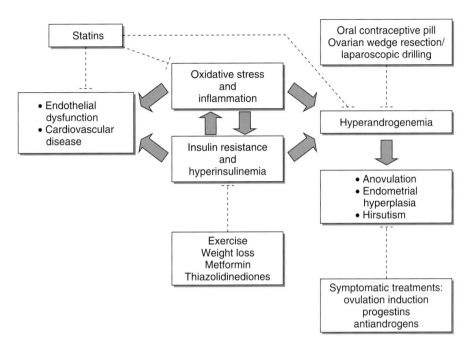

Figure 12.1 Proposed paradigm for the management of polycystic ovarian syndrome (PCOS) and its sequelae

and multiple gestations. Various approaches have been described to avoid these risks, including the step-down[25,26] and step-up[27,28] protocols in which high or low starting doses, respectively, of gonadotropins are initiated and then adjusted according to response. A recent comparative randomized trial of these two protocols demonstrated that the cumulative rate of clinical gestations did not differ between the two groups; however, the step-up protocol was more effective at producing monofollicular development in women with clomiphene citrate-resistant PCOS.[28] While a disadvantage of the step-up protocol was the longer duration of stimulation, the rate of OHSS was much lower, and the total amounts of exogenous gonadotropin used were similar in both groups.[29]

Pulsatile gonadotropin releasing hormone (GnRH) represents another alternative for ovulation induction. A recent study of pulsatile GnRH therapy of women with PCOS demonstrated a 56% ovulation rate and a 40% pregnancy rate; success correlated with lower body mass index, higher baseline FSH levels, and lower fasting insulin levels, suggesting that this treatment may be preferable for lean women with PCOS, who are less insulin resistant.[30] In vitro fertilization with embryo transfer (IVF–ET) usually represents a last resort for the treatment of PCOS-related infertility, as these women are at increased risk for the complications of controlled ovarian hyperstimulation, including OHSS and its sequelae. One advantage of IVF–ET is that the multiple gestation rate can be controlled by transferring fewer embryos.

Endometrial hyperplasia

In addition to infertility, a consequence of the chronic anovulation associated with PCOS is endometrial hyperplasia, which can progress to endometrial adenocarcinoma. Endometrial hyperplasia has been reported to occur in up to 35% of untreated women with PCOS. Risk factors include less than four menses per year and an endometrial thickness of greater than 7 mm on ultrasound.[31] Unopposed estrogen exposure leads to hyperplasia of the endometrium, and given that insulin receptors are present in the endometrium,[32] hyperinsulinemia may also have a potential role in the pathophysiology of endometrial hyperplasia and cancer.[33] In fact, in vitro treatment with insulin stimulates cellular proliferation of both estrogen receptor negative and positive endometrial cancer cells.[34]

Cyclic progestin treatment, typically medroxyprogesterone acetate 10 mg daily for 10 days per month, is sufficient to counteract the proliferative effects of estrogen on the uterine endometrium. Other options for the prevention of endometrial hyperplasia, particularly when contraception is desired, include the levonorgestrel-releasing intrauterine system, oral contraceptive pills (OCPs), or depot medroxyprogesterone acetate. While restoration of ovulation with metformin treatment, which will be further discussed below, may limit the occurrence and sequelae of endometrial hyperplasia, it should not be used for this indication as its efficacy has not been demonstrated in this regard.

Women who have been anovulatory for 6 months or more should have an endometrial biopsy to rule out endometrial hyperplasia or cancer. If hyperplasia is identified, more intensive treatment with high-dose progestin, for instance megestrol 40–160 mg daily for 3 months, is instituted prior to a repeat endometrial biopsy to assess resolution of the hyperplasia.

Symptoms of androgen excess

Hyperandrogenemia or clinical manifestations of hyperandrogenism, such as hirsutism, male-pattern balding, and acne, are common among women with PCOS. In fact, up to 90% of women with PCOS have elevated androgen levels.[35] As mentioned above, increased LH promotes thecal steroidogenesis, and thus hyperandrogenism. In addition, there is a strong association between insulin resistance and hyperandrogenism, and most evidence indicates that insulin causes hyperandrogenism.[36,37]

With respect to hirsutism, androgens are involved in the irreversible transformation of fine vellus hairs into coarse terminal hairs.[38] Androgens also contribute to the pathogenesis of acne vulgaris in that androgen receptors and 5α-reductase, the enzyme that transforms testosterone to the more potent dihydrotestosterone (DHT), are both present within the sebaceous follicle.[39,40] Still, the complex nature of androgen action is underscored by the fact that androgen levels are frequently within normal limits among women with acne or hirsutism, and these conditions do not always occur together.[41] DHT metabolism differs with regard to acne and hirsutism, which may explain some of the differences in the pathophysiology of these two androgen-mediated conditions.[42]

Symptomatic treatment of hirsutism

Various options exist for the treatment of symptomatic hyperandrogenemia, and as with most other aspects of PCOS, the choice of therapy depends on the individual's desire for fertility or lack thereof. With respect to hirsutism, non-pharmacological options include shaving, bleaching, wax depilation, electrolysis, and laser treatments. Even if medical management is instituted, cosmetic measures are often required, since medications have only a partial therapeutic effect on already terminalized hairs.[43]

A relatively new topical drug, eflornithine, inhibits hair growth and is one of the few licensed medications for the treatment of facial hirsutism.[44] Its mechanism of action involves the irreversible inhibition of ornithine decarboxylase, an androgen-modulated enzyme that regulates hair growth.[41] The medication is available in a 13.9% cream that is used twice daily. Initial effects are seen within 1–2 months; such a delay is not unusual in the treatment of hirsutism, given that hair follicles have a half-life of up to 6 months. Eflornithine must be used indefinitely, otherwise facial hair recurs within a few weeks of discontinuation of therapy.[44] Another disadvantage of this cream is its pregnancy class C designation.

Antiandrogens, such as spironolactone and flutamide, both of which bind and block the androgen receptor, are effective treatments for hyperandrogenism; however, they also cannot be used in women at risk for pregnancy due to their potential teratogenic effects. Therefore, these medications are coadministered with an oral contraceptive or another reliable form of contraception. Spironolactone at a dose of 100 mg daily significantly improves hirsutism as demonstrated by a recent meta-analysis.[45] One study of women with moderate to severe hirsutism showed an initial effect at 2 months, followed by maximal effect at 6 months, which was maintained thereafter.[46]

As will be discussed below, OCPs used alone can also improve symptomatic hyperandrogenism as they directly treat the underlying hyperandrogenemia. For this reason, OCPs are frequently used as a first-line treatment for hyperandrogenism, particularly among women who want to be on a single medication. The combination of an OCP with spironolactone is an effective therapy for hirsutism.[47,48]

Second-line treatment of hirsutism may include flutamide, which is another androgen receptor blocker, and the usual dose of flutamide is 250 mg twice daily. One randomized controlled trial (RCT) demonstrated that this antiandrogen has greater potency than spironolactone in the treatment of hirsutism,[49] while another RCT showed similar efficacies of the two drugs.[50] Flutamide may offer additional benefits in the treatment of hyperandrogenism, since it not only acts as a competitive androgen receptor antagonist, but may also reduce serum androgen levels,[51] though no significant effect of flutamide on free or total testosterone levels was found in a study of the drug in women with PCOS.[51] Yet, in these women, flutamide has been shown to decrease visceral fat and improve dyslipidemia.[52,53] While flutamide is generally well tolerated, it carries the uncommon, but potentially life-threatening risk of hepatotoxicity, and therefore must be used with caution and close monitoring of liver function.[54]

Finasteride, which blocks the 5α-reductase type 2-mediated conversion of testosterone to the more potent DHT, represents another option for the treatment of hirsutism,[55] and is used at a dose of 5 mg per day. Although finasteride inhibits the type 2 5α-reductase, and it is type 1 5α-reductase enzyme activity that is increased in the skin of hirsute women, at therapeutic doses, finasteride appears to have an effect on both isoenzymes.[41] While one prospective RCT demonstrated its inferior efficacy compared to spironolactone,[56] other studies comparing finasteride to the various treatments for hirsutism, including spironolactone and flutamide, have shown comparable effects of all therapies.[50,57] The inconsistencies among the studies of drug therapies for hirsutism may be secondary to the heterogeneity of the condition itself. However, at this time, spironolactone is usually the antiandrogen of choice in the USA, largely due to clinical experience and a quite favorable side-effect profile.[41]

Symptomatic treatment of acne

While the above-discussed antiandrogens may additionally have favorable effects on acne vulgaris, they are not usually first-line treatments for this condition. The initial approach to acne typically involves topical treatments, with progression to systemic therapy as required. Treatment delays should be avoided, since facial scarring from acne lesions affects almost 95% of individuals and can lead to long-term psychosocial sequelae.[41] Topical treatments consist of retinoids, such as tretinoin and isotretinoin, to control hyperkeratosis as well as antibacterial agents, such as benzoyl peroxide or antibiotics, to inhibit the proliferation of *Propionibacterium acnes*, the bacteria involved in the pathogenesis of acne vulgaris. Oral antibiotics, such as tetracycline, doxycycline, and erythromycin, may have an additional benefit for severe acne, though antibiotic resistance with prolonged use of systemic antibiotics has become a significant issue.[58] Systemic retinoids are very effective for severe acne in that they have anti-inflammatory actions and also block sebum production and *P. acnes* proliferation. The use of these medications, however, is limited by their side-effects, including hepatotoxicity, desquamation, and dyslipidemia, as well as their potential teratogenicity.[41,59]

HYPERANDROGENEMIA

While the previous discussion focused on the treatment of symptomatic hyperandrogenism, the following will address the treatment of the underlying hyperandrogenemia of PCOS. First and foremost, in women with PCOS who are not interested in conceiving,

combined OCPs represent a first-line therapeutic choice in that they inhibit hyperandrogenemia and thus hyperandrogenism by a variety of mechanisms, including suppression of the hypothalamic–pituitary–gonadal axis such that the theca cells lose their stimulatory LH signal for continued steroidogenesis. In addition, circulating levels of sex hormone binding globulin (SHBG), which is produced by the liver, increase in response to the estrogen in combined OCPs, and thereby serum levels of free, bioavailable androgens are reduced.[60] OCPs also inhibit adrenal androgen production of dehydroepiandrosterone.[61]

One caveat with respect to the choice of OCPs is that a formulation containing a progestin with minimal androgenic activity, such as norgestimate or desogestrel, should be selected. Androgenic progestins, including norgestrel and levonorgestrel block the estrogen-mediated hepatic production of SHBG and therefore inhibit one of the key antiandrogenic mechanisms of OCPs. Though not available in the USA, a particularly useful OCP for the treatment of hyperandrogenemia (Diane®) contains the antiandrogen cyproterone acetate. This synthetic steroid not only binds the androgen receptor, but also has progestational and weak glucocorticoid activities. The efficacy of cyproterone acetate with respect to the treatment of hirsutism has been clearly established.[62,63] OCP formulations containing drosperinone, a newer progestin with antimineralocorticoid activity derived from 17α-spirolactone, may also have a specific benefit in the treatment of hirsutism, though the limited studies published to date are inconclusive in this regard.[64-66]

Additional treatments for hyperandrogenemia include GnRH analogs[67] and the antifungal agent ketoconazole. The latter has antisteroidogenic actions that reduce both ovarian and adrenal androgen production; however, the potential hepatotoxicity of ketoconazole limits its widespread use.[57] GnRH analogs, such as leuprolide acetate, effectively block ovarian androgen production, but they also inhibit estrogen synthesis, which leads to symptoms and sequelae of estrogen deficiency, including hot flashes, vaginal atrophy, and bone loss; furthermore, the long-term use of these medications is also limited by their cost.[67]

While not the focus of this chapter, an alternative treatment for the underlying hyperandrogenemia of PCOS is ovarian wedge resection or another form of partial destruction of ovarian tissue, which was first proposed in 1935 by Stein and Leventhal as a surgical approach to ovulation induction in women with PCOS.[68] By removing a significant portion of ovarian tissue, this method leads to a subsequent reduction of circulating androgen levels.[69] While ovarian wedge resection as described by Stein and Leventhal lost favor due to post-surgical adhesion formation with subsequent infertility,[70] as well as the introduction of medical treatments for anovulation, the concept of debulking excess ovarian tissue has been reintroduced with the development of laparoscopy.

Various methods of laparoscopic ovarian wedge resection and drilling (LOD) have been described, including those using laser,[71] electrocautery,[72] and harmonic scalpel,[73] which also lead to a decrease in androgen excess.[74,75] A recent meta-analysis demonstrated that LOD resulted in a pregnancy rate similar to that with gonadotropin treatment, but the multiple gestation rate was significantly lower with LOD.[76] This represents a significant benefit of surgery, since gonadotropin treatment of women with PCOS leads to a multiple pregnancy rate of between 10 and 30%, including high-order multiples.[76–78]

While LOD represents a reasonable, but invasive, approach for the treatment of anovulation, its use for other symptoms of hyperandrogenemia, such as hirsutism, cannot be recommended at this time due to a lack of supportive data.[79] LOD does decrease total and free testosterone levels by approximately 40–50% of the preoperative values.[80] Yet, one limited meta-analysis on the effects of ovarian wedge resection or LOD on hyperandrogenism among women with PCOS showed only a trend towards decreasing serum androgen levels, and there were no clear improvements with respect to hirsutism or acne.[81]

INSULIN RESISTANCE AND HYPERINSULINEMIA

One of the driving factors of ovarian androgen production is insulin,[36,37] and therefore, targeting the effects of insulin on the ovary represents an alternative approach to the treatment of the hyperandrogenemia of PCOS. Insulin stimulates the production of androgens by ovarian thecal and stromal cells.[82] PCOS is also associated with increased levels of bioavailable insulin-like growth factor I (IGF-I),[83–86] and both insulin and IGF-I not only induce proliferation of theca-interstitial cells,[87–90] but also prevent these cells from undergoing apoptosis.[91] Thus, excessive androgen production in PCOS may be due, in part, to stimulation of the growth of the theca-interstitial compartment by insulin and IGF-I.

In addition to stimulating ovarian steroidogenesis, elevated insulin levels inhibit hepatic production of SHBG and thereby further increase bioavailable androgens.[92] Excess insulin has other untoward metabolic effects, including those on muscle, fat, and the vasculature; in fact, insulin resistance appears to be intimately involved in the etiology of the metabolic syndrome, an entity to be further discussed below, which predisposes affected individuals to cardiovascular disease and type 2 diabetes.[93]

The molecular basis for insulin resistance, though not yet fully understood, may be related to a post-receptor defect involving oxidative stress-mediated phosphorylation of the insulin receptor substrates 1 and 2 (IRS-1, IRS-2), which leads to an abrogation of insulin signaling via its receptor.[94,95] Specifically, phosphorylated IRS molecules lose efficacy in binding to the insulin receptor as well as downstream targets, and this leads to impaired insulin action with compensatory hyperinsulinemia.[96,97] In addition, when phosphorylated, IRS molecules are more susceptible to degradation.[96,97] The alterations in IRS function and integrity result in impaired metabolic effects of insulin, specifically with respect to glucose transport, but paradoxically, the mitogenic effects of insulin persist.[98] In fact, certain mitogenic pathways, including those involving the mitogen activated protein kinase (MAPK), are constitutively activated in PCOS, and may potentiate the resistance to insulin since MAPK activity leads to phosphorylation of IRS-1.[99]

Insulin resistance with resulting hyperinsulinemia is common among both lean and obese women with PCOS, and glucose intolerance rates of up to 40% have been reported.[100–102] Furthermore, type 2 diabetes is diagnosed in approximately 10% of women with PCOS,[100–102] and while impaired glucose tolerance and type 2 diabetes are most common among women with PCOS who are in their 30s or 40s, a significant percentage of adolescents with PCOS are also affected.[103] The diagnostic criteria for PCOS do not require evaluation for insulin resistance; however, screening for impaired glucose tolerance or frank type 2 diabetes is strongly recommended given the prevalence of these conditions among women with PCOS. A 2-hour oral glucose tolerance test (75-g load) is more effective than measuring fasting levels of glucose, since many women with PCOS, who have impaired glucose tolerance, maintain fasting euglycemia.[101] Furthermore, determinations of insulin levels during a glucose tolerance test may be helpful in the identification and quantification of hyperinsulinemia.

Weight loss

The initial management of insulin resistance and hyperinsulinemia should involve weight loss, as this approach not only improves insulin resistance, but can also restore ovulation and improve hirsutism among women with PCOS.[104–106] While various dietary approaches, including low carbohydrate/high protein and low protein/high carbohydrate diets, have been studied, at present there is no evidence to support one over the other among women with PCOS.[107] Implicit in weight loss therapy is exercise, as physical inactivity is associated with insulin resistance and an increased risk of developing the metabolic syndrome.[108]

Metformin

If weight loss and exercise are insufficient, or if a lean woman with PCOS has insulin resistance, insulin-sensitizing agents can be added. The biguanide, metformin, has been studied extensively among women with PCOS,[109,110] and currently represents the most frequently used insulin-sensitizer employed in this setting.[111] Metformin has a pleiotropic mechanism of action, which includes a decrease in gluconeogenesis, inhibition of intestinal glucose absorption, increased glucose uptake, and blockade of lipolysis.[112,113] One specific advantage of metformin among the other insulin-sensitizing agents is its ability to potentiate weight loss,[114–116] likely by suppressing appetite.[117] In fact, one clinical trial demonstrated that weight loss associated with the use of metformin was comparable to that resulting from sibutramine and orlistat, two medications specifically approved for weight reduction.[114]

Metformin is initiated using a step-up regimen to reach a target dose of 1500–2550 mg daily. This allows for gradual adjustment to the medication's substantial gastrointestinal side-effects, which include nausea, vomiting, cramping, bloating, diarrhea, and flatulence. Extended release formulations may result in fewer side-effects, and are usually reserved for the subset of patients who have intolerable side-effects on the regular formulation. Lactic acidosis is a rare, but serious complication of metformin. Since metformin is excreted via the kidneys, patients should be screened with respect to their renal function prior to initiating metformin, and they should be instructed to hold the medication during periods of actual or potential dehydration, such as pre-operatively or during a significant medical illness, and prior to an imaging procedure involving iodinated contrast dye, which may negatively affect renal function.[118]

In women with PCOS, metformin not only improves insulin resistance, but also leads to a reduction in serum androgens and gonadotropins. Metformin as well as other insulin-sensitizing agents, such as the thiazolidinediones, have modest, but significant effects on

hirsutism among women with PCOS.[119,120] In addition, metformin reverses metabolic abnormalities, including hyperinsulinemia, dyslipidemia, and elevation of the prothrombotic factor plasminogen activator inhibitor type 1 (PAI-1).[121,122] Increased expression of the latter has been suggested as a possible etiology for the increased frequency of spontaneous abortion,[123,124] which affects up to 50% of all conceptions in women with PCOS.[5] Studies have indicated that the use of metformin during the first trimester may lower the incidence of early pregnancy loss among women with PCOS,[125,126] though, to date, there is no randomized, prospective trial addressing this issue.

Continuation of metformin during pregnancy also appears to have a favorable effect on the incidence of gestational diabetes.[127,128] Women with PCOS are at increased risk for this pregnancy complication as well as others, including preeclampsia and preterm labor.[129–132] The effect of metformin, a class B drug, on neonatal outcomes has been studied, and while the data seem reassuring,[128,133] there are no long-term data available, and one recent study showed a small decrease in birth weight with metformin use that was of marginal significance.[134] Due to insufficient evidence, metformin use during pregnancy cannot be recommended at this time as a first-line treatment for gestational diabetes, or for the prevention of this complication in women with PCOS.

One of the more common uses of metformin in women with PCOS is to aid in ovulation induction. Metformin can restore ovulation in up to 50% of women with PCOS.[135] Multiple RCTs suggest a beneficial effect of metformin coadministration with clomiphene citrate on ovulation induction, specifically in women who are clomiphene-resistant.[136–139] However, a recent randomized, double blinded trial demonstrated that there is no advantage of combined clomiphene citrate and metformin therapy with respect to live birth rates, and metformin alone was less effective than clomiphene citrate.[140]

Even among women who do not ovulate in response to metformin alone, this medication may nevertheless exert favorable effects; for example, it may improve oocyte quality[141] and promote monofollicular development,[142] though the use of metformin for these purposes remains controversial.[143] Similarly, studies of metformin pretreatment of women with PCOS undergoing IVF have also reported conflicting results, with some showing a benefit in terms of number of oocytes retrieved[144] and pregnancy rates,[144–146] while others found no differences with respect to either of these parameters.[147] A recent meta-analysis of metformin coadministration during ovulation induction with gonadotropins or IVF in women with PCOS failed to show a significant effect with respect to ovulation, pregnancy, or live birth rates.[148] There was, however, a significant decrease in the incidence of OHSS.[148] Some of the conflicting data with respect to metformin use in PCOS may be a result of the heterogeneous nature of PCOS itself that may render certain studies incomparable.

Other insulin sensitizers

Thiazolidinediones represent another class of insulin-sensitizers and include rosiglitazone, pioglitazone, and troglitazone. The last agent is no longer available in the USA and UK due to its significant hepatotoxicity, including liver failure. The mechanism of action of thiazolidinediones involves their binding to the peroxisome proliferator-activated receptor γ (PPAR-γ), which mediates the transcription of various factors involved in the regulation of glucose and lipid metabolism.[149,150] In effect, thiazolidinediones promote fatty acid uptake and storage in adipose tissue and increase the expression of adiponectin, a cytokine that mediates insulin sensitivity.[151]

Like metformin, these medications have a favorable effect on women with PCOS, including improved glucose tolerance and insulin resistance, a reduction in PAI-1 levels, and, as mentioned above, decreased hyperandrogenemia.[120,152,153] The latter effect appears to be mediated, at least in part, by an increase in SHBG.[153] Furthermore, both rosiglitazone and pioglitazone have been shown to significantly improve ovulatory rates in women with PCOS.[153,154] When compared directly to metformin, pioglitazone, at a dose of 30 mg a day, resulted in similar improvements with respect to insulin resistance and hyperandrogenemia among obese, insulin-resistant women with PCOS.[155] However, due to the propensity of thiazolidinediones to induce weight gain and because of their potential association with hepatotoxicity, metformin remains the first-line medical treatment for insulin resistance among women with PCOS.

D-chiro-inositol is another insulin sensitizer, which appears to restore deficiency in a phosphoglycan that mediates insulin action. While this medication is not currently available in the USA, it has been shown to significantly decrease hyperinsulinemia and free testosterone levels in women with PCOS.[156]

OXIDATIVE STRESS AND INFLAMMATION

Oxidative stress, which is an imbalance between the production of reactive oxygen species (ROS) and antioxidant defenses favoring the former, is associated with a variety of pathological conditions including diabetes, cancer, and cardiovascular disease.[157–159] PCOS is also associated with increased oxidative stress and systemic inflammation.[160–162] Furthermore, antioxidant reserve appears to be compromised in women with PCOS.[160] Even lean women with PCOS exhibit increased oxidative stress, as measured by levels of malonyldialdehyde, a marker of lipid peroxidation, and they have decreased serum total antioxidant levels compared to controls.[163] Recent evidence suggests that oxidative stress and inflammatory cytokines, such as tumor necrosis factor α (TNF-α) and C-reactive protein (CRP),[164,165] may mediate the dysregulation of the theca-interstitial compartment, and both of these factors are elevated in PCOS.[160,161,166,167]

ROS have a bimodal effect on theca-interstitial cells such that modest oxidative stress induced by xanthine oxidase stimulates proliferation of these cells in vitro, while greater oxidative stress and antioxidants such as vitamin E succinate inhibit their proliferation.[164] TNF-α and insulin also stimulate theca-interstitial cell proliferation,[87,89,165] and several in vitro and in vivo studies have shown that insulin and TNF-α also induce oxidative stress.[168–170] It is well known that ROS mediate proliferation of various other cell types, including fibroblasts and aortic endothelial cells,[171] while antioxidants, such as α-tocopherol, inhibit proliferation of vascular smooth muscle, fibroblasts, and many cancer cell lines.[172–175]

In addition to simulating proliferation of the cainterstitial cells, moderate oxidative stress also induces testosterone and progesterone production by enhancing theca-interstitial cell expression of key steroidogenic enzymes, such as CYP17, CYP11A1, and 3β-HSD (hydroxysteroid dehydrogenase).[176] Thus, the excess androgen production in PCOS may be due not only to increased numbers of theca cells, but also to an induction of their steroidogenic capability. Furthermore, oxidative stress, as discussed above, impairs insulin signaling, resulting in a compensatory hyperinsulinemia, which, in turn, further stimulates thecal steroidogenesis.[96,97]

Antioxidants represent a potential treatment for the increased oxidative stress and associated insulin resistance of PCOS. There are in vivo data showing that antioxidants, and α-lipoic acid (LA) in particular, improve insulin sensitivity in animal models of diabetes.[177,178] This finding is supported by several clinical trials involving subjects with insulin resistance or diabetes, who were treated with various antioxidants, including LA,[179] vitamin E,[180] vitamin C,[181,182] glutathione,[183] or N-acetylcysteine.[184] The latter was specifically evaluated in insulin-resistant women with PCOS

Table 12.3 Diagnostic criteria for the metabolic syndrome in women. From the Third Report of the National Cholesterol Education Program (NCEP) Expert Panel on Detection, Evaluation, and Treatment of High Blood Cholesterol in Adults (Adult Treatment Panel III (ATPIII))[193]

NCEP/ATPIII Criteria (at least 3 of 5 of the following)

Waist circumference ≥ 88 cm
Serum triglyceride levels ≥ 150 mg/dl
HDL cholesterol < 50 mg/dl
Systolic blood pressure ≥ 130 mmHg or diastolic blood pressure ≥ 85 mmHg
Fasting blood glucose ≥ 100 mg/dl

and shown to have a benefit.[184] A recent study comparing rosiglitazone and metformin treatment of lean women with PCOS demonstrated that rosiglitazone decreased malonyldialdehyde levels and increased total antioxidant status, while metformin did not significantly affect these parameters.[163] In addition, a novel approach for the treatment of oxidative stress may be statin therapy, as these drugs, which will be discussed in further detail below, have a pleiotropic mechanism of action that includes a direct antioxidant activity.

CARDIOVASCULAR DISEASE AND THE METABOLIC SYNDROME

One of the significant sequelae of oxidative stress is endothelial dysfunction and the subsequent development of cardiovascular disease, which is the leading cause of death in women.[185] One study reported that women with PCOS have a sevenfold increased risk for myocardial infarction.[186] Although increased mortality due to cardiovascular disease has not been demonstrated among this group,[187] long-term data are lacking, and given that PCOS affects women of reproductive age, the increased risk for cardiovascular disease is concerning.

Both symptomatic and asymptomatic women with PCOS have signs of significant vascular impairment. For example, common carotid artery vascular compliance is decreased while arterial stiffness is increased,[188] and endothelial dysfunction detected as impaired vasodilatation has been shown in hyperandrogenic, insulin-resistant women with PCOS compared with age- and weight-matched controls.[189] PCOS is also associated with increased thickness of arterial intima–media and greater prevalence of subclinical

atherosclerosis.[190,191] Cardiac catheterization of women with PCOS demonstrated significant occlusion in more arterial segments compared to women with normal-appearing ovaries.[192]

A major risk factor for the development of cardiovascular disease is the metabolic syndrome, which consists of a combination of factors, including obesity, dyslipidemia, hypertension, and glucose intolerance (Table 12.3).[93] The prevalence of the metabolic syndrome in women with PCOS is approximately 43%, which is twofold higher than that for age-matched controls.[194] The most prominent metabolic syndrome features among women with PCOS are, in decreasing order, decreased high density lipoprotein (HDL) levels, obesity, and hypertension.[194] Notably, serum free testosterone is higher and SHBG is lower in women who have both PCOS and the metabolic syndrome compared to those who have PCOS alone.[194] Insulin resistance, one of the major causative factors involved in the development of the metabolic syndrome,[195] is prevalent in both lean and obese women with PCOS and potentiates dyslipidemia, obesity, and glucose intolerance.

Homocysteine levels are higher in women with PCOS compared to healthy subjects,[163,196–198] and hyperhomocysteinemia represents another independent risk factor for the development of cardiovascular disease.[199] Moderate hyperhomocysteinemia predisposes individuals to endothelial dysfunction via a mechanism involving increased oxidative stress.[200] While not yet fully understood, the increased oxidative stress may be due to an increased production of ROS, an inhibition of antioxidant enzyme expression or activity, or a combination of these two mechanisms.[201–203] In women with PCOS, regular exercise lowers plasma homocysteine levels[197] as does the administration of B-group vitamins and folic acid.[204] There is no evidence that the treatment of insulin resistance with metformin or thiazolidinediones improves hyperhomocysteinemia;[163] in fact, homocysteine levels may increase.[198,205]

The dyslipidemia in PCOS is characterized by elevated plasma levels of cholesterol, low density lipoprotein (LDL), very low density lipoprotein (VLDL), and triglycerides with concomitantly reduced concentrations of HDL.[7,186,206,207] Dyslipidemia correlates with the hyperinsulinemia and hyperandrogenemia of PCOS,[208] and treatment of these conditions can lead to improvements in the lipid profile.[52,53] The use of statins to treat women with PCOS may represent a novel therapeutic option with additional benefits, as will be discussed below.

Statins

Statins are selective inhibitors of 3-hydroxy-3-methyl-glutaryl-coenzyme A (HMG-CoA) reductase, the rate-limiting enzyme in the cholesterol biosynthetic pathway. Statins improve the lipid profile primarily by decreasing total cholesterol and LDL levels,[209,210] and these medications also decrease both cardiovascular morbidity and mortality.[209,211] Statins significantly reduce both fatal and non-fatal cardiovascular disease events in primary and secondary prevention trials.[209,212,213] Statins appear to stabilize atherosclerotic plaques by decreasing levels of metalloproteases and reducing oxidized-LDL levels,[214,215] thereby preventing plaque rupture, which is the direct cause of most acute coronary events.

The pleiotropic actions of statins also include their inhibitory effect on N-linked glycosylation,[216] which may inhibit the maturation of insulin and type I IGF receptors.[217] In addition, statins possess both indirect and direct antioxidant activity.[218] The antioxidant actions of statins include inhibition of NADPH (reduced nicotinamide adenine dinucleotide phosphate) oxidase activity, preservation of relative levels of vitamins C and E, and inhibition of the uptake and generation of oxidized LDL.[219,220] Statins' intrinsic antioxidant activity involves both antihydroxyl and antiperoxyl radical activity.[218] In vitro, simvastatin is the most effective antihydroxyl radical antioxidant, while fluvastatin is the most effective antiperoxyl radical antioxidant.[218] In vivo, statins reduce plasma levels of nitrotyrosine and chlorotyrosine,[221] and they also exert anti-inflammatory effects by lowering C-reactive protein levels and suppressing proinflammatory agents, such as TNF-α.[222]

The rationale for the use of statins in women with PCOS is based not only on the dyslipidemia frequently associated with this endocrinopathy, but also the recent finding that the dysregulation of theca-interstitial growth and stimulation of steroidogenesis appear to be mediated by oxidative stress. By lowering the production of cholesterol, a substrate for testosterone production, statins may also improve hyperandrogenemia in women with PCOS, and given the inhibitory actions of statins on N-linked glycosylation of the insulin and IGF-I receptors, the sequelae of hyperinsulinemia may be abrogated.

In vitro, the statin mevastatin inhibits the proliferation of theca-interstitial cells and also inhibits LH-stimulated production of both progesterone and testosterone by these cells through a mechanism that is independent of its effect on cell number.[223] The inhibitory effects of mevastatin on ovarian cell proliferation are consistent with previous reports regarding other mesenchymal cell types, including vascular smooth muscle,[224–226] cardiomyocytes,[227] and mesangial cells.[228]

The effects of statins on ovarian steroidogenesis may be due to several mechanisms. Besides impairing the availability of the substrate cholesterol, statins also decrease the expression of several key enzymes involved in testosterone production including P450scc, P450c17, and 3β-HSD as demonstrated in adrenocortical cells,[229,230] and similar findings have been observed in ovarian cells.[231] It has been established previously that oxidative stress increases the expression of these same steroidogenic enzymes in the ovary.[176] A major source of ROS is the enzyme NADPH oxidase, which is activated by various cytokines.[71] Mevastatin and simvastatin, in the presence of LH, inhibit the expression of p22phox, a membrane-bound subunit essential for the function of NADPH oxidase in theca-interstitial cells.[232] The expression of another NADPH oxidase subunit, p47phox, is also decreased by these statins.[232] In addition, mevastatin blocks basal and insulin-dependent activation of the MAPK pathway in vitro as measured by phosphorylation of Erk1/2, a downstream kinase.[233]

Thus, in summary, the in vitro studies on ovarian theca-interstitial cells demonstrate that statins decrease cell proliferation and testosterone production, inhibit the expression of steroidogenic enzymes, decrease expression of NADPH oxidase subunits, and block MAPK-dependent phosphorylation. Taken together, these finding raise the possibility that the use of statins in women with PCOS could decrease thecal hyperplasia, hyperandrogenism, and oxidative stress.

Recently, a randomized, prospective clinical trial investigated the effects of simvastatin on women with PCOS,[234] and was followed by a cross-over study comparing the effects of simvastatin and a combined OCP on PCOS.[235] Women with PCOS were treated with simvastatin and OCP or the OCP alone. Testosterone levels declined more in the statin plus OCP group compared to the OCP-alone group; simvastatin also had a modest but statistically significant inhibitory effect on hirsutism. In contrast to the effects on testosterone, simvastatin had no effect on dehydroepiandrosterone sulfate (DHEAS) levels, suggesting that the actions of statins are selective and may not alter adrenal steroidogenesis.

However, simvastatin did affect the hypothalamic–pituitary axis, since, between the groups, there were distinctly different responses noted with respect to gonadotropin levels. LH levels decreased more in the statin plus OCP group compared to the OCP-alone group, and as FSH levels did not significantly change, the net effect was a statin-induced reduction in the LH/FSH ratio. Neither of the treatments had a significant effect on body mass index (BMI). The improvements in testosterone and LH by simvastatin were not mediated by improved insulin sensitivity, as determined by fasting and post-glucose challenge levels of insulin and glucose. This finding points to the different pathways of insulin with respect to its actions on glucose transport and other cellular functions, such as cellular proliferation, as discussed earlier.

As expected, statin use resulted in a decrease of total cholesterol and LDL, while OCP alone induced a small increase of total cholesterol. There was a small, but significant increase in HDL in both groups, and triglyceride levels were not affected in the statin plus OCP group, while they increased in the OCP-alone group. The improvement of lipid profile by simvastatin is of particular value in PCOS, a condition characterized by dyslipidemia and other cardiovascular risk factors. In addition, CRP was slightly increased by OCP, but reduced by simvastatin. Taken together, these data suggest that the use of statins in women with PCOS is likely to offer significant protection from long-term cardiovascular morbidity. However, further studies of this potentially promising therapy are needed before it can be recommended in routine clinical practice. One limitation of this therapy is the potential teratogenicity of statins, which are pregnancy category X, and therefore should not be used in women who are at risk of conceiving.

CONCLUSIONS

PCOS is a complex, heterogeneous endocrinopathy affecting a significant proportion of women in the reproductive age group. The primary treatment of this disorder should involve a medical approach that is tailored to the individual patient. With respect to symptomatic therapy, anovulatory infertility is usually first treated with clomiphene citrate, while gonadotropins and other therapies for ovulation induction may be reserved as second-line treatments. Spironolactone and OCPs are first-line treatments for symptomatic hirsutism, but cosmetic hair removal is also frequently required, given the lack of significant drug effect on already terminalized hairs. Eflornithine is a new and effective therapy that is approved for facial hirsutism, but like other treatments for this disorder, it must be used indefinitely. Women with PCOS should be monitored for endometrial hyperplasia, a condition that can

be prevented by the use of cyclic or prolonged progestin therapy to counteract the predominantly estrogen-rich milieu of PCOS.

The underlying hyperandrogenemia of PCOS is primarily treated with combined OCPs. GnRH analogs, ketoconazole, and ovarian wedge resection or LOD should be reserved for selected circumstances. Metformin is an effective medical therapy for the hyperinsulinemia and insulin resistance of PCOS, and also has additional benefits with respect to restoration of ovulation, weight loss, and the treatment of androgen excess. The other insulin sensitizers, namely the thiazolidinediones, are used less frequently due to side-effects.

Finally, as women with PCOS are at significant risk for cardiovascular morbiditiy and potentially mortality, it is imperative to diagnose and manage cardiovascular risk factors, including those constituting the metabolic syndrome and hyperhomocysteinemia, which are prevalent among women with PCOS. Statins represent an exciting, potential, new approach to the medical management not only of the dyslipidemia of PCOS, but also of the increased oxidative stress and hyperandrogenemia associated with this disorder; however, further studies are needed before the routine use of statins can be recommended.

REFERENCES

1. Azziz R, Woods KS, Reyna R et al. The prevalence and features of the polycystic ovary syndrome in an unselected population. J Clin Endocrinol Metab 2004; 89: 2745–9.
2. Rotterdam ESHRE/ASRM-Sponsored PCOS Consensus Workshop Group. Revised 2003 consensus on diagnostic criteria and long-term health risks related to polycystic ovary syndrome. Fertil Steril 2004; 81: 19–25.
3. Azziz R, Carmina E, Dewailly D et al. Positions statement: criteria for defining polycystic ovary syndrome as a predominantly hyperandrogenic syndrome: an Androgen Excess Society guideline. J Endocrinol Metab 2006; 91: 4237–45.
4. Homburg R, Armar NA, Eshel A, Adams J, Jacobs HS. Influence of serum luteinising hormone concentrations on ovulation, conception and early pregnancy loss in polycystic ovary syndrome. Br Med J 1988; 297: 1024–6.
5. Sagle M, Bishop K, Ridley N et al. Recurrent early miscarriage and polycystic ovaries. Br Med J 1988; 297: 1027–8.
6. Wild RA, Applebaum-Bowden D, Demers LM et al. Lipoprotein lipids in women with androgen excess: independent associations with increased insulin and androgens. Clin Chem 1990; 36: 283–9.
7. Mahabeer S, Naidoo C, Norman RJ et al. Metabolic profiles and lipoprotein lipid concentrations in non-obese and obese patients with polycystic ovarian disease. Horm Metab Res 1990; 22: 537–40.
8. Dahlgren E, Johansson S, Lindstedt G et al. Women with polycystic ovary syndrome wedge resected in 1956 to 1965: a long-term follow-up focusing on natural history and circulating hormones. Fertil Steril 1992; 57: 505–13.

9. Dahlgren E, Janson PO, Johansson S, Lapidus L, Oden A. Polycystic ovary syndrome and risk for myocardial infarction. Acta Obstet Gynecol Scand 1992; 71: 599–604.

10. Vermeulen A, Verdonck L, Kaufman JM. A critical evaluation of simple methods for the estimation of free testosterone in serum. J Clin Endocrinol Metab 1999; 84: 3666–72.

11. Yen SS, Vela P, Rankin J Inappropriate secretion of follicle-stimulating hormone and luteinizing hormone in polycystic ovarian disease. J Clin Endocrinol Metab 1970; 30: 435–42.

12. Jakimiuk AJ, Weitsman SR, Brzechffa PR, Magoffin DA. Aromatase messenger ribonucleic acid expression in individual follicles from polycystic ovaries. Mol Hum Reprod 1998; 4: 1–8.

13. Jakimiuk AJ, Weitsman SR, Navab A, Magoffin DA. Luteinizing hormone receptor, steroidogenesis acute regulatory protein and steroidogenic enzyme messenger ribonucleic acids are overexpressed in theca and granulosa cells from polycystic ovaries. J Clin Endocrinol Metab 2001; 86: 1318–23.

14. Kousta E, White DM, Franks S. Modern use of clomiphene citrate in induction of ovulation. Hum Reprod Update 1997; 3: 359–65.

15. Hughes E, Collins J, Vandekerckhove P, Lilford R. Clomiphene citrate for ovulation induction in women with oligo-amenorrhea. Cochrane Database Syst Rev 2000; (2): CD000056.

16. Pritts EA. Treatment of the infertile patient with polycystic ovarian syndrome. Obstet Gynecol Surv 2002; 57: 587–97.

17. Mitwally MFM, Casper RF. Use of an aromatase inhibitor for induction of ovulation in patients with an inadequate response to clomiphene citrate. Fertil Steril 2001; 75: 305–9.

18. Mitwally MFM, Casper RF. Aromatase inhibition for ovarian stimulation: future avenues for infertility management. Curr Opinion Obstet Gynecol 2002; 14: 255–63.

19. Bayar U, Basaran M, Kiran S, Coskun A, Gezer S. Use of an aromatase inhibitor in patients with polycystic ovary syndrome: a prospective randomized trial. Fertil Steril 2006; 86: 1447–51.

20. Biljan MM, Hemmings R, Brassard N. The outcome of 150 babies following the treatment with letrozole or letrozole and gonadotropins. Fertil Steril 2005; 84 (Suppl 1): O–231, Abstr 1033.

21. Mitwally MFM, Biljan MM, Casper RF. Pregnancy outcome after the use of an aromatase inhibitor for ovarian stimulation. Am J Obstet Gynecol 2005; 192: 381–6.

22. Sohrabvand F, Ansari S, Bagheri M. Efficacy of combined metformin-letrozole in comparison with metformin-clomiphene citrate in clomiphene-resistant infertile women with polycystic ovarian disease. Hum Reprod 2006; 21: 1432–5.

23. Tulandi T, Martin J, Al-Fadhli R et al. Congenital malformations among 911 newborns conceived after infertility treatment with letrozole or clomiphene citrate. Fertil Steril 2006; 85: 1761–5.

24. White DM, Polson DW, Kiddy D et al. Induction of ovulation with low-dose gonadotropins in polycystic ovary syndrome: an analysis of 109 pregnancies in 225 women. J Clin Endocrinol Metab 1996; 81: 3821–4.

25. Mizunuma H, Takagi T, Yamada K et al. Ovulation induction by step-down administration of purified urinary follicle-stimulation hormone in patients with polycystic ovarian syndrome. Fertil Steril 1991; 55: 1195–6.

26. van Santbrink E, Fauser BCJM. Urinary follicle stimulating hormone for normogonadotropic clomiphene-resistant anovulatory infertility: prospective randomized comparison between low dose step-up and step-down dose regimens. J Clin Endocrinol Metab 1997; 82: 3597–602.

27. Buvat J, Buvat HM, Marcolin G et al. Purified follicle-stimulating hormone in polycystic ovary syndrome: slow administration is safer and more effective. Fertil Steril 1989; 52: 553–9.

28. Kamrava M, Seibel MM, Berger MJ, Thompson I, Taymore ML. Reversal of persistent anovulation in polycystic ovarian disease by administration of chronic low-dose follicle-stimulating hormone. Fertil Steril 1982; 37: 520–3.

29. Christin-Maitre S, Hugues JN. A comparative randomized multicentric study comparing the step-up versus step-down protocol in polycystic ovary syndrome. Hum Reprod 2003; 18: 1626–31.

30. Gill S, Taylor AE, Martin KA et al. Specific factors predict the response to pulsatile gonadotropin-releasing hormone therapy in polycystic ovarian syndrome. J Clin Endocrinol Metab 2001; 86: 2428–36.

31. Cheung AP. Ultrasound and menstrual history in predicting endometrial hyperplasia in polycystic ovary syndrome. Obstet Gynecol 2001; 98: 325–31.

32. Talbi S, Hamilton AE, Vo KC et al. Molecular phenotyping of human endometrium distinguishes menstrual cycle phases and underlying biological processes in normo-ovulatory women. Endocrinology 2006; 147: 1097–121.

33. Giudice LC. Endometrium in PCOS: implantation and predisposition to endocrine cancer. Best Pract Res Clin Endocrinol Metab 2006; 20: 235–44.

34. Nagamani M, Stuart CA. Specific binding and growth-promoting activity of insulin in endometrial cancer cells in culture. Am J Obstet Gynecol 1998; 179: 6–12.

35. DeVane GW, Czekala NM, Judd HL, Yen SS. Circulating gonadotropins, estrogens, and androgens in polycystic ovarian disease. Am J Obstet Gynecol 1975; 121: 496–500.

36. Dunaif A, Green G, Futterweit W, Dobrjansky A. Suppression of hyperandrogenism does not improve peripheral or hepatic insulin resistance in the polycystic ovary syndrome. J Clin Endocrinol Metab 1990; 70: 699–704.

37. Nestler JE, Barlascini CO, Matt DW et al. Suppression of serum insulin by diazoxide reduces serum testosterone levels in obese women with polycystic ovary syndrome. J Clin Endocrinol Metab 1989; 68: 1027–32.

38. Azziz R, Carmina E, Sawaya ME. Idiopathic hirsutism. Endocr Rev 2000; 21: 347–62.

39. Choudhry R, Hodgins MB, Van der Kwast T, Brinkman AO, Boersma WJ. Localization of androgen receptors in human skin by immunohistochemistry: implications for the hormonal regulation of hair grown, sebacious glands, and sweat glands. J Endocrinol 1992; 133: 467–75.

40. Baille A, Calman K, Milne J. Histochemical distribution of hydroxysteroid dehydrogenases in human skin. Br J Dermatol 1965; 7: 610–16.

41. Moghetti P, Toscano V. Treatment of hirsutism and acne in hyperandrogenism. Best Pract Res Clin Endocrinol Metab 2006; 20: 221–34.

42. Toscano V, Balducci R, Bianchi P et al. Two different pathogenetic mechanisms may play a role in acne and in hirsutism. Clin Endocrinol 1993; 39: 551–6.

43. Azziz R. The evaluation and management of hirsutism. Obstet Gynecol 2003; 101: 995–1007.

44. Eflornithine: new drug overview. Am J Health System Pharm 2001; 58: 2244.

45. Farquhar C, Lee O, Toomath R, Jepson R. Spironolactone versus placebo or in combination with steroids for hirsutism and/or acne. Cochrane Database Syst Rev 2003; (4): CD000194.

46. Cumming DC, Yang JC, Rebar RW, Yen SSC. Treatment of hirsutism with spironolactone. JAMA 1982; 247: 1295–8.

47. Pittaway DE, Maxson WS, Wentz AC. Spironolactone in combination drugy therapy for unresponsive hirsutism. Fertil Steril 1985; 43: 878–82.

48. Board JA, Rosenberg SM, Smeltzer JS. Spironolacotne and estrogen-progestin therapy for hirsutism. South Med J 1987; 80: 483–6.

49. Cusan L, Dupont A, Gomez J-L, Tremblay RR, Labrie F. Comparison of flutamide and spironolactone in the treatment of hirsutism: a randomized controlled trial. Fertil Steril 1994; 61: 281–7.

50. Moghetti P, Tosi F, Tosti A et al. Comparison of spironolactone, flutamide, and finasteride efficacy in the treatment of hirsutism: a randomized, double blind, placebo-controlled trial. J Clin Endocrinol Metab 2000; 85: 89–94.

51. Cusan L, Dupont A, Belanger A et al. Treatment of hirsutism with the pure anti-androgen flutamide. J Am Acad Dermatol 1990; 23: 462–9.

52. Diamanti-Kandarakis E, Mitrakou A, Raptis S, Tolis G, Duleba AJ. The effect of a pure anti-androgen receptor blocker flutamide on the lipid profile in the polycystic ovary syndrome. J Clin Endocrinol Metab 1998; 83: 2699–705.

53. Gambineri A, Pelusi C, Genghini S et al. Effect of flutamide and metformin administered alone or in combination in dieting obese women with polycystic ovary syndrome. Clin Endocrinol 2004; 60: 241–9.

54. Wysowski DK, Freiman JP, Tourtelot JB, Horton ML. Fatal and nonfatal hepatotoxicity associated with flutamide. Ann Intern Med 1993; 118: 860–4.

55. Faloia E, Fillipponi S, Mancini V, Di Marco S, Mantero F. Effect of finasteride in idiopathic hirsutism. J Endocrinol Invest 1998; 21: 694–8.

56. Wong IL, Morris RS, Chang L et al. A prospective randomized trial comparing finasteride to spironolactone in the treatment of hirsute women. J Clin Endocrinol Metab 1995; 80: 233–8.

57. Veturoli S, Marescalchi O, Colombo FM et al. A prospective randomized trial comparing low dose flutamide, finasteride, ketoconazole, and cyproterone acetate-estrogen regimens in the treatment of hirsutism. J Clin Endocrinol Metab 1999; 84: 1304–10.

58. Cooper AJ. Systemic review of Propionibacterium acnes resistance to systemic antibiotics. Med J Aust 1998; 169: 259–61.

59. Hurwits S. Acne vulgaris: its pathogenesis and management. Adolesc Med 1990; 1: 301–14.

60. Granger LR, Roy S, Mishell DR. Changes in unbound sex steroids and sex hormone binding globulin-binding capacity during oral and vaginal progestogen administration. Am J Obstet Gynecol 1982; 144: 578–84.

61. Madden JD, Milewich L, Parker CR et al. The effect of oral contraceptive treatment on the serum concentration of dehydroisoandrosterone sulfate. Am J Obstet Gynecol 1978; 132: 380–4.

62. Barth JH, Cherry CA, Wojnarowska F, Dawber RP. Cyproterone acetate for severe hirsutism: results of a double-blind, dose-ranging study. Clin Endocrinol 1991; 35: 5–10.

63. Van der Spuy ZM, Le Roux PA. Cyproterone acetate for hirsutism. Cochrane Database Syst Rev 2003; (4): CD001125.

64. Guido M, Romualdi D, Giuliani M et al. Drosperinone for the treatment of hirsute women with polycystic ovary syndrome: a clinical, endocrinological, metabolic pilot study. J Clin Endocrinol Metab 2004; 89: 2817–23.

65. Palep-Singh M, Mook K, Barth JH, Balen A. An observational study of Yasmin in the management of women with polycystic ovary syndrome. J Fam Plann Reprod Health Care 2004; 30: 163–5.

66. Ibanez L, de Zegher F. Flutamide-metformin plus an oral contraceptive for young women with polycystic ovary syndrome: switch from third to fourth generation OC reduces body adiposity. Hum Reprod 2004; 19: 1725–7.

67. Azziz R, Ochoa TM, Bradley ELJ, Potter HD, Boots LR. Leuprolide and estrogen versus oral contraceptive pills for the treatment of hirsutism: a prospective randomized study. J Clin Endocrinol Metab 1995; 80: 3406–11.

68. Stein IF, Leventhal ML. Amenorrhea associated with bilateral polycystic ovaries. Am J Obstet Gynecol 1935; 29: 181–91.

69. Katz M, Carr PJ, Cohen BM, Millar RP. Hormonal effects of wedge resection of polycystic ovaries. Obstet Gynecol 1978; 23: 98–9.

70. Toaff R, Toaff ME, Peyser MR. Infertility following wedge resection of the ovaries. Am J Obstet Gynecol 1976; 124: 94–6.

71. Felemban A, Tulandi T. Laparoscopic treatment of polycystic ovarian syndrome-related infertility. Infertil Reprod Med Clin North Am 2000; 11: 49–60.

72. Gjonnaess H. Polycystic ovarian syndrome treated by ovarian electrocautery through the laparoscope. Fertil Steril 1984; 4: 20–5.

73. Duleba AJ, Banaszewska B, Spaczynski RZ, Pawelczyk L. Success of laparoscopic ovarian wedge resection is related to obesity, lipid profile, and insulin levels. Fertil Steril 2003; 79: 1008–14.

74. Greenblatt E, Casper RF. Endocrine changes after laparoscopic ovarian cautery in polycystic ovarian syndrome. Am J Obstet Gynecol 1987; 156: 279–85.

75. Armar NA, McGarrible H, Honour J et al. Laparoscopic ovarian surgery in the management of anovulatory infertility in women with polycystic ovaries: endocrine changes and clinical outcomes. Fertil Steril 1990; 53: 45–9.

76. Farquhar C, Vandekerckhove P, Lilford R. Laparoscopic drilling by diathermy or laser for ovulation induction in anovulatory polycystic ovary syndrome. Cochrane Database Syst Rev 2005; (3): CD001122.

77. Bayram N, van Wely M, van der Veen F. Recombinant FSH versus urinary gonadotrophins or recombinant FSH for ovulation induction in subfertility associated with polycystic ovary syndrome. Cochrane Database Syst Rev 2001; (2): CD002121.

78. Nugent D, Vandekerckhove P, Hughes E, Arnot M, Lilford R. Gonadotrophin therapy for ovulation induction in subfertility associated with polycystic ovary syndrome. Cochrane Database Syst Rev 2000; (4): CD000410.

79. Unlu C, Atabekoglu CS. Surgical treatment in polycystic ovary syndrome. Curr Opin Obstet Gynecol 2006; 18: 286–92.

80. Rossmanith WG, Keckstein J, Spatzier K, Lauritzen C. The impact of ovarian laser surgery on the gonadotrophin secretion in women with polycystic ovarian disease. Clin Endocrinol 1991; 34: 23–30.

81. Johnson NP, Wang K. Is ovarian surgery effective for androgenic symptoms of polycystic ovarian syndrome? J Obstet Gynecol 2003; 23: 599–606.

82. Barbieri RL, Makris A, Ryan KJ. Insulin stimulates androgen accumulation in incubations of human ovarian stroma and theca. Obstet Gynecol 1984; 64: 74S–80S.

83. Iwashita M, Mimuro T, Watanabe M et al. Plasma levels of insulin-like growth factor-I and its binding protein in polycystic ovary syndrome. Horm Res 1990; 33 (Suppl 2): 21–6.

84. Homburg R, Pariente C, Lunenfeld B, Jacobs HS. The role of insulin-like growth factor-I (IGF-I) and IGF binding protein in patients with polycystic ovarian disease. Hum Reprod 1992; 7: 1379–83.

85. Suikkari AM, Ruutiainen K, Erkkola R, Seppala M. Low levels of low molecular weight insulin like growth factor binding protein in patients with polycystic ovarian disease. Hum Reprod 1989; 4: 136–9.

86. Thierry van Dessel HJ, Lee PD, Faessen G, Fauser BC, Giudice L. Elevated serum levels of free insulin-like growth factor I in polycystic ovary syndrome. J Clin Endocrinol Metab 1999; 84: 3030–5.

87. Duleba AJ, Spaczynski RZ, Olive DL, Behrman HR. Effects of insulin and insulin-like growth factors on proliferation of rat ovarian theca-interstitial cells. Biol Reprod 1997; 56: 891–7.

88. Duleba AJ, Spaczynski RZ, Olive DL. Insulin and insulin-like growth factor I stimulate the proliferation of human ovarian theca-interstitial cells. Fertil Steril 1998; 69: 335–40.

89. Duleba AJ, Spaczynski RZ, Arici A, Carbone R, Behrman HR. Proliferation and differentiation of rat theca-interstitial cells: comparison of effects induced by platelet-derived growth factor and insulin-like growth factor-I. Biol Reprod 1999; 60: 546–50.

90. Duleba AJ, Spaczynski RZ, Olive DL, Behrman HR. Divergent mechanism regulate proliferation/survival and steroidogenesis of theca-interstitial cells. Mol Hum Reprod 1999; 5: 193–8.

91. Duleba AJ, Spaczynski RZ, Tilly JL, Olive DL. Insulin and insulin-like growth factors protect ovarian theca-interstitial cells from apoptosis. Presented at 45th Annual Meeting of the Society for Gynecologic Investigation 1998, Atlanta, GA.

92. Nestler JE, Powers LP, Matt DW et al. A direct effect of hyperinsulinemia on serum sex hormone-binding globulin levels in obese women with the polycystic ovary syndrome. J Clin Endocrinol Metab 1991; 72: 83–9.

93. Schneider JG, Tompkins C, Blumenthal RS, Mora S. The metabolic syndrome in women. Cardiol Rev 2006; 14: 286–91.

94. Potashnik R, Bloch-Damti A, Bashan N, Rudich A. IRS-1 degradation and increased serine phosphorylation cannot predict the degree of metabolic insulin resistance induced by oxidative stress. Diabetologia 2003; 46: 639–48.

95. Evans J, Maddux BA, Goldfine ID. The molecular basis for oxidative stress-induced insulin resistance. Antioxid Redox Signal 2005; 7: 1040–52.

96. Paz K, Voliovitch H, Hadari YR et al. Interaction between the insulin receptor and its downstream effectors. Use of individually expressed receptor domains for structure/function analysis. J Biol Chem 1996; 271: 6998–7003.

97. Paz K, Hemi R, LeRoith D et al. A molecular basis for insulin resistance. Elevated serine/threonine phosphorylation of IRS-1 and IRS-2 inhibits their binding to the juxtamembrane region of the insulin receptor and impairs their ability to undergo insulin-induced tryosine phosphoryalation. J Biol Chem 1997; 272: 29911–18.

98. Book CB, Dunaif A. Selective insulin resistance in the polycystic ovary syndrome. J Clin Endocrinol Metab 1999; 84: 3110–16.

99. Corbould A, Zhao H, Mirzoeva S, Aird F, Dunaif A. Enhanced mitogenic signaling in skeletal muscle of women with polycystic ovary syndrome. Diabetes 2006; 55: 751–9.

100. Ehrmann DA, Barnes RB, Rosenfield RL, Cavaghan MK, Imperial J. Prevalence of impaired glucose tolerance and diabetes in women with polycystic ovary syndrome. Diabetes Care 1999; 22: 141–6.

101. Legro RS, Kunselman AR, Dodson WC, Dunaif A. Prevalence and predictors of risk for type 2 diabetes mellitus and impaired glucose tolerance in polycystic ovary syndrome: a prospective, controlled study in 254 affected women. J Clin Endocrinol Metab 1999; 84: 165–9.

102. Ehrmann DA, Kasza K, Azziz R, Legro RS, Ghazzi MN. Effect of race and family history of type 2 diabetes on metabolic status of women with polycystic ovary syndrome. J Clin Endocrinol Metab 2005; 90: 66–71.

103. Palmert MR, Gordon CM, Kartashov AI et al. Screening for abnormal glucose tolerance in adolescents with polycystic ovary syndrome. J Clin Endocrinol Metab 2002; 87: 1017–23.

104. Pasquali R, Antenucci D, Casimirri F et al. Clinical and hormonal characteristics of obese amenorrheic hyperandrogenic women before and after weight loss. J Clin Endocrinol Metab 1989; 68: 173–9.

105. Kiddy DS, Hamilton-Fairley D, Bush A et al. Improvement in endocrine and ovarian function during dietary treatment of obese women with polycystic ovary syndrome. Clin Endocrinol 1992; 36: 105–11.

106. Huber-Buchholz MM, Carey DG, Norman RJ. Restoration of reproductive potential by lifestyle modification in obese polycystic ovary syndrome: role of insulin sensitivity and luteinizing hormone. J Clin Endocrinol Metab 1999; 84: 1470–4.

107. Moran LJ, Noakes M, Clifton PM. Dietary composition in restoring reproductive and metabolic physiology in overweight women with polycystic ovary syndrome. J Clin Endocrinol Metab 2003; 88: 812–19.

108. LaMonte MJ, Barlow CE, Jurca R et al. Cardiorespiratory fitness is inversely associated with the incidence of metabolic syndrome. Circulation 2005; 112: 505–12.

109. Harborne L, Fleming R, Lyall H, Norman RJ, Sattar N. Descriptive review of the evidence for the use of metformin in polycystic ovary syndrome. Lancet 2003; 361: 1894–901.

110. Lord JM, Flight IH, Norman RJ. Insulin-sensitizing drugs (metformin, troglitazone, rosiglitazone, pioglitazone, D-chiro-inositol) for polycystic ovary syndrome. Cochrane Database Syst Rev 2003; (3): CD003053.

111. De Leo V, La Marca A, Petraglia F. Insulin lowering agents in the management of the polycystic ovary syndrome. Endocr Rev 2003; 24: 633–67.

112. Bailey CJ, Turner RC. Metformin N Engl J Med 1996; 334: 574–9.

113. Patane G, Piro S, Rabuazzo AM et al. Metformin restores insulin secretion altered by chronic exposure to free fatty acids or high glucose: a direct metformin effect on pancreatic beta cells. Diabetes 2000; 49: 735–40.

114. Gokcel A, Gumurdulu Y, Karakose H et al. Evaluation of the safety and efficacy of sibutramine, orlistat, and metformin in the treatment of obesity. Diabetes Obes Metab 2002; 4: 49–55.

115. Pasquali R, Gambineri A, Biscotti D et al. Effect of long-term treatment with metformin added to hypocaloric diet on body composition, fat distribution, and androgen and insulin levels in abdominally obese women with and without the polycystic ovary syndrome. J Clin Endocrinol Metab 2000; 85: 2767–74.

116. Jayagopal V, Kilpatrick ES, Holding S, Jennings PE, Atkin SL. Orlistat is as beneficial as metformin in the treatment of polycystic ovarian syndrome. J Clin Endocrinol Metab 2005; 90: 729–33.

117. Yki-Jarvinen H, Nikkila K, Makimattila S. Metformin prevents weight gain by reducing dietary intake during insulin therapy in patients with type 2 diabetes mellitus. Drugs 1999; 58 (Suppl 1): 53–4.

118. Barbieri RL. Metformin for the treatment of polycystic ovary syndrome. Obstet Gynecol 2003; 101: 785–93.

119. Harborne L, Fleming R, Lyall H, Sattar N, Norman J. Metformin or anti-androgen in the treatment of hirsutism in polycystic ovary syndrome. J Clin Endocrinol Metab 2003; 88: 4116–23.

120. Azziz R, Ehrmann DA, Legro RS, Fereshetian AG, Ghazzi MN; PCOS/Troglitazone Study Group. Troglitazone improves ovulation and hirsutism in the polycystic ovary syndrome: a multicenter, double-blind, placebo-controlled trial. J Clin Endocrinol Metab 2001; 86: 1626–32.

121. Lord JM, Flight IH, Norman RJ. Metformin in polycystic ovary syndrome: systematic review and meta-analysis. BMJ 2003; 327: 951–7.

122. Kashyap S, Wells GA, Rosenwaks Z. Insulin-sensitizing agents as primary therapy for patients with polycystic ovary syndrome. Hum Reprod 2004; 19: 2474–83.

123. Glueck CJ, Wang P, Fontaine RN et al. Plasminogen activator inhibitor activity: an independent risk factor for the high miscarriage rate during pregnancy in women with polycystic ovary syndrome. Metabolism 1999; 48: 1589–95.

124. Glueck CJ, Awadalla SG, Phillips H et al. Polycystic ovary syndrome, infertility, familial thrombophilia, familial hypofibrinolysis, recurrent loss of in vitro fertilized embryos, and miscarriage. Fertil Steril 2000; 74: 394–7.

125. Jakubowicz DJ, Iuorno MJ, Jakubowicz S, Roberts KA, Nestler JE. Effects of metformin on early pregnancy loss in the polycystic ovary syndrome. J Clin Endocrinol Metab 2002; 87: 524–9.

126. Glueck CJ, Phillips H, Cameron D, Sieve-Smith L, Wang P. Continuing metformin throughout pregnancy in women with polycystic ovary syndrome appears to safely reduce first-trimester spontaneous abortion: a pilot study. Fertil Steril 2001; 75: 46–52.

127. Glueck CJ, Wang P, Kobayashi K, Phillips H, Sieve-Smith L. Metformin therapy throughout pregnancy reduces the development of gestational diabetes in women with polycystic ovary syndrome. Fertil Steril 2002; 77: 520–5.

128. Glueck CJ, Goldenberg N, Pranikoff J et al. Height, weight, and motor-social development during the first 18 months of life in 126 infants born to 109 mothers with polycystic ovary syndrome who conceived on and continued metformin through pregnancy. Hum Reprod 2004; 19: 1323–30.

129. Mikola M, Hiilesmaa V, Halttunen M, Suhonen L, Tiitinen A. Obstetric outcome in women with polycystic ovarian syndrome. Hum Reprod 2001; 16: 226–9.

130. deVries MJ, Dekker GA, Schoemaker J. Higher risk of preeclampsia in the polycystic ovary syndrome. A case control study. Eur J Obstet Gynecol Reprod Biol 1998; 76: 91–5.

131. Bjercke S, Dale PO, Tanbo T et al. Impact of insulin resistance on pregnancy complications and outcome in women with polycystic ovary syndrome. Gynecol Obstet Invest 2002; 54: 94–8.

132. Radon PA, McMahon MJ, Meyer WR. Impaired glucose tolerance in pregnant women with polycystic ovary syndrome. Obstet Gynecol 1999; 94: 194–7.

133. Vanky E, Salvesen KA, Heimstad R et al. Metformin reduces pregnancy complications without affecting androgen levels in pregnant polycystic ovary syndrome women: results of a randomized study. Hum Reprod 2004; 19: 1734–40.

134. Kovo M, Weissman A, Gur D et al. Neonatal outcome in polycystic ovarian syndrome patients treated with metformin during pregnancy. J Matern Fetal Neonatal Med 2006; 19: 415–19.

135. Moghetti P, Castello R, Negri C et al. Metformin effects on clinical features, endocrine and metabolic profiles, and insulin sensitivity in polycystic ovary syndrome: a randomized, double-blind, placebo-controlled 6-month trial, followed by open, long-term clinical evaluation. J Endocrinol Metab 2000; 85: 139–46.

136. Kocak M, Caliskan E, Simsir C, Haberal A. Metformin therapy improves ovulatory rates, cervical scores, and pregnancy rates in clomiphene citrate-resistant women with polycystic ovary syndrome. Fertil Steril 2002; 77: 101–6.

137. Vandermolen DT, Ratts VS, Evans WS et al. Metformin increases the ovulatory rate and pregnancy rate from clomiphene citrate in patients with polycystic ovary syndrome who are resistant to clomiphene citrate alone. Fertil Steril 2001; 75: 310–15.

138. George SS, George K, Irwin C et al. Sequential treatment of metformin and clomiphene citrate in clomiphene-resistant women with polycystic ovary syndrome: a randomized, controlled trial. Hum Reprod 2003; 18: 299–304.

139. Nestler JE, Jakubowicz DJ, Evans WS, Pasquali R. Effects of metformin on spontaneous and clomiphene-induced ovulation in polycystic ovary syndrome. N Engl J Med 1998: 1876–80.

140. Legro RS, Myers ER, Schlaff WD, Carr BR, Diamond MP. Improvement in live births with clomiphene citrate and metformin, alone and in combination in infetile women with polycystic ovary syndrome. Abstract presented at ASRM 62nd Annual Meeting, 21–25 October, 2006, New Orleans, LA, abstr On2.

141. De Leo V, La Marca A, Ditto A, Morgante G, Cianci A. Effects of metformin on gonadotropin-induced ovulation in women with polycystic ovary syndrome. Fertil Steril 1999; 72: 282–5.

142. Palomba S, Falbo A, Orio FJ et al. A randomized controlled trial evaluating metformin pretreatment and co-administration in non-obese insulin-resistant women with polycystic ovary syndrome treated with controlled ovarian stimulation plus timed intercourse or intrauterine insemination. Hum Reprod 2005; 20: 2879–86.

143. Yarali H, Yildiz BO, Demirol A et al. Co-administration of metformin during rFSH treatment in patients with clomiphene citrate resistant polycystic ovary syndrome: a prospective randomized trial. Hum Reprod 2002; 17: 289–94.

144. Fedorcsak P, Dale PO, Storeng R, Abyholm T, Tanbo T. The effect of metformin on ovarian stimulation and in vitro fertilization in insulin-resistant women with polycystic ovary syndrome: an open label randomized cross-over trial. Gynecol Endocrinol 2003; 17: 207–14.

145. Stadtmauer LA, Toma SK, Riehl RM, Talbert LM. Metformin treatment of patients with polycystic ovary syndrome undergoing in vitro fertilization improves outcomes and is associated with modulation of the insulin-like growth factors. Fertil Steril 2001; 75: 505–9.

146. Stadtmauer LA, Toma SK, Riehl RM, Talbert LM. Impact of metformin therapy on ovarian stimulation and outcome in 'coasted' patients with polycystic ovary syndrome undergoing in-vitro fertilization. Reprod Biomed Online 2002; 5: 112–16.

147. Kjotrod SB, von During V, Carlsen SM. Metformin treatment before IVF/ICSI in women with polycystic ovary syndrome: a prospective, randomized, double-blind study. Hum Reprod 2004; 19: 1315–22.

148. Costello M, Chapman M, Conway U. A systematic review and meta-analysis of randomized controlled trials on metformin co-administration during gonadotrophin ovulation induction or IVF in women with polycystic ovary syndrome. Hum Reprod 2006; 21: 1387–99.

149. Camp HS, Li O, Wise SC et al. Differential activation of peroxisome proliferator activated receptor-gamma by troglitazone and rosiglitazone. Diabetes 2000; 49: 539–47.

150. Hsueh WA, Law R. The central role of fat and effect of peroxisome proliferator-activated receptor-gamma on progression of insulin resistance and cardiovascular disease. Am J Cardiol 2003; 92: 3J–9J.

151. Yki-Jarvinen H. Thiazolidinediones. N Engl J Med 2004; 351: 1106–18.

152. Belli SH, Graffigna MN, Oneto A et al. Effect of rosiglitazone on insulin resistance, growth factors, and reproductive disturbances in women with polycystic ovary syndrome. Fertil Steril 2004; 81: 624–9.

153. Brettenthaler N, De Geyter C, Huber PR, Keller U. Effect of the insulin sensitizer pioglitazone on insulin resistance, hyperandrogenism, and ovulatory dysfunction in women with polycystic ovary syndrome. J Clin Endocrinol Metab 2004; 89: 3835–40.

154. Ghazeeri G, Kutteh WH, Bryer-Ash M, Haas D. Effect of rosiglitazone on spontaneous and clomiphene citrate-induced ovulation in women with polycystic ovary syndrome. Fertil Steril 2003; 79: 562–6.

155. Ortega-Gonzalez C, Luna S, Hernandez L et al. Responses of serum androgen and insulin resistance to metformin and pioglitazone in obese, insulin-resistant women with polycystic ovary syndrome. J Clin Endocrinol Metab 2005; 90: 1360–5.

156. Nestler JE, Jakubowicz DJ, Reamer P, Gunn RD, Allan G. Ovulatory and metabolic effects of D-chiro-inositol in the polycystic ovary syndrome. N Engl J Med 1999; 430: 1314–20.

157. Halliwell B, Gutteridge JM. Free Radicals in Biology and Medicine. Oxford: Clarendon Press, 1999.

158. Paolisso G, Esposito R, D'Alessio MA, Barbieri M. Primary and secondary prevention of atherosclerosis: is there a role for antioxidants? Diabetes Metab 2002; 25: 298–306.

159. Rosen P, Nawroth PP, King G et al. The role of oxidative stress in the onset and progression of diabetes and its complications: a summary of a Congress Series sponsored by UNESCO-MCBN, the American Diabetes Association, and the German Diabetes Society. Diabetes Metab Res Rev 2001; 17: 189–212.

160. Sabuncu T, Vural H, Harma M. Oxidative stress in polycystic ovary syndrome and its contribution to the risk of cardiovascular disease. Clin Biochem 2001; 34: 407–13.

161. Kelly CC, Lyall H, Petrie JR et al. Low grade chronic inflammation in women with polycystic ovarian syndrome. J Clin Endocrinol Metab 2001; 86: 2453–5.

162. Orio FJ, Palomba S, Cascela T et al. The increase of leukocytes as a new putative marker of low-grade chronic inflammation and early cardiovascular risk in polycystic ovary syndrome. J Clin Endocrinol Metab 2004; 90: 2–5.

163. Yilmaz M, Bukan N, Ayvaz G et al. The effects of rosiglitazone and metformin on oxidative stress and homocysteine levels in lean patients with polycystic ovary syndrome. Hum Reprod 2005; 20: 3333–40.

164. Duleba AJ, Foyouzi N, Karaca M et al. Proliferation of ovarian theca-interstitial cells is modulated by antioxidants and oxidative stress. Hum Reprod 2004; 19: 1519–24.

165. Spaczynski RZ, Arici A, Duleba AJ. Tumor necrosis factor-alpha stimulates proliferation of rat ovarian theca-interstitial cells. Biol Reprod 1999; 61: 993–8.

166. Naz RK, Thurston D, Santoro N. Circulating tumor necrosis factor (TNF)-alpha in normally cycling women and patients with premature ovarian failure and polycystic ovaries. Am J Reprod Immunol 1995; 34: 170–5.

167. Gonzalez F, Thusu K, Abdel-Rahman E et al. Elevated serum levels of tumor necrosis factor alpha in normal-weight women with polycystic ovary syndrome. Metabolism 1999; 48: 437–41.

168. Adamson GM, Billings RE. Tumor necrosis factor induced oxidative stress in isolated mouse hepatocytes. Arch Biochem Biophys 1992; 294: 223–9.

169. Krieger-Brauer HI, Kather H. Human fat cells possess a plasma membrane-bound H_2O_2 generating system that is activated by insulin via a mechanism bypassing the receptor kinase. J Clin Invest 1992; 89: 1006–13.

170. Rifici VA, Schneider SH, Khachadurian AK. Stimulation of low-density lipoprotein oxidation by insulin and insulin like growth factor I. Atherosclerosis 1994; 107: 99–108.

171. Ruiz-Gines JA, Lopez-Ongil S, Gonzalez-Rubio M et al. Reactive oxygen species induce proliferation of bovine aortic endothelial cells. J Cardiovasc Pharmacol 2000; 35: 109–13.

172. Ivanov VO, Ivanova SV, Niedzwiecki A. Ascorbate affects proliferation of guinea pig vascular smooth muscle cells by direct and extracellular matrix-mediated effects. J Mol Cell Cardiol 1997; 29: 3293–303.

173. Azzi A, Aratri E, Boscoboinik D et al. Molecular basis of alpha-tocopherol control of smooth muscle cell proliferation. Biofactors 1998; 7: 3–14.

174. Nesaretnam K, Stephen R, Dils R, Darbre P. Tocotrienols inhibit the growth of human breast cancer cells irrespective of estrogen receptor status. Lipids 1998; 33: 461–9.

175. Onat D, Boscoboinik D, Azzi A, Basaga H. Effects of alpha-tocopherol and silibin dihemisuccinate on the proliferation of human skin fibroblasts. Biotechnol Appl Biochem 1999; 29: 213–15.

176. Piotrowski P, Rzepczynska I, Kwintkiewicz J, Duleba AJ. Oxidative stress induces expression of CYP11A, CYP17,

177. Henriksen EJ. Oxidative stress and antioxidant treatment: effects on muscle glucose transport in animal models of type 1 and type 2 diabetes. In: Packer L, Rosen P, Tritschler HJ, King GL, eds. Antioxidants in Diabetes Management. New York: Marcel Dekker, 2000:

178. Henriksen EJ, Saengsirisuwan V. Exercise training and antioxidants: relief from oxidative stress and insulin resistance. Exerc Sport Sci Rev 2003; 31: 79–84.

179. Jacob S, Ruus P, Hermann R et al. Oral administration of RAC-alpha-lipoic acid modulates insulin sensitivity in patients with type 2 diabetes mellitus: a placebo-controlled pilot trial. Free Radic Biol Med 1999; 27: 309–14.

180. Cabellero B. Vitamin E improves the action of insulin. Nutr Rev 1993; 51: 339–40.

181. Hirai N, Kawano H, Hirashima O et al. Insulin resistance and endothelial dysfunction in smokers: effects of vitamin C. Am J Physiol 2000; 279: H1172–8.

182. Hirashima O, Kawano H, Motoyama T et al. Improvement of endothelial function and insulin sensitivity with vitamin C in patients with coronary spastic angina: possible role of reactive oxygen species. J Am Coll Cardol 2000; 35: 1860–6.

183. Paolisso G, Di Maro G, Pizza G et al. Plasma GSH/GSSG affects glucose homeostasis in healthy subjects and non-insulin dependent diabetics. Am J Physiol 1992; 263: E435–40.

184. Fulghesu AM, Ciampelli M, Muzj G et al. N-acetylcysteine treatment improves insulin sensitivity in women with polycystic ovary syndrome. Fertil Steril 2002; 77: 1128–35.

185. Anderson RN, Smith BL. Deaths: leading causes for 2002. Natl Vital Stat 2005; 53: 17.

186. Wild RA, Painter PC, Coulson PB, Carruth KB, Ranney GB. Lipoprotein lipid concentrations and cardiovascular risk in women with polycystic ovary syndrome. J Clin Endocrinol Metab 1985; 61: 946–51.

187. Pierpoint T, McKeigue P, Isaacs AJ, Wild SH, Jacobs H. Mortality of women with polycystic ovary syndrome at long-term follow-up. J Clin Epidemiol 1998; 51: 581–6.

188. Lakhani K, Seifalian AM, Hardiman P. Impaired carotid viscoelastic properties in women with polycystic ovaries. Circulation 2002; 106: 81–5.

189. Paradisi G, Steinberg HO, Hempfling A et al. Polycystic ovary syndrome is associated with endothelial dysfunction. Circulation 2001; 103: 1410–15.

190. Guzick DS, Talbott EO, Sutton-Tyrrell K et al. Carotid atherosclerosis in women with polycystic ovary syndrome: initial results from a case-control study. Am J Obstet Gynecol 1996; 174: 1224–9.

191. Talbott EO, Guzick DS, Clerici A et al. Coronary heart disease risk factors in women with polycystic ovary syndrome. Arterioscler Thromb Vasc Biol 1995; 15: 821–6.

192. Birdsall MA, Farquhar CM, White HD. Association between polycystic ovaries and extent of coronary artery disease in women having cardiac catheterization. Ann Intern Med 1997; 126: 32–5.

193. National Cholesterol Education Program (NCEP) Expert Panel on Detection, Evaluation, and Treatment of High Blood Cholesterol in Adults (Adult Treatment Panel III). Third Report of the National Cholesterol Education Program (NCEP) Expert Panel on Detection, Evaluation, and Treatment of High Blood Cholesterol in Adults (Adult Treatment Panel III) final report. Circulation 2002; 106: 3143–421.

194. Apridonidze T, Essah PA, Iuorno MJ, Nestler JE. Prevalence and characteristics of the metabolic syndrome in women with polycystic ovary syndrome. J Clin Endocrinol Metab 2005; 90: 1929–35.

195. Reaven GM. Banting lecture: Role of insulin resistance in human disease. Diabetes 1988; 37: 1597–607.

StAR and 3bHSD in rat theca-interstitial cells. Presented at 52nd Annual Meeting of the Society for Gynecologic Investigation, 23–26 March, 2005, Los Angeles, CA.

196. Loverro G, Lorusso F, Mei L et al. The plasma homocysteine levels are increased in polycystic ovary syndrome. Gynecol Obstet Invest 2002; 53: 157–62.

197. Randeva H, Lewandowski KC, Drzewoski J et al. Exercise decreases plasma total homocysteine in overweight young women with polycystic ovary syndrome. J Clin Endocrinol Metab 2002; 87: 4496–501.

198. Vrbikova J, Bicikova M, Tallova J, Hill M, Starka L. Homocysteine and steroid levels in metformin-treated women with polycystic ovary syndrome. Exp Clin Endocrinol Diabetes 2002; 110: 74–7.

199. Clark R, Daly L, Robinson K et al. Hyperhomocysteinemia: an independent risk factor for vascular disease. N Engl J Med 1991; 324: 1149–55.

200. Kanani P, Sinkey C, Browning R et al. Role of oxidant stress in endothelial dysfunction produced by experimental hyperhomocysteinemia in humans. Circulation 1999; 100: 1161–8.

201. Eberhardt RT, Forgione MA, Cap A et al. Endothelial dysfunction in a murine model of mild hyperhomocysteinemia. J Clin Invest 2000; 106: 483–91.

202. Loscalzo J. Oxidant stress: a key determinant of atherothrombosis. Biochem Soc Trans 2003; 31: 1059–61.

203. Ungvari Z, Csiszar A, Edwards JG et al. Increased superoxide production in coronary arteries in hyperhomocysteinemia: role of TNF-a, NADPH oxidase, and iNOS. Arterioscler Thromb Vasc Biol 2003; 23: 418–24.

204. Kilicdag EB, Bagheri M, Tarim E et al. Administration of B-group vitamins reduces circulating homocysteine in polycystic ovary syndrome patients treated with metformin: a randomized trial. Hum Reprod 2005; 20: 1521–8.

205. Kilicdag EB, Bagis T, Zeyneloglu HB et al. Homocysteine levels in women with polycystic ovary syndrome treated with metformin versus rosiglitazone: a randomized study. Hum Reprod 2005; 20: 894–9.

206. Conway GS, Agrawal R, Betteridge DJ, Jacobs HS. Risk factors for coronary artery disease in lean and obese women with the polycystic ovary syndrome. Clin Endocrinol 1992; 37: 119–25.

207. Holte J, Bergh T, Berne C, Lithell H. Serum lipoprotein lipid profile in women with the polycystic ovary syndrome: relation to anthropometric, endocrine, and metabolic variables. Clin Endocrinol 1994; 41: 463–71.

208. Amowitz LL, Sobel BE. Cardiovascular consequences of polycystic ovary syndrome. Endocrinol Metab Clin North Am 1999; 28: 439–58.

209. Randomised trial of cholesterol lowering in 4444 patients with coronary heart disease: the Scandinavian Simvastatin Survival Study (4S). Lancet 1994; 344: 1383–9.

210. Goldstein JL, Brown MS. Regulation of the mevalonate pathway. Nature 1990; 343: 425–30.

211. Sacks FM, Pfeffer MA, Moye LA et al. The effect of pravastatin on coronary events after myocardial infarction in patients with average cholesterol levels. N Engl J Med 1996; 335: 1001–9.

212. Shepard J, Cobbe SM, Ford I et al. Prevention of coronary heart disease with pravastatin in men with hypercholesterolemia. West of Scotland Coronary Prevention Study Group. N Engl J Med 1995; 333: 1301–7.

213. Downs JR, Clearfield M, Weis S et al. Primary prevention of acute coronary events with lovastatin in men and women with average cholesterol levels: results of AFCAPS/TexCAPS. Air Force/Texas Coronary Atherosclerosis Prevention Study. JAMA 1998; 279: 1615–22.

214. McFarlane SI, Muniyappa R, Francisco R, Sowers JR. Clinical review 145: Pleiotropic effects of statins: lipid reduction and beyond. J Clin Endocrinol Metab 2002; 87: 1451–8.

215. Crisby M, Nordin-Fredriksson G, Shah PK et al. Pravastatin treatment increases collagen content and decreases lipid content, inflammation, metalloproteinases, and cell death in human carotid plaques: implications for plaque stabilization. Circulation 2001; 103: 926–33.

216. Siddals KW, Marshman E, Westwood M, Gibson JM. Abrogation of insulin-like growth factor-I (IGF-I) and insulin action by mevalonic acid depletion; synergy between protein prenylation and receptor glycosylation pathways. J Biol Chem 2004; 279: 38353–9.

217. Carlberg M, Dricu A, Blegen H et al. Mevalonic acid is limiting for N-linked glycosylation and translocation of the insulin-like growth factor-I receptor to the cell surface. Evidence for a new link between 3-hydroxy-3-methylglutaryl coenzyme A reductase and cell growth. J Biol Chem 1996; 271: 17453–62.

218. Franzoni F, Quinones-Galvan A, Regoli F, Ferrannini E, Galetta F. A comparative study of the in vitro antioxidant activity of statins. Int J Cardiol 2003; 90: 317–21.

219. Wassmann S, Laufs U, Muller K et al. Cellular antioxidant effects of atorvastatin in vitro and in vivo. Arterioscler Thromb Vasc Biol 2002; 22: 300–5.

220. Avram M, Dankner G, Cogan U, Hochgraf E, Brook JGW. Lovastatin inhibits low-density lipoprotein oxidation and alters its fluidity and uptake by macrophages: in vitro and in vivo studies. Metabolism 1992; 41: 229–35.

221. Shishehbor MH, Brennan ML, Aviles RJ, Fu X, Sprecher DL, Hazen SL. Statins promote potent systemic antioxidant effects through specific inflammatory pathways. Circulation 2003; 108: 426–31.

222. Ando H, Takamura T, Ota T, Nagai Y, Kobayashi K. Cerivastatin improves survival of mice with lipopolysaccharide-induced sepsis. J Pharmacol Exp Ther 2000; 294: 1043–6.

223. Izquierdo D, Foyouzi N, Kwintkiewicz J, Duleba AJ. Mevastatin inhibits ovarian theca-interstitial cell proliferation and steroidogenesis. Fertil Steril 2004; 82: 1193–7.

224. O'Driscoll G, Green D, Taylor RR. Simvastatin, an HMG coenzyme A reductase inhibitor, improves endothelial function within 1 month. Circulation 1997; 95: 1126–31.

225. Axel DI, Riessen R, Runge H, Viebahn R, Karsch KR. Effects of cerivastatin on human arterial smooth muscle cell proliferation and migration in transfilter cocultures. J Cardiovasc Pharmacol 2000; 35: 619–29.

226. Buemi M, Allegra A, Senatore M et al. Pro-apoptotic effect of fluvastatin on human smooth muscle cells. Eur J Pharmacol 1999; 370: 201–3.

227. El-Ani D, Zimlichman R. Simvastatin induces apoptosis of cultured rat cardiomyocytes. J Basic Clin Physiol Pharmacol 2001; 12: 325–38.

228. Danesh FR, Sadeghi MM, Amro N et al. 3-Hydroxy-3-methylglutaryl CoA reductase inhibitors prevent high glucose-induced proliferation of mesangial cells via modulation of Rho GTPase/p21 signaling pathway: implications for diabetic nephropathy. Proc Natl Acad Sci USA 2002; 99: 8301–5.

229. Wu CH, Lee SC, Chiu HH et al. Morphologic change and elevation of cortisol secretion in cultured human normal adrenocortical cells caused by mutant p21K-ras protein. DNA Cell Biol 2002; 21: 21–9.

230. Dobs AS, Schrott H, Davidson MH et al. Effects of high-dose simvastatin on adrenal and gonadal steroidogenesis in men with hypercholesterolemia. Metabolism 2000; 49: 1234–8.

231. Rzepczynska I, Piotrowski P, Kwintkiewicz J, Duleba AJ. Effect of mevastatin on expression of CYP17, 3bHSD, CYP11A and StAR in rat theca-interstitial cells. Presented at 52nd Annual Meeting of the Society for Gynecologic Investigation, 23–26 March, 2005, Los Angeles, CA.

232. Piotrowski P, Kwintkiewicz J, Rzepczynska I, Duleba AJ. Simvastatin and mevastatin inhibit expression of NADPH

oxidase subunits: p22phox and p47phox in rat theca-interstitial cells. Presented at 52nd Annual Meeting of the Society for Gynecologic Investigation, 23–26 March, 2005, Los Angeles, CA.

233. Kwintkiewicz J, Foyouzi N, Piotrowski P, Rzepczynska I, Duleba AJ. Mevastatin inhibits proliferation of rat ovarian theca-interstitial cells by blocking the mitogen activated protein kinase pathway. Fertil Steril 2006; 86: 1053–8.

234. Duleba AJ, Banaszweska B, Spaczynski RZ, Pawelczyk L. Simvastatin improves biochemical parameters of polycystic ovary syndrome: results of a prospective randomized trial. Fertil Steril 2006; 85: 996–1001.

235. Banaszewska B, Pawelczyk L, Spaczynski RZ, Dziura J, Duleba AJ. Effects of simvastatin and oral contraceptive agent on polycystic ovary syndrome: prospective randomized crossover trial. J Clin Endocrinol Metab 2007; 92: 456–61.

13 Hyperprolactinemia and its medical management

John K Park and Sarah L Berga

INTRODUCTION

Hyperprolactinemia is one of the most frequently diagnosed endocrine disorders in women. It is defined as the consistent presence of an abnormally high level of prolactin in the blood when physiological causes have been excluded. Normal prolactin levels are typically between 10 and 28 ng/ml in a woman who is not pregnant or breastfeeding. Prolactin is secreted from lactotrophs of the anterior pituitary, and its main physiological role is to promote milk secretion. It is normal for serum prolactin levels to rise during pregnancy and breastfeeding. There are a variety of mechanisms by which prolactin may be present in excess, and these can generally be broken down into physiologic, pathologic, and medication-induced causes (Table 13.1). The most significant regulatory substance for prolactin secretion is dopamine, which is tonically secreted from the hypothalamus. Anything that interferes with dopamine synthesis, its transport to the pituitary gland, or the binding and activation of the dopamine receptor on the lactotroph can result in hyperprolactinemia.

EPIDEMIOLOGY/PREVALENCE

Hyperprolactinemia is most frequently caused by a prolactinoma, which is the most common type of benign pituitary adenoma.[1] Prolactinomas <10 mm are microprolactinomas, and those ≥10 mm are macroprolactinomas. Prolactinomas are categorized based on size because their size predicts their behavior. Microadenomas rarely progress in size, while macroadenomas may grow to a considerable size and invade tissue planes. This fits with the finding that macroprolactinomas have a vascular density that is significantly higher than that of microprolactinomas, which suggests they are products of different pathological processes.[2] Prolactinomas account for up to 45% of pituitary tumors, occurring with an incidence of 6–10 cases per million annually and a prevalence of 60–100 cases per million.[3] Prolactinomas occur more frequently in women during the second through fifth and decade, but the gender disparity disappears in the

Table 13.1 Causes of hyperprolactinemia

Physiological
Pregnancy
Breastfeeding
Food ingestion
Stress (physical or psychological)
Exercise
Sleep
Sexual activity/breast stimulation

Pharmacological
Antipsychotics
Antidepressants
Antihypertensives
Gastrointestinal medications
Opiates
Estrogen

Pathological
Pituitary
  microprolactinoma
  macroprolactinoma
  hypophysitis
  stalk interruption/displacement
  pituitary adenoma
  acromegaly
  cushing's syndrome
  empty sella syndrome
  rathke cysts
  infiltrative diseases (tuberculosis, sarcoidosis, Langerhans cell histiocytosis)
Hypothalamic
  primary hypothyroidism
  adrenal insufficiency
  tumors (craniopharyngioma, germinoma)
  pseudotumor cerebri
  cranial irradiation
Neurogenic
  chest wall injury/surgery
  spinal cord lesions
Reduced prolactin elimination
  renal failure
  hepatic insufficiency

fifth decade. The peak incidence occurs during the third decade of life, where the female to male ratio is 14.5:1.[1]

The gender disparity in the incidence of prolactinomas may be somewhat fallacious. Men may not seek immediate medical attention for signs of hyperprolactinemia, such as impotence and decreased libido. This may explain why men have a higher frequency of more advanced lesions, such as macroadenomas and tumors with mass effects. Women, on the other hand, most commonly experience problems such as infertility, amenorrhea, or galactorrhea: signs that are more likely to prompt a visit to the clinician. It is possible that these differences account for some of the gender disparity in the incidence of the disease.

REGULATION OF PROLACTIN SYNTHESIS AND SECRETION

Prolactin is a single-chain peptide hormone consisting of 199 amino acids and has a molecular weight of 23 kDa. The amino acid sequence bears a striking resemblance to those of growth hormone and human placental lactogen.[4] Prolactin is synthesized and secreted from lactotrophs located in the posterior lateral aspect of the anterior pituitary. It is released in pulses of varying amplitude superimposed on continuous basal secretion, which is also likely pulsatile. There are 13–14 peaks per day in young subjects.[5] The circulating levels of prolactin follow a circadian rhythm, with peak levels during sleep and troughs during waking hours. The synthesis and secretion is influenced by certain physiologic states and external factors, whose effects are translated through various neurotransmitters and substances in the circulation that act as either prolactin inhibitory factors or prolactin releasing factors.

Prolactin inhibitory factors

Prolactin is primarily regulated by dopamine. Dopamine provides tonic inhibition of prolactin release, and if endogenous dopamine receptors are blocked, a prolactin increase will follow. Dopamine is released from axons that originate in the dorsal portion of the arcuate nucleus and the inferior portion of the ventromedial nucleus of the hypothalamus. Dopamine binds to the type 2 dopamine (D_2) receptors on the lactotroph cell membrane. These receptors belong to the G protein-coupled receptor family that has a single polypeptide chain containing seven hydrophobic transmembrane domains. The binding of dopamine to the D_2 receptors causes the inhibition of adenyl cyclase activity and consequently reduces intracellular cyclic adenosine monophosphate (cAMP) levels. The inhibition of cAMP is a key step in the inhibition

of prolactin synthesis and secretion. Anything that prohibits dopamine from binding to the D_2 receptor on the lactotroph, such as pituitary stalk transection or a hypothalamic tumor, will cause an increase in prolactin secretion.

Of all the pituitary hormones, only prolactin is under tonic inhibition by the hypothalamus. All of the other pituitary hormones require excitatory input for their secretion. Thus, when an organic condition is present that impairs hypothalamic or median eminence input to the pituitary, prolactin levels rise while levels of the other pituitary hormones decline. In contrast, any direct damage to the pituitary will cause all of the pituitary hormones, including prolactin, to fall.

Another prolactin inhibitory factor is γ–aminobutyric acid (GABA), which has a relatively minor role in prolactin regulation. GABA is secreted into the portal circulation, and it binds to GABA receptors on the lactotroph. Increases in GABAergic tone reduce basal and breast-stimulated prolactin release.[6]

Prolactin releasing factors

Thyrotropin releasing hormone (TRH) causes prolactin gene transcription and an acute release of prolactin. This rapid effect is mediated by the binding of TRH to TRH receptors on the lactotrophs. Lactotrophs appear to be quite sensitive to TRH, because the smallest dose of TRH that releases thyroid stimulating hormone (TSH) also releases prolactin.[7] Given that suckling causes a rise in prolactin but not TSH, it does not appear that TRH is a prolactin releasing factor of major importance.

Vasoactive intestinal polypeptide (VIP) also stimulates prolactin release through cAMP.[8] The precise physiologic role of VIP is still not clear, but it appears that VIP has autocrine and paracrine effects on prolactin and growth hormone.[9]

More than one mechanism exists for the positive influence of estrogen on the synthesis and release of prolactin. Estrogen acts on the lactotroph to activate gene transcription and accumulation of prolactin mRNA.[10] Furthermore, estrogen stimulates lactotroph proliferation.[11] These actions account for the large increases in prolactin levels during pregnancy.

Serotonin also appears to act as a prolactin releasing factor. Prolactin levels increase when 5-hydroxytryptophan is infused,[12] or when serotonin-reuptake inhibitors are used.[13] Opioids have a role in prolactin regulation. Opioid peptides appear to stimulate prolactin release by inhibiting dopamine turnover and release from hypothalamic neurons.[14] Growth hormone releasing hormone increases prolactin release in vivo in humans.[15] Angiotensin II appears to be a potent secretagog, and its action can be blocked by the angiotensin II antagonist, saralasin.[16]

CLINICAL MANIFESTATIONS OF HYPERPROLACTINEMIA

Although prolactin receptors have been identified in many organs, the clinical manifestations of excess prolactin most commonly relate to the hypothalamic–pituitary–gonadal axis and the breast. In the breast, excess prolactin causes the inappropriate stimulation of milk production, leading to galactorrhea. In the hypothalamus, hyperprolactinemia disturbs the pattern of gonadotropin releasing hormone secretion, which in turn alters pituitary gonadotropin secretion. This problem manifests as ovarian dysfunction, with irregular ovulation, oligo/amenorrhea, infertility, and decreased sex steroid production.

Decreased sex steroid production may present as decreased libido and osteopenia or osteoporosis. The bone loss associated with hyperprolactinemia is attributable to reduced sex steroid exposure and prolactin per se does not induce bone loss or prevent accretion.[17,18] The degree of bone loss is ultimately related to the duration and severity of hypogonadism, and therapy is recommended for osteopenia to prevent further bone loss and improve bone density.

If a pituitary tumor is present, such as a macroadenoma, the mass effect of the tumor can cause symptoms such as headache, visual field defects due to compression of the optic chiasm, or cranial nerve palsies if the cavernous sinus is affected. Other symptoms of a pituitary tumor include hypopituitarism, seizures, or cerebrospinal fluid rhinorrhea.

DIAGNOSIS OF HYPERPROLACTINEMIA

Hyperprolactinemia is diagnosed when two separate serum prolactin levels are found to be elevated. In order to minimize the potential for confounding physiologic factors that can increase prolactin levels, the sample should be obtained in the morning while the patient is fasting and at least 2 hours following coitus, nipple stimulation, sleep, exercise, and physical or emotional stress. Any of these activities may cause a transient increase in prolactin. It may also be helpful to obtain the measurement during the early follicular phase of the menstrual cycle, as prolactin is known to increase with luteinizing hormone (LH) just prior to ovulation.[19] Painful venipuncture can provoke a prolactin elevation in some women. For these patients, a more accurate measurement may be obtained by inserting a venous catheter and taking a sample 60–90 minutes later. Although sexual activity, including breast and nipple stimulation, can transiently increase prolactin levels, routine breast examination does not acutely increase levels.[20]

Diagnostic considerations

Hook effect

The 'hook effect' refers to the phenomenon whereby a two-site immunological assay grossly underestimates the amount of the substance being measured. This effect has been observed in both radioimmunometric assays and chemiluminescence assays.[21,22] The principle of these types of assays is that the patient's serum and a labeled signal antibody are simultaneously added to a solid surface to which a capture antibody is fixed. The antigen being measured becomes sandwiched between the capture and signal antibody. After the unbound signal antibodies are washed away, the amount of signal antibody that remains is proportional to the amount of antigen that is present in the sample.

The hook effect is seen when the ligand concentration is high enough that many signal antibody binding sites are occupied by free ligand, and are therefore unable to bind to antigen complexed to capture antibody. The signal antibodies that are free or bound to free antigen are washed away, which results in a decreased measurement of the antigen.

There are two simple strategies to prevent the miscalculation of prolactin concentration. A 1/50 to 1/200 dilution of the serum sample can be measured in parallel with the original sample when there is a high suspicion of hyperprolactinemia, such as when there is a macroadenoma.[22] If the concentration of prolactin is high enough to result in the hook effect, a detectable amount of prolactin should be present in the dilutions. Another approach is to switch to an assay that uses a two-step process. Instead of simultaneously adding the patient's serum and signal antibody to the capture antibody, the serum is added first and the excess antigen is washed away prior to addition of the signal antibody. This approach is more time-consuming, but it prevents the formation of free antigen–signal antibody complexes that can be washed away.

Circulating variants of prolactin

Molecular variants of prolactin should be suspected in patients with asymptomatic hyperprolactinemia. Variants of prolactin can have normal immunoactivity but reduced bioactivity. Some patients with asymptomatic hyperprolactinemia have normal levels of monomeric prolactin with elevated levels of either glycosylated prolactin or high molecular weight post-translational variants.[23] The reduced bioactivity prevents the patient from developing symptoms. Unnecessary treatment of these patients can be avoided by the identification of such prolactin variants.

Glycosylated prolactin   During prolactin synthesis, the final product exhibits some heterogeneity due to various forms of post-translational modification and glycosylation. The major circulating form of prolactin is a 23-kDa monomeric protein, which constitutes up to 80% of the total prolactin in serum from normal subjects and the majority of patients with hyperprolactinemia. Glycosylation yields a molecule of 25 kDa, which constitutes 16–24% of total circulating plasma prolactin.[24] Alterations in the glycosylation pattern of secreted prolactin do not occur with prolactinomas.[25] The biological activity of glycosylated prolactin is lower than that of non-glycosylated prolactin, and in vitro studies have shown that glycosylation reduces the ability of prolactin to bind to lactogenic receptors.[23,26]

Macroprolactin   There are two isoforms of prolactin that have much higher molecular weights: big prolactin has a molecular mass of 45–60 kDa, and big big prolactin (macroprolactin) has a molecular mass > 100 kDa. Big prolactin is derived from covalently or non-covalently bound dimers or monomeric prolactin bound to another serum component, possibly prolactin-binding protein, which is identical to the extracellular domain of the prolactin receptor.[27] Macroprolactin consists of monomeric prolactin bound to antiprolactin autoantibodies. The larger isoforms are rarely physiologically active but are detectable in prolactin immunoassays. The decreased bioactivity is likely due to the high molecular weight preventing the molecule from crossing through the capillary wall. This may also explain the reduced rate of clearance of the larger isoforms.

Macroprolactinemia is characterized by the presence of significant levels of macroprolactin, with or without elevated levels of monomeric prolactin. This condition was initially recognized in asymptomatic patients with idiopathic hyperprolactinemia.[28] Their prolactin elevation was the result of macroprolactinemia in the presence of normal monomeric prolactin levels, and the patients were asymptomatic due to the lack of bioactivity of the macroprolactin. More recent studies have discovered that symptomatic hyperprolactinemic patients can also have significant macroprolactin. One study reported that 46% of patients with macroprolactinemia suffered from galactorrhea and 39% experienced menstrual disorders.[29] The overall prevalence of macroprolactinemia in hyperprolactinemic patients is approximately 26%. Leslie et al examined 1225 hyperprolactinemic patients and found that 322 (26%) had macroprolactinemia.[30] Although macroprolactin is commonly found in patients with hyperprolactinemia, neither symptoms nor magnetic resonance imaging (MRI) findings are useful in predicting its presence. Patients with macroprolactinemia often have symptoms similar to those in patients with elevation in monomeric prolactin.[31]

Macroprolactin does not appear to be formed in the pituitary, as the culture media of two pituitary adenomas removed from patients with macroprolactinemia demonstrated normal prolactin elution patterns.[29] This suggests that macroprolactin is formed in and confined to the vascular compartment. The mechanisms that trigger production of antiprolactin antibodies remain to be elucidated. It also appears that the presence of antiprolactin antibody is independent of whether there is a pituitary adenoma causing the overproduction of little prolactin. Thus, a pituitary lesion should still be ruled out by neuroradiological imaging when macroprolactinemia is present.

Recently, investigators began recommending routine screening for the presence of macroprolactin in all hyperprolactinemic patients.[32–36] Routine screening is advocated to avoid misdiagnosis and unnecessary medical and surgical intervention. Implementing routine testing can be cost-effective because repeated hormone, neuroradiological examinations, and unnecessary treatments with dopamine agonists can be avoided if the source of hyperprolactinemia is solely attributed to the presence of macroprolactin.[36] The recommendation for screening all hyperprolactinemic patients has not been adopted universally. However, there are groups of patients who could certainly benefit from macroprolactin screening. If macroprolactin is identified as the cause of hyperprolactinemia in an asymptomatic patient, observation would be appropriate rather than therapy and intensive monitoring. Macroprolactin screening would also be helpful for patients undergoing therapy who do not experience complete normalization of prolactin levels despite having resolution of symptoms. Macroprolactin may be present, but no additional therapy would be required because the therapy may actually be successful in normalizing monomeric prolactin.

Currently, the only means to screen hyperprolactinemic sera for macroprolactin is to repeat a prolactin assay after macroprolactin has been depleted from the sample. The two most commonly used methods of macroprolactin depletion include gel filtration chromatography (GFC) or polyethylene glycol (PEG) precipitation. Gel filtration chromatography is the gold standard, but it is more time-consuming and more costly, and thus its widespread use is precluded. Results from PEG precipitation correlate very well with GFC, and it has become the method of choice for the simultaneous removal of both macroprolactin and big prolactin from hyperprolactinemic sera.[37] Recently it has been proposed that the diagnosis of macroprolactinemia requires monomeric prolactin levels to fall within a normal range following removal of macroprolactin by PEG.[38]

EVALUATION OF HYPERPROLACTINEMIA

Once the presence of hyperprolactinemia is confirmed, an investigation to identify the source should be initiated. Evaluation begins with ruling out physiologic and pharmacologic causes of hyperprolactinemia. This starts with a detailed history, including a current list of medications. A pregnancy test is required, along with thyroid function tests to rule out primary hypothyroidism. Renal function tests are needed to rule out kidney failure. An imaging study of the pituitary is then indicated, even when the prolactin level is not significantly elevated.

A prolactin level greater than 200 ng/ml is thought to be pathognomonic of a pituitary adenoma in non-pregnant women.[39] However, prolactinomas are also very common when prolactin levels are < 100 ng/ml. When over 100 women with infertility were found to have hyperprolactinemia, 74% of patients had a pituitary tumor by MRI.[40] Of those with microadenomas, 52% had prolactin levels < 100 ng/ml.

Although the prolactinoma is the most likely lesion to be found on MRI, other sellar masses may be identified, such as craniopharyngiomas, germinomas, or meningiomas. These lesions cause a mild to moderate hyperprolactinemia by interrupting the flow of dopamine from the hypothalamus to the pituitary. The treatment for these mass lesions is surgical rather than medical, which highlights the importance of pituitary imaging even in the presence of mildly elevated prolactin levels. MRI with gadolinium contrast is the preferred method for pituitary imaging, as it provides the greatest detail. A computed tomography (CT) scan may be performed if MRI is unavailable, but X-ray studies with views of the sella turcica are no longer adequate.

If a large sellar mass or a mass near the optic chiasm is identified, a formal neuro-ophthalmologic evaluation should be performed to determine whether there are any visual or cranial nerve defects. A formal endocrine evaluation is also recommended to determine whether there is evidence of hypopituitarism. A patient with hypogonadism requires a dual-energy X-ray absorptiometry (DEXA) scan to evaluate her bone density.

Physiologic causes

The presence of physiologic causes of hyperprolactinemia can be determined with a detailed history and a few serum tests. The most obvious physiologic stimuli that can increase pituitary prolactin secretion include pregnancy and suckling. Although prolactin receptors are widely expressed throughout the body, the main physiologic role of pituitary prolactin is to promote milk production and secretion. With this function in mind, it is normal to see a gradual increase in prolactin levels during pregnancy, and at term there may be a 10-fold increase, reaching levels > 200 ng/ml. This increase in prolactin is attributed to estrogenic stimulation of the lactotrophs, causing replication of lactotrophs and secretion of prolactin. However, high estrogen levels inhibit prolactin action at the breast, and, as a result, lactation does not begin until the estrogen levels decline postpartum. During the postpartum period, prolactin remains elevated in lactating women, with each suckling episode causing a rapid release of pituitary prolactin. As long as frequent nursing behavior is maintained, basal prolactin levels remain elevated and amenorrhea often persists.[41]

There are several physiologic factors that can cause mild, transient elevations in serum prolactin. These factors should be considered during the evaluation of hyperprolactinemia, so that prolactin levels may be measured at a time with the fewest confounding factors. For example, food ingestion, sleep, coitus, and nipple stimulation can increase prolactin secretion. Taken together, these physiologic factors dictate that the best time to assess prolactin status would be during a fasting state in the late morning. Stress, both physical and emotional, may also increase prolactin levels. Venipuncture can be a stressful event for some patients, and these may benefit from having a venous catheter inserted in order to measure prolactin 60–90 minutes later.

Pharmacologic induced hyperprolactinemia

There is an extensive list of medications that can increase prolactin (Table 13.2). A detailed patient history is important in the consideration of medication induced hyperprolactinemia. It may be discovered that symptoms of hyperprolactinemia surfaced shortly after initiating a medication. It is important to obtain MRI to ensure that hyperprolactinemia is caused by a medication and not a lesion in the area of the hypothalamus or pituitary. The most straightforward approach to confirming that a particular pharmacologic agent is causing hyperprolactinemia is to temporarily eliminate the medication and repeat a prolactin measurement.

The special case is the patient on neuroleptics for psychiatric illness. It may not be practical to eliminate a psychiatric medication as this may precipitate a psychosis. The alternative to discontinuing a medication is to temporarily provide a substitute agent that does not cause hyperprolactinemia, and repeat a prolactin measurement. It is prudent to obtain MRI prior to undertaking either of these approaches. A lesion on MRI would obviate the need to rule out pharmacologic induced hyperprolactinemia. If the MRI is negative, one should realize the risk of psychiatric destabilization and decide whether it is worth medication discontinuation or alteration. Manipulation of any psychoactive medication should be done with the assistance of a psychiatrist or prescribing physician to avoid a sudden exacerbation of the underlying psychiatric disorder.

Antipsychotic medications (neuroleptics)

Antipsychotic agents are the medications that most commonly cause hyperprolactinemia. These drugs are dopamine receptor blockers that affect dopamine D_2 and D_4 receptors in the brain. Prolactin levels with these medications are generally < 100 ng/ml, and they usually decline to normal within 48–96 hours after discontinuation.[42] The atypical antipsychotic agents are newer medications in this class. Risperidone is a combined serotonin/dopamine receptor antagonist that can cause significantly higher prolactin elevations compared to the typical antipsychotics.[43]

Antidepressant medications

There are a few reports that tricyclic antidepressants and monoamine oxidase inhibitors can cause mild hyperprolactinemia. Clomipramine, for example, has reportedly caused hyperprolactinemia in 60% of men and 87.5% of women.[44] Selective serotonin reuptake

Table 13.2 Medications that may cause hyperprolactinemia

Antipsychotics (neuroleptics)
- Phenothiazines
- Thioxanthenes
- Butyrophenones
- Atypical antipsychotics

Antidepressants
- Tricyclic antidepressants
- Monoamine oxidase inhibitors
- Selective serotonin reuptake inhibitors

Antihypertensive medications
- Verapamil
- Methyldopa
- Reserpine

Gastrointestinal medications
- Metoclopramide
- Domperidone

Opiates
- Cocaine
- Heroin
- Morphine

Estrogens

inhibitors (SSRIs) have also been reported to increase prolactin. Out of 80 patients with major depressive disorder and normal baseline prolactin levels, 10 (12.5%) developed hyperprolactinemia after fluoxetine treatment for 12 weeks.[45] This effect was more profound in women, where 22% developed hyperprolactinemia. The largest prolactin increase in this study was 26.2 ng/ml.[45] Though unlikely, it remains to be seen whether hyperprolactinemia from SSRIs will compromise the hypothalamic–pituitary–gonadal axis.

Antihypertensive medications

Verapamil is the only calcium channel blocker to cause hyperprolactinemia. Verapamil causes short-term and long-term increases in basal prolactin secretion. It is believed to cause hyperprolactinemia by blocking the hypothalamic generation of dopamine.[46] Other calcium channel blockers do not affect prolactin secretion. Methyldopa also increases prolactin by decreasing dopamine synthesis.[47]

Gastrointestinal medications

Metoclopramide is used to stimulate gastrointestinal motility for patients with nausea or diabetic gastroparesis. Metoclopramide can cause acute hyperprolactinemia because it is a dopamine receptor blocker.[48]

Opiates

Morphine, heroin, and cocaine use have been associated with mild hyperprolactinemia.[49–51] These substances appear to stimulate prolactin secretion by inhibiting hypothalamic dopamine release.

Estrogens

The dramatic increase in serum prolactin during pregnancy is the result of estrogen stimulation of the lactotrophs. This estrogen-induced prolactin elevation has raised concerns that estrogens in oral contraceptives or postmenopausal hormonal therapy may also increase prolactin. There have been conflicting studies on the issue, and at this point it is unclear whether there is a relationship between oral contraceptives or hormone replacement therapy and hyperprolactinemia. With negative MRI, it is reasonable to continue estrogen containing medication with periodic surveillance.

If a medication is found to cause hyperprolactinemia, the degree of symptomatology will dictate the treatment approach. As long as the hypothalamic–pituitary–gonadal axis is not disrupted by the hyperprolactinemia, the patient may only require reassurance. On the other hand, hypoestrogenism may occur when the gonadal function is perturbed. This should prompt an evaluation into the necessity of the offending medication and determine a course of action that will either restore gonadal function or replace steroid hormones. If the medication is required, gonadal function may be restored by switching to another drug in the same class that does not cause hyperprolactinemia. Another approach is to continue the medication and replace gonadal hormones with oral contraceptives or hormone replacement therapy.

Pathologic causes

Pathologic causes of hyperprolactinemia include any condition that interferes with dopamine reaching the lactotrophs and thus loss of the tonic inhibition of prolactin secretion. Common conditions include pituitary tumors, such as prolactinomas, but can also include hypothalamic and pituitary lesions, such as craniopharyngiomas, lymphocytic hypophysitis, or pituitary stalk transaction, damage, or displacement. Pathological causes also include primary hypothyroidism, renal failure, seizures, and chest wall trauma. In primary hypothyroidism, thyrotropin releasing hormone from the hypothalamus can stimulate lactotroph secretion of prolactin. Renal failure can affect the clearance of prolactin, resulting in elevated serum levels. Seizures are associated with prolactin secretion, and a prolactin measurement can be used to help differentiate a seizure from a pseudoseizure. Any chest wall trauma along the dermatome of the nipple, such as surgery, herpes zoster, or breast augmentation, can elicit prolactin secretion.

The most common cause of hyperprolactinemia is the prolactinoma, which is a predominantly benign tumor.[52] The prolactinoma may escape the inhibitory control of dopamine and constitutively express high levels of prolactin. Some prolactin secreting tumors cosecrete growth hormone, which is why hyperprolactinemia can be found in some acromegalics.[53] If a patient has any symptoms or signs of acromegaly, such as enlarged hands and feet and coarsening of the face, a serum level for insulin-like growth factor I should be obtained.

MANAGEMENT OF PROLACTINOMAS

Regardless of the mode of treatment, whether it involves medication, surgery, or radiotherapy, the treatment goal should be individualized for each patient. If a large tumor is not present, the treatment goal may be the suppression of prolactin to prevent unwanted effects such as infertility and osteoporosis. If a large prolactinoma is present, the goal may be to control or reduce the tumor mass to prevent visual field defects resulting from compression of the optic chiasm, hypopituitarism resulting from pituitary stalk compression, or cranial nerve dysfunction resulting from compression of the cavernous sinus. For some patients, the treatment goal is the prevention of disease recurrence or progression.

Observation

It is reasonable for some patients with hyperprolactinemia to forgo any intervention and, instead, be followed by observation. This population would include those do not have a macroadenoma, do not wish to conceive, are eugonadal, are asymptomatic, and have stable prolactin levels. Patients with microadenomas do not necessarily require treatment because the majority of these will not enlarge. One study followed untreated patients with microadenomas for up to 8 years. Of 139 women, only nine (7%) had evidence for growth.[54] Similar results were found for patients with idiopathic hyperprolactinemia. After an average of 5.5 years of follow-up for 41 patients with idiopathic hyperprolactinemia, only 17% of patients had serum prolactin levels increase by >50% of their baseline value, and only one developed a prolactinoma.[55] In either situation, serum prolactin levels should be periodically measured to determine whether a prolactinoma is developing, or enlarging if one is already present. It is unlikely for a prolactinoma to grow significantly without an increase in serum prolactin levels, but periodic MRI can verify the absence of tumor growth and ensure that serum prolactin is a reliable indicator of tumor size. There is no consensus on the frequency of pituitary imaging for these patients. Observation is not recommended for the macroprolactinoma, given the increased likelihood for a macroprolactinoma to continue to grow.[54] Furthermore, most macroadenomas are associated with prolactin levels high enough to elicit symptoms that warrant treatment.

Treatment of hypogonadism

Estrogen therapy in the form of combined oral contraceptives or hormone replacement therapy may be employed as an alternative for women with idiopathic hyperprolactinemia or microadenoma who do not wish to become pregnant and in whom estrogen deficiency is the major concern. Hormone replacement is necessary to reduce the risk of bone loss. There does not appear to be a substantial risk for tumor enlargement in patients with prolactinomas who are treated with oral contraceptives or hormone replacement therapy for hypogonadism.[56] Rare cases of tumor growth during estrogen therapy have been reported, but it is not known whether estrogen played a role or the tumors progressed on their own.[57,58] Nevertheless, prolactin levels should be monitored annually.[59]

Medical management: dopamine agonists

Dopamine agonist therapy is the primary treatment for almost all patients, while surgery and radiotherapy have very limited use. In most cases, dopamine agonists are capable of suppressing prolactin secretion, reducing the size of prolactinomas, and restoring gonadal function. The dopamine agonists inhibit prolactin secretion at the level of the lactotroph. Their effects are mediated by the D_2 dopamine receptor, which belongs to the family of G protein-coupled receptors. The D_2 receptor inhibits adenyl cyclase activity, and consequently reduces intracellular cAMP

levels. This inhibition of cAMP is a key step in the inhibition of prolactin synthesis and secretion.

Bromocriptine

Bromocriptine is the first dopamine agonist used in clinical practice for prolactinomas. It has become the reference compound against which newer dopamine agonists are compared. It is a D_2 receptor agonist and a D_1 receptor antagonist. For patients with microprolactinomas, bromocriptine is 80–90% successful in normalizing serum prolactin, restoring gonadal function, and shrinking tumor mass.[60] For patients with macroprolactinomas, bromocriptine is approximately 70% successful in normalizing prolactin levels and shrinking tumor mass.[60] Bromocriptine has a short half-life of 3.3 hours, so this medication must be administered 2–3 times daily. Therapeutic doses are in the range of 2.5–15 mg/day, but resistant patients may require doses up to 30 mg/day.[54] The effects of treatment are rapid, with most patients experiencing dramatic improvement in headache and visual field defects within days after initiating therapy. If bromocriptine is discontinued, a rebound hyperprolactinemia may occur, along with tumor regrowth.

Approximately 12% of patients cannot tolerate bromocriptine due to the side-effects.[61] The most common side-effects include: nausea, vomiting, postural hypotension, and headache. Administration via the intravaginal route has been shown to improve the nausea and vomiting and maintain clinical effectiveness.[62] Postural hypotension is a common side-effect during the initiation of therapy, and can result in dizziness or even syncope.[61] For this reason, it is recommended that the medication be initiated at bedtime. To further minimize side-effects, it may be helpful to introduce the medication at a low dose and titrate the dosage until it is effective. The medication can be started at 1.25 mg at bedtime, and the dose and frequency can gradually be increased. Fortunately, tolerance to postural hypotension develops after just a few days. Adverse psychiatric effects are rare with the doses used for hyperprolactinemia, but there have been a few cases of mania in the postpartum period.[61]

Cabergoline

Cabergoline has superseded bromocriptine as the agent of choice for the treatment of hyperprolactinemia. It is the most effective compound to treat prolactinomas and has very good patient compliance. Cabergoline is a D_2 selective agonist, with a long

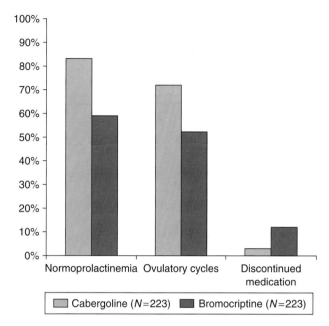

Figure 13.1   Comparison of cabergoline and bromocriptine for hyperprolactinemic amenorrhea. Cabergoline was more successful than bromocriptine in restoring normoprolactinemia (83% vs 59%, $p < 0.001$) and ovulatory cycles (72% vs 52%, $p < 0.001$). Fewer subjects discontinued cabergoline compared to bromocriptine (3% vs 12%, $p < 0.001$)[63]

plasma half-life of 65 hours. This allows for once- or twice-weekly dosing, instead of the twice- or three times-daily dosing for bromocriptine. Therapeutic doses are in the range of 0.25–1.0 mg twice weekly.

In a randomized, multicenter, 24-week, partially double-blind trial comparing cabergoline with bromocriptine in 459 women with hyperprolactinemic amenorrhea, cabergoline induced normoprolactinemia in 83% compared with 59% for bromocriptine (Figure 13.1).[63] Ovulatory cycles occurred in 72% of women treated with cabergoline, and 52% of those treated with bromocriptine. Cabergoline was also better tolerated, with adverse effects recorded in 68% of women taking cabergoline and 78% of those taking bromocriptine. Only 3% discontinued cabergoline, while 12% stopped bromocriptine.

The high efficacy and tolerability of cabergoline for hyperprolactinemia was also confirmed in a retrospective cohort study of 455 patients.[64] Prolactin levels normalized in 86% of all patients. For those with idiopathic hyperprolactinemia or microprolactinoma, prolactin normalized in 92% of patients, and for those with macroadenomas prolactin normalized in 77% of patients. Only 3.9% discontinued cabergoline secondary to side-effects. It is also important to note that 70% of the bromocriptine resistant patients in the study were eventually controlled with cabergoline.

Cabergoline is also very effective in shrinking macroprolactinomas. After 12–24 months of treatment with cabergoline, > 90% of patients had at least a 25% reduction in maximal tumor diameter.[65] Furthermore, 21% of patients had complete resolution of the macroprolactinoma. The ability to shrink tumor volume is even greater when cabergoline is used in naive patients rather than patients previously treated with other dopamine agonists.[66] Patients with macroprolactinomas who were given cabergoline as the first-line treatment achieved a lower prolactin level and a higher percentage tumor volume reduction than patients previously treated with bromocriptine or quinagolide before starting cabergoline treatment. Out of 26 naive patients, 92% achieved tumor shrinkage, compared to 59% of patients previously responsive to bromocriptine or quinagolide. Therefore, cabergoline should be employed as first-line therapy in macroprolactinomas.

Side-effects are similar to those with bromocriptine, but generally less frequent, less severe, and of shorter duration. Like bromocriptine, the most common side-effects are nausea, vomiting, dizziness, and headache.[61] The low incidence of side-effects is likely owed to the long plasma half-life, which results in a flat plasma drug concentration. Discontinuation of cabergoline due to side-effects is reported in fewer than 3% of patients.[61]

Recently, some reports have surfaced that describe the occurrence of fibrotic valvular heart disease in patients treated with high doses of cabergoline and pergolide for Parkinson's disease.[67,68] Causality has not been proven, but there appears to be a strong association for high doses of dopamine agonists used in Parkinson's disease. Doses for Parkinson's disease are at least four times those used for hyperprolactinemia. Caution should be exercised in titrating patients to high doses of dopamine agonists for hyperprolactinemia.

Pergolide

Pergolide is a dopamine agonist with long-acting D_1 and D_2 agonist properties. It is approximately 100 times more potent than bromocriptine, which allows for once-daily dosing. It is approved in the United States only for Parkinson's disease, but investigators using it for prolactinomas demonstrate effectiveness equal to bromocriptine for lowering prolactin levels and inducing tumor shrinkage.[69] The optimal median dose in this study was 0.075–0.1 mg/day. In contrast, doses for Parkinson's disease can reach 1 mg three times daily. Pergolide has some attractive advantages over bromocriptine: the dosing is once daily and its cost is 20% of bromocriptine's.[54]

In general, the nature and incidence of most side-effects are similar to those of bromocriptine, which include nausea, vomiting, dizziness, postural hypotension, and headache.[69] As mentioned above, pergolide-associated valvular heart disease has been reported in Parkinson's patients. The growing number of reported cases of valvular heart disease in Parkinson's patients warrants routine cardiac evaluation for patients using these higher doses.[67,68]

Quinagolide

Quinagolide is a dopamine agonist with specific D_2 receptor activity. It is available in Europe and Canada but not in the United States. Quinagolide has a half-life of 22 hours, which allows for once-daily administration. There are fewer studies in the effectiveness of quinagolide in hyperprolactinemia, but the evidence consistently shows clinical efficacy that is similar to that of cabergoline. Di Sarno et al compared the outcomes of quinagolide and cabergoline in a sequential treatment with a cross-over design.[70] Treatment with quinagolide for 12 months was followed by a 12-month washout period, followed by 12 months of cabergoline and another 12-month washout. Both quinagolide and cabergoline induced the normalization of serum prolactin levels in the great majority of patients with prolactinoma. Both medications also induced tumor shrinkage; however, cabergoline induced further shrinkage in patients who had partial tumor shrinkage after quinagolide. Cabergoline was also better tolerated than quinagolide. The most common side-effects were similar to those with the other dopamine agonists. Nausea and postural hypotension were experienced by approximately 30% of subjects.

Following patients on dopamine agonists

Serum prolactin levels should be repeated at 3, 6, and 12 months after initiating or changing medical therapy, and yearly thereafter, in the absence of an increase in prolactin levels or symptoms. Repeat MRI is not necessary in patients with microadenomas unless there is an increase in prolactin levels or symptoms. On the other hand, annual imaging is appropriate for those with macroadenomas. Imaging can be repeated even earlier if there is an increase in symptoms or prolactin levels.

The dose of dopamine agonist can be decreased once prolactin levels have been normal for at least 2 years and the tumor size has decreased by more than 50%.[59] At this stage prolactin levels and tumor size are usually maintained by low doses of dopamine agonists. Suspension of medical therapy can also be attempted, but this may lead to tumor expansion and recurrence of hyperprolactinemia. Recurrence rates are highest during the first year of withdrawal, so follow-up should be very strict during this time.[54]

The continuing need for dopamine agonist therapy should be evaluated when a patient experiences either pregnancy or menopause. Both of these events are associated with remission of hyperprolactinemia.[71–73]

Dopamine agonist resistance

For any of the dopamine agonists there are a percentage of patients who show resistance, which is defined as the failure to achieve normal prolactin levels or at least a 50% reduction in tumor size.[74] The inability to achieve normoprolactinemia occurs in about 25% of patients using bromocriptine, 13% of patients using pergolide, and 11% using cabergoline.[74] The failure to achieve at least a 50% reduction in tumor size occurs in about 36% of patients using bromocriptine, 15% of patients using pergolide, and 5–10% of those using cabergoline.[74] A more clinically relevant endpoint to express dopamine agonist resistance might be the percentage of patients who do not experience restoration of the hypothalamic–pituitary–gonadal axis, as evidenced by anovulation. In the study by the Cabergoline Comparative Study Group, 28% of patients on cabergoline failed to ovulate compared to 48% taking bromocriptine.[63]

Resistance to dopamine agonists involves a decrease in D_2 receptors on the membranes of tumor cells, yet the binding affinity is unchanged.[75] It was also discovered that dopamine agonist resistant adenomas had a fourfold decreased expression of D_2 mRNA when compared to bromocriptine sensitive adenomas.[76] In addition, there is a decrease in G-proteins that are coupled to the D_2 receptor, reducing the ability of the receptor to inhibit adenyl cyclase activity.[77]

There are several ways to approach the treatment of a dopamine agonist-resistant patient. If a patient does not demonstrate any response to a dopamine agonist, the patient should be switched to another agonist. Because bromocriptine was the first dopamine agonist used for prolactinomas, most of the data regarding treatment of dopamine agonist resistance involve this medication. There are many studies that examined whether another dopamine agonist might be effective in patients resistant to bromocriptine. The greatest efficacy in bromocriptine resistant patients has been shown with cabergoline. Approximately 70–80% achieve normal prolactin levels.[64,78] Cabergoline may be highly effective in resistant patients due to the higher affinity for D_2 binding sites, a longer time occupying the receptor, and a slower elimination from the pituitary.[78]

If a patient experiences a weak response to a dopamine agonist, one treatment approach would be to increase the dose of the agonist beyond the conventional dose. The vast majority of patients who respond to dopamine agonists will respond rapidly with low doses. However, about 5% of patients will respond in a stepwise fashion with increasing doses of agonist.[74] It is appropriate to increase the dose as long as there is no adverse effect and the patient continues to respond. Doses of cabergoline up to 3 mg/day have been reported in the treatment of a giant prolactinoma.[79]

Trans-sphenoidal surgery and radiotherapy are also options for the dopamine agonist-resistant patient. These options are considered for those who do not respond to having their medication changed or having their dose increased.

Surgical management

Trans-sphenoidal surgery was the preferred therapy for prolactinomas before dopamine agonists became available in the 1970s. Surgery is now reserved for a select population, which includes those who fail to restore gonadal function with medical therapy, those who have unstable pituitary apoplexy, those who experience cerebrospinal fluid rhinorrhea, or those who desire tumor debulking prior to pregnancy (Table 13.3). Surgery could also be considered in the psychotic patient with a macroadenoma who cannot take a dopamine agonist as it may precipitate a psychotic episode.

Pituitary apoplexy is a rare, potentially life-threatening neuroendocrine emergency. This occurs when there is infarction or hemorrhage into a pituitary tumor, but can also occur as a complication of pituitary surgery.[80–82] These patients may develop visual disturbance, severe headache, altered consciousness, and vascular collapse. Surgical intervention should be performed expeditiously for those with progressive neurologic deficits, while those with stable symptoms may be managed medically under careful monitoring.[83]

Cerebrospinal fluid (CSF) rhinorrhea is a complication of dopamine agonist treatment in patients with invasive macroprolactinomas. This is an uncommon complication that is the result of rapid tumor shrinkage that causes a tear in the dura mater. This should be

Table 13.3 Indications for surgery. Adapted from reference[54]

- Failure of medical therapy:
  - Inadequate reduction of prolactin to restore gonadal function
  - Tumor enlargement
- Unstable pituitary apoplexy
- Cerebrospinal fluid rhinorrhea
- Desire for pregnancy:
  - Prior pregnancy complicated by symptomatic tumor enlargement
  - Patient opts for surgery instead of dopamine agonist therapy during pregnancy
- Symptomatic tumor enlargement (e.g. bitemporal hemianopsia) during pregnancy that does not respond to reinstitution of dopamine agonist treatment

surgically repaired as soon as possible to stop the leakage of CSF and prevent complications, such as meningitis.[84]

It is difficult to quantify surgical success rates because outcomes are highly dependent upon the experience of the neurosurgeon and the size of the tumor. A recent review pointed out that surgical success rates are highly variable between studies.[54] Surgical remission rates varied from 38 to 100% for microadenomas and from 6.7 to 80% for macroadenomas. Remission was defined as having normal prolactin levels by 12 weeks after surgery. It is also difficult to assess recurrence rates after surgery. Like success rates, recurrence rates are dependent on the skill of the surgeon, and different definitions of recurrence are used throughout the literature. The reported rates are highly variable, ranging from 0 to 50%.[54]

Complications from trans-sphenoidal surgery are greater for larger tumors. For macroadenomas, the mortality rate is approximately 0.9%, and the major morbidity rate is about 6.5%, which includes vision loss, stroke, meningitis, and oculomotor palsy.[85,86] For microadenomas, the mortality rate is about 0.6%, with a major morbidity rate at 3.4%.[85,86] One of the most common complications of trans-sphenoidal surgery is hypopituitarism.[87]

Radiotherapy

In most cases, radiotherapy is used after medical therapy and trans-sphenoidal surgery has failed. Conventional radiotherapy involves multiple external X-ray beams concentrated on the pituitary fossa while the patient is immobilized. This radiotherapy is delivered daily over

6 weeks. More recently, gamma knife radiotherapy has been developed. This uses a single dose of radiation focused at the treatment field, with reduced radiation exposure to the surrounding normal tissue.

The efficacy of conventional radiotherapy is rather modest. Overall prolactin normalization is approximately 34%, but it is much lower for patients who have failed surgery (approximately 11%).[54] Gamma knife radiotherapy appears to have a slightly better outcome. In a recent series of 23 patients who failed medical or surgical therapy, 26% experienced normalization of prolactin levels with gamma knife radiotherapy.[88] The variables that were associated with remission by gamma knife radiotherapy were: (1) pre-procedure volume of $<3\,cm^3$; and (2) not taking a dopamine agonist at the time of the procedure.

The most frequent long-term morbidity of conventional radiotherapy is radiation induced hypopituitarism, which occurs in approximately 50% of patients by 20 years.[89] Hypopituitarism also appears to be a common complication for gamma knife radiotherapy. In a series of 28 patients treated by gamma knife, eight (29%) developed at least one new pituitary hormone deficiency.[88] The deficiencies included thyroid stimulating hormone, growth hormone, and adrenocorticotropic hormone. The average time to onset of a deficiency was 44 months. Cranial neuropathies can also develop. Extraocular movement difficulties developed in two out of 28 patients treated with gamma knife radiotherapy.[88] One patient had a cranial nerve (CN) III palsy and another had a CN VI palsy.

Conventional radiotherapy is also associated with an increased risk of secondary radiation-induced intracranial malignancies, with a cumulative risk of 2.4% at 20 years.[54] Given the relatively recent development of gamma knife technology, there is limited follow-up to determine the risk of secondary intracranial malignancies. It is also worth mentioning that irradiation of the hypothalamus can damage dopaminergic neurons, creating a secondary cause for hyperprolactinemia.

Radiotherapy has a very limited yet well-defined role in the management of prolactinomas. The few patients who require radiotherapy are those who do not respond to dopamine agonists and cannot be cured by surgery.

Prolactinoma in pregnancy

MRI studies show that the size of the normal pituitary more than doubles in pregnancy.[90] The pituitary is largest during the 3 days immediately postpartum, and the gland returns to normal size within 6 months. This normal pituitary gland enlargement is predominantly the effect of estrogen on the lactotrophs causing hypertrophy and hyperplasia.[91] When a prolactinoma is present, it is possible that the estrogenic stimulation during pregnancy will cause tumor enlargement.

A review by Molitch combined data from several studies to determine the rate of tumor progression during pregnancy.[92] There were 363 women with microadenomas who were followed during pregnancy. Only five (1.4%) had symptoms of tumor enlargement, such as headaches or visual disturbances. Surgical intervention was not necessary for any of the cases. There were 84 patients with macroadenomas who did not have prior surgery or irradiation. Symptomatic tumor enlargement was experienced by 22 (26.2%). Four patients required surgery and 15 required treatment with bromocriptine. There were 67 women with macroadenomas who had been treated with irradiation or surgery before pregnancy. Only two of the 67 (3%) had symptomatic tumor enlargement[92] (Table 13.4).

Management of the patient desiring pregnancy

Despite the favorable efficacy and side-effect profile of cabergoline, bromocriptine is the preferred dopamine agonist when the patient desires fertility. Although both bromocriptine and cabergoline appear safe when taken during the first few weeks of pregnancy, the data supporting the safety for bromocriptine are more robust. Outcome data from over 6000 pregnancies where bromocriptine was taken for the first few weeks of gestation have not shown any increase in spontaneous abortions, ectopic pregnancies, trophoblastic disease, multiple pregnancies, or congenital malformations.[93] The effects of cabergoline on pregnancy outcome have only been reported in several hundred pregnancies.[64,94,95] Based on the relatively limited information reported, cabergoline does not appear to increase the likelihood of fetal malformations, miscarriage, preterm birth, or low birth weight.

Although there is no strong evidence that dopamine agonists may be harmful during pregnancy, there is little information on their effect when they are used throughout the gestation. Except for rare situations, dopamine agonists should be discontinued when a patient becomes pregnant.

Management of the pregnant patient

With a low incidence of tumor enlargement in microprolactinomas, these patients can be followed at each trimester for the development of symptoms, such as

Table 13.4   Effect of pregnancy on prolactinomas. From reference[92]

Tumor type	Prior therapy	Number of patients	Symptomatic tumor enlargement[a]
Microadenoma	None	363	5 (1.4%)
Macroadenoma	None	84	22 (26.2%)
Macroadenoma	Yes	67	2 (3%)

[a]Defined as headaches or visual disturbances or both

headache or visual symptoms.[92] Any symptoms should be evaluated with MRI and visual field testing. On the other hand, patients with macroadenomas should have visual fields tested at each trimester, with MRI whenever there are symptoms of tumor enlargement or visual field defect.[92] Whenever the MRI confirms tumor enlargement, bromocriptine therapy should be reinstituted immediately. When bromocriptine does not work, more drastic measures should be taken, such as transsphenoidal surgery or labor induction, if possible.

There is little value in following prolactin levels in the hyperprolactinemic patient who becomes pregnant. Prolactin levels normally increase during pregnancy, but they do not always increase in the hyperprolactinemic patient or in those who experience pregnancy-induced tumor enlargement.[96,97]

If a large macroadenoma is present prior to conception, one should consider trans-sphenoidal surgery prior to pregnancy to debulk the tumor. If surgery is not performed, one should be cognizant that the risk of tumor enlargement is greater than 25%.[92] Reinstitution of bromocriptine in patients with tumor enlargement during pregnancy is effective in most cases, and one can consider bromocriptine maintenance throughout pregnancy to prevent tumor enlargement. Otherwise, surgery should be strongly considered.

Suckling during breastfeeding can stimulate prolactin secretion. However, breastfeeding does not appear to stimulate tumor growth in patients with a prolactinoma.[97] It may, however, be prudent to discourage breastfeeding in the patient who develops signs of tumor growth.

Interestingly, pregnancy appears to have a beneficial effect on the prolactinoma. In one series, 60% and 72% of patients with micro- and macroprolactinomas, respectively, showed a decrease in prolactin levels after delivery when compared to pre-gestational levels.[72] Another series showed a normalization of prolactin levels in 29% of patients after pregnancy.[71] The explanation for the paradoxical effect of pregnancy on prolactinomas is not clear. One possibility is that there is necrosis or microinfarction of the tumor resulting from the estrogen stimulus of the lactotrophs. Another possibility is remodeling of the sinusoids within the microvascular network of the anterior pituitary that supplies dopamine to the lactotrophs.

CONCLUSION

There are a myriad of causes of hyperprolactinemia. The evaluation should begin with a detailed history and physical examination to begin ruling out physiological and pharmacological causes of hyperprolactinemia. MRI of the brain should follow, even if prolactin levels are modestly elevated, as a tumor may still be present. Most prolactinomas are successfully treated using medical therapy with minimal morbidity. Cabergoline is the first-line agent, except in the patient desiring conception, where bromocriptine should be used. A small proportion of patients do not respond to dopamine agonists, and these may need surgery or radiotherapy. Unfortunately these treatment approaches are associated with a suboptimal response and higher morbidity. Dopamine agonists should be discontinued upon conception, but they may be reinstituted if symptoms of tumor growth recur during pregnancy. Fortunately, close to a third of patients will have normal prolactin levels after pregnancy.

REFERENCES

1. Mindermann T, Wilson C. Age-related and gender-related occurrence of pituitary adenomas. Clin Endocrinol 1994; 41: 359–64.
2. Turner H, Nagy Z, Gatter K et al. Angiogenesis in pituitary adenomas and the normal pituitary gland. J Clin Endocrinol Metab 2000; 85: 1159–62.
3. Davis J, Farrell W, Clayton R. Pituitary tumours. Reproduction 2001; 121: 363–71.
4. Niall H, Hogan M, Sauer R, Rosenblum I, Greenwood F. Sequences of pituitary and placental lactogenic and growth hormones: evolution from a primordial peptide by gene reduplication. Proc Natl Acad Sci USA 1971; 68: 866–9.
5. Veldhuis J, Johnson L. Operating characteristics of the hypothalamo-pituitary-gonadal axis in men: circadian, ultradian, and pulsatile release of prolactin and its temporal coupling with luteinizing hormone. J Clin Endocrinol Metab 1988; 67: 116–23.

6. Melis G, Fruzetti F, Paoletti A et al. Pharmacological activation of γ-aminobutyric acid-system blunts prolactin response to mechanical breast stimulation in puerperal women. J Clin Endocrinol Metab 1984; 58: 201–5.

7. Noel G, Dimond R, Wartofsky L, Earll J, Frantz A. Studies of prolactin and TSH secretion by continuous infusion of small amounts of thyrotropin-releasing hormone (TRH). J Clin Endocrinol Metab 1974; 39: 6–17.

8. Kato Y, Shimatusu A, Matsushita N, Ohta H, Imura H. Role of vasoactive intestinal polypeptide (VIP) in regulating the pituitary function in man. Peptides 1984; 5: 389–94.

9. Fazekas I, Bacsy E, Varga I et al. Effect of vasoactive intestinal polypeptide (VIP) on growth hormone (GH) and prolactin (PRL) release and cell morphology in human pituitary adenoma cell cultures. Folia Histochem Cytobiol 2000; 38: 119–27.

10. Lieberman M, Maurer R, Claude P et al. Regulation of pituitary growth and prolactin gene expression by estrogen. Adv Exp Med Biol 1981; 138: 151–63.

11. Spady T, McComb R, Shull J. Estrogen action in the regulation of cell proliferation, cell survivial, and tumorigenesis in the rat anterior pituitary gland. Endocrine 1999; 11: 217–33.

12. Kato Y, Nakai Y, Imura H, Chihara K, Ogo S. Effect of 5-hydroxytryptophan (5-HTP) on plasma prolactin levels in man. J Clin Endocrinol Metab 1974; 38: 695–7.

13. Urban R, Veldhuis J. A selective serotonin reuptake inhibitor, fluoxetine hydrochloride, modulates the pulsatile release of prolactin in postmenopausal women. Am J Obstet Gynecol 1991; 164: 147–52.

14. Gudelsky G, Porter J. Morphine- and opioid peptide-induced inhibition of the release of dopamine from tuberoinfundibular neurons. Life Sci 1979; 25: 1697–702.

15. Goldman J, Molitch M, Thorner M et al. Growth hormone and prolactin responses to bolus and sustained infusions of GRH-1-40-OH in man. J Endocrinol Invest 1987; 10: 397–406.

16. Aguilera G, Hyde C, Catt K. Angiotensin II receptors and prolactin release in pituitary lactotrophs. Endocrinology 1982; 111: 1045–50.

17. Schlechte J, Walkner L, Kathol M. A longitudinal analysis of premenopausal bone loss in healthy women and women with hyperprolactinemia. J Clin Endocrinol Metab 1992; 75: 698–703.

18. Biller B, Baum H, Rosenthal D et al. Progressive trabecular osteopenia in women with hyperprolactinemic amenorrhea. J Clin Endocrinol Metab 1992; 75: 692–7.

19. Vekemans M, Delvoye P, L'Hermite M, Robyn C. Serum prolactin levels during the menstrual cycle. J Clin Endocrinol Metab 1977; 44: 989–93.

20. Hammond K, Steinkampf M, Boots L, Blackwell R. The effect of routine breast examination on serum prolactin levels. Fertil Steril 1996; 65: 869–70.

21. St-Jean E, Blain F, Comtois R. High prolactin levels may be missed by immunoradiometric assay in patients with macroprolactinomas. Clin Endocrinol 1996; 44: 305–9.

22. Unnikrishnan A, Rajaratnam S, Seshadri M, Kanagasapabathy A, Stephen D. The 'hook effect' on serum prolactin estimation in a patient wth macroprolactinoma. Neurol India 2001; 49: 78–80.

23. Guitelman M, Colombani-Vidal M, Zylbersztein C et al. Hyperprolactinemia in asymptomatic patients is related to high molecular weight posttranslational variants or glycosylated forms. Pituitary 2002; 5: 255–60.

24. Brue T, Caruso E, Morange I et al. Immunoradiometric analysis of circulating human glycosylated and nonglycosylated prolactin forms: spontaneous and stimulated secretions. J Clin Endocrinol Metab 1992; 75: 1338–44.

25. Gambino G, Beck-Peccoz P, Borgato S et al. Bioactivity and glycosylation of circulating prolactin in various physiological and pathological conditions. Pituitary 1999; 2: 225–31.

26. Markoff E, Sigel M, Lacour N et al. Glycosylation selectively alters the biological activity of prolactin. Endocrinology 1988; 123: 1303–6.

27. Kline J, Clevenger C. Identification and characterization of the prolactin-binding protein in human serum and milk. J Biol Chem 2001; 276: 24760–6.

28. Hattori N, Ikekubo K, Ishihara T et al. Correlation of the antibody titers with serum prolactin levels and their clinical course in patients with anti-prolactin autoantibody. Eur J Endocrinol 1994; 130: 438–45.

29. Vallette-Kasic S, Morange-Ramos I, Selim A et al. Macroprolactinemia revisited: a study on 106 patients. J Clin Endocrinol Metab 2002; 87: 581–8.

30. Leslie H, Courtney C, Bell P et al. Laboratory and clinical experience in 55 patients with macroprolactinemia identified by a simple polyethylene glycol precipitation method. J Clin Endocrinol Metab 2001; 86: 2743–6.

31. Alfonso A, Rieniets K, Vigersky R. Incidence and clinical significance of elevated macroprolactin levels in patients with hyperprolactinemia. Endocr Pract 2006; 12: 275–80.

32. Hattori N. Macroprolactinemia: a new cause of hyperprolactinemia. J Pharmacol Sci 2003; 92: 171–7.

33. Escobar-Morreale H. Macroprolactinemia in women presenting with hyperandrogenic symptoms: implications for the management of polycystic ovary syndrome. Fertil Steril 2004; 82: 1697–9.

34. Fahie-Wilson M. In hyperprolactinemia, testing for macroprolactin is essential. Clin Chem 2003; 49: 1434–6.

35. Schlechte J. The macroprolactin problem [Editorial]. J Clin Endocrinol Metab 2002; 87: 5408–9.

36. Gibney J, Smith P, McKenna T. The impact on clinical practice of routine screening for macroprolactin. J Clin Endocrinol Metab 2005; 90: 3927–32.

37. Kavanagh L, McKenna T, Fahie-Wilson M, Gibney J, Smith T. Specificity and clinical utility of methods for the detection of macroprolactin. Clin Chem 2006; 52: 1366–72.

38. Suliman A, Smith T, Gibney J, McKenna T. Frequent misdiagnosis and mismanagement of hyperprolactinemic patients before the introduction of macroprolactin screening: application of a new strict laboratory definition of macroprolactinemia. Clin Chem 2003; 49: 1504–9.

39. Kleinberg D, Noel G, Frantz A. Galactorrhea: a study of 235 cases, including 48 with pituitary tumors. N Engl J Med 1977; 296: 589–600.

40. Bayrak A, Saadat P, Mor E et al. Pituitary imaging is indicated for the evaluation of hyperprolactinemia. Fertil Steril 2005; 84: 181–5.

41. Stern J, Konner M, Herman T, Reichlin S. Nursing behaviour, prolactin and postpartum amenorrhoea during prolonged lactation in American and Kung mothers. Clin Endocrinol 1986; 25: 247–58.

42. Meltzer H, Fang V. Serum prolactin levels in schizophrenia – effect of antipsychotic drugs: a preliminary report. In: Sachar E, ed. Hormones, Behavior, and Psychopathology. New York: Raven Press, 1976: 177–90.

43. Kinon B, Gilmore J, Liu H, Halbreich U. Prevalence of hyperprolactinemia in schizophrenic patients treated with conventional antipsychotic medications or risperidone. Psychoneuroendocrinology 2003; 28 (Suppl 2): 55–68.

44. Jones R, Luscombe D, Groom G. Plasma prolactin concentrations in normal subjects and depressive patients following oral clomipramine. Postgrad Med J 1977; 53 (Suppl 4): 166–71.

45. Papakostas G, Miller K, Petersen T et al. Serum prolactin levels among outpatients with major depressive disorder during the acute phase of treatment with fluoxetine. J Clin Psychol 2006; 67: 952–7.

46. Kelley S, Kamal T, Molitch M. Mechanism of verapamil calcium channel blockade-induced hyperprolactinemia. Am J Physiol 1996; 270: E96–100.

47. Steiner J, Cassar J, Mashiter K et al. Effect of methyldopa on prolactin and growth hormone. BMJ 1976; 1: 1186–8.

48. Tamagna E, Lane W, Hershman J et al. Effect of chronic metoclopramide therapy on serum pituitary hormone concentrations. Horm Res 1979; 11: 161–9.

49. Zis A, Haskett R, Albala A, Carroll B. Morphine inhibits cortisol and stimulates prolactin secretion in man. Psychoneuroendocrinology 1984; 9: 423–7.

50. Chan V, Wang C, Yeung R. Effects of heroin addiction on thyrotrophin, thyroid hormones and prolactin secretion in men. Clin Endocrinol 1979; 10: 557–65.

51. Mendelson J, Mello N, Teoh S, Ellingoe J, Cochin J. Cocaine effects on pulsatile secretion of anterior pituitary, gonadal, and adrenal hormones. J Clin Endocrinol Metab 1989; 69: 1256–60.

52. Mah P, Webster J. Hyperprolactinemia: etiology, diagnosis, and management. Semin Reprod Med 2002; 20: 365–74.

53. Asa S, Ezzat S. The pathogenesis of pituitary tumours. Nat Rev Cancer 2002; 2: 836–49.

54. Gillam M, Molitch M, Lombardi G, Colao A. Advances in the treatment of prolactinomas. Endocr Rev 2006; 27: 485–534.

55. Martin T, Kim M, Malarkey W. The natural history of idiopathic hyperprolactinemia. J Clin Endocrinol Metab 1985; 60: 855–8.

56. Corenblum B, Donovan L. The safety of physiological estrogen plus progestin replacement therapy and with oral contraceptive therapy in women with pathological hyperprolactinemia. Fertil Steril 1993; 59: 671–3.

57. Fahy U, Foster P, Torode H, Hartog M, Hull M. The effect of combined estrogen/progestogen treatment in women with hyperprolactinemic amenorrhea. Gynecol Endocrinol 1992; 6: 183–8.

58. Garcia M, Kapcala L. Growth of a microprolactinoma to a macroprolactinoma during estrogen therapy. J Endocrinol Invest 1995; 18: 450–5.

59. Casanueva F, Molitch M, Schlechte J et al. Guidelines of the Pituitary Society for the diagnosis and management of prolactinomas. Clin Endocrinol 2006; 65: 265–73.

60. Colao A, Di Sarno A, Pivonello R, di Somma C, Lombardi G. Dopamine receptor agonists for treating prolactinomas. Expert Opin Investig Drugs 2002; 11: 787–800.

61. Webster J. A comparative review of the tolerability profiles of dopamine agonists in the treatment of hyperprolactinaemia and inhibition of lactation. Drug Saf 1996; 14: 228–38.

62. Kletzky O, Vermesh M. Effectiveness of vaginal bromocriptine in treating women with hyperprolactinemia. Fertil Steril 1989; 51: 269–72.

63. Webster J, Piscitelli G, Polli A et al. A comparison of cabergoline and bromocriptine in the treatment of hyperprolactinemic amenorrhea. Cabergoline Comparative Study Group. N Engl J Med 1994; 331: 904–9.

64. Verhelst J, Abs R, Maiter D et al. Cabergoline in the treatment of hyperprolactinemia: a study in 455 patients. J Clin Endocrinol Metab 1999; 84: 2518–22.

65. Colao A, Di Sarno A, Landi M et al. Long-term and low-dose treatment with cabergoline induces macroprolactinoma shrinkage. J Clin Endocrinol Metab 1997; 82: 3574–9.

66. Colao A, Di Sarno A, Landi M et al. Macroprolactinoma shrinkage during cabergoline treatment is greater in naive patients than in patients pretreated with other dopamine agonists: a prospective study in 100 patients. J Clin Endocrinol Metab 2000; 85: 2247–52.

67. Junghanns S, Fuhrmann J, Simonis G et al. Valvular heart disease in Parkinson's disease patients treated with dopamine agonists: a reader-blinded monocenter echocardiography study. Mov Disord 2007; 22: 234–7.

68. Zanettini R, Antonini A, Gatto G et al. Valvular heart disease and the use of dopamine agonists for Parkinson's disease. N Engl J Med 2007; 356: 39–46.

69. Lamberts S, Quik R. A comparison of the efficacy and safety of pergolide and bromocriptine in the treatment of hyperprolactinemia. J Clin Endocrinol Metab 1991; 72: 635–41.

70. Di Sarno A, Landi M, Marzullo P et al. The effect of quinagolide and cabergoline, two selective dopamine receptor type 2 agonists, in the treatment of prolactinomas. Clin Endocrinol 2000; 53: 53–60.

71. Crosignani P, Mattei A, Severini V et al. Long-term effects of time, medical treatment and pregnancy in 176 hyperprolactinemic women. Eur J Obstet Gynecol Reprod Biol 1992; 44: 175–80.

72. Musolino N, Bronstein M. Prolactinomas and pregnancy. In: Bronstein M, ed. Pituitary Tumors in Pregnancy. Boston: Kluwer Academic Publishers, 2001: 91–108.

73. Karunakaran S, Page R, Wass J. The effect of the menopause on prolactin levels in patients with hyperprolactinemia. Clin Endocrinol 2001; 54: 295–300.

74. Molitch M. Pharmacologic resistance in prolactinoma patients. Pituitary 2005; 8: 43–52.

75. Pellegrini I, Rasolonjanahary R, Gunz G et al. Resistance to bromocriptine in prolactinomas. J Clin Endocrinol Metab 1989; 69: 500–9.

76. Caccavelli L, Feron F, Morange I et al. Decreased expression of the two D2 dopamine receptor isoforms in bromocriptine-resistant prolactinomas. Neuroendocrinol 1994; 60: 314–22.

77. Caccavelli L, Morange-Ramos I, Kordon C, Jaquet P, Enjalbert A. Alteration of Gα subunits mRNA levels in bromocriptine resistant adenomas. J Neuroendocrinol 1996; 8: 737–46.

78. Colao A, Di Sarno A, Sarnacchiaro F et al. Prolactinomas resistant to standard dopamine agonists respond to chronic cabergoline treatment. J Clin Endocrinol Metab 1997; 82: 876–83.

79. Gillam M, Middler S, Freed D, Molitch M. The novel use of very high doses of cabergoline and a combination of testosterone and an aromatase inhibitor in the treatment of a giant prolactinoma. J Clin Endocrinol Metab 2002; 87: 4447–51.

80. Rovit R, Fien J. Pituitary apoplexy: a review and reappraisal. J Neurosurg 1972; 37: 280–8.

81. Goel A, Doegaonkar M, Desai K. Fatal postoperative pituitary apoplexy: its cause and management. Br J Neurosurg 1995; 9: 37–40.

82. Ahmad F, Pandey P, Mahapatra A. Post operative pituitary apoplexy in giant pituitary adenomas: a series of cases. Neurol India 2005; 53: 326–8.

83. Maccagnan P, Macedo C, Kayath M, Nogueira R, Abucham J. Conservative management of pituitary apoplexy: a prospective study. J Clin Endocrinol Metab 1995; 80: 2190–7.

84. Leong K, Foy P, Swift A et al. CSF rhinorrhoea following treatment with dopamine agonists for massive invasive prolactinomas. Clin Endocrinol 2000; 52: 43–9.

85. Barker F, Klibanski A, Swearingen B. Transsphenoidal surgery for pituitary tumors in the United States, 1996–2000: mortality, morbidity, and the effects of hospital and surgeon volume. J Clin Endocrinol Metab 2003; 88: 4709–19.

86. Sudhakar N, Ray A, Vafidis J. Complications after transsphenoidal surgery: our experience and a review of the literature. Br J Neurosurg 2004; 18: 507–12.

87. Nelson A, Tucker H, Becker D. Residual anterior pituitary function following transsphenoidal resection of pituitary macroadenomas. J Neurosurg 1984; 61: 577–80.

88. Pouratian N, Sheehan J, Jagannathan J et al. Gamma knife radiosurgery for medically and surgically refractory prolactinomas. Neurosurgery 2006; 59: 255–66.

89. Snyder P, Fowble B, Schatz N, Savino P, Gennarelli T. Hypopituitarism following radiation therapy of pituitary adenomas. Am J Med 1986; 81: 457–62.

90. Dinc H, Esen F, Demirci A, Sari A, Resit Gumele H. Pituitary dimensions and volume measurements in pregnancy and post partum. Acta Radiol 1998; 39: 64–9.

91. Scheithauer B, Sano T, Kovacs K et al. The pituitary gland in pregnancy. A clinicopathologic and immunohistochemical study of 69 cases. Mayo Clin Proc 1990; 65: 461–74.
92. Molitch M. Pituitary tumors and pregnancy. Growth Horm IGF Res 2003; 13 (Suppl A): S38–44.
93. Krupp P, Monka C, Richter K. The safety aspects of infertility treatments. In: Program of the Second World Congress of Gynecology and Obstetrics, 1988, Rio de Janeiro, Brazil, 9.
94. Robert E, Musatti L, Piscitelli G, Ferrari C. Pregnancy outcome after treatment with the ergot derivative, cabergoline. Reprod Toxicol 1996; 10: 333–7.
95. Ricci E, Parazzini F, Motta T et al. Pregnancy outcome after cabergoline treatment in early weeks of gestation. Reprod Toxicol 2002; 16: 791–3.
96. Divers W Jr, Yen S. Prolactin-producing microadenomas in pregnancy. Obstet Gynecol 1983; 62: 425–9.
97. Holmgren U, Bergstrand G, Hagenfeldt K, Werner S. Women with prolactinoma – effect of pregnancy and lactation on serum prolactin and on tumour growth. Acta Endocrinol (Copenh) 1986; 111: 452–9.

14 Non-surgical management of Mullerian anomalies

Bala Bhagavath and Karen D Bradshaw

Non-surgical management of vaginal agenesis was first advocated by Amussat in 1835, and it has taken more than 150 years for the technique to be accepted as the most effective. The aim of this chapter is to review the evidence for non-surgical management of Mullerian anomalies. In some instances the evidence is strong for non-surgical management and in others the evidence is very much against such an approach.

EMBRYOLOGY

The genital organs and the urinary organs develop from the intermediate mesoderm.[1] The genital organs consist of the gonads, the ductal system, and the external genitalia. The urinary organs consist of the kidney, the ureters, the bladder, and the urethra. A longitudinal ridge of the intermediate mesoderm, called the urogenital ridge, develops on either side of the primitive aorta. The urogenital ridge further differentiates into the nephrogenic and genital ridges.

The nephrogenic ridges develop into mesonephric ducts (Wolffian ducts) which connect the mesonephric kidneys to the cloaca. The cloaca is the common opening into which the embryonic urinary, genital, and alimentary tracts join. The ureteric bud (fifth week) then arises from the mesonephric duct, lengthens, and induces formation of the metanephros (final functional kidney). The mesonephric kidneys degenerate at 10 weeks.

Invagination of the coelomic epithelium (sixth week) on either side of the developing gonad and mesonephric duct gives rise to the paramesonephric (Mullerian) ducts. The caudal parts of these ducts meet in the midline behind the cloaca. By the seventh week, the urorectal septum has divided the cloaca into the rectum and the urogenital sinus. The cephalad part of the urogenital sinus gives rise to the urinary bladder. The middle part of the urogenital sinus develops into the female urethra whereas the distal part of the sinus develops into the distal vagina, Bartholin glands, urethra, and Skene glands.

The undifferentiated genital ridge consists of the coelomic epithelium with the underlying mesenchyme.

Large polyhedral cells in the yolk sac give rise to germ cells and are called primordial germ cells. They migrate into the undifferentiated genital ridge by passing through the dorsal mesentery. Though gonadal sex correlates to a large extent with sex chromosomal complement, the presence or absence of certain transcription factors (e.g. SRY for males and RSPO1 for females) is more critical for gonadal differentiation. Gonadal differentiation is one of the crucial factors that determine phenotypic sex. The presence of functional SRY and SOX9 allows differentiation of the gonads to testes.[2] Sertoli cells in the testes secrete anti-Mullerian hormone (AMH) by around 7–8 weeks. AMH causes regression of ipsilateral Mullerian duct by 9–10 weeks.[3] Leydig cell differentiation in the testes occurs about a week after Sertoli cell development. Testosterone acts on the ipsilateral mesonephric duct resulting in the formation of the epididymis, vas deferens, and seminal vesicle. Testosterone and its metabolite dihydrotestosterone induce formation of the male external genitalia.

On the other hand, in the presence of RSPO1 and the absence of SRY, the undifferentiated gonad develops into the ovary.[4] Differentiation into the ovary occurs 2 weeks later than that of the testis. In the absence of AMH, the Mullerian ducts persist, fuse, and then resorb in the midline to form the uterus and the upper part of the vagina. In the absence of testosterone, the mesonephric ducts degenerate and the external genitalia differentiate into the female phenotype.

CLASSIFICATION

The American Society for Reproductive Medicine (ASRM) classification of Mullerian anomalies is the most commonly used classification system (Table 14.1).[5] The disadvantage in using this classification is that most vaginal anomalies and other rare uterine anomalies are not included in the classification. Attempts have been made by many clinicians to introduce classifications to address this deficiency.[6-8] These classifications serve to compare patients from different studies. However, in

Table 14.1 ASRM classification of Mullerian anomalies

Class		Anomaly
Class	I	Hypoplasia/agenesis
	a	Vaginal
	b	Cervical
	c	Fundal
	d	Tubal
	e	Combined
Class	II	Unicornuate
	a	Communicating
	b	Non-communicating
	c	No cavity
	d	No horn
Class	III	Didelphus
Class	IV	Bicornuate
	a	Complete
	b	Partial
Class	V	Septate
	a	Complete
	b	Partial
Class	VI	Arcuate
Class	VII	DES related

DES, diethylstilbestrol

our opinion, the classification used has little bearing on the principles behind the diagnosis and management of the conditions. Clear understanding of the embryology combined with thorough investigation using appropriate diagnostic modalities before formulating a treatment plan is of paramount importance. Unfortunately, many of the anomalies are so uncommon or rare that one has to formulate a management plan based on case series, case reports, and personal experience.

ANOMALIES OF EXTERNAL GENITALIA

Anomalies of the external genitalia are relatively rare in the general population. The most common cause of ambiguous genitalia is congenital adrenal hyperplasia (CAH) which accounts for about 80% of cases. Gonadal dysgenesis and partial androgen insensitivity syndrome (PAIS) are the next most common causes of ambiguous genitalia at birth. In complete androgen insensitivity syndrome (CAIS), patients have a normal external female phenotype with a blind-ending vagina and intra-abdominal testes. The management of gonads in intersex is discussed under 'Gonads in disorders of sex development' later in this chapter.

Ambiguous genitalia, diagnosed at birth, should be approached as a medical emergency. Detailed family and

prenatal history must be taken. Palpation of the groin and the labioscrotal folds is crucial, as the presence of a gonad, even on one side, makes it highly likely to be a testis. The length of the phallus, if any, is noted. In addition to detailed history taking and physical examination, the following laboratory tests should be ordered: serum electrolytes (to rule out salt-wasting CAH), testosterone (to rule out androgen insensitivity syndrome), dihydrotestosterone (to rule out 5α-reductase deficiency), 17-OH progesterone (to rule out CAH), and karyotype analysis (to rule out gonadal dysgenesis). Pelvic and abdominal ultrasound scans will help to determine the presence of the uterus and both kidneys.

In addition to diagnosing potential life-threatening disorders, determining the sex of rearing expeditiously is of paramount importance to parents. Almost all cultures in the world do not recognize a place for sex-indeterminate or gender-neutral children.

A major pitfall in the management of these patients has been the way in which the conditions have been classified in the literature: male pseudohermaphrodite, female pseudohermaphrodite, and true hermaphrodite. The thinking was that if the underlying chromosomal make-up is 46,XY then the person is male and is classified as a male pseudohermaphrodite, and if the underlying chromosomal make-up is 46,XX then the person is female and is classified as a female pseudohermaphrodite. However, the above classification not withstanding, there was consensus that the appearance of external genitalia and the sex of rearing determine the gender role or gender identity that the person assumes later in childhood/adolescent/adult life. The problem was perhaps compounded by our inability to reconstruct male genitalia from female-appearing genitals. We now believe that exposure to androgens, chromosomal make-up, and brain structure all play a part in determining gender identity and role.[9]

Some progress has been made in the management of ambiguous genitalia in recent years. It has been recognized that male chromosomal make-up does not necessarily mean male identity (e.g. CAIS). We understand now that the appearance of the external genitalia and the sex of rearing have minimal bearing on the gender identity assumed by the child, adolescent, or adult. Simultaneously, improvements in surgical technique have allowed reconstruction of certain ambiguous genitalia to the male phenotype which, in the past, would have been converted to female. Recently, consensus was arrived at regarding the classification of ambiguous genitalia. It has been proposed that 'pseudohermaphroditism' be replaced by the term 'disorder of sex development' (Table 14.2).[9]

Table 14.2 Proposed revised classification of intersex. Modified from reference 9

Previous	Proposed
Intersex	DSD
Male pseudohermaphrodite	46,XY DSD
Female pseudohermaphrodite	46,XX DSD
True hermaphrodite	Ovotesticular DSD
XX sex reversal	46,XX testicular DSD
XY sex reversal	46,XY complete gonadal dysgenesis

DSD, disorder of sex development

The consensus statement on intersex disorders and their management advocates gender assignment to all babies at birth based on certain outcome data.[10] All patients with CAIS identify with the female gender and more than 90% of 46,XX CAH patients identify as females in adult life. In contrast, about 60% of 5α-reductase deficient patients assigned as female in infancy virilize during puberty and live as males. Dissatisfaction with sex of assignment is about 25% in partial androgen insensitivity and incomplete gonadal dysgenesis patients.

There is a great deal of controversy regarding the timing of feminizing and masculinizing genital surgery in children with ambiguous genitalia. In 46,XX children with ambiguous genitalia, feminizing genitoplasty (except in the extreme cases) is not recommended in infancy.[11] Clitoral reduction surgery carries has a high risk of dissatisfaction in adult life due to lack of clitoral sensation with inability to achieve orgasm. The focus should be on function rather than cosmetic appearance.[9] The American Academy of Pediatrics policy statement on elective surgery in male infants recommends masculinizing genitoplasty to be carried out between 6 weeks and 15 months of age.[12] The ideal scenario would be to rear the child in a gender-neutral fashion until the child is capable of deciding on a gender for itself. However, as mentioned earlier, there are very few cultures in the world today that would accept a gender-neutral child. Consequently, many physicians argue that most parents cannot cope with bringing up their children in a gender-neutral fashion and advocate gender assignment and surgery in infancy. However, there is no evidence for the belief that cosmetic surgery in infancy relieves parental distress and improves the attachment between child and parents.[9]

In conclusion, female genitoplasty is better deferred until later ages, whereas male genitoplasty is currently recommended to be performed in infancy. The management of these conditions is constantly evolving, and our ability to assign gender with accuracy will hold the key to satisfactory outcomes for affected children in the future.

VAGINAL AGENESIS

It is estimated that one in 5000 females has vaginal agenesis. Patients with vaginal agenesis are phenotypically normal and go through normal pubertal development except for the delay in attaining menarche. When an apparent absence of the vagina is noted, four possible diagnoses must be entertained: imperforate hymen, low transverse vaginal septum, androgen insensitivity syndrome, and Mullerian agenesis.

Differential diagnosis

Imperforate hymen can usually be differentiated from low transverse vaginal septum by the absence of hymenal fronds and by the bulging of the membrane due to hematocolpos. Complete androgen insensitivity syndrome is suspected when there is no axillary or pubic hair. Unfortunately, partial androgen insensitivity syndrome (PAIS) presents with a wide phenotypic spectrum, and it may be difficult to distinguish PAIS from Mullerian agenesis. In any case, karyotype analysis should be performed to establish the diagnosis. Patients with androgen insensitivity syndrome will have a 46,XY karyotype and those with Mullerian agenesis will have a 46,XX karyotype. Mullerian agenesis may be associated with renal and/or skeletal abnormalities and cardiac abnormalities. Determination of the extent of Mullerian agenesis can be accomplished using ultrasound examination of the pelvis or magnetic resonance imaging (MRI). A rectal probe may have to be used to perform the pelvic sonogram. Occasionally, laparoscopy is needed to diagnose pelvic pain and to biopsy gonadal tissue for confirmation of the diagnosis.

Timing of therapy

In patients with vaginal agenesis, attempts at creating a vagina should be made only when the child reaches emotional maturity, usually around the age of 16 years.[12,13] Attempts at an earlier age will invariably fail, as the patient rarely has the motivation to regularly dilate the vagina. On the other hand, dilatation is better attempted when she is still at home, to avoid embarrassment when she starts living with other girls upon joining college.

Vaginal dilatation method

Amussat is credited with proposing strong digital pressure on the vaginal dimple to create a neovagina.[14] Today, vaginal agenesis is the only Mullerian defect for which the management of choice is non-surgical intervention. In all other cases, the decision hinges on whether or not and when to perform surgery. The American College of Obstetricians and Gynecologists' Committee Opinion Number 355 strongly recommends non-surgical management in all vaginal agenesis patients before attempting a surgical correction.[13]

Ingram's modification of Frank's method is better, as it avoids fatigue to the hands, allows the patient to perform other activities while she is using the dilator, allows the patient to be fully clothed at the time, and allows the patient's body weight to exert force, which is far better than force exerted by the hand.[15]

Williams and colleagues published their original series on the use of Ingram's method in 1985.[16] They achieved successful vaginal dilatation in 37 of 45 (82.2%) patients. Ingram advocated extensive nursing participation and the use of a former patient as motivator. However, the need for a patient motivator is not universal.[17]

Roberts and colleagues published the results of a retrospective analysis of vaginal dilatation to create a neovagina.[17] Of 47 patients analyzed retrospectively, 10 had refused vaginal dilatation. Some 91.9% of the 37 patients who underwent vaginal dilatation succeeded in creating a neovagina. The time taken to succeed varied from 3 to 33 months with a mean of 11.8 ± 1.6 months. Patients who failed dilatation subsequently underwent McIndoe vaginoplasty successfully. Previous attempts at surgery and vaginal length less than 1 cm were potential risk factors for failure. However, success was demonstrated even in patients with only a vaginal dimple, and also in patients with prior attempts at hymenotomy (six of seven patients).

The observation that coitus alone can result in neovagina is not new, and D'Alberton and Santi proposed coitus as a technique for creating a neovagina in 1972.[18] Lappohn slightly modified this advice, and advocated the use of interfemoral coitus for the creation of a neovagina.[19] Patients were instructed to have coitus between lubricated thighs aiming to exert pressure on the vaginal dimple by the tip of the penis. In his series, nine of 11 women who used interfemoral coitus alone achieved satisfactory vaginal lengths of greater than 8 cm between 4 and 6 months from beginning therapy. In the same series, all nine women who used a combination of intercourse and vaginal mold achieved a vaginal length of greater than 8 cm between 2 and 4 months from beginning therapy. The complication that can ensue with interfemoral coitus is urethral dilatation due to inadvertent urethral coitus. All patients with this complication managed to create a neovagina after correction of their technique. However, no mention is made of the long-term consequence of urethral dilatation. Of the nine patients who chose mold therapy alone (due to lack of a sexual partner), only three achieved a vaginal length of greater than 8 cm. However, two of the six failures had Klippel–Feil syndrome, and there is no mention of other associated anomalies that could have resulted in failure of therapy. One patient had a rigid perineum. These three patients achieved a vaginal depth of 5–6 cm. One other patient had severe amelia, with no legs and only one arm, for whom an appropriate mold could not be manufactured. If these patients were excluded, Lappohn achieved successful dilatation with mold alone in three of five patients.

Ingram's method

The patient should be advised to carefully choose two 20-minute slots in the day when she will be free to apply the vaginal dilators. She will be able to read a book or work on the computer or any other task that can be accomplished while she is seated. The importance of discipline in achieving success should be stressed to her.

As mentioned earlier, Ingram's method has advantages over Frank's method of vaginal dilatation. Traditionally, Lucite dilators have been advocated. However, a large selection of vaginal dilators are available on the market today. The choice of dilator is entirely up to the patient and the physician. One should start with the narrowest and shortest dilator. The aim is to achieve comfortable insertion with one size within 2 weeks, and then to move on to the next size. Naturally, the time taken to achieve adequate vaginal dilatation that allows comfortable coitus is very variable, and is dependent upon the individual patient.

A lubricant must be applied to the perineum or vagina and on the dilators at the start of each session. The choice of lubricant is not important as any vaginal cream can be used. A water based lubricant is probably the best as it will not stain clothing. The dilator is placed in the vagina while the patient is in a supine position with knees bent and thighs abducted. Initially the patient is advised to direct the pressure towards her coccyx in order to avoid urethral dilatation. Once a vaginal length of a few centimeters is formed, the direction is determined by posture on a saddle seat. She should then wear tight fitting underwear to hold the dilator in place while she is sitting down for the next 20 minutes. If the patient has only a perineal dimple, she may have to start dilating with pressure exerted by hand (Frank's method) before progressing to sit on the stool. If a patient feels that sitting on a saddle seat is too uncomfortable, she should be encouraged to use Frank's method.

The key principles are to let gravity assist by sitting on the perineum and to exert maximum pressure on the perineum in the right direction by leaning forward. While Ingram advocated the bicycle seat stool, the intended effect of gravity assisting in applying the pressure can be achieved even by sitting on a chair. However, the bicycle seat stool (or saddle seat stool) achieves the stated principles better by facilitating a forward leaning posture. The amount of pressure exerted should be enough to cause discomfort but not pain.

The frequency of clinic appointments to assess progress is dictated by individual patients. Initially, patients can be seen every month. In addition to providing objective feedback to the patient, this serves to reinforce correct use of the dilators. Patient access to counselors is most critical, as lack of encouragement and perceived lack of progress by patients is most likely to lead to frustration and failure of therapy.

Length of the neovagina

The minimum vaginal length needed to achieve satisfactory coitus was studied in one postoperative study and was found to be at least 6 cm.[20] It is generally accepted that 6–8 cm vaginal length is necessary for satisfactory coitus.

Histology of neovagina

The histological features of the neovagina have been studied by many investigators. No study has been conducted to compare the vagina created by dilatation with that created by surgical means. However, the study by Fedele and colleagues showed that the histological and ultrastructural features were not different between women who had undergone Vecchietti's procedure and those who had a undergone normal vagina.[21] Vecchietti's procedure can be considered a surgically assisted, accelerated creation of a neovagina.

This group of patients, therefore, bears the closest resemblance to dilating the vagina with Lucite dilators. It is encouraging to note how closely this resembles a normal vagina as opposed to a vagina from a sigmoid colon or from skin of the buttock.

Sexual function

Sexual function in patients who underwent vaginal dilatation between 1984 and 2001 was evaluated by questionnaire.[22] A control group of 131 women from the general population with normal sexual function were administered the questionnaire as well. In the treatment group, 79 of 145 patients responded to the invitation, and eventually only 60 patients took part in the study. The mean age at which these patients underwent therapy was 20.5 years, with a range of 16–44 years. The mean age at the time of filling out the questionnaire was 26.5 years, with a range of 17–46 years. The study patients reported similar sexual desire, arousal, and sexual satisfaction as compared with the control population. However, they reported significantly decreased vaginal lubrication during coitus, decreased orgasmic frequency, and increased dyspareunia as compared with the control population.

In comparison, 83 patients who had surgical creation of a vagina between 1971 and 1991 were identified to be evaluated by questionnaire.[20] Only 44 patients eventually took part in the study. The mean age at which these patients underwent therapy was 19.5 years with a range of 15–51 years. Only 36 women had sexual partners at the time of study, and 30 of them claimed to have satisfactory to optimal sexual intercourse. Thirty-six women reported orgasm during coitus and 24 claimed to have an orgasm every time. Fifty per cent of the women complained of pain and extreme discomfort in the first 3–6 months after surgery. It is not clear how many patients were totally pain free at the time of the questionnaire.

Counseling

Adequate counseling is important before attempting vaginal dilatation. If necessary, a psychiatric consultation should be requested. Counseling should include use of visual material including a set of dilators. A mirror should be used to demonstrate the perineal anatomy and the dimple between the urethra and anus where she should start the dilatation.

Summary

Attempts at creation of a neovagina should not be made until emotional maturity is attained which is usually around 16 years of age. Dilatation methods should be the method of choice (success rate 82–92%), and Ingram's method is to be favored. Adequate teaching, written instructions, and support from physicians, nurses, and patient motivators (if necessary) are critical in achieving success. Histologically, the vagina created by the dilatation method most closely resembles the normal vagina. Sexual function is similar in patients who have non-surgical management compared with surgical management. It is therefore important to adequately counsel the patient when she is initially considering the mode of therapy to choose.

LONGITUDINAL VAGINAL SEPTUM

The longitudinal vaginal septum accounts for 12% of all vaginal anomalies.[23] The largest case series published to date is of 202 patients with longitudinal vaginal septum.[23] In 56.4% of the patients, the diagnosis was made incidentally. The rest of the patients presented with dyspareunia (29.7%), apareunia or bleeding with intercourse (8.9%), and difficulty using a tampon (9.4%). In 45.6% of cases, the septum was complete and in the rest it was incomplete, being present mainly in the upper part of the vagina. The vast majority (87.8%) of these patients had associated uterine anomalies. Almost all (99.4%) complete or partial high longitudinal vaginal septa were associated with a uterine malformation, whereas only 30.3% of partial medium or low vaginal septa had associated uterine anomalies. Approximately three of four (73.2%) patients with complete or high partial vaginal septum had septate uterus and the rest had uterus didelphys. Only two patients in this group had bicornuate uterus and one had a normal uterus. In contrast, 69.7% of patients with medium or low vaginal septum had a normal uterus. The rest of the patients had septate uterus. Only one patient in this group had a bicornuate uterus. Although rare, normal uterus associated with cervical and vaginal septa has also been reported by others.[24–26] Dystocia or tear of the longitudinal vaginal septum associated with labor and delivery is reportedly rare.

In another series, only 53.7% of 67 patients with complete uterine, cervical, and vaginal septum had the vaginal septum divided. Dyspareunia was the most common indication for division of the vaginal septum.[27]

Unless the patient is symptomatic, it is not necessary to surgically correct the longitudinal vaginal septum. The possibility of encountering a uterine anomaly is small in the case of a low/medium longitudinal vaginal septum. The possibility of coexistent uterine malformation is high with high vaginal septum. If an associated uterine septum has to be resected, it is safe to divide the vaginal septum. Dividing the vaginal septum makes it technically easier and safer to perform resection of the cervical and uterine septum.

CERVICAL SEPTUM

Isolated cervical septum has not been described in the literature. Cervical septum is always found in association with vaginal septum, uterine septum, or bicornuate uterus. It is generally believed that duplication of the uterine cervix has occurred in such cases and there is functional cervical tissue in the cervical septum. It is therefore frequently described as duplication of the uterine cervix. The classical teaching, thus, has been to preserve the cervical septum when dividing the uterine septum.[28] However, multiple reports have confirmed the advantage and safety of resecting the cervical septum.[29–32] In addition to decreasing the operating time, division of the cervical septum reduces the associated complications of fluid overload, pulmonary edema, and intraoperative bleeding. Moreover, retaining the cervical septum results in increased cesarean delivery rates.[32] The need for cervical cerclage is similar in patients with retained cervical septum and in those who have had it resected. If resection of the uterine septum is considered necessary (see section below on 'Uterine septum'), any existing cervical septum should be resected as well.

UTERINE SEPTUM

The incidence of uterine anomalies in the asymptomatic general population is unknown. Uterine septum is the most common uterine anomaly seen in practice. Of 404 women with uterine anomalies seen in a Finnish hospital, 48% were septate, 17% bicornuate, 10% unicornuate, and 10% didelphys.[33] Recurrent miscarriages and dysmenorrhea are the possible presenting complaints. The management of these patients has been very controversial, as some argue for resection of the septum in all patients and others maintain that only a select few should undergo metroplasty.

Miscarriage, fetal loss, and operative delivery

A high-risk obstetric team followed 101 pregnancies in 42 women with previously diagnosed but uncorrected uterine malformations.[34] Twenty-five of these pregnancies occurred in women with uterine septum. The term pregnancy rate was 48% and the fetal survival rate was 65% with high-risk obstetric care (fetal survival rate was 53% prior to inclusion in the study). Tocolysis for preterm labor was required in 15% of pregnancies. The investigators concluded that high-risk obstetric care did not statistically improve the outcome in these patients.

In another retrospective analysis of 62 women with uterine malformations, 127 pregnancies were noted with a 36% miscarriage rate, 26% preterm delivery rate, and 42% term delivery rate.[35] Complete septate uterus was associated with a higher miscarriage rate. Cervical cerclage had to be performed in 23 cases and breech presentation occurred in 46%. The cesarean delivery rate was 63%.

The reproductive performance in women with septate or bicornuate uteri was retrospectively analyzed in a Finnish hospital population.[36] Fifty-two patients had metroplasty (32 hysteroscopic and 20 abdominal) and 140 did not have surgery. One hundred and sixteen of the 140 women achieved a total of 264 pregnancies and the fetal survival rate was 67%. The women who had metroplasty were chosen to undergo the procedure because of a history of recurrent miscarriage, and they had a combined fetal survival rate of 9% prior to surgery. After surgery, the fetal survival rate improved to 84%. Nineteen patients from the surgery group were matched for age, gravidity, and type of uterine anomaly with patients from the non-surgical group. The fetal survival was 86% in the surgery group compared with 68% in the non-surgical group. This investigator arrived at the same conclusion as Michalas[35] that resection of the uterine septum decreases breech presentation and cesarean delivery rates while improving fetal survival rates.

The same Finnish investigator has recently published results of pregnancies in 53 women with complete uterine, cervical, and vaginal septum.[27] Forty-nine women did not have metroplasty and suffered a 27% miscarriage rate in a total of 115 pregnancies. Twelve per cent of deliveries were preterm and 61% were born at term, with a total survival rate of 82%. The cesarean delivery rate was 72% and the breech presentation rate was 40%. In contrast, the four patients who underwent metroplasty had an 87% miscarriage rate and 13% live birth rate prior to surgery, which improved to 25% miscarriage rate and 75% live birth rate after surgery. No preterm births were noted in this group.

One hundred and two women with a history of recurrent pregnancy loss and uterine septum had hysteroscopic resection of the septum.[37] Of these, 23 women had complete uterine septa and 79 had incomplete septa. They were followed for 36 months after surgery. The cumulative pregnancy and birth rates were 89% and 75% in the complete septum group and 80% and 67% in the incomplete septum group.

Venturoli et al reported that 52.7% of 72 patients with recurrent miscarriage and uterine septum became pregnant after resection of the uterine septum. The outcome was 25% miscarriage, 15.4% preterm delivery, 46.2% term delivery, and 11.5% ongoing pregnancies.[38]

Fairly similar outcomes were reported by Colacurci and colleagues in their series of 69 patients with septate uteri. Forty-eight of these patients had a history of recurrent abortion.[39] Forty of the 48 patients became pregnant after metroplasty. The miscarriage rate was 12.5%, preterm delivery rate was 8.3%, and 58.3% were carried to term, while 5% were ongoing at the time of report.

Zabak and colleagues reported a miscarriage rate of 79% in 1601 pregnancies in women with uterine septum (the paper is in French and this report is based on the abstract only). This decreased to 15% after resection of the uterine septum.[40] Yet another retrospective analysis of 78 patients with septate uterus studied the effect of metroplasty on fetal survival rate which improved from 4.4% preoperatively to 87.5% postoperatively.[41] Patton and colleagues reported nine patients with 75% miscarriage and 25% preterm delivery rates prior to metroplasty whose outcome improved postoperatively to 25% miscarriage and 75% term delivery rates.[42] Grimbizis et al noted an 88.9% term delivery rate with 11.1% abortion rate in patients with a history of recurrent pregnancy loss.[43]

Dysmenorrhea and endometriosis

Patients with dysmenorrhea, uterine septum, and no other associated anomaly respond well to resection of the uterine septum. The incidence of dysmenorrhea dropped from 54.8 to 17.7% after hysteroscopic metroplasty.[44]

A recent report of increased incidence (25.8%) of endometriosis in 120 patients with septate uterus contradicts previous reports.[45,46]

Infertility

It is generally agreed that the incidence of infertility is not correlated with the presence of a uterine anomaly.[27,35,40] In a small series of 21 patients who had undergone metroplasty and had a diagnosis of infertility, only six pregnancies resulted. There were three term deliveries, one preterm delivery, and two ongoing pregnancies.[39]

In contrast, Venturoli et al reported that 52.1% of 69 patients with infertility became pregnant after resection of the uterine septum, while 15% ended in miscarriage, 10% preterm delivery, and 52.5% term deliveries, and 20% were ongoing.[38] Compiling a series of such case reports, Pabuccu and Gomel estimated that the crude pregnancy rate after metroplasty in patients with primary infertility is 48%.[47]

Summary

Non-surgical management of uterine septum is associated with a 42–61% term delivery rate and a fetal survival rate of only 65–82% with high-risk obstetric care. Malpresentation rates are high (40–46%), and the risk of cesarean delivery is 63–72%.

Resection of uterine septum decreases the miscarriage rate to 25% in patients with a history of recurrent miscarriage. The fetal survival rate improves to 75–88.9%. The malpresentation and cesarean delivery rates decrease.

The association of uterine septum in causing primary infertility is unclear, though there is some evidence that the length of time taken for these patients to become pregnant may be prolonged. It is clear, however, that the pregnancy outcome in these patients is poorer without surgical correction of the septum. Hysteroscopic metroplasty is relatively safe and easy to perform in experienced hands. It can therefore be argued that patients with a history of infertility or miscarriage should be offered hysteroscopic metroplasty.

BICORNUATE UTERUS

Sixty-one of 101 pregnancies reported by Ludmir and colleagues occurred in women with a bicornuate uterus.[34] The term pregnancy rate was 39% and the fetal survival rate was 58% with high-risk obstetric care (52% prior to inclusion in the study). Tocolysis for preterm labor was required in 21% of patients and 5% needed cervical cerclage. The investigators concluded that high-risk obstetric care did not statistically improve the outcome in these patients.

Bicornuate uterus was reported in six of 36 patients of a series from an Italian university hospital.[48] Data were available in five patients regarding pregnancy. Two were infertile and one had an abortion. Two patients delivered after 34 weeks.

The pregnancy outcome is rather poor with bicornuate uterus. However, the surgical correction of this anomaly has to be either by laparotomy or by laparoscopy. This increases the morbidity associated with the condition. In view of this, surgical correction is generally advocated only if there is recurrent pregnancy loss or preterm delivery.

UTERUS DIDELPHYS

Uterus didelphys may be associated with longitudinal vaginal septum and patent hemivagina on both sides or with obstructed hemivagina. Patients with obstructed hemivagina invariably present after puberty with abdominal pain and vaginal/pelvic mass, and require removal of the vaginal septum. However, the role of surgery (if any) in the former group with bilateral patent hemivaginas will be debated in this section.

Ten of 101 pregnancies occurred in women with uterus didelphys in the series reported by Ludmir and colleagues.[34] The term pregnancy rate was 60%.

Thirty women with uterus didelphys were managed at an Italian university hospital over a period of 30 years.[48] Three of these cases were categorized on the basis of hysterosalpingography alone, whereas the remaining 27 were confirmed didelphys by laparoscopy or laparotomy. Apparently, only 15 women were interested in becoming pregnant. Two patients had a hysterectomy and the pregnancy status of one was unknown. Two were infertile, two had first trimester abortions, four preterm deliveries (all >34 weeks), and four term deliveries, making the term pregnancy rate 40%. Seven were cesarean deliveries and one was a vaginal delivery. Endometriosis was noted in 26.7% of the patients.

As is the case with bicornuate uterus, surgical correction of uterus didelphys is more complex than correction of a uterine septum. In addition, the pregnancy outcome is reasonable, with 80% of deliveries occurring after 34 weeks. It is therefore prudent to perform any surgery only when there are symptoms such as dysmenorrhea, pelvic pain, or coital difficulty. No data are available, except as rare case reports, regarding uterine unification surgery in these patients.

Table 14.3   Risk of germ cell malignancy according to diagnosis. Modified from reference 9

Risk Group	Disorder	Malignancy risk (%)	Recommended action
High	Gonadal dysgenesis (+Y), intra-abdominal	15–35	Gonadectomy upon diagnosis
	PAIS, non-scrotal	50	Gonadectomy upon diagnosis
	Frasier	60	Gonadectomy upon diagnosis
	Denys–Drash (+Y)	40	Gonadectomy upon diagnosis
Intermediate	17β–hydroxysteroid	28	Watchful waiting
	Turner syndrome (+Y)	12	Gonadectomy upon diagnosis
	Gonadal dysgenesis (+Y), scrotal	Unknown	Biopsy and irradiation?
	PAIS, scrotal	Unknown	Biopsy and irradiation?
Low	CAIS	2	Biopsy and ???
	Ovotesticular DSD	3	Testicular tissue removal
	Turner syndrome (–Y)	1	None
No	5α-reductase, type 2 deficiency	0	Unresolved
	Leydig cell hypoplasia	0	Unresolved

PAIS, partial androgen insensitivity syndrome; CAIS, complete androgen insensitivity syndrome

GONADS IN DISORDERS OF SEX DEVELOPMENT

The gonads in many disorders of sex development carry a risk of malignancy. The risk of malignancy varies with the disorder, and removal of the gonads was advocated as a blanket policy in the past. There are advantages to retaining the gonads in cases with a low risk of malignancy, as natural pubertal development can be maintained (e.g. CAIS). A summary of the risk of gonadal malignancy and the recommended management is given in Table 14.3.[9]

CONCLUSIONS

The management of ambiguous genitalia remains controversial. Gender assignment remains difficult in many cases. When possible, feminizing genitoplasty should be deferred to adult life. Vaginal agenesis is best managed by vaginal dilatation. Low or intermediate longitudinal vaginal septum that is not associated with a uterine anomaly need not be corrected in the asymptomatic patient. The high longitudinal vaginal septum has a high incidence of coexistent uterine septum or bicornuate uterus. It is recommended that uterine septum is divided in patients with a history of infertility or miscarriage, and division of the cervical and vaginal septum (if present) makes the operation safer and shorter in duration. Bicornuate uterus is associated with an increased risk of poor obstetric outcome, but surgery has to be abdominal metroplasty. It is therefore recommended that surgery should be undertaken only in those patients with a history of poor obstetric outcome. Uterus didelphys has a good obstetric outcome, and surgery to unify the uterus is not recommended. Disorders of sex development that are associated with a low risk of gonadal malignancy should have the gonads conserved.

REFERENCES

1. Moore K. The urogenital system. In: MacNamara-Barnett J, ed. The Developing Human 1998: 246.
2. Viger RS, Silversides DW, Tremblay JJ. New insights into the regulation of mammalian sex determination and male sex differentiation. Vitam Horm 2005; 70: 387–413.
3. Marshall FF. Vaginal abnormalities. Urol Clin North Am 1978; 5: 155–9.
4. Parma P, Radi O, Vidal V et al. R-spondin1 is essential in sex determination, skin differentiation and malignancy. Nat Genet 2006; 38: 1304–9.
5. Classification of Mullerian anomalies. Fertil Steril 1989; 51: 199–201.
6. Acien P. Embryological observations on the female genital tract. Hum Reprod 1992; 7: 437–45.
7. Acien P, Acien M, Sanchez-Ferrer M. Complex malformations of the female genital tract. New types and revision of classification. Hum Reprod 2004; 19: 2377–84.
8. Oppelt P, Renner SP, Brucker S et al. The VCUAM (Vagina Cervix Uterus Adnex-associated Malformation) classification: a new classification for genital malformations. Fertil Steril 2005; 84: 1493–7.
9. Lee PA, Houk CP, Ahmed SF, Hughes IA. Consensus statement on management of intersex disorders. International Consensus Conference on Intersex. Pediatrics 2006; 118: e488–500.
10. Houk CP, Hughes IA, Ahmed SF, Lee PA. Summary of consensus statement on intersex disorders and their management. International Intersex Consensus Conference. Pediatrics. 2006; 118: 753–7.
11. Migeon CJ, Wisniewski AB. Human sex differentiation and its abnormalities. Best Pract Res Clin Obstet Gynaecol 2003; 17: 1–18.
12. Timing of elective surgery on the genitalia of male children with particular reference to the risks, benefits, and psychological effects of surgery and anesthesia. American Academy of Pediatrics. Pediatrics 1996; 97: 590–4.

13. ACOG Committee on Adolescent Health Care. ACOG Committee Opinion No. 355: Vaginal agenesis: diagnosis, management and routine care. Obstet Gynecol 2006; 108: 1605–9.

14. Edmonds DK. Congenital malformations of the genital tract and their management. Best Pract Res Clin Obstet Gynaecol 2003; 17: 19–40.

15. Ingram JM. The bicycle seat stool in the treatment of vaginal agenesis and stenosis: a preliminary report. Am J Obstet Gynecol 1981; 140: 867–73.

16. Williams JK, Lake M, Ingram JM. The bicycle seat stool in the treatment of vaginal agenesis and stenosis. J Obstet Gynecol Neonatal Nurs 1985; 14: 147–50.

17. Roberts CP, Haber MJ, Rock JA. Vaginal creation for mullerian agenesis. Am J Obstet Gynecol. 2001; 185: 1349–52; discussion 1352–43.

18. D'Alberton A, Santi F. Formation of a neovagina by coitus. Obstet Gynecol 1972; 40: 763–4.

19. Lappohn RE. Congenital absence of the vagina – results of conservative treatment. Eur J Obstet Gynecol Reprod Biol 1995; 59: 183–6.

20. Mobus VJ, Kortenhorn K, Kreienberg R, Friedberg V. Long-term results after operative correction of vaginal aplasia. Am J Obstet Gynecol 1996; 175: 617–24.

21. Fedele L, Bianchi S, Berlanda N et al. Neovaginal mucosa after Vecchietti's laparoscopic operation for Rokitansky syndrome: structural and ultrastructural study. Am J Obstet Gynecol 2006; 195: 56–61.

22. Nadarajah S, Quek J, Rose GL, Edmonds DK. Sexual function in women treated with dilators for vaginal agenesis. J Pediatr Adolesc Gynecol 2005; 18: 39–42.

23. Haddad B, Louis-Sylvestre C, Poitout P, Paniel BJ. Longitudinal vaginal septum: a retrospective study of 202 cases. Eur J Obstet Gynecol Reprod Biol 1997; 74: 197–9.

24. Goldberg JM, Falcone T. Double cervix and vagina with a normal uterus: an unusual Mullerian anomaly. Hum Reprod 1996; 11: 1350–1.

25. Dunn R, Hantes J. Double cervix and vagina with a normal uterus and blind cervical pouch: a rare mullerian anomaly. Fertil Steril 2004; 82: 458–9.

26. Candiani M, Busacca M, Natale A, Sambruni I. Bicervical uterus and septate vagina: report of a previously undescribed Mullerian anomaly. Hum Reprod 1996; 11: 218–19.

27. Heinonen PK. Complete septate uterus with longitudinal vaginal septum. Fertil Steril 2006; 85: 700–5.

28. Rock JA, Roberts CP, Hesla JS. Hysteroscopic metroplasty of the Class Va uterus with preservation of the cervical septum. Fertil Steril 1999; 72: 942–5.

29. Sirbu P, Niculescu M, Marinescu B, Titiriga L. The improvement of fertility at women with bicervical bicornuate uterus and double vagina. Acta Eur Fertil 1981; 12: 199–212.

30. Valle RF. Hysteroscopic treatment of partial and complete uterine septum. Int J Fertil Menopausal Stud 1996; 41: 310–15.

31. Parsanezhad ME, Alborzi S. Hysteroscopic metroplasty: section of the cervical septum does not impair reproductive outcome. Int J Gynaecol Obstet 2000; 69: 165–6.

32. Parsanezhad ME, Alborzi S, Zarei A et al. Hysteroscopic metroplasty of the complete uterine septum, duplicate cervix, and vaginal septum. Fertil Steril 2006; 85: 1473–7.

33. Heinonen PK. Reproductive performance of women with uterine anomalies after abdominal or hysteroscopic metroplasty or no surgical treatment. J Am Assoc Gynecol Laparosc 1996; 3 (Suppl): S17.

34. Ludmir J, Samuels P, Brooks S, Mennuti MT. Pregnancy outcome of patients with uncorrected uterine anomalies managed in a high-risk obstetric setting. Obstet Gynecol 1990; 75: 906–10.

35. Michalas SP. Outcome of pregnancy in women with uterine malformation: evaluation of 62 cases. Int J Gynaecol Obstet 1991; 35: 215–19.

36. Heinonen PK. Reproductive performance of women with uterine anomalies after abdominal or hysteroscopic metroplasty or no surgical treatment. J Am Assoc Gynecol Laparosc 1997; 4: 311–17.

37. Fedele L, Arcaini L, Parazzini F, Vercellini P, Di Nola G. Reproductive prognosis after hysteroscopic metroplasty in 102 women: life-table analysis. Fertil Steril 1993; 59: 768–72.

38. Venturoli S, Colombo FM, Vianello F et al. A study of hysteroscopic metroplasty in 141 women with a septate uterus. Arch Gynecol Obstet 2002; 266: 157–9.

39. Colacurci N, De Placido G, Mollo A, Carravetta C, De Franciscis P. Reproductive outcome after hysteroscopic metroplasty. Eur J Obstet Gynecol Reprod Biol 1996; 66: 147–50.

40. Zabak K, Benifla JL, Uzan S. [Septate uterus and reproduction disorders: current results of hysteroscopic septoplasty]. Gynecol Obstet Fertil 2001; 29: 829–40. [in French]

41. Gaucherand P, Awada A, Rudigoz RC, Dargent D. Obstetrical prognosis of the septate uterus: a plea for treatment of the septum. Eur J Obstet Gynecol Reprod Biol 1994; 54: 109–12.

42. Patton PE, Novy MJ, Lee DM, Hickok LR. The diagnosis and reproductive outcome after surgical treatment of the complete septate uterus, duplicated cervix and vaginal septum. Am J Obstet Gynecol 2004; 190: 1669–75; discussion 1675–68.

43. Grimbizis G, Camus M, Clasen K et al. Hysteroscopic septum resection in patients with recurrent abortions or infertility. Hum Reprod 1998; 13: 1188–93.

44. Fedele L, Bianchi S, Bocciolone L et al. Relief of dysmenorrhea associated with septate uteri after abdominal or hysteroscopic metroplasty. Acta Obstet Gynecol Scand 1994; 73: 56–8.

45. Fedele L, Bianchi S, Di Nola G, Franchi D, Candiani GB. Endometriosis and nonobstructive Mullerian anomalies. Obstet Gynecol 1992; 79: 515–17.

46. Ugur M, Turan C, Mungan T et al. Endometriosis in association with mullerian anomalies. Gynecol Obstet Invest 1995; 40: 261–4.

47. Pabuccu R, Gomel V. Reproductive outcome after hysteroscopic metroplasty in women with septate uterus and otherwise unexplained infertility. Fertil Steril 2004; 81: 1675–8.

48. Candiani GB, Fedele L, Candiani M. Double uterus, blind hemivagina, and ipsilateral renal agenesis: 36 cases and long-term follow-up. Obstet Gynecol 1997; 90: 26–32.

15 Non-invasive management of urinary incontinence

Jerry L Lowder and Anne M Weber

INTRODUCTION

Urinary incontinence is a deceptively simple term as it is generally understood: the inappropriate passage of urine from the bladder through the urethra. 'Inappropriate' is the key word; of course, urine must be passed from the bladder through the urethra at regular intervals, which constitutes normal voiding. Incontinence, then, is defined by urine passage (often called leakage) apart from normal voiding. It is simple, yes?

Unfortunately, it is not. There are a number of issues that arise between this seemingly simple definition and what becomes a clinical entity in women who we strive to treat, such as duration of symptoms; frequency and severity; and life impact of urinary incontinence. Urinary incontinence is a chronic condition. If it occurs acutely, an acute explanation can usually be found; for example, urine loss sometimes accompanies the painful urgency of acute cystitis. Acute conditions will not be covered here.

The amount of incontinence must be considered, commonly captured as frequency (how often leakage occurs) and severity (how much, or volume, with each episode). Although perfect continence may be the ideal, the reality is that incontinence occurs in women where it might be least expected: for example, in young, otherwise healthy, nulliparous women, including athletes and soldiers (especially related to high-impact activities such as in gymnasts and paratroopers). Do these women have incontinence? By the definition above, yes they do. This is one reason why the reported prevalence of urinary incontinence varies so widely. The question of incontinence 'ever' casts a very broad net that will mark a high proportion of any group of women as incontinent. Frequency of incontinence narrows the field, as does the related characteristic of severity. However, what level of frequency and severity constitutes a standard definition of incontinence has been notoriously elusive. When women present for clinical care, it is because something about their symptoms has crossed their own personal threshold between what is acceptable and what is unacceptable. Attempts have been made to quantify this threshold in

terms of life impact using condition-specific health-related quality of life measures; yet even that varies from woman to woman, by age, by culture, and by factors unmeasured.

Clinicians are accustomed to seeing women who present for care with different levels of incontinence, although usually at the more severe end of the spectrum. Clearly, many more women experience incontinence but do not seek care. In addition to the threshold issue, unfortunately, there remain powerful issues of stigma, fear, and lack of knowledge. Stigma is perhaps weaker now than in the past although it is still potent, particularly in older women. Women are afraid, sometimes because they think surgery is the only treatment. Unfortunately, some women and even some clinicians are unaware that incontinence can always be treated, almost always with non-surgical means first, and improvement can be achieved in virtually all women. While incontinence is common, it is never 'normal.' Across the lifespan, at every age, more women are continent than are incontinent. However, it is impractical to think of 'cure' for incontinence, as impractical as it is for essential hypertension or adult-onset diabetes. As with these other chronic conditions, incontinence can be successfully managed, to reduce its life impact and improve quality of life. In many (if not most) cases, successful management can be achieved with non-invasive (non-surgical) treatments.

Much attention has been directed at the different 'types' of urinary incontinence symptoms, commonly categorized into urge, stress, and mixed (urge and stress) incontinence. (Other, less common types of incontinence will not be considered here.) Urge incontinence, along with urgency and frequency, is characterized by the now infamous 'gotta go, gotta go' of television commercials, direct-to-consumer advertising promoting various pharmaceutical products. Stress incontinence is perhaps less famous, but its symptoms of urine loss with coughing, sneezing, and other physical types of stress are classic. Mixed incontinence is a combination of both types of symptoms.

This categorization of incontinence symptoms carries over into diagnoses that can be assigned only after urodynamic testing: detrusor overactivity (DO, previously called detrusor instability; also known commonly as overactive bladder (OAB) or the overactive bladder syndrome); urodynamic stress incontinence (USI, previously genuine stress incontinence); and mixed, which is still mixed. However, these tidy categories belie the unfortunate fact that symptoms do not correspond neatly with urodynamic diagnoses, which serves to emphasize that we do not fully understand the cause of urinary incontinence. In addition, women do not usually experience their symptoms in distinctly different categories; there is a good deal of overlap in how and why symptoms occur that can include environmental triggers and exacerbating factors. Nevertheless, much effort has been expended in trying to develop techniques that reliably distinguish between the types of incontinence as if they exist independently; techniques in common use range from so-called 'subjective' measures (e.g. questionnaires, voiding diaries) to so-called 'objective' measures (e.g. electronic urodynamics). For our purposes in this chapter, non-invasive management options applicable to all types of urinary incontinence will be described first, followed by those options geared to a specific 'type' of incontinence.

Etiologic theories for incontinence by type will be reviewed briefly. Detrusor overactivity or overactive bladder is commonly attributed to some malfunction in the detrusor muscle of the bladder, which ordinarily should be quiescent (through accommodation, as bladder volume increases but pressure does not) during bladder filling and active when voluntary voiding is initiated by urethral relaxation. Therefore, abnormal detrusor contractions are held responsible for symptoms of urgency (feeling the overwhelming need to urinate for fear of leakage) and frequency (voiding too often). Therefore, therapy has been directed at 'quieting' the detrusor muscle enough to relieve symptoms, but not so much as to interfere with normal bladder emptying. Urgency and frequency symptoms without urge incontinence, 'OAB-dry' as shorthand, is distinguished from 'OAB-wet', urgency and urge incontinence, with or without frequency. (Nocturia, excessive frequency of night-time voiding, is sometimes included in the combination of symptoms that constitute OAB or OAB syndrome.) Exactly what role is played by the urethra in detrusor overactivity is not understood. It is plausible that detrusor overactivity in a woman with relatively intact urethral function could result in 'OAB-dry' symptoms, while 'OAB-wet' represents the combination of detrusor overactivity with urethral dysfunction.

Stress incontinence has been blamed on various problems associated with the urethra. When surgery that 'corrected' urethral hypermobility (e.g. Burch colposuspension) was found to be a successful treatment for stress incontinence, a theory was developed to fit that observation, and it was held that deficient urethral support (urethral hypermobility) leads to stress incontinence. When not all cases of stress incontinence responded to suspension-type surgery, another type of stress incontinence was named: intrinsic sphincter deficiency (ISD). ISD was often seen after surgery had 'fixed' urethral support but not the incontinence symptoms. At its worst, the urethra in ISD was vividly described as a 'drainpipe' – so unable to maintain closure, it was as if an open pipe led from the bladder. Traditional slings attempted to create enough obstruction (compression) to alleviate such severe incontinence, but too often led to urinary retention or lesser forms of voiding dysfunction. Then came a new kind of sling surgery that was effective despite the fact that it did not 'fix' urethral support or cause compression: 'tension-free' mid-urethral slings. Once again, the etiologic theories backtracked to explain clinical observations. Now, the etiologic theory is simpler: all stress incontinence is a result of adversely altered urethral function. In other words, all stress incontinence reflects some degree of intrinsic sphincter deficiency. Incontinence symptoms vary, not necessarily due to the presence or absence of urethral support, but due to the severity of the underlying urethral dysfunction. Please note that this simplification is no doubt an oversimplification; the comprehensive explanation of incontinence, whether stress, urge, or mixed, still remains to be fully elucidated.

In the meantime, clinicians need to care for many, many women with urinary incontinence. After briefly commenting on important features of evaluation, the remainder of this chapter will be devoted to the discussion of non-invasive management strategies that can be used to improve incontinence symptoms in virtually all women.

EVALUATION

A full discussion regarding the evaluation of women with urinary incontinence is beyond the scope of this chapter. Nevertheless, a few key points deserve emphasis before the discussion of non-invasive management.

What is the goal of therapy? This is the most important information to obtain from patients in the course of evaluation before deciding on appropriate

Table 15.1 Information obtained in the evaluation of women with urinary incontinence

Fluid intake

Type of fluid, especially containing:

   caffeine

   carbonation

   alcohol

   acid

Amount of fluid

   overall amount per 24-hour period

   amount per serving

   amount in relation to daily schedule, bedtime

Lifestyle and environment

Access to toileting at home

   home environment: single level, two-story, etc.

Type of work

Access to toileting at work

Smoking

Exercise

Dietary restrictions or excesses

Vegetarian

Dieting

Medications

Over-the-counter

   supplements

Prescription

Medical history

Diabetes

Table 15.2 Mnemonic to remember important contributing factors to urinary incontinence in elderly women. Adapted from Resnick and Yalla, 1985

DIAPERS

Delirium

Infection

Atrophy

Pharmaceuticals

Excess urine output

Restricted mobility

Stool impaction

---

recommendations for management. It might seem obvious that the goal of therapy for incontinence would be to achieve continence. However, as discussed above, a 'cure' for incontinence is not necessarily achievable; and it is never wise to make assumptions about what a patient wants from therapy, especially for chronic conditions. In addition, incontinence often occurs in the setting of a combination of other urinary symptoms such as urgency and frequency in 'OAB-wet'. In such cases, women can often identify what specific aspect of their symptoms is most bothersome (noting that this will be different for different women) and this should usually be the primary target for therapy.

Features of the personal, social, and medical history will be important in many women when considering different non-invasive management strategies. Specific examples will be discussed in more detail with each type of management; however, some information should be obtained routinely from most or all women with incontinence (Table 15.1). For example, information on fluid intake (type and amount) will be important in virtually all women with incontinence. Such

information may help the clinician understand factors potentially contributing to the woman's symptoms, and form the basis for certain types of intervention.

Medical history will reveal some key issues related to urinary function. Poorly controlled diabetes is well known for symptoms of polydipsia and polyuria; perhaps less well known, symptoms of urgency, frequency, and urge incontinence are commonly exacerbated. Indeed, improving urinary symptoms is difficult if not impossible without first achieving adequate diabetic control that eliminates glucosuria. A comprehensive list of medications (including over-the-counter and herbal products, supplements, and prescription drugs) should be carefully reviewed to determine which may be adversely affecting urinary symptoms.

It is important to remember that urinary symptoms are more commonly exacerbated by factors outside the urinary tract in elderly women than in younger women. Issues of no consequence in younger women can assume great importance in older women. In order to be able to make effective recommendations for management of urinary symptoms, clinicians need to obtain information about such disparate issues as cognitive impairment, living arrangements (e.g. bathroom access related to stairs), and limitations on physical mobility (e.g. severe arthritis impairing ability to move quickly to the bathroom). To aid in remembering important contributing factors to urinary symptoms in the elderly, a mnemonic 'DIAPERS' has been developed (Table 15.2).

There is no consensus as to what constitutes a standard evaluation for women with urinary incontinence, with controversy particularly as to when urodynamic testing is indicated before initiating management. Nevertheless, there are two conditions that should be considered in virtually all women with incontinence before assigning a diagnosis and planning treatment: (1) urinary tract infection (UTI); and (2) overflow incontinence. The symptoms of acute cystitis are usually obvious in younger women; however, this is not necessarily the case in older women. Urine screening for UTI should be performed liberally in women with incontinence, including follow-up visits, since a new UTI may manifest only as a change in pre-existing urgency.

Testing for overflow incontinence consists of measuring the post-void residual (PVR) after spontaneous voiding. Ideally, the patient will have the sensation of bladder fullness before voiding in private with a measuring container placed in the toilet; PVR measures are less reliable when the voided volume is less than 150 ml. While no standard cut-off exists for 'normal' versus 'abnormal' PVR measures, clearly lower is better and serves to indicate the efficiency of bladder emptying. In general, bladder emptying is considered adequate when the PVR is less than 100 ml and/or less than one-half the voided volume. Equivocal results or results inconsistent with the clinical picture should be repeated. The further evaluation and management of a patient with suspected impaired bladder emptying is beyond the scope of this chapter; the most important point for the purposes of this chapter is to rule out the possibility of overflow incontinence in virtually all women who present with incontinence.

When confirming the symptom of stress incontinence will provide information important in assigning a diagnosis and initiating management, many clinicians perform a bladder 'stress test'. The principle involves observing transurethral urine leakage coincident with a cough or Valsalva effort. There is no consensus as to the 'best' bladder volume for stress testing; in general, leakage at lower bladder volumes implies more severe urethral dysfunction. In addition, position and perhaps type of stress effort may affect the likelihood of obtaining a positive stress test. Women are usually more likely to leak when standing versus sitting versus lying down or positioned in gynecologic stirrups; and for many women, cough will provoke leaking while Valsalva may not. This suggests a useful step-wise progression for testing: first supine with Valsalva, then cough, and then sitting or standing with Valsalva, then cough. As soon as a positive test is observed, no further testing is necessary. Some women will have negative stress testing despite a history consistent with stress incontinence; this usually means mild urethral dysfunction or stress conditions that are not easily replicated by testing (such as sneezing or maximal effort associated with specific exercise). In this case, it is appropriate to initiate non-invasive management with the presumed diagnosis of stress incontinence; if symptoms do not improve as expected, consider further evaluation before altering management.

MANAGEMENT OPTIONS

Non-invasive management of urinary incontinence comprises behavioral therapy, pelvic muscle exercises, medication, and devices. It is possible and often beneficial to combine different types of non-invasive management in the same patient; this will be addressed in the presentation of typical cases in the last section of this chapter. Many recommendations for non-invasive management of urinary incontinence and particularly those regarding combinations are not based on rigorous evidence of benefit. Even for treatments that have been studied, such as pelvic muscle exercises and medications, results of research are usually limited by focusing on very short-term effects (weeks or months) of single therapies. Since such results are not sufficient to provide a strong evidence base to guide management in the setting of a chronic condition like urinary incontinence, clinicians must use their judgment to fill in the gaps when caring for women over many years.

Non-invasive management for urinary incontinence offers many advantages when compared with invasive (i.e. surgical) management. Non-invasive management is widely applicable, low-risk, and low-cost. One or more forms of non-invasive management are appropriate for all common types (stress, urge, and mixed) and all levels of severity (mild, moderate, severe) of incontinence. Several forms of non-invasive management can be combined to be implemented together or in series, depending on the goals of therapy. One of the strongest advantages of non-invasive therapy is that, even in all its forms, success or failure with one form of non-invasive management never precludes a different form of management, whether another non-invasive or an invasive (surgical) option. Even after women have been treated with surgery for incontinence, all non-invasive forms of management remain potentially applicable.

Other advantages of non-invasive management are its low risk and low cost when compared with surgery. With the exception of medications, non-invasive management has virtually no risks; and medications used for incontinence are generally low in risk when recommended to appropriate candidates. Some forms of non-invasive management have no direct medical costs, except for the time it takes to explain the therapy and provide follow-up to the patient. Other forms of management carry a low one-time cost for a device, such as a pessary, plus clinician time. Often, detailed instructions and follow-up can be efficiently provided by allied healthcare professionals such as nurses or nurse practitioners. Medications for incontinence vary widely in cost; when appropriate, cost savings may be realized by using generic drugs.

Day, date:	Fluids	Voiding	Urgency	Leaking episode	Comments
Please record the time of day for each event in the columns	How much, what type	Estimate small or large amount	*Place '√' for urgency without leaking*	*Place '√' for each leaking episode**	*Describe activities associated with events*
Example: Wake up, 8:00 am Breakfast, 8:30 am 9:00 am 9:15 am 10:00 am ...	2 cups coffee	Large Small	√	√ – urge	Watching TV Watching TV

Please record the time you get up from sleeping and the time you go to sleep each day

Figure 15.1   Voiding diary. Instruct the patient as follow: 'Please record the time you get up from sleeping and the time you go to sleep each day.'

*If this information is important for reaching a diagnosis or planning management, the patient can be asked to characterize leaking episodes as 'stress-related' (i.e. related to physical stress of coughing, sneezing, jumping, etc.), 'urge-related' (i.e. related to the overwhelming urge to void), or 'other' when it is not possible to characterize an episode as stress or urge.

There are some disadvantages associated with non-invasive management strategies. Most require a high level of involvement from patients. While many women appreciate the opportunity to play a key role in their healthcare, this may not be possible for all. Various medical conditions may interfere with the likelihood of success for some non-invasive strategies; for example, women with severe cognitive impairment will not be able to follow complex instructions independently. For other women, they may not have the time or the motivation to participate in an ongoing exercise program at an optimal level. It is important to note that these are not contraindications to the use of non-invasive management; rather, they are features that may influence the likelihood of symptom improvement.

Behavioral therapy

Behavioral therapy is a broad term encompassing a variety of interventions, with the common element of altering some aspect(s) of a patient's behavior to achieve an improvement in her urinary symptoms. For the purposes of this chapter, behavioral therapy for urinary incontinence will focus on voiding diaries, fluid management, and timed voiding. Much of behavioral therapy for incontinence is not evidence-based; nevertheless, accumulated experience of both clinicians and patients suggests that these therapies are important in the overall plan of management.

Voiding diary

A voiding diary has two distinct uses in the evaluation and management of urinary incontinence: (1) as a means of gathering more information about a woman's voiding habits as well as lifestyle features that may be influencing her incontinence symptoms; and (2) as a means of reinforcing behavioral change by recording. Much of the information typically gathered when taking the patient's history is only the patient's best guess regarding items she may not have previously considered important. Provided that the voiding diary is completed correctly and concurrent with daily events, it provides more accurate information on fluid intake, number of voids per day and night, and number and pattern of incontinence episodes and their potential triggers. An example of a typical voiding diary is shown in Figure 15.1. A 3-day diary is probably sufficient for most patients; consider asking the patient to complete the voiding diary for 7 days if she experiences high variation in her symptoms from day to day.

When such information would be helpful, the patient can be asked to measure voided volumes as well. This can be important if bladder testing suggested low bladder capacity; a record of voided volumes can help distinguish between a false positive if bladder capacity was artificially low due to the testing itself (e.g. requirement for voiding in an unnatural environment) versus a true positive of low bladder capacity due to restrictive bladder disease.

Another valuable aspect of voiding diaries is their use to help set goals of therapy and then to demonstrate change with time. Clinicians often ask patients to complete a voiding diary in advance of their first appointment. In this way, the voiding diary complements the information obtained as part of the patient's history. Particularly in the setting of a chronic condition such as incontinence, it is sometimes difficult for patients to remember the level of symptoms that preceded therapy. Completing voiding diaries at intervals can more clearly demonstrate whether therapy is effective or ineffective at addressing the patient's symptoms.

Recording information in a voiding diary may have a potential therapeutic effect as well. When voiding diaries are used to measure outcomes in clinical research, part of the improvement seen in groups receiving placebo has been attributed to the effect of voiding diaries. Similar to the way a food diary enables dieters to recognize patterns of behavior linked with eating, a voiding diary can identify previously unrecognized patterns between fluid intake, activities that precede or accompany incontinence episodes, and voiding habits that may contribute to the severity of incontinence symptoms. As noted above, the patient and clinician can work together to recognize these patterns and plan ways to change behavior accordingly.

Fluid management

Using information obtained during the patient's history and ideally complemented with a voiding diary, the clinician can identify patterns of fluid intake that may be influencing the patient's symptoms. The overall amount of fluids should be assessed. On occasion, patients misunderstand the common advice of drinking 6–8 (8-ounce) glasses of fluid each day to mean that 48–64 ounces of *water* should be consumed each day. This amount of water combined with other fluids usually leads to an unnecessarily high fluid intake, easily remedied by helping the patient understand that the 48–64-ounce goal for fluid intake includes all fluids, not just water. At the other extreme, some women severely limit their fluids to reduce their incontinence. However, concentrated urine can aggravate urgency and urge incontinence, thereby provoking the very symptoms that women are trying to avoid. In that event, it is useful to advise a judicious increase in fluid intake along with timed voiding (discussed below).

The pattern of fluid intake may exacerbate some symptoms. For example, drinking a large quantity of fluid over a short time results in a large volume of urine filling the bladder quickly. Rapid bladder filling may produce worsening of urgency and urge incontinence in some women. If such a pattern is evident, suggest that the patient drink smaller amounts over a longer period of time. As another example, fluid intake with or after the evening meal can result in bothersome nocturia. If this is the case, suggest to the patient that she limit her beverages after some time in the early evening, such as 6 or 8 pm.

Certain fluids have acquired a reputation for aggravating bladder symptoms, particularly urgency and urge incontinence. This includes beverages that contain alcohol, caffeine, and/or carbonation. In addition to its possible effect on urge symptoms, caffeine has a well-known diuretic effect that can cause rapid bladder filling and large urine volumes. Carbonation produces fluids of high acid content; other acidic fluids include cranberry, citrus, and tomato juices. Some women describe a strong association between sugar intake and urinary symptoms. Not all women will be affected by the same things; especially when patterns on voiding diaries suggest an association, clinicians can encourage women to experiment by withdrawing specific items from their diet and monitoring for a potential effect on symptoms. In some cases, it will be clear that an improvement occurred when an offending fluid has been avoided; in other cases, it is only when the fluid is reintroduced that an association with symptoms is confirmed. In addition, other fluids will be found not to worsen symptoms and thus can be safely enjoyed.

Many women and clinicians are aware of the beneficial effect of cranberry in reducing recurrent or persistent urinary tract infections. For women who cannot tolerate cranberry juice for its adverse effect on urgency and urge incontinence (perhaps due to high sugar and acid content), cranberry extract in pill form can usually be substituted.

Timed voiding

Timed voiding, also known as bladder training or retraining, is perhaps best known for its beneficial effect on overactive bladder symptoms; less well known is its effect in reducing the frequency and amount of urine lost from episodes of stress incontinence. As its name implies, timed voiding imposes a schedule on daytime voiding that is otherwise dominated by symptoms of urgency, frequency, and urge and/or stress incontinence. The theoretical background to timed voiding proposes that voluntary voiding reestablishes the elements of cortical control over unwanted detrusor activity. On a more pragmatic note, voiding on schedule limits the amount of time the bladder spends at volumes close to fullness where an episode of urgency may become an episode of urge incontinence and where coughing or sneezing may trigger stress incontinent episodes that might not occur at lower bladder volumes.

Although evidence supports the effectiveness of timed voiding as an intervention for incontinence, specific details of instituting a schedule for voiding are not evidence-based. A common strategy is to identify the voiding interval associated with incontinence episodes and choose an interval of time below that to initiate scheduled voiding. For example, by history ideally corroborated by a voiding diary, a woman

Table 15.3   Urge suppression strategies

Perform a pelvic muscle contraction
Avoid triggers with full bladder:
   key-in-door
   running water
   sudden exposure to cold
If standing, sit. If sitting, cross your legs
Distract yourself mentally until the urge passes:
   count backwards from 10
   say the alphabet backwards
Do not try to run to the toilet when the feeling of urge begins.
   Using the above strategies, wait until the urge passes and
   then walk, do not run, to the toilet

experiences urgency and urge incontinence when she voids about every 2 hours. Thus, her schedule for voiding can begin at intervals of every hour. Some women find it beneficial to set a timer to help in remembering to follow the schedule. In order to cope with sensations of urgency that may occur before the scheduled time to void, women can be taught several urge suppression strategies (Table 15.3). At the scheduled time, women should be encouraged to void whether they perceive bladder fullness or not. Women should not try to force voiding by excessive straining.

Once symptoms are improved or, with an optimal response, avoided with the initial schedule of voiding, the interval can be gradually increased every 2–3 weeks by increments of 15–30 minutes. If symptoms recur at a certain interval, advise the woman to drop back to the previous level where her symptoms were controlled; with more time, it may be possible to attempt another increase in voiding interval. The goal is to reach a voiding interval of every 3 hours or so without symptoms. Women can also be advised to use the strategy of timed voiding when symptoms are intermittent, for example, when stress incontinence symptoms are exacerbated by coughing due to bronchitis.

Women must have relatively intact cognitive function in order to implement timed voiding independently. An effective alternative for women with cognitive impairment is prompted voiding. Rather than requiring a woman to keep track of scheduled voiding herself, a family member or staff member prompts the woman to void at regular intervals. Assistance with toileting is provided as necessary.

Pelvic muscle exercises

Pelvic muscle exercises are commonly known as Kegel exercises, in tribute to the gynecologist who first published the use of such exercises for women with prolapse and urinary incontinence. Although the usefulness of pelvic muscle exercises for prolapse has not been established, pelvic muscle exercises have become a mainstay of non-invasive management for urinary incontinence (as well as fecal incontinence). Despite the passage of almost 60 years since Kegel's description, the mechanism of action is not fully known through which pelvic muscle exercises exert their beneficial effect.

It might seem intuitive that improving pelvic muscle function should improve incontinence symptoms, but this has been remarkably difficult to explain in detail. One problem is the lack of tools that can adequately measure pelvic muscle function; even more fundamental is a lack of understanding of what aspects of muscle function should be targeted to result in symptom improvement. Nevertheless, many experienced physical therapists focus on training to improve power and endurance in pelvic muscles. More muscle power can be achieved by increasing muscle work (e.g. moving from supine to sitting to standing when performing exercises) and by decreasing the time needed to produce the same work (e.g. performing more contractions in less time). Endurance is enhanced by increasing the number of contractions and/or by sustaining contractions for a longer time.

In practical terms, although the best pelvic muscle exercise program remains a topic of some controversy, many regimens are available for clinicians and patients to choose from. Some basic principles can be applied (Table 15.4). Before attempting to instruct a woman in pelvic muscle exercises, the clinician should use vaginal palpation to assess her ability to identify and contract the correct muscles. It is not safe to assume that women will understand verbal instructions alone. Some women, when attempting a pelvic muscle contraction, inadvertently contract their abdominal muscles instead of or in addition to their pelvic muscles. The clinician can identify this by resting one hand lightly on the woman's abdomen while using the vaginal hand to palpate the pelvic muscles. If abdominal muscle contraction occurs, the woman should be alerted to avoid this; it is often helpful to remind the woman to avoid holding her breath and to continue breathing evenly.

Women should be specifically queried about whether they are contracting their pelvic muscles while voiding in order to interrupt their urine stream. If so, explain that this practice is not advisable especially for women with urgency and urge incontinence, who instead will be trying to train their bladders to empty only under appropriate circumstances and no

Table 15.4   Basic principles of pelvic muscle exercise programs

Using vaginal palpation, determine whether the patient can correctly identify and contract her pelvic muscles (without simultaneously contracting her abdominal muscles)

NO → Consider immediate referral to an experienced physical therapist for individualized instruction, with or without biofeedback
YES → Discuss with the patient what her preferences are regarding different pelvic muscle exercise programs and which she will feel most confident about incorporating effectively into her daily routine

Direct methods of pelvic muscle exercises:
  exercise program independently implemented and supervised by the clinician

- instruct the woman's baseline activities
- position: lying down, sitting, standing (in order of difficulty)
- repetitions: begin with low number and gradually increase at intervals
- duration: begin with short duration and gradually increase at intervals
- rest: relax completely between contractions for duration equal to previous contraction
- sets of exercises: at least daily, up to three times daily

  exercise program with instruction and supervision by experienced physical therapist

Indirect methods of pelvic muscle exercises:

  biofeedback

Women should not experience pain during or after pelvic muscle exercises
Women should not try to identify their pelvic muscles by contracting them to interrupt voiding

---

others. Interrupting normal voiding could conceivably be counterproductive, and is certainly not beneficial, for such women. In general, women should relax between pelvic muscle contractions, for roughly the same length of time as the preceding contraction. Women should not experience pain either during or after performing pelvic muscle exercises; if pain does occur, women should be advised to notify their clinicians promptly and discontinue exercising until evaluation takes place.

As noted, no consensus exists as to the best combination of repetitions and the exact type of pelvic muscle contractions: an example of an exercise program is discussed in the last section of the chapter. Indeed, whether strengthening the pelvic muscles is even necessary to obtain symptom improvement with pelvic muscle exercises has been challenged. Women commonly report improved symptoms shortly after instruction in pelvic muscle exercises, far sooner than could be attributed to a true change in muscle strength. Termed 'the knack', this early improvement may be due to enhanced awareness of pelvic muscles and the (sometimes newly found) ability to augment pelvic muscle tone with voluntary contraction. To take advantage of this observation, advise women to contract their pelvic muscles right before a sneeze or cough. In addition, as noted earlier under urge suppression strategies, pelvic muscle contractions can be used to suppress the sensation of urgency and ideally prevent episodes of urge incontinence.

Despite the reported effectiveness of pelvic muscle exercises in the setting of research protocols, such impressive results may not be replicated in clinical practice. Unfortunately, a number of factors interfere with the full realization of the promise of pelvic muscle exercises. Perhaps of greatest importance, patients need sufficient time, effort, and motivation to participate in not only an intensive exercise program for initial symptom improvement, but also an ongoing exercise program that ideally maintains that level of improvement. In an effort to bypass the ongoing patient effort required for traditional pelvic muscle exercises, different strategies have been developed that aim to achieve the effect of pelvic muscle exercises without such a high level of patient involvement. These strategies may also be useful for women who initially have difficulty identifying and contracting the correct muscles. These strategies include biofeedback, vaginal cones (or weights), electrical stimulation, and magnetic stimulation.

Biofeedback is often used in conjunction with a pelvic muscle exercise program to help the patient learn to contract the pelvic floor muscles appropriately. To verify correct muscle contraction, digital palpation, vaginal manometry, or vaginal or anal electromyography (EMG) is used to give the patient feedback on her efforts at pelvic muscle contraction. For digital palpation, the healthcare provider places the first two digits of their dominant gloved hand into the vagina or rectum and palpates the pelvic muscles during a contraction to assess strength and duration of the contraction; in addition, the provider looks for extraneous recruitment of surrounding gluteal and lower extremity muscles, and/or abdominal wall muscles (which may be perceived as a Valsalva or bearing-down effort). Different scales (e.g. Brink, Oxford) have been developed to provide a semiquantitative assessment of pelvic muscle function although these are not in wide use in clinical practice.

Manometry or EMG can be used in evaluation (although standards for 'normal' pelvic muscle function have not been established) and/or in training to provide feedback. Vaginal manometry, or perineometry, is performed by placing a probe in the vagina to record the force or pressure generated by pelvic muscle contraction. When using a balloon perineometer to measure pressure, the shape of the device helps to insure that a proper contraction is being performed as a Valsalva would expel the balloon from the vagina. This modality allows the patient to learn proper muscle awareness and contraction, as well as develop muscle strength, without the invasive nature of an examiner actually palpating the muscle groups. Both handheld personal and larger computer-based devices are available.

Vaginal or anal EMG involves detecting electrical activity of the pelvic (skeletal) muscles via a vaginal or anal probe or a skin patch electrode placed perianally. For vaginal manometry and vaginal or anal EMG, the device used to measure the contraction provides visual, auditory, and/or tactile feedback to the patient. These modalities can help teach the patient, who may have been unaware and/or unable, to contract the pelvic muscles so that leakage of urine with a physical stress (coughing/laughing/sneezing) can be prevented, and/or so that unwanted detrusor contractions associated with overactive bladder symptoms can be inhibited.

Vaginal cones (ball- or cone-shaped weights) are a form of behavioral therapy often recommended in conjunction with pelvic muscle exercises. Cones can help patients identify and contract the pelvic muscles even during everyday activities. The theory behind vaginal cones is that a correct and sustained contraction of the pelvic muscles is necessary to maintain them in place. Vaginal cones are sold in sets with varying weights (i.e. ranging from 20 to 100 g that increase by 20-g increments). Women are instructed to start with the heaviest cone that can be held in place and then to insert the cones and retain them for 20–30 minutes twice daily. As success with each cone is achieved, the patient will advance to the next heavier cone. Vaginal cones may be most helpful as adjunct

therapy in stress urinary incontinence, especially in highly motivated patients.

Electrical stimulation is another method to stimulate awareness of the pelvic muscles as well as to develop contraction strength, either independently or in combination with formal pelvic muscle exercise and behavior modification programs. Usually, non-implantable vaginal or anal electrodes are used to stimulate a contraction of the pelvic muscles by contact through the vaginal or rectal epithelium or indirectly by stimulation of the pudendal nerve. The electrodes are cone- or hourglass-shaped for easy insertion into the vaginal or anal canal. Electrical stimulation can be performed in a healthcare provider's office or at home with a personal electrical stimulation unit. Treatment sessions usually last 15–20 minutes, once or twice daily, for a period of 6–12 weeks. Stimulation parameters that can be varied are frequency, pulse duration, duty cycle ('on-off' time), and amplitude. Side-effects appear to occur infrequently and are mild, including vaginal irritation, pain, bleeding, and vaginal and urinary tract infections.

Magnetic stimulation therapy, also known as extracorporeal magnetic innervation, is performed using electromagnetic stimulation 'chairs' that allow a patient to be fully clothed during treatment. The stimulation chair has a surface electrode built into the seat of the chair that generates pulsed electromagnetic fields when a high voltage electrical current is applied. The pulsed electromagnetic fields induce action potentials in the lumbosacral nerve roots innervating the pelvic muscles, thereby initiating a muscle contraction. While electrical stimulation activates a nerve directly and magnetic stimulation indirectly, there appears to be no difference in the nerve depolarization and propagation of action potentials along the nerve axon. In theory, electromagnetic stimulation may modulate both the autonomic and somatic nervous systems. It is thought that improvement of overactive bladder symptoms occurs due to activation of pudendal nerve afferents that 'block' parasympathetic detrusor motor fibers at the spinal reflex arc and activation of inhibitory hypogastric sympathetic neurons. For stress urinary incontinence, repetitive stimulation of the pudendal nerve and pelvic muscles is thought to act as a passive Kegel exercise, and may result in improved strength of pelvic muscles. Treatment regimens usually involve biweekly treatments, 20 minutes in length, and lasting 6–12 weeks. Unfortunately, only office-based treatment can be provided, which may limit its acceptance by patients unwilling or unable to comply with these requirements.

Table 15.5 Currently available pharmacologic agents indicated for overactive bladder symptoms

Drug name: brand (generic)	Recommended dosing	Comments
Ditropan® (oxybutynin)	Ditropan® tablets (immediate-release): 5 mg three times daily	Immediate-release tablets can be cut in half by the patient to obtain dosing of approximately 2.5 mg
	Ditropan XL® tablets (extended-release): 5 or 10 mg once daily	Dose of Ditropan XL® can be increased by 5-mg increments to a maximum of 30 mg daily
	Oxytrol® patch: applied twice weekly	Oxytrol® patch provides approximately 3.9 mg oxybutynin per day
Detrol® (tolterodine)	Detrol® tablets (short-acting): 2 mg twice daily	Short-acting tablet dose may be lowered to 1 mg twice daily
	Detrol LA® capsules (long-acting): 4 mg once daily	Long-acting capsule dose may be lowered to 2 mg once daily
Sanctura® (trospium)	20 mg twice daily	Due to impaired absorption when taken with fat, take each dose on an empty stomach or at least 1 hour before meals
VESIcare® (solifenacin)	5 mg once daily	Dose of VESIcare® can be increased to 10 mg once daily
Enablex® Extended Release (darifenacin)	7.5 mg once daily	Dose of Enablex® Extended Release can be increased to 15 mg once daily

Medication

For patients with overactive bladder (OAB) symptoms, with and without incontinence, medication is often offered in conjunction with behavioral modification. The goal of pharmacologic therapy is to reduce the symptoms of urgency, frequency of micturition, and number of urge incontinence episodes. OAB is a chronic medical condition in most instances, and compliance with drug therapy is often an issue for patients, especially elderly women in whom polypharmacy is common. The ideal medication would have high efficacy, few side-effects, and a good safety profile. Antimuscarinic agents are the primary class of drugs used in pharmacologic management of OAB. Antimuscarinic agents suppress detrusor muscle contractions by binding to muscarinic receptors and blocking the activity of acetylcholine, thereby reducing detrusor muscle contractions. Muscarinic receptors in the bladder are found in the detrusor muscle, urothelium, and parasympathetic and sympathetic nerve endings. Muscarinic receptors are found in other parts of the body, including the parotid glands, gastrointestinal tract, brain, and eye, and are responsible for the common side-effects reported with virtually all antimuscarinic agents (dry mouth, constipation, cognitive impairment, and blurred vision). Of importance,

antimuscarinic drugs are contraindicated in women with narrow-angle glaucoma. If a patient with glaucoma is unsure of her type, it is necessary to review the type of eye drop medication she uses and/or to contact her ophthalmologist.

Currently available antimuscarinic agents are listed in Table 15.5. Tolterodine (Detrol®, Detrol LA®: Pharmacia & Upjohn) and oxybutynin (Ditropan®, Ditropan XL®: Ortho) are the most-studied oral OAB drugs on the market. Early formulations of tolterodine and oxybutynin were short-acting (4–6 hours), and required multiple doses per day. Drug discontinuation was common due to the frequency of side-effects. Long-acting formulations allow once-a-day dosing, with potential for improved compliance and decreased side-effects. The oxybutynin transdermal patch (Oxytrol®: Watson) allows for twice-weekly dosing and has a theoretic advantage in avoiding the first-pass effect of the liver, thereby using a lower dose of oxybutynin. Trospium (Sanctura®: Espirit) is promoted as having fewer central nervous side-effects due to its large molecular structure; it has the least muscarinic receptor selectivity and the strongest receptor binding of all the available agents. Two drugs are promoted with the potential for less severe side-effects of dry mouth: solifenacin (VESIcare®: Astellas), with stronger binding to muscarinic receptors in the bladder than in the salivary glands; and darifenacin (Enablex® Extended Release: Novartis), with selectively greater binding for receptors in the bladder than in the salivary glands.

Imipramine, a tricyclic antidepressant, is another medication that has been used for treatment of OAB. As with other tricyclic antidepressants, it has both anticholinergic and α-agonist properties, which may make it effective for patients with mixed urinary incontinence. The side-effect profile limits use of imipramine, with both sedation and other typical anticholinergic symptoms increasing if dose escalation is necessary. Because of its sedative side-effects, imipramine may be useful in women with a primary complaint of nocturia.

Once drug therapy is initiated, close patient follow-up is mandatory. Typically, a medication is prescribed on a trial basis for 4 weeks, with a return visit scheduled at that point or sooner if significant problems develop. The patient should be instructed to notify the physician sooner if any intolerable side-effects occur and if the medication is discontinued or changed. It is reasonable to initiate treatment with one of the older agents (oxybutynin or tolterodine) as these medications are covered by most prescription plans. Frequently, a patient will not respond to one medication but will to another, or will have side-effects with one medication but not another. A trial of different medications should be considered before abandoning drug therapy. Drug discontinuation, usually due to perceived lack of benefit and side-effects, is the greatest impediment to patient compliance for long-term treatment.

Devices

Numerous devices have been developed over the years in attempts to reduce the symptoms of urinary incontinence. While traditionally used for pelvic organ prolapse, vaginal pessaries can improve stress incontinence symptoms in some women. Use of a vaginal pessary may be particularly well suited for women who experience intermittent symptoms, for example associated with a particular exercise such as tennis. Although pessaries for prolapse come in numerous shapes, pessaries designed to address stress incontinence symptoms are typically circular, such as the incontinence ring (ring pessary with knob; Figure 15.2) and incontinence dish, both with and without platform. Both the incontinence ring and dish have a knob, an enlarged area that is positioned underneath the urethra. In theory, the knob provides additional support to the urethra and helps compress the urethra during stress activities such as

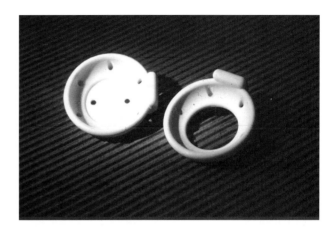

Figure 15.2   Incontinence rings.

coughing or the Valsalva maneuver (bearing down). Patients should undergo pessary fitting with the appropriate size selected to avoid discomfort, urethral obstruction, and vaginal irritation or ulceration. Pessary care includes scheduled follow-up, initially monthly then perhaps every 3 months, at which time a pelvic examination should be performed to assess vaginal irritation or ulceration, and the pessary should be cleaned with water. Depending on the pessary type and patient comfort level, patients can be taught to remove their pessary on a more frequent basis for cleaning. Sexual activity is not precluded by pessary use (although the pessary is not effective for contraception); women can determine whether they are more comfortable with or without the pessary during sexual activity.

Urethral devices are designed to be inserted into the urethra by the patient, and provide continence by obstructing the urethra. To void, the patient removes the device, voids, and then reinserts a new device for continued protection. Early enthusiasm for urethral devices as a non-surgical management of incontinence dwindled as many patients developed urinary tract infections, hematuria, and urethral irritation. While several devices are still available in Europe, no products are currently marketed in the United States.

DISCUSSION OF CASES

Case 1

A 45-year-old woman presents for well-woman preventive care. On review of systems, she acknowledges that stress incontinence symptoms, present intermittently since the birth of her third child 12 years ago, are now more frequent and becoming bothersome. She is especially bothered by incontinence of larger volumes when she plays tennis twice a week. She is otherwise healthy and taking no medications.

Evaluation

History You complete her history with particular attention to her fluid intake, voiding habits, the presence or absence of other lower urinary tract symptoms, and other aspects of functional impact of her stress incontinence symptoms. She denies other symptoms. She has not experienced incontinence during sexual activity, although from long habit, she voids before and after intercourse. She knows of Kegel exercises and she has tried 'a few' to no effect.

Physical examination Her general examination is normal and her body mass index (BMI) shows her to be of normal weight. Her pelvic examination is consistent with her vaginal parity without clinically significant prolapse. On request, she can contract her pelvic muscles strongly but the contraction duration is brief (less than 3 seconds). You ask her to cough while she is positioned in gynecologic stirrups and you note a spurt of urine from the urethra immediately following the cough. You ask her to void; her measured void is 325 ml and her post-void residual is less than 5 ml. Dip urinalysis is negative.

Further testing You have already performed a cough stress test that established transurethral leakage with cough. Her voiding efficiency is excellent. Given that her history, examination, and limited testing are all consistent with the presumed diagnosis of stress incontinence, it is controversial whether any additional testing is beneficial in clarifying the diagnosis or in improving her outcome with standard treatment. Certainly, it is acceptable clinical practice to proceed with non-surgical treatment based on information acquired so far.

Management

You discuss with her the condition of stress incontinence and options for management. She feels that she would have trouble incorporating a physical therapy program for pelvic muscle exercises, plus the need for maintenance exercises, into her busy lifestyle. She does not want to consider surgery at this time, considering the relative infrequency of bothersome symptoms. She agrees to a trial of an incontinence pessary that she can wear in anticipation of vigorous exercise, including tennis. You fit her with an incontinence ring; since her vaginal tissue is well-estrogenized, you suggest that she can use a water-based lubricant (such as K-Y Jelly®)

as needed for pessary insertion (although not too much or the pessary may not stay in place as desired). You review healthy bladder habits and fluid intake with her.

Follow-up

She returns for follow-up in 1 month. She reports sufficient improvement of her stress incontinence symptoms while wearing the pessary, and no other symptoms or difficulties in using it. Her examination remains normal. You recommend that she returns for follow-up in 3 months, or sooner if any difficulties arise. If all remains well at her next visit, you may suggest resuming care at yearly intervals, with instructions for her to contact you if anything changes between visits.

Case 2

A middle-aged daughter brings her 82-year-old mother in for a visit because of more frequent episodes of urinary incontinence during the day. The patient lives alone, with her daughter nearby and visiting daily. The patient's medical problems include severe arthritis with joint pain limiting her mobility and mild cognitive impairment associated with dementia. She takes nine prescription medications.

Evaluation

History In reviewing her symptoms, you find it difficult to evaluate her patterns of fluid intake, voiding, and incontinence. She wears large sanitary napkins on a continuous basis.

Physical examination Her pelvic examination shows moderate irritation of the vulvar tissues consistent with chronic wetness. Her pelvic support is adequate. She cannot perform a pelvic muscle contraction.

Testing Clean-catch urinalysis is positive for white blood cells and nitrites. The patient voids 300 ml with a post-void residual of 100 ml. Dip urinalysis of a catheterized urine specimen still shows white blood cells and nitrites. You order urine culture with antibiotic sensitivities.

Management

Because of difficulty ascertaining her symptoms as well as other important information including fluid intake and voiding pattern, you recommend that the patient completes a voiding diary for 3 days. In discussing this with the patient and her daughter, you note the possibility that the patient may have difficulty in completing the diary, and the daughter agrees to stay with her mother during the day to provide help if needed. In the meantime, you prescribe an antibiotic appropriate for the organism(s) likely to cause urinary tract infections in your community. You advise use of incontinence pads rather than sanitary napkins, and use of zinc oxide on the vulvar skin after each voiding and incontinence episode. Since night-time incontinence is not an issue, you suggest the patient goes without wearing pads at night.

Follow-up

The patient and her daughter return in 2 weeks. The patient completed the antibiotic as prescribed and noted improvement, although not resolution, of her incontinence. Urinalysis today is negative and the vulvar skin is improved in appearance. The patient did have some difficulty in remembering to complete the voiding diary and ultimately her daughter helped her complete it over a span of 3 days. (This experience prompted the daughter to initiate an evaluation for home-care services for her mother and to consider changing living arrangements in the future to provide more support as her mother's needs change over time.) The patient's fluid intake was low at about four cups per day, and consisted primarily of coffee and cola products. You recommend a judicious and gradual increase in fluids, to five and then six cups per day, and avoidance of caffeinated and carbonated beverages. By the voiding diary, it appears that the patient may have diminished awareness of bladder fullness until an episode of overwhelming urgency and urge incontinence occurs. You recommend scheduled voiding, initially 1 hour apart during the day, with prompts (for example, using a digital watch set to hourly intervals) to help the patient remember to void on schedule, without waiting for the sensation of bladder fullness or urgency. Considering the number of prescription drugs she already takes and the increased risk associated with polypharmacy, you decide to hold pharmacologic treatment at this point. You ask that another 3-day voiding diary be completed before the next visit.

The patient and her daughter return in about 1 month, with the voiding diary completed for 2 days. The patient reports very few episodes of incontinence, with the most help obtained with scheduled voiding. (On the one day that she forgot to wear the watch with pre-set alarms, she voided spontaneously only once and experienced several incontinent episodes.) Urinalysis is again negative, and on examination her

vulvar skin appears healthy. You encourage the patient (and her daughter) to continue with the current management plan with adequate fluid intake, avoiding caffeine and carbonated beverages, scheduled voiding now up to 2 hours apart with continued use of the watch, and vulvar care with zinc oxide as needed. You suggest follow-up in 6 months or sooner if anything changes.

Case 3

A 50-year-old woman presents on referral from her family doctor for persistent urinary incontinence. Her family doctor had initiated evaluation, determined that she had mixed stress and urge incontinence, and started management with Detrol LA 4 mg once a day. The patient reports that she responded initially but experienced such severe constipation that she stopped after 2 weeks of treatment. Her medical problems include obesity, type 2 diabetes managed with diet, and hypertension managed with a diuretic.

Evaluation

History You review her incontinence history in detail and agree with the initial assessment of mixed stress and urge incontinence symptoms. The patient experiences her urge incontinence symptoms as much more bothersome because of their unpredictable timing and larger volume of urine lost. She has gained about 50 pounds, 10 pounds per year for the past 5 years, without a strong effort at weight loss. She acknowledges that she does not follow her diabetic diet 'perfectly'.

Physical examination Her BMI is 35 kg/m². The remainder of her examination is normal, including adequate pelvic support, except that her voluntary pelvic muscle contraction is weak and not sustained.

Testing She voids 400 ml with a post-void residual of 25 ml. Cough stress testing is negative at bladder volume 400 ml. Dip urinalysis is positive only for glucose.

Management

You review with her the likely contribution of her medical problems (obesity, uncontrolled diabetes), and their treatment (diuretic for hypertension), to her urinary symptoms. You emphasize the importance of achieving adequate control of her diabetes, indicating that urge incontinence is very difficult to improve with standard treatment in the presence of glucosuria.

You strongly recommend weight loss under medical supervision, both to improve her stress incontinence symptoms and to ideally improve the likelihood of adequately controlling her diabetes. You plan to discuss an alternative non-diuretic hypertension treatment with her family doctor. For specific treatment of her incontinence symptoms, you recommend a physical therapy program for pelvic muscle exercises and urge suppression strategies; fluid management and scheduled voiding; and a different anticholinergic drug with preventive management to avoid constipation. Since she has already had a trial with Detrol LA, you recommend Ditropan XL at a starting dose of 5 mg once daily.

Follow-up

The patient returns for follow-up in 1 month. She has seen her family doctor several times in the meantime and she has started a weight loss regimen in conjunction with closer attention to diabetes management. In addition, she no longer takes the diuretic and her family doctor has suggested watchful waiting for her blood pressure as long as she continues to lose weight toward her goal. She has started the physical therapy program and has completed two of eight planned visits. She reports that with scheduled voiding and fluid management, her incontinence episodes are somewhat less frequent but, most important, greatly diminished in volume. She has not experienced constipation or other significant side-effects with Ditropan XL at 5 mg daily. Urinalysis today is negative. You encourage her to continue with her programs for weight loss, diabetes management, and physical therapy. In addition to continuing with fluid management and scheduled voiding, you recommend that she increase the dose of Ditropan XL to 10 mg once daily, again with emphasis on avoiding constipation. You ask her to return for follow-up in 2 months or sooner if any new problems should arise.

BIBLIOGRAPHY

Resnick NM, Yalla SV. Management of urinary incontinence in the elderly. N Engl J Med 1985; 313: 800–5.

Resnick NM, Yalla SV. Geriatric incontinence and voiding dysfunction. In: Walsh P, ed. Campbell's Urology, 8th edn. Philadelphia: Saunders, 2002.

Miller JM, Ashton-Miller JA, DeLancey JO. A pelvic muscle pre-contraction can reduce cough-related urine loss in selected women with mild stress urinary incontinence. J Am Geriatr Soc 1998; 46: 870–4.

16 Non-surgical management of interstitial cystitis

Mat H Ho and Narender N Bhatia

INTRODUCTION

Interstitial cystitis (IC) is a poorly defined clinical syndrome that manifests as urinary frequency, urgency, nocturia, and bladder pain without an identifiable etiology. Until recently, most of the women with these symptoms were presumed to have a urinary tract infection (UTI), overactive bladder, or chronic pelvic pain, and were often treated accordingly. IC is now gaining recognition, and the diagnostic methods as well as treatment modalities are emerging.

Despite recent advances, the epidemiology of IC remains incompletely understood. IC affects mainly women, with a female to male ratio of approximately 10:1.[1] Reports on the prevalence of IC are conflicting, depending on the criteria used for the diagnosis and method of study. In a population-based study, the estimated prevalence of IC was 66 per 100 000 adult American females.[2] By using validated questionnaires, other studies demonstrated that the estimated prevalence of IC can range from 0.23 to 12.6%.[3,4] Parsons and co-workers[5] suggested that the prevalence of IC may be as high as 20%. By using the potassium sensitive test as a diagnostic method, IC prevalence rates of 81–85% in gynecologic patients with a complaint of pelvic pain were also reported.[6,7] Although prevalence estimates vary greatly, IC is obviously much more common than traditionally believed.

Recently, several studies have reported associations between IC and other disorders, such as endometriosis, vulvodynia, chronic pelvic pain, irritable bowel syndrome, inflammatory bowel disease, fibromyalgia, chronic fatigue syndrome, systemic lupus erythematosus, Sjogren's syndrome, and allergies.[8] These associations suggest that IC may be a systemic syndrome or a genetically predisposed disease. The suggestion of the genetic predisposition to IC is further supported by the observation that the concordance rate of IC among monozygotic twins was greater than among dizygotic twins.[9]

PATHOPHYSIOLOGY

Currently, there are no proven etiologies for IC, and the pathophysiology of this disease is not completely understood. The etiology of IC is probably multifactorial rather than a single entity because a variety of etiologies has been proposed, but none adequately explains the variable presentations, clinical courses, or responses to therapies. It is also possible that different patients may have different etiologies.

One of the earliest theories suggested that IC could result from a 'leaky' urothelium in the bladder caused by a deficiency of the glycosaminoglycan (GAG) layer. The presence of a GAG layer in the urothelium helps to protect the bladder against both bacteria and urinary toxins, such as potassium.[10] If bladder urothelium becomes more permeable to these agents, IC may develop. This theory, which forms a basis for the potassium sensitive test (PST) and pentosan polysulfate therapy in IC, was derived from several studies in animal models and in humans using protamine to induce increased permeability of the urothelium by stripping the GAG layer.[11] However, whether there is an increase in permeability of the urothelium in IC patients and whether the penetration of bacteria and urinary toxins can be prevented by the GAG layer are still being debated.[12]

Another proposed etiology is augmentation of the release of adenosine triphosphate (ATP) in the urothelium, which subsequently enhances bladder hypersensitivity in IC patients.[13] Altering the production of growth factors, such as antiproliferative factor (APF) and heparin-binding epidermal growth factor, in the urothelium was also proposed to explain the etiology of IC.[14] These factors may inhibit the growth or regeneration of normal bladder urothelium. Although more investigations are needed to elucidate the mechanism, these growth factors may provide the basis to develop a urinary test for IC.

The degranulation of mast cells causing the release of neuroactive and vasoactive agents in the bladder is also believed to play an important role in IC.[15] This proposed mechanism forms a basis for the use of antihistamines, such as hydroxyzine, in the treatment of IC. Because studies to date strongly suggest that IC is a syndrome caused by multiple mechanisms, the degranulation of mast cells could be a common final pathway of these mechanisms. Chronic bladder infection with a poorly characterized agent that triggers IC is another proposed theory.[15] Currently, there are few data to support the role of an infectious etiology. Other suggested theories include neurogenic hypersensitivity, neurogenic inflammation, and autoimmunity which occur in the bladder causing pain and urinary symptoms.[15]

EVALUATION AND DIAGNOSIS

Clinical presentation

The symptoms of IC, such as urinary frequency, urgency, and bladder pain, overlap with the symptoms of overactive bladder or chronic pelvic pain. The main differences between these conditions are that overactive bladder does not include bladder pain, and chronic pelvic pain may not be associated with urinary frequency and urgency. The presentation of IC symptoms is highly variable from one patient to another, and does not necessarily follow a set pattern. Generally, IC patients complain of urinary frequency, urgency, nocturia, and pelvic pain, which do not have identifiable etiologies. Other patients may complain of vague symptoms of pain and incomplete bladder emptying, or a constant sensation to void. These symptoms can wax and wane during the course of the disease and one symptomatic component may predominate over the others. IC is characterized by periods of exacerbation followed by variable periods of remission, and the spontaneous remissions, although temporary, occur in as many as 50% of patients at a mean of 8 months.[15]

The pain component of IC is non-specific, because the bladder is autonomically innervated and patients often have difficulty in locating or describing the pain. The typical pain over the bladder (suprapubic) area that can be relieved by voiding is described only by a small number of patients, while the majority of women with IC may complain of referral pains, such as urethral pain, back pain, vulvar pain, rectal pain, dyspareunia, dysuria, constant burning sensation, or general pelvic pain. Nocturia and urinary frequency and urgency are other components of IC. These symptoms are difficult to separate from each other and from the pain complaint, because urinary frequency

can be a result of urgency or bladder pain. IC patients may also have a constant strong urge to void, despite low bladder volume, which may often be described as pain. The typical patient may void 16 times a day and two or more times at night; however, in severe cases, the patient may urinate as often as 60 times a day and every half hour at night.[5] Voided volumes are usually small. Quality of life is severely impaired in these women. The patient may be anxious, depressed, angry, and sleep-deprived, which can exacerbate the pain and urinary symptoms. Certain foods or beverages can also exacerbate symptoms.

Because of its possible association and overlapping symptoms, IC should be suspected in all patients who present with the following: (1) complaint of chronic pelvic pain, especially with the coexistence of urinary frequency or urgency; (2) symptoms of overactive bladder that do not respond to anticholinergic agents; (3) recurrent UTI; (4) dyspareunia; and (5) history of or symptoms suggesting endometriosis.

Diagnosis

The ability to diagnose IC definitively does not exist, because proven etiology, typical physical examination findings, and conclusive tests or markers are not available. The key is to have a high clinical suspicion, exclude other identifiable conditions, and quantify the symptoms as objectively as possible. Currently, the clinical diagnosis of IC is made primarily by the combination of symptomatic features and exclusionary criteria. Although a dilemma still exists in the diagnosis of IC, the studies described below can be employed together with the National Institute of Diabetes and Digestive and Kidney Diseases (NIDDK) exclusionary criteria and validated questionnaires to guide the evaluation and treatment while awaiting further understanding of the pathophysiology of IC.

The NIDDK criteria

In 1988, a list of criteria was formulated by the NIDDK of the National Institutes of Health (NIH) to standardize subject selection for research purposes.[16] These criteria are summarized in Table 16.1. Although these criteria were not designed as a diagnostic tool, they can provide clinicians with a useful guideline. However, some studies showed that 60% of IC cases may be missed if the diagnosis relies only on these criteria.[17] Furthermore, early IC may not show the presence of glomerulation or Hunner's ulcer, thus excluding these cases from the NIDDK criteria. The

Table 16.1 NIDDK (National Institute of Diabetes and Digestive and Kidney Diseases) Diagnostic Criteria for Interstitial Cystitis

Inclusion criteria
- Symptoms of urinary frequency/urgency or bladder pain
- Presence of glomerulations (in at least 3 quadrants with at least 10 glomerulations per quadrant) and/or Hunner's ulcers on cystoscopy and hydrodistention

Exclusion criteria
- Maximal bladder capacity greater than 350 ml on cystometry while patient is awake
- Absence of an intense urge to void with the bladder filled to 150 ml of water during cystometry using a fill rate of 30 to 100 ml/min
- Demonstration of phasic involuntary bladder contractions on cystometry using the fill rate of 30 to 100 ml/min
- Duration of symptoms less than 9 months
- Absence of nocturia
- Symptoms relieved by antimicrobials, urinary antiseptics, anticholinergics, or antispasmodics
- Frequency of urination while awake of less than 8 times a day
- Diagnosis of bacterial cystitis in the past 3 months
- Bladder, ureteral or urethral calculi
- Active genital herpes
- Uterine, cervical, vaginal, or urethral cancer
- Urethral diverticulum
- Cyclophosphamide or any type of chemical cystitis
- Tuberculous cystitis
- Radiation cystitis
- Benign or malignant bladder tumors
- Active vaginitis
- Age less than 18 years

challenge to clinicians is to diagnose and treat IC early, because the more severe and advanced stages of IC are more resistant to current therapies.[8,15,18] The usefulness of the NIDDK criteria in clinical practice is, therefore, limited.

Physical examination and laboratory studies

General and pelvic examinations are performed to rule out other diseases and pelvic pathologies. Typically, the pelvic examination is negative in IC patients, except for suprapubic and/or trigonal tenderness. Sexually transmitted diseases, urinary tract infections, urethral diverticulum, and pelvic masses should be ruled out. During the pelvic examination, specimens are collected for the determination of sexually transmitted diseases if clinically indicated. Urinalysis and urine culture are warranted, although the results are usually negative. Urine cytology should be obtained if microscopic hematuria is present, or if the patient has other risk factors such as a history of smoking and age over 40 years.

Voiding diary and symptoms scales

A voiding diary as described in Chapter 15 is very helpful in establishing baseline frequency, urgency, and bladder capacity in IC patients. These patients should also keep a voiding diary before and after treatment, as well as during any flare-up, to document improvements and identify triggers.

Several patient symptoms scales have been developed and validated for IC symptoms quantification. These instruments include the O'Leary–Sant IC Indices, the University of Wisconsin IC Scale (UW-ICS), and the Pelvic Pain and Urinary Urgency and Frequency Scale (PUF). The O'Leary-Sant IC Indices (Table 16.1) have two components: the IC Symptom Index (ICSI), which quantifies the symptoms, and the IC Problem Index (ICPI), which quantifies the quality of life.[19] Using cystoscopic and hydrodistension findings and the NIDDK criteria for the objective diagnosis of IC, the sensitivity, specificity, positive predictive value, and negative predictive value of ICSI and ICPI were found to be 94%, 50%, 53%, and 93%, respectively.[20] The UW-ICS (Table 16.2), based on how much patients experience the symptoms, was also developed and validated for IC.[21] Recently, the PUF scale (Table 16.3) has become more popular as a simple, but reliable symptom index for IC screening.[5] This scale has been validated, and higher scores are strongly correlated with a more positive PST. Consequently, a high PUF score (10 or above), in combination with a history and physical examination suggesting IC, is considered by many clinicians to be sufficient to make a presumptive diagnosis.[5] Any of these validated instruments can be used to quantify patient symptoms and help in the evaluation and treatment of IC, as well as in following patient improvement as objectively as possible.

Cystoscopy and hydrodistension

Cystoscopy is generally recommended for ruling out bladder neoplasm and other pathologies. The bladder capacity under anesthesia can also be determined and its reduction suggests the presence of IC, although this criterion is not reliable because many IC patients may have a normal anesthetic bladder capacity. Although a number of investigators advocate bladder biopsies to rule out carcinoma in situ (CIS) and to confirm the presence of inflammation, the morbidity of the procedure outweighs any potential benefits because CIS is very rare in the bladder, and histologic findings are not specific for IC.[18]

Table 16.2   The Symptom Index and Problem Index for interstitial cystitis

Interstitial Cystitis Symptom Index (ICSI)	Interstitial Cystitis Problem Index (ICPI)
1. During the past month, how often have you felt the strong need to urinate with little or no warning? 0. not at all 1. less than 1 time in 5 2. less than half the time 3. about half the time 4. more than half the time 5. almost always	1. During the past month, how much has each of the following been a problem for you: 0. Frequent urination during the day? 1. no problem 2. very small problem 3. small problem 4. medium problem 5. big problem
2. During the past month, have you had to urinate less than 2 hours after you finished urinating? 0. not at all 1. less than 1 time in 5 2. less than half the time 3. about half the time 4. more than half the time 5. almost always	2. Getting up at night to urinate? 0. no problem 1. very small problem 2. small problem 3. medium problem 4. big problem
3. During the past month, how often did you most typically get up at night to urinate? 0. none 1. once 2. 2 times 3. 3 times 4. 4 times 5. 5 or more times	3. Need to urinate with little warning? 0. no problem 1. very small problem 2. small problem 3. medium problem 4. big problem
4. During the past month, have you experienced pain or burning in your bladder? 0. not at all 2. a few times 3. almost always 4. fairly often 5. usually	4. Burning, pain, discomfort, or pressure in your bladder? 0. no problem 1. very small problem 2. small problem 3. medium problem 4. big problem

(Adapted from O'Leary MP, Sant GR, Fowler FJ Jr, Whitmore KE, Spolarich-Kroll J. The interstitial cystitis symptom index and problem index. Urology. 1997; 49(5A Suppl): 58–63.)

Hydrodistension can be carried out at the time of cytoscopy under general or regional anesthesia. The bladder is fully examined first with cystoscopy to rule out any abnormal lesions. The bladder is then distended with sterile water or normal saline at a pressure of 80–100 cmH₂O for 2–5 minutes. After that the bladder is emptied, and bloody efflux of irrigant suggests the presence of IC. Repeat cystoscopy is performed to re-examine the bladder epithelium, and any glomerulation and/or Hunner's ulcers are noted (Figure 16.1). Careful inspection during filling and avoiding overdistension are crucial because bladder rupture can occur in these patients. The presence of glomerulations and/or Hunner's ulcer in the bladder on hydrodistension is the specific NIDDK criterion for the diagnosis of IC. In the United States, Hunner's ulcer (ulcerative form) only occurred in fewer than 10% of IC patients, and is considered to be more resistant to therapy.[15] The appearance of glomerulation after hydrodistension is more common; however, its specificity for the diagnosis of IC is subject to debate because the incidences of glomerulation between IC patients and asymptomatic controls were not significantly different, as reported by one study.[22] The sensitivity of glomerulation findings in the diagnosis of IC is also questionable.[15]

Hydrodistension may have a therapeutic effect on IC symptoms, although a randomized trial to compare hydrodistension with sham cystoscopy (without hydrodistension) has not been performed. Before improving, some patients may have a temporary worsening of symptoms after hydrodistension. Chai and co-workers[23] suggested that bladder stretching during hydrodistension can normalize the abnormally expressed growth factors in IC patients. Hunner's ulcer may be treated at the time of cystoscopy by laser fulguration.[24]

Table 16.3   University of Wisconsin Interstitial Cystitis Scale

Interstitial Cystitis Items

How much have you experienced the following symptoms today? (0: not at all; 6: a lot)	0	1	2	3	4	5	6
1. Bladder pain							
2. Bladder discomfort							
3. Getting up at night to go to the bathroom							
4. Going to the bathroom frequently in the day							
5. Urgency to urinate							
6. Difficulty sleeping because of bladder problems							
7. Burning sensation in the bladder							

Reference Items

How much have you experienced the following symptoms today? (0: not at all; 6: a lot)	0	1	2	3	4	5	6
8. Other pelvic discomfort							
9. Backache							
10. Abdominal cramps							
11. Dizziness							
12. Aches in joints							
13. Heart pounding							
14. Chest pain							
15. Headache							
16. Nausea							
17. Numbness, tingling							
18. Blind spots, blurry vision							
19. Sore throat							
20. Swollen ankles							
21. Nasal congestion							
22. Coughing							
23. Suffocation							
24. Ringing in ears							
25. Flu							

(Adapted from Goin JE, Olaleye D, Peters KM, Steinert B, Habicht K, Wynant G. Psychometric analysis of the University of Wisconsin Interstitial Cystitis Scale: implications for use in randomized clinical trials. J Urol. 1998; 159: 1085–1090.)

Potassium sensitive test

The potassium sensitive test (PST) is based on the theory that the bladder epithelium in IC patients is 'leaky' because of a deficiency in the GAG layer.[5,25] If potassium is present in the urine, it will cross the leaky urothelium to activate the sensory nerve endings in the suburothelium and thus cause pain. This test is performed while the patient is awake and without anesthesia. About 40 ml of sterile water is infused into the bladder at a rate of 15–20 ml/min, and 5 minutes after completion of the infusion the patient rates her pain and urgency using a visual scale from 0 to 5, with 5 being the worst. The bladder is then emptied and 40 ml of a solution of 0.4 mol/l potassium chloride (KCl) is instilled into the bladder and kept there for 5 minutes, in the same fashion as with sterile water. The patient then rates her pain and urgency, using the same visual scale, before voiding. The test is considered positive if the patient is asymptomatic with water instillation and has a score of ≥2 in either pain or urgency with the KCl solution.[5] This test is quite painful in IC patients, and the bladder should be emptied immediately after completion of the test. Subsequent irrigation with sterile water or rescue therapy may be necessary.

A positive PST was obtained in 75–78% of patients with IC and in 4% of controls.[5,25] However, a negative PST does not rule out IC, because up to 46% of patients with a negative PST meet the NIDDK criteria for IC.[26] In gynecologic patients with chronic pelvic pain, 81–85% had a positive PST[6,7] while only 38% had positive findings for IC with cystoscopy and hydrodistension.[20] The data suggest that PST may be more sensitive for IC, and most gynecologic patients with chronic pelvic pain may have this condition. However, in another study of a population who had symptoms suggestive of IC, the positive predictive values of PST and

Table 16.4 Pelvic pain and urgency/frequency (PUF) Scale for interstitial cystitis

Please circle the answer that best describes how you feel for each question

		Score 0	Score 1	Score 2	Score 3	Score 4
1	How many times do you go to the bathroom during the day?	3–6	7–10	11–14	15–19	20+
2	a. How many times do you go to the bathroom at night?	0	1	2	3	4+
	b. If you get up at night to go the bathroom, does it bother you?	Never	Occasionally	Usually	Always	
3	Are you sexually active? Yes____ No____					
4	a. If you are sexually active, do you now or have you ever had pain or symptoms during or after sexual intercourse?	Never	Occasionally	Usually	Always	
	b. If you have pain, does it make you avoid sexual activity?	Never	Occasionally	Usually	Always	
5	Do you have pain associated with your bladder or in your pelvis (vagina, labia, lower abdomen, urethra, perineum, testes, or scrotum)?	Never	Occasionally	Usually	Always	
6	a. If you have pain, is it usually		Mild	Moderate	Severe	
	b. Does your pain bother you?	Never	Occasionally	Usually	Always	
7	Do you still have urgency after going to the bathroom?	Never	Occasionally	Usually	Always	
8	a. If you have urgency, is it usually		Mild	Moderate	Severe	
	b. Does your urgency bother you?	Never	Occasionally	Usually	Always	

Symptom Score (1, 2a, 4a, 5, 6, 7a, 8a) =
Bother Score (2b, 4b, 7b, 8b) =
Total Score (Symptom Score + Bother Score) =

PUF Symptom Scale. ©2000 C. Lowell Parsons, MD
(From Parsons CL. Diagnosing chronic pelvic pain of bladder origin. J Reprod Med 2004; 49 (Suppl): 235–242.)

cystoscopy with hydrodistension were not significantly different (56% and 66%, respectively).[26] A false-positive result can be caused by infection or prior exposure to radiation or chemotherapy. This test may help to predict the response to pentosan polysulfate therapy, because patients with positive PST seem to have a better response than those who demonstrate negative results.[27]

Urodynamics

In general, urodynamic studies are not necessary in the evaluation of IC because voiding diaries can provide adequate information. However, some investigators believe that urodynamics will allow determination of detrusor instability and urethral dysfunction that can be treated differently. If urinary incontinence is present, urodynamic investigations are recommended.

Urinary markers

An attractive approach is to find a sensitive and specific maker in the urine that might serve as a non-invasive diagnostic tool for IC. Among many urinary substances

that have been investigated, antiproliferative factor (APF)[14] and glycoprotein-51 (GP-51)[28] are potentially useful. Both of these markers have been evaluated, and there was no overlap in the urinary levels of APF and GP-51 in those who met the NIDDK diagnostic criteria and in controls. Recently, the alteration of APF levels in IC patients has been confirmed, and this marker is the most likely candidate to become a diagnostic test.[29] However, the alteration of these markers in patients who do not fulfill the NIDDK criteria remains unknown. Although attractive, the usefulness of these urinary markers in the diagnosis of IC requires more investigation.

NON-SURGICAL TREATMENT

Because the etiology of IC is not completely understood, effective treatment for this disease does not exist. Currently there is no cure for this condition, and clinicians should carefully counsel patients on the best form of therapy and realistic expectation of the out-

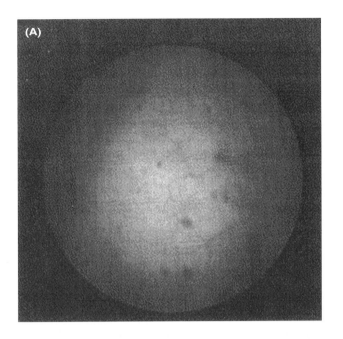

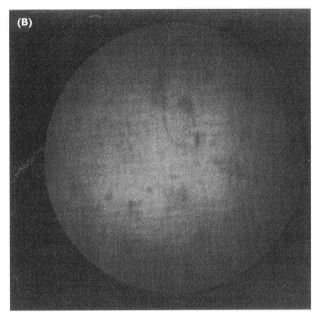

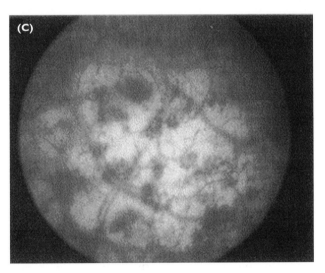

Figure 16.1   Glomerulations in interstitial cystitis. (A) Mild glomerulations. (B) Moderate glomerulations. (C) Severe glomerulations. (Adapted from Evans RJ, Sant GR. Current diagnosis of interstitial cystitis: an evolving paradigm. Urol 2007; 69: 69).

come. The current treatments of IC are empirical, and can only alleviate symptoms. Most of the employed modalities have not been studied in prospective, randomized, and placebo-controlled trials. However, there are some ongoing studies being carried out by the NIH-sponsored Interstitial Cystitis Clinical Trial Group and the results are pending. Besides the therapeutic effects of hydrodistension, the current treatments of IC include supportive management, oral therapy, intravesical instillation, and surgical approach. Non-steroidal anti-inflammatory drugs (NSAIDs) can be used adjunctively to reduce pain and inflammation. It should be noted that anticholinergic and antispasmodic agents are ineffective in women with IC, because these medications block the motor pathway while IC is primarily a hypersensory condition.

Supportive management

Supportive management consists of dietary modification, stress management, pelvic floor exercises, bladder training programs, and other behavioral measures. Although the link between dietary factors and IC symptoms has not been fully established, some foods and beverages may exacerbate the symptoms. It has been shown that about 53% of IC patients associate symptom aggravation with acidic foods and beverages.[30] Another study demonstrated that urinary levels of tryptophan metabolites were elevated in women with hypersensitive bladder as compared to controls.[31] This increase in tryptophan metabolites may disrupt the GAG layer of the urothelium, thus predisposing to the development of IC or exacerbating its symptoms.

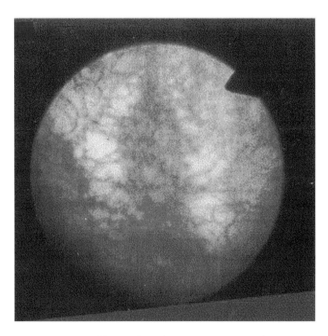

Figure 16.2 Hunner's ulcer in interstitial cystitis. (Adapted from Evans RJ, Sant GR. Current diagnosis of interstitial cystitis: an evolving paradigm. Urol 2007; 69:69).

However, more studies are needed to investigate the role of dietary factors, and dogmatic restrictions should be avoided unless certain diets are shown to improve symptoms in a particular patient.

Stress management and behavioral modification also play a role in the treatment of IC. Distraction techniques can be employed to increase the time between voids. Contracting the pelvic floor muscles and over-riding the first urge to void are very helpful for this purpose. Pelvic floor exercises and bladder training programs as described in Chapter 15 can be employed in IC patients. These are good initial or adjunctive interventions and have been used with some success.

Oral therapy

Sodium pentosan polysulfate (Elmiron®)

Sodium pentosan polysulfate is a weak heparinoid that supposedly reverses the GAG layer deficiency in the urothelium, thus correcting the defect in the permeability barrier of the bladder surface. This medication has been approved by the US Food and Drug Administration (FDA) for oral use in the treatment of IC. Hanno[32] reported that pain relief occurred in approximately 40–60% of patients after 3 months of treatment with 100 mg, three times per day. In other prospective, randomized, and placebo-controlled trials, the improvement of certain IC symptoms was significant with pentosan polysulfate (28% of treated subjects

versus 13% of placebo controls), although the degree of improvement was not dramatic from a clinical standpoint.[33] A recent study showed that the response rates to pentosan polysulfate at 32 weeks of treatment range from 45 to 49%, and these responses are not dose dependent, but the duration of therapy appears to be more important.[34] Since pentosan polysulfate may take 3–6 months to achieve maximal benefit,[32] adequate time should be allowed for the treatment to become effective. Long-term efficacy studies demonstrated that the benefit was maintained for 1–2 years in those who responded to the therapy.[32] Although this medication is well tolerated, gastrointestinal side-effects and reversible alopecia occur in 4% of patients.

Amitriptyline (Elavil®)

This medication has been used to decrease the chronic pain component of IC.[35,36] In addition to its inhibiting properties in noradrenaline and serotonin reuptakes, amitryptyline also has analgesic, sedative, anticholinergic, and antihistaminic effects. Amitryptyline is usually given at night to obtain additional benefit of improving sleep disturbance and decreasing nocturia. The starting dose is 10–25 mg at bedtime, then it is gradually increased to 75 mg or until the side-effects are intolerable, in order to achieve maximal benefit. Weight gain, sedation, and anticholinergic side-effects, such as dry mouth and constipation, occur in 20–80% of patients.[35] When compared with placebo, amitryptyline significantly improved pain and urgency in patients with IC, and a long-term efficacy study (mean of 17 months) revealed a 64% improvement rate using the global assessment questionnaire.[36] When used in conjunction with pentosan polysulfate, amitryptyline can be tapered off once remission is attained. Other tricyclic antidepressants have not been studied in the treatment of IC.

Hydroxyzine (Atarax®)

Hydroxyzine, which is an antihistamine that prevents mast cell degranulation, has been employed in the treatment of IC. The degranulation of mast cells causing the release of neuroactive and vasoactive agents is believed to be responsible for the symptoms of IC. In an open-label investigation with hydroxyzine, 40% reductions in IC symptoms were reported.[37] This improvement increased to 55% in patients with a history of allergies. For these patients and for those in whom mast cell degranulation is confirmed on bladder biopsy, an antihistamine such as hydroxyzine is a good choice. Hydroxyzine can be taken alone, or given together with pentosan polysulfate, at a dose of 10–25 mg at bedtime for 1 week, then gradually increased to 50–75 mg. Hydroxyzine also has sedative and anxiolytic side-effects, which are beneficial for nocturia and other IC symptoms.

Gabapentin (Neurontin®)

Gabapentin is an antileptic medication that can hyperpolarize the neurons involved in pain transduction and thus increase their sensory thresholds. Because of this action, gabapentin has been tried for chronic urogenital pain and in IC patients. About 50% of treated patients reported subjective improvement of their pain while the remaining 50% did not perceive any change in their symptoms.[38] Although half of the patients improved with gabapentin, it should be noted that this cohort included only subjects with refractory pain that failed other treatments.

Intravesical instillation

As compared to oral therapy, intravesical instillation is an attractive approach in the treatment of IC for three main reasons. First, the side-effects can be minimized in intravesical therapy because of less systemic absorption. Second, the therapy may be more effective because it targets the urothelium directly where the abnormalities are believed to occur. Finally, a 'cocktail' mixture of multiple medications can be employed in intravesical instillation to provide the synergistic effect. Several agents, either single or as a mixture, have been used; however, the selection of these agents is empirical, and data on prospective and randomized studies of these agents are limited.

These medications are instilled through a urethral catheter and left in the bladder for 20–30 minutes or as long as the patient can tolerate. Although the schedule of treatment varies with each agent, the instillation is usually carried out once per week for a total 6-week period. After this initial treatment, some patients may need a maintenance schedule of instillations, usually biweekly or monthly. Intravesical instillation can also be used as an adjunct to oral therapy. A potential risk for urinary tract infections via catheterization and transient chemical cystitis, which exacerbates the symptoms, can occur.

Dimethyl sulfoxide

Besides the oral form of pentosan polysulfate, dimethyl sulfoxide (DMSO) is the only other drug approved by the FDA for the treatment of IC. DMSO is thought to improve IC symptoms through its anti-inflammatory action, mast cell inhibition, muscle relaxant effect, and sensory neuropeptide depletion of the afferent nerves. About 50 ml of a 50% DMSO solution is instilled into the bladder and held for 15–30 minutes before voiding. Instillations are performed every 1–2 weeks for a total of 4–8 treatments. Some patients may need a maintenance schedule of instillations because of relapsed symptoms. A garlic-like odor may occur in the skin or breath because DMSO is secreted through the skin and lungs. A placebo-controlled study reported a 93% objective improvement and 53% subjective improvement with DMSO compared to 35% and 18%, respectively, with saline solution.[39] DMSO is well tolerated and can induce remission in 50–70% of patients for up to 24 months. If patients do not respond to DMSO initially, the combination of DMSO with hydrocortisone, heparin, and sodium bicarbonate in the instilled solution has been recommended.[15]

Sodium pentosan polysulfate (Elmiron)

The action of sodium pentosan polysulfate is to replenish the defective GAG layer in the bladder urothelium. Because sodium pentosan polysulfate is poorly excreted in the urine (only 3%), intravesical application of this medication is expected to be more effective than the oral route. However, this effect has not been observed clinically. This agent is administered as a solution of 300 mg in 50 ml of normal saline, twice weekly for 12 weeks.[40] It has been shown that intravesical instillation of pentosan polysulfate increases the bladder capacity and improves the symptoms of IC. These improvements are similar to the oral route, but symptoms are relieved quicker with the instillation.

Steroids

Steroids such as hydrocortisone, methylprednisolone, or triamcinolone can be reconstituted in a small volume (10–15 ml) and instilled intravesically, usually in a mixture with other agents such as DMSO, heparin, or lidocaine. Steroids are thought to improve IC symptoms through their immunosuppression and anti-inflammatory properties.

Heparin

Heparin is thought to help replenish the GAG layer in the bladder urothelium, thus improving IC symptoms. In addition to this surface protective action, heparin is believed to have anti-inflammatory effects in the bladder. Heparin solution can be used alone or in a mixture with other agents. Because this medication has been shown to reduce relapses in patients who responded to DMSO, it is common for heparin and DMSO to be instilled together into the bladder. The instillation can be carried out three times per week, at a dose of 10 000 units in 10 ml of sterile water each time. When administered for 3 months, remission of symptoms was reported in 56% of patients.[41] The remission was maintained for up to 1 year in 80–90% of patients, if the treatment was continued. Recently, bladder instillation of a mixture of 40 000 units of heparin and 2% alkalinized lidocaine (lidocaine and bicarbonate) has been shown to produce immediate symptom relief in 94% of patients before heparin reaches its full effect.[42]

Local anesthetics

Local anesthetics, such as lidocaine (1%) or bupivacaine (Marcaine®, 0.5%), can be used intravesically, either as a single solution or in a mixture with other agents. These agents are administered in bicarbonate buffered solutions. The responses to lidocaine and bupivacaine are significant; however, lidocaine requires frequent instillation due to its short duration of action. Lidocaine and the longer-acting bupivacaine have been used in a variety of mixtures with other agents for bladder instillation to provide quicker relief of symptoms before these agents reach their full effect.[15,42]

Hyaluronic acid (Cystistat®)

Hyaluronic acid, which occurs naturally in human connective tissue, is another agent for intravesical therapy. When instilled into the bladder, hyaluronic acid is believed to coat the lining of the bladder and protect it from irritating substances in the urine. Hyaluronic acid can be instilled, as a 40-mg in 40 ml normal saline solution, weekly for 4–6 weeks followed by every month for 6 months, or twice weekly and then monthly when an improvement in symptoms occurs. In a small study involving 20 patients, weekly administration of hyaluronic acid decreased pain and nocturia in 30% and 40% of patients, respectively, while improving the IC symptoms in 65% of patients.[43]

Capsaicin/resiniferatoxin

Capsaicin is an extract of chili pepper that can desensitize C-fiber afferent neurons. Symptoms of IC are thought to involve the C-fibers in the bladder.[8,15] If the sensation of bladder pain mediated by these fibers can be reduced or blocked by capsaicin, then the symptoms of IC may be improved. Resiniferatoxin (RTX) is a potent analog of capsaicin that has a similar effect.

In previous studies, intravesical instillations of capsaicin or RTX have been shown to improve symptoms of IC.[15] RTX has an advantage over capsaicin because it does not cause a burning sensation with the instillation. However, a recent prospective, randomized, and placebo-controlled clinical trial involving 163 patients demonstrated that RTX is not effective for IC.[44]

Bacillus Calmette–Guérin

Bacillus Calmette–Guérin (BCG) is currently approved by the FDA for bladder cancer treatment. The mechanism of BCG action in the treatment of IC is unknown, although modulation of the host immune response by this agent has been proposed. This agent has been employed intravesically in a prospective study involving 30 patients, and showed a 60% improvement in IC symptoms versus 27% for placebo.[45] However, another study was unable to reproduce these results.[46] Recently, a prospective, randomized, and placebo-controlled study involving 248 patients showed response rates (in global assessment) of 21% for BCG and 12% for placebo.[47] Although the safety profile of BCG is acceptable and the effectiveness of this agent is confirmed, the response rate is not dramatic from a clinical standpoint.

Multimodal therapeutic strategies

More emphasis is now being placed on multimodal therapeutic approaches. Several 'cocktail' regimens, which are mixtures of different agents, have been employed empirically for bladder instillations.[15] These solutions involve lidocaine (or bupivacaine), bicarbonate, hydrocortisone (or triamcinolone), heparin, and DMSO, in a variety of mixtures, to provide immediate symptom relief as well as long-term effects. The common 'cocktail' solutions are: (1) a mixture of 50 ml of DMSO, 10 000 units of heparin, 10 mg of triamcinolone, and 44 mmol of bicarbonate that can be administered weekly for 6 weeks;[15] and (2) a mixture of 40 000 units of heparin, 8 ml of 2% lidocaine, 3 ml of 8.4% bicarbonate, and 5 ml of sterile water that can be administered three times per week for 2–3 weeks.[42] Alternatively, an oral medication can be added for a patient who has already started with intravesical therapy to enhance the effects.

Other therapies

Transcutaneous electrical nerve stimulation (TENS) has been described for the treatment of IC with some benefit.[50] This treatment modality supposedly stimulates the afferent nerves, thereby activating the inhibitory circuits and decreasing the sensation of pain. However, its exact mechanism remains unclear. Other approaches under investigation include intravesical injection of botulinum toxin and gene therapy.[51] Botulinum toxin has been shown to have some benefit in the treatment of IC;[51] however, a recent report demonstrated that intravesical injection of botulinum toxin A was not effective in eight patients who had refractory IC.[52]

REFERENCES

1. Simon LJ, Landis JR, Erickson DR, Nyberg LM. The Interstitial Cystitis Data Base Study: concepts and preliminary baseline descriptive statistics. Urology 1997; 49 (5A Suppl): 64–75.
2. Curhan GC, Speizer FE, Hunter DJ, Curhan SG, Stampfer MJ. Epidemiology of interstitial cystitis: a population based study. J Urol 1999; 161: 549–52.
3. Leppilahti M, Sairanen J, Tammela TL et al. Finnish Interstitial Cystitis-Pelvic Pain Syndrome Study Group. Prevalence of clinically confirmed interstitial cystitis in women: a population based study in Finland. J Urol 2005; 174: 581–3.
4. Rosenberg MT, Hazzard M. Prevalence of interstitial cystitis symptoms in women: a population based study in the primary care office. J Urol 2005; 174: 2231–4.
5. Parsons CL. Diagnosing chronic pelvic pain of bladder origin. J Reprod Med 2004; 49 (Suppl): 235–42.
6. Parsons CL, Dell J, Stanford EJ et al. The prevalence of interstitial cystitis in gynecologic patients with pelvic pain, as detected by intravesical potassium sensitivity. Am J Obstet Gynecol 2002; 187: 1395–400.
7. Parsons CL, Bullen M, Kahn BS, Stanford EJ, Willems JJ. Gynecologic presentation of interstitial cystitis as detected by intravesical potassium sensitivity. Obstet Gynecol 2001; 98: 127–32.
8. Chai TC. Interstitial cystitis. In: Bent AE, Ostergard DR, Cundiff GW, Swift SE, eds. Ostergard's Urogynecology and Pelvic Floor Dysfunction, 5th edn. Philadelphia: Lippincott Williams & Wilkins, 2003: 307–23.
9. Warren JW, Keay SK, Meyers D, Xu J. Concordance of interstitial cystitis in monozygotic and dizygotic twin pairs. Urology 2001; 57 (Suppl 1): 22–5.
10. Parsons CL. A model for the function of glycosaminoglycans in the urinary tract. World J Urol 1994; 12: 38–42.
11. Lilly JD, Parsons CL. Bladder surface glycosaminoglycans is a human epithelial permeability barrier. Surg Gynecol Obstet 1990; 171: 493–6.
12. Chelsky MJ, Rosen SI, Knight LC et al. Bladder permeability in interstitial cystitis is similar to that of normal volunteers: direct measurement by transvesical absorption of 99mtechnetium-diethylenetriaminepentaacetic acid. J Urol 1994; 151: 346–9.
13. Sun Y, Keay S, De Deyne PG, Chai TC. Augmented stretch activated adenosine triphosphate release from bladder uroepithelial cells in patients with interstitial cystitis. J Urol 2001; 166: 1951–6.
14. Keay SK, Zhang CO, Shoenfelt J et al. Sensitivity and specificity of antiproliferative factor, heparin-binding epidermal growth factor-like growth factor, and epidermal growth factor as urine markers for interstitial cystitis. Urology 2001; 57 (Suppl 1): 9–14.
15. Hanno PM. Interstitial cystitis and related disorders. In: Campbell MF, Walsh PC, Alan B, Retik AB, eds. Campbell's Urology, 8th edn. Philadelphia: WB Saunders, 2002: 631–70.
16. Gillenwater JY, Wein AJ. Summary of the National Institute of Arthritis, Diabetes, Digestive and Kidney Diseases Workshop on Interstitial Cystitis, National Institutes of Health, Bethesda, Maryland, August 28–29, 1987. J Urol 1988; 140: 203–6.
17. Hanno PM, Landis JR, Matthews-Cook Y, Kusek J, Nyberg L Jr. The diagnosis of interstitial cystitis revisited: lessons learned from the National Institutes of Health Interstitial Cystitis Database study. J Urol 1999; 161: 553–7.
18. Nickel JC. Interstitial cystitis: a chronic pelvic pain syndrome. Med Clin North Am 2004; 88: 467–81, xii.
19. O'Leary MP, Sant GR, Fowler FJ Jr, Whitmore KE, Spolarich-Kroll J. The interstitial cystitis symptom index and problem index. Urology 1997; 49 (5A Suppl): 58–63.
20. Clemons JL, Arya LA, Myers DL. Diagnosing interstitial cystitis in women with chronic pelvic pain. Obstet Gynecol 2002; 100: 337–41.
21. Goin JE, Olaleye D, Peters KM et al. Psychometric analysis of the University of Wisconsin Interstitial Cystitis Scale: implications for use in randomized clinical trials. J Urol 1998; 159: 1085–90.
22. Waxman JA, Sulak PJ, Kuehl TJ. Cystoscopic findings consistent with interstitial cystitis in normal women undergoing tubal ligation. J Urol 1998; 160: 1663–7.
23. Chai TC, Zhang CO, Shoenfelt JL et al. Bladder stretch alters urinary heparin-binding epidermal growth factor and antiproliferative factor in patients with interstitial cystitis. J Urol 2000; 163: 1440–4.
24. Rofeim O, Hom D, Freid RM, Moldwin RM. Use of the neodymium: YAG laser for interstitial cystitis: a prospective study. J Urol 2001; 166: 134–6.
25. Parsons CL, Greenberger M, Gabal L, Bidair M, Barme G. The role of urinary potassium in the pathogenesis and diagnosis of interstitial cystitis. J Urol 1998; 159: 1862–6; discussion 1866–7.
26. Chambers GK, Fenster HN, Cripps S, Jens M, Taylor D. An assessment of the use of intravesical potassium in the diagnosis of interstitial cystitis. J Urol 1999; 162: 699–701.
27. Teichman JM, Nielsen-Omeis BJ. Potassium leak test predicts outcome in interstitial cystitis. J Urol 1999; 161: 1791–4; discussion 1794–6. Erratum in: J Urol 1999; 162: 503.
28. Byrne DS, Sedor JF, Estojak J et al. The urinary glycoprotein GP51 as a clinical marker for interstitial cystitis. J Urol 1999; 161: 1786–90.
29. Erickson DR, Xie SX, Bhavanandan VP et al. A comparison of multiple urine markers for interstitial cystitis. J Urol 2002; 167: 2461–9.
30. Whitmore KE. Self-care regimens for patients with interstitial cystitis. Urol Clin North Am 1994; 21: 121–30.
31. Gillespie L. Metabolic appraisal of the effects of dietary modification on hypersensitive bladder symptoms. Br J Urol 1993; 72: 293–7.
32. Hanno PM. Analysis of long-term Elmiron therapy for interstitial cystitis. Urology 1997; 49 (5A Suppl): 93–9.
33. Mulholland SG, Hanno P, Parsons CL, Sant GR, Staskin DR. Pentosan polysulfate sodium for therapy of interstitial cystitis. A double-blind placebo-controlled clinical study. Urology 1990; 35: 552–8.
34. Nickel JC, Barkin J, Forrest J et al. Elmiron Study Group. Randomized, double-blind, dose-ranging study of pentosan polysulfate sodium for interstitial cystitis. Urology 2005; 65: 654–8.
35. van Ophoven A, Pokupic S, Heinecke A, Hertle L. A prospective, randomized, placebo controlled, double-blind study of amitriptyline for the treatment of interstitial cystitis. J Urol 2004; 172: 533–6.
36. van Ophoven A, Hertle L. Long-term results of amitriptyline treatment for interstitial cystitis. J Urol 2005; 174: 1837–40.
37. Theoharides TC, Sant GR. Hydroxyzine therapy for interstitial cystitis. Urology 1997; 49 (5A Suppl): 108–10.
38. Sasaki K, Smith CP, Chuang YC et al. Oral gabapentin (neurontin) treatment of refractory genitourinary tract pain. Tech Urol 2001; 7: 47–9.

39. Perez-Marrero R, Emerson LE, Feltis JT. A controlled study of dimethyl sulfoxide in interstitial cystitis. J Urol 1988; 140: 36–9.

40. Bade JJ, Laseur M, Nieuwenburg A, van der Weele LT, Mensink HJ. A placebo-controlled study of intravesical pentosanpolysulphate for the treatment of interstitial cystitis. Br J Urol 1997; 79: 168–71.

41. Parsons CL, Housley T, Schmidt JD, Lebow D. Treatment of interstitial cystitis with intravesical heparin. Br J Urol 1994; 73: 504–7.

42. Parsons CL. Successful downregulation of bladder sensory nerves with combination of heparin and alkalinized lidocaine in patients with interstitial cystitis. Urology 2005; 65: 45–8.

43. Kallestrup EB, Jorgensen SS, Nordling J, Hald T. Treatment of interstitial cystitis with Cystistat: a hyaluronic acid product. Scand J Urol Nephrol 2005; 39: 143–7.

44. Payne CK, Mosbaugh PG, Forrest JB et al. ICOS RTX Study Group (Resiniferatoxin Treatment for Interstitial Cystitis). Intravesical resiniferatoxin for the treatment of interstitial cystitis: a randomized, double-blind, placebo controlled trial. J Urol 2005; 173: 1590–4.

45. Peters K, Diokno A, Steinert B et al. The efficacy of intravesical Tice strain bacillus Calmette-Guerin in the treatment of interstitial cystitis: a double-blind, prospective, placebo controlled trial. J Urol 1997; 157: 2090–4.

46. Peeker R, Haghsheno MA, Holmang S, Fall M. Intravesical bacillus Calmette-Guerin and dimethyl sulfoxide for treatment of classic and nonulcer interstitial cystitis: a prospective, randomized double-blind study. J Urol 2000; 164: 1912–15; discussion 1915–16.

47. Mayer R, Propert KJ, Peters KM et al. Interstitial Cystitis Clinical Trials Group. A randomized controlled trial of intravesical bacillus calmette-guerin for treatment refractory interstitial cystitis. J Urol 2005; 173: 1186–91.

48. Comiter CV. Sacral neuromodulation for the symptomatic treatment of refractory interstitial cystitis: a prospective study. J Urol 2003; 169: 1369–73.

49. Whitmore KE, Payne CK, Diokno AC, Lukban JC. Sacral neuromodulation in patients with interstitial cystitis: a multicenter clinical trial. Int Urogynecol J Pelvic Floor Dysfunct 2003; 14: 305–8; discussion 308–9.

50. Fall M, Lindstrom S. Transcutaneous electrical nerve stimulation in classic and nonulcer interstitial cystitis. Urol Clin North Am 1994; 21: 131–9.

51. Chancellor MB, Yoshimura N. Treatment of interstitial cystitis. Urology 2004; 63 (Suppl 1): 85–92.

52. Kuo HC. Preliminary results of suburothelial injection of botulinum a toxin in the treatment of chronic interstitial cystitis. Urol Int 2005; 75: 170–4.

17 Non-invasive management of pelvic organ prolapse

Mat H Ho and Narender N Bhatia

INTRODUCTION

In the United States and other developed countries, women are expected to spend a significant part of their life in the postmenopausal years, a period when pelvic organ prolapses (POPs) are more likely to occur.[1] POP is the abnormal protrusion of the pelvic organs from their normal locations into or out of the vaginal canal. These abnormalities, which result from defects of the pelvic support, include anterior compartment prolapse such as cystocele or urethrocele, posterior compartment prolapse such as rectocele or enterocele, and apical problems such as uterine or vaginal vault prolapse. Enterocele can also occur with defects of the anterior and apical compartments. These conditions often occur in combinations of various defects and/or in coexistence with urinary incontinence.

Although POP seldom leads to serious medical illness, it may have a major impact on the patient's quality of life. Significant morbidity can occur with POP, including alterations in bladder, bowel, or sexual function. These patients often suffer from urinary frequency, urgency, and/or incontinence, fecal incontinence, constipation, and decrease in sexual activity. The POP conditions are also associated with loss of self-esteem, social isolation, depression, and other psychological burdens.

CLASSIFICATION AND QUANTIFICATION OF PELVIC ORGAN PROLAPSE

Standardized description and classification of POP are important in the documentation and communication of the problem as well as in establishing guidelines for treatment. Although the traditional descriptions of POP have been widely used, compartmental and site-specific descriptions are now advocated. Methods for clinical grading or staging of POP, which include the halfway system, the modification system, and the Pelvic Organ Prolapse Quantification (POPQ) system, are also critical in the evaluation and treatment of these problems.

Classification and description of pelvic organ prolapse

Traditional classification

Traditionally, POP referred to displacement of the bladder, urethra, uterus, vaginal vault, rectum, or bowel from its normal position into or out of the vaginal canal. *Cystocele* is protrusion of the bladder into or out of the vaginal canal that results from tearing or weakening of the supporting structure in the anterior vaginal wall. The bladder bulging should be beyond its normal limit, which is usually the mid-portion of the vagina. *Urethrocele* results from protrusion of the urethra into the vaginal canal and is also associated with anterior vaginal wall defects. *Cystourethrocele* is the term used when it is difficult to discriminate between prolapse of the urethra and of the bladder. It is also used for a cystocele that includes the urethra as part of the prolapsing complex. *Rectocele* is protrusion of the rectum into or out of the vaginal canal and associated with posterior vaginal wall defects. *Enterocele* involves protrusion of bowel into or out of the vagina, in which the peritoneum is in contact with the vaginal mucosa and the normal intervening endopelvic fascia is absent. Upper posterior vaginal wall prolapse is nearly always associated with herniation of the pouch of Douglas containing loops of bowel, thus forming an enterocele. Defects in the upper anterior wall and apex of the vagina also predispose to enterocele.

Uterine prolapse is protrusion of the cervix/uterus into or out of the vaginal canal and associated with apical defects of the vagina. Since the uterus cannot descend without carrying some parts of the upper, anterior, or posterior vaginal walls with it, concomitant defects of these compartments can occur. *Procidentia* (or total uterine prolapse) represents failure of all the pelvic supports and the uterus protrudes completely out of the vaginal canal. Hypertrophy, elongation, congestion, and edema of the cervix may sometimes cause a large protrusion of tissue beyond the introitus, which may be mistaken for a procidentia. *Vaginal vault prolapse* occurs in post-hysterectomy patients and results

Table 17.1   Different Types of Pelvic Organ Prolapse

Anterior compartment prolapse
- Cystocele
- Urethrocele
- Cystourethrocele
- Anterior enterocele

Apical prolapse
- Uterovaginal prolapse/uterine prolapse
- Vaginal vault prolapse
- Apical enterocele

Posterior compartment prolapse
- Rectocele
- Enterocele

from protrusion of the vaginal apex into the vaginal canal or total inversion through the vagina.

Compartmental classification

The traditional descriptive terms for POP are convenient, but can be inaccurate and misleading because they imply an unrealistic certainty as to the prolapsing structures underneath the bulging vaginal wall. For example, it is often difficult to discriminate between a high rectocele and an enterocele or to distinguish an anterior enterocele from a high cystocele on physical examination. The traditional terms focus on the bladder, urethra, uterus, or rectum rather than on the site-specific defects responsible for the prolapse. Descriptions of POP based on compartmental defects are, therefore, being advocated in order to avoid erroneous assumptions regarding the prolapsing ogans, unless the involved organs are identified by ancillary tests. In the compartmental classification, anterior vaginal wall (or anterior compartment) prolapse is used instead of cystocele, urethrocele, or anterior enterocele (Table 17.1). Likewise, posterior vaginal wall (or posterior compartment) prolapse is preferable to rectocele or enterocele, and apical prolapse is used instead of vaginal vault prolapse or apical enterocele.

According to the International Continence Society (ICS) standardization of terminology,[6] anterior vaginal wall prolapse is defined as any descent of the anterior vagina so that the urethrovesical junction, or any midline point on the anterior vaginal wall proximal to this junction, is less than 3 cm above the plane of the hymen. Posterior vaginal wall prolapse is defined as any descent of the posterior vagina so that a midline point on the posterior vaginal wall is 3 cm above the level of the hymen, or any point proximal to this is less than 3 cm above the plane of the hymen. Prolapse

of the apical segment of the vagina is defined as any descent of the cervix, or vaginal cuff scar (for posthysterectomy), below a point which is 2 cm less than the total vaginal length above the hymenal plane. These definitions and use of the Pelvic Organ Prolapse Quantification (POPQ) system described below provide a more accurate way to describe POP problems.

Quantification of pelvic organ prolapse

Grading or staging of POP is important for documentation, communication, correlation of symptoms with severity of the prolapse, following the patient longitudinally, and assessment of treatment outcomes. Although multiple grading schemes have been proposed, two widely used methods are the halfway system[7] and the modification system.[8] Recently, the Pelvic Organ Prolapse Quantification system was developed for staging the problem more accurately and reproducibly.[8,9]

The halfway system

The halfway system was developed by Baden and Walker in 1968 and revised in 1992.[7] This grading system has been widely employed in clinical practice for describing the severity of POP. The hymen is chosen as a reference, and the most dependent position of the pelvic organs during maximal straining is used for grading. Grade 0 represents normal position and grade 4 is the maximum possible descent of the prolapse (Table 17.2). Prolapse halfway to the hymen is considered to be grade 1, at the hymen is grade 2, and halfway past the hymen is grade 3. If there is any doubt the patient should be regraded in a standing position, and when a decision has to be made between two grades, the greater grade should be used. If multiple sites of defects occur together, the worst grade of the worst site is employed for quantification. This system is simple and useful in the grading of POP for clinical practice; however, it does not provide an exact measurement of the prolapse but rather an estimate of

Table 17.2   The Halfway System for Clinical Grading of Pelvic Organ Prolapse

Grade	Description
0	No descent (normal position for each respective site)
1	Descent halfway to the hymen
2	Descent to the hymen
3	Descent halfway past the hymen
4	Maximum of possible descent for each site

descent of the involved structures proximal or distal to the hymen.

The modification system

The Beecham system for grading POP was introduced in 1980.[10] The reference for this system is the introitus and the prolapse is expressed as first degree, second degree, and third degree. Prolapse above or to the introitus is considered to be first degree, between the introitus and complete eversion is second degree, and at complete eversion is third degree. In this system, the prolapse that is visible at the introitus by depressing the perineum should be considered first degree. The major drawback of this system is that the patient is not allowed to strain during the examination. All other grading systems require maximal straining or standing position to reproduce the prolapse. The use of introitus for a reference point is also not as reproducible as the hymen ring.

In order to avoid these problems but keep the simplicity of the grading system, several modifications have been made over the years. One proposed system, which was modified from the Beecham and Baden–Walker methods, is simple to use and has reasonable interobserver variability.[8] This system classifies cystocele, uterine or vaginal vault prolapse, and rectocele into first degree, second degree, and third degree as explained in Table 17.3. The most dependent position of the pelvic organs during maximal straining or standing is used, and the hymen is employed as a reference point. First degree is when the prolapse descends halfway to the hymen, second degree is when it extends to the hymen, and third degree is when it protrudes beyond the hymen. The classification of rectocele is aided by performing a rectovaginal examination. For enterocele, the presence and depth of the enterocele sac, relative to the hymen, is described. The terms grade and degree are sometimes used interchangeably in this system.

The POPQ system

The Pelvic Organ Prolapse Quantification (POPQ) system,[8,9] which has been adopted by the ICS, the American Urogynecologic Society (AUGS), and the Society of Gynecologic Surgeons (SGS), provides a precise description of the prolapse; however, it is complicated for routine use. There are six points within the vaginal canal (two on the anterior wall, two on the apex, and two on the posterior wall) to be located and measured with reference to the plane of the hymen (Figure 17.1). On the midline of the anterior vaginal

Table 17.3 The Modification System for Clinical Grading of Pelvic Organ Prolapse

A. Modification with grades 0 to 4

Grade	Description
0	No descent
1	Descent between normal position and ischial spines
2	Descent between ischial spines and hymen
3	Descent within hymen
4	Descent through hymen

B. Modification with degrees 1 to 3

1. Cystocele, rectocele, uterine prolapse, or vaginal vault prolapse

First degree: Descent halfway to the hymen
Second degree: Descent to the hymen
Third degree: Descent beyond the hymen

2. Enterocele

The presence and depth of the enterocele sac, relative to the hymen, should be described anatomically, with the patient in the supine and standing positions during Valsalva maneuver

wall, point Aa is 3 cm proximal to the external urethral meatus and point Ba is the most distal (or most dependent) position of any part of the anterior vaginal wall segment between the anterior vaginal fornix (or vaginal cuff) and point Aa. On the midline of the posterior vaginal wall, point Ap is 3 cm proximal to the hymen, and point Bp represents the most distal (or most dependent) position of any part of the posterior vaginal wall segment between the posterior vaginal fornix (or vaginal cuff) and point Ap. By definition, the ranges of points Aa and Ap relative to the hymen are from −3 cm for normal support to +3 cm for complete eversion of the vagina.

On the vaginal apex, point C is the most distal (or most dependent) edge of the cervix or the leading edge of the vaginal cuff (in patients who have had a hysterectomy), and point D represents the location of the posterior vaginal fornix. Point D is omitted in the absence of the cervix. Genital hiatus (gh) is measured from the middle of the external urethral meatus to the posterior midline of the hymen. The perineal body (pb) is measured from the posterior margin of the vagina to the middle of the anal opening. The total vaginal length (tvl) is the greatest depth of the vagina when point C or D is reduced to its full normal position.

All measurements of points Aa, Ba, C, D, Ap, and Bp are in centimeters and expressed as negative if above (proximal) and positive if below (distal) to the hymen ring. The lengths of gh, pb, and tvl are also measured

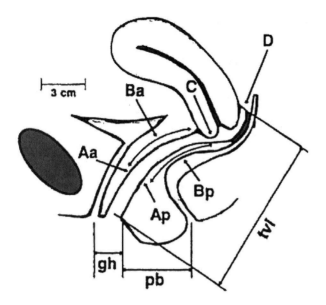

Figure 17.1 Diagrammatic representation of the Pelvic Organ Prolapse Quantification (POPQ) System. Six sites (Aa, Ba, C, D, Bp, and Ap), genital hiatus (gh), perineal body (pb), and total vaginal length (tvl) are used for pelvic organ prolapse quantification. (Reproduced from Bump RC, Mattiasson A, Bo K, Brubaker LP, DeLancey JO, Klarskov P, Shull BL, Smith AR. The standardization of terminology of female pelvic organ prolapse and pelvic floor dysfunction. Am J Obstet Gynecol. 1996; 175: 10–17).

Table 17.4 The Pelvic Organ Prolapse Quantification (POPQ) System for Clinical Staging of Pelvic Organ Prolapse

Stage	Description
0	No prolapse is demonstrated. Points Aa, Ap, Ba, and Bp are all at -3 cm and either point C or D is at no more than $-(X-2)$ cm (a)
I	The most distal portion (leading edge) of the prolapse is less than -1 cm (b) and the criteria for stage 0 are not met
II	The most distal portion of the prolapse is at least -1 cm but no more than $+1$ cm (c)
III	The most distal portion of the prolapse is greater than $+1$ cm but less than $+ (X-2)$ cm (a, d)
IV	The most distal portion of the prolapse is at least $+ (X-2)$ cm (a, e)

(From Bump RC, Mattiasson A, Bo K, Brubaker LP, DeLancey JO, Klarskov P, Shull BL, Smith AR. The standardization of terminology of female pelvic organ prolapse and pelvic floor dysfunction. Am J Obstet Gynecol. 1996; 175: 10-17.)

Note: (a) X is the total vaginal length in centimeter; (b) The leading edge of the prolapse locates more than 1 cm above the level of the hymen; (c) The leading edge of the prolapse locates between the points of less than 1 cm proximal to 1 cm distal to the level of the hymen; (d) The leading edge of the prolapse locates at more than 1 cm below the plane of the hymen but protrudes no further than 2 cm less than the total vaginal length; (e) The leading edge of the prolapse protrudes to at least 2 cm less than the total vaginal length.

in centimeters. A diagram and grid are used to describe the result showing normal support or defects (Figure 17.2). These measurements can also be converted to a staging system from 0 to IV as shown in Table 17.4. An easy way to remember this staging system is that grade 0 represents no descensus while stage IV is completely everted. A prolapse where its leading edge is at or between 1 cm above and 1 cm below the hymen ring represents stage II. Grades I and III are in between. The good reproducibility of the POPQ system is reflected by a highly significant correlation between interobserver and intraobserver examinations.[11] Although a valuable tool for the quantification of POP in both research and patient care, the POPQ system tends to be complicated and confusing for general use in clinical practice.

PATHOPHYSIOLOGY

Pelvic support defects

The problems of pelvic support are often referred to as pelvic floor defects, which is more accurate than the term pelvic relaxation that has been used previously.

Pelvic support defects can occur secondary to damage to the pelvic floor structures including muscles, endopelvic fascia, and their innervations. When the pelvic floor structures are damaged or weakened, pelvic organs can descend and cause further attenuation in the endopelvic fasciae. Eventually, these fasciae and their connections can break, allowing the pelvic organs to protrude through and contact the vaginal mucosa, thus causing prolapses in the apex, anterior, or posterior compartments. Most women with POP have multiple defects; however, these defects can be described separately for the apex, anterior, and posterior compartments.

Apical defects

Defects in the apical compartment can produce uterine prolapse or vaginal vault prolapse. These defects are usually located at the insertions of the cardinal–uterosacral ligament complex, pubocervical fascia, and rectovaginal fascia to the pericervical ring. In post-hysterectomy, the defects can also occur at the connection of the pubocervical and rectovaginal fasciae in the vaginal cuff. Although vaginal prolapse can occur without uterine prolapse, the uterus cannot descend

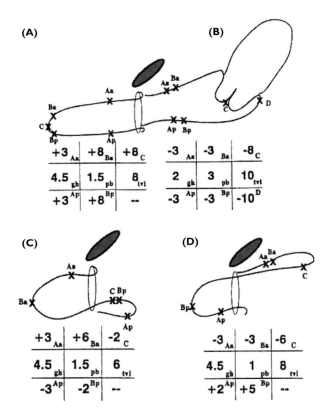

(A)   (B)

(C)   (D)

Figure 17.2 Line and grid diagram for description of pelvic organ prolapse (A) Line and grid diagram of complete eversion of vagina. Most distal point of anterior wall (Ba), vaginal cuff scar (C), and most distal point of the posterior wall (Bp) are all at the same position (+8). (B) Line and grid diagram of normal support. Points Aa and Ba and points Ap and Bp are all –3 because there is no anterior or posterior wall descent. (C) Line and grid diagram of predominant anterior support defect. Leading point of prolapse is upper anterior vaginal wall, point Ba (+6). (D) Line and grid)diagram of predominant posterior support defect. Leading point of prolapse is upper posterior vaginal wall, point Bp (+5). (Reproduced from Bump RC, Mattiasson A, Bo K, Brubaker LP, DeLancey JO, Klarskov P, Shull BL, Smith AR. The standardization of terminology of female pelvic organ prolapse and pelvic floor dysfunction. Am J Obstet Gynecol. 1996; 175: 10–17.)

without carrying some parts of the anterior or posterior vaginal walls with it. Due to these associations, uterine prolapse is probably the most troubling type of POP. These patients may have some degree of high cystocele, high rectocele, and enterocele together with the apical prolapse.

In patients whose uterus remains intact, apical enterocele usually occurs secondary to the detachment of rectovaginal fascia from the pericervical ring. The peritoneum is in contact with the vaginal mucosa, which can be stretched with time, forming an enterocele. The enterocele bulges out from the top of vagina, when the patient is in the upright position, and the entrapped

Table 17.5 Pessary Selection for Pelvic Organ Prolapse

For anterior vaginal wall prolapse such as cystocele
- Ring with/without support
- Hodge
- Gehrung
- Donut

For apical prolapse such as vaginal vault prolapse or uterine prolapse
A. First and second degrees
  - Ring with/without support
  - Shaatz
B. Third degree and procidentia
  - Gellhorn
  - Donut
  - Cube
  - Infl atoball

For posterior vaginal wall prolapse such as rectocele
- Donut
- Ring
- Risser
- Gehrung
- Gellhorn

loops of small intestine can cause pain and pressure. These enterocele sacs are located posterior to the cervix and anterior to the rectum. For patients who have had a hysterectomy, an enterocele develops when the pubocervical and rectovaginal fasciae are separated, thus allowing peritoneum and bowel to protrude through. Enteroceles in these patients can occur anterior to, posterior to, or at the vaginal apex.

Anterior vaginal wall defects

The intact pubocervical fascia and its attachments, which support the bladder and urethra, prevent anterior vaginal wall prolapse, such as cystocele or urethrocele, occurring. Anterior compartment defects can be a result of overstretching and attenuation, which are often referred as distension of the anterior vaginal wall. The underlying pubocervical fascia are usually very thin throughout or lost in the midline, resulting in an absence of rugal folds of the vaginal epithelium. Another type are site-specific defects, which can be paravaginal, transverse, or midline (Table 17.5). Site-specific defects often coexist with some degree of distension in the anterior vaginal wall.

The underlying breaks in the pubocervical fascia occur more commonly at peripheral attachments than at central locations. Paravaginal defects occur at the attachments of the pubocervical fascia to the arcus tendineus fascia pelvis, and can be a partial disruption or complete detachment from the fascial white lines. They can also occur unilaterally or bilaterally. Transverse defects occur when the pubocervical fascia is separated from its insertion into the pericervical ring and/or its connection to the cardinal–uterosacral ligament complex. Midline defects represent an anteroposterior break in the pubocervical fascia and usually occur around the bladder neck and proximal urethra. The vaginal epithelium is often smooth without rugae because there is no underlying pubocervical fascia. Defects in the anterior vaginal wall are often associated with stress urinary incontinence.

An anterior enterocele due to prolapse of the upper anterior wall can occur. This is usually seen in patients who have had a hysterectomy and retropubic colposuspension or sacrospinous fixation without attention to reconstruction of the pericervical ring.

Posterior vaginal wall defects

The rectovaginal fascia connects to the pericervical ring superiorly and extends downward from the cardinal–uterosacral ligament complex to the perineal body inferiorly and the fascial white line laterally. Rectocele is bulging in the posterior vaginal wall, and is caused by breaks in the rectovaginal fascia and/or its connections, with the anterior wall of the rectum in direct apposition to the vaginal epithelium. It is basically a defect of the rectovaginal fascia, not the rectum. Similar to the anterior compartment, the vaginal epithelium is smooth without rugae if there is no underlying rectovaginal fascia.

The rectovaginal fascia is normally fused with the perineal body at the lower end, and the vast majority of rectoceles occur secondary to the tear along this attachment. In addition to midline defects in the posterior vaginal wall, detachments of the rectovaginal fascia along the arcus tendineus fasciae rectovaginalis and breaks at the pericervical ring insertion are responsible for lateral and transverse defects, respectively. All of these defects can form rectoceles. However, detachment of the rectovaginal fascia from its posterior insertion into the pericervical ring also allows the peritoneum to herniate into the upper third of the vagina, resulting in an enterocele which can mimic high rectocele and should be differentiated with a rectovaginal examination.

EVALUATION AND DIAGNOSIS

Clinical presentation

Mild degrees of POP are usually asymptomatic, although their signs are frequently observed.[12] In general, patients with POP may complain of symptoms directly caused by vaginal protrusions or symptoms related to the prolapse. Direct symptoms include vaginal mass or bulge, pelvic pressure, low abdominal or back pain, and coital difficulty. Associated symptoms can be urinary frequency, urgency, or incontinence, voiding difficulty, constipation, fecal incontinence, or inability to evacuate the rectum completely without straining or splinting. In many patients, the symptoms of POP are non-specific. Often there is a feeling of heaviness or fullness in the pelvis, or feeling of something protruding from the vagina. Patients may describe something falling out or a bearing-down discomfort. Characteristic of nearly all symptoms is that they are less noticeable in the morning, worsen as the day progresses or after prolonged standing or walking, and are relieved by lying down.

Although symptoms associated with a specific type of POP are not well characterized, defects in the anterior vaginal wall often lead to bladder neck and urethral hypermobility, which may cause stress urinary incontinence. A large anterior vaginal prolapse can also compress the urethra causing obstructional, incomplete, or intermittent bladder emptying. Some patients may require manual displacement of the prolapse in order to void. These patients may have recurrent urinary tract infections. Other patients may describe that their urinary incontinence has been resolved since the time their prolapse became worse. The resolution of urinary incontinence is secondary to the urethral kinking caused by advanced prolapse.

Defects in the apical compartment of the vagina can also cause stress urinary incontinence because uterine prolapse and vaginal vault eversion often have a concomitant descent of the anterior vaginal wall. Obstructive voiding and urinary retention as well as masking of urinary incontinence may occur with uterine or vaginal vault prolapses. The protruding cervix or vagina can cause vaginal spotting or purulent discharge from their ulceration. Neglected cases of procidentia may be complicated by bleeding and, rarely, carcinoma of the cervix. In posterior vaginal wall defects, patients with a rectocele may have difficulty in emptying the rectum and complain of the need to splint the posterior vagina in order to evacuate the trapped stool.

Examination

General and vaginal examinations

The general physical examination should include height and weight for body mass index calculation, because obesity is a promoting factor for POP. The examination should also include evaluations of the cardiac, pulmonary, abdominal, extremities, skin, and neurologic systems to detect medical conditions such as musculoskeletal disorders, connective tissue diseases, neurologic disorders, and pulmonary diseases that may affect the pelvic floor support.

Vaginal examinations are conducted with the patient in the lithotomy position. External genitalia, estrogen status, and caliber of the introitus and the vagina are assessed. Signs of hypoestrogenism, such as loss of rugae in the vaginal mucosa, decreased secretions, thin perineal skin, and easy perineal tearing should be investigated. Vaginal rugae are the irregular surface of the epithelium due to variations in its thickness caused by contraction and tension of the smooth muscles and elastin fibers within the collagen matrix of the underlying visceral fascia. In addition to the demonstration of a well estrogenized epithelium, vaginal rugations also reflect intact and healthy underlying endopelvic fascia. In postmenopausal women or patients with marked vaginal atrophy, topical estrogen can be used for 4–6 weeks to restore prominent rugae before determining the status of the underlying endopelvic fascia. In a bimanual examination, the uterus and adnexa are palpated for masses, mobility, and tenderness.

Pelvic organ prolapse examinations

Systematic evaluation   A systemic pelvic support examination should be part of the evaluation. The examination is usually carried out first in the dorsal lithotomy position. The prolapse is inspected, and if no bulging is apparent, the labia are spread to expose the vestibule and the hymen. After evaluation in the resting condition, the patient is asked to strain vigorously, because observing the maximal amount of prolapse is critical in the staging of POP and planning treatment. It is useful to ask the patient to confirm the maximal extent of her prolapse with a handheld mirror during the examination. The patient is then examined in the standing position, because the degree of prolapse is almost invariably worse when the patient is upright. Standing is also a position when symptoms of the prolapse occur in the patient's daily life. A standing pelvic examination can be conducted quickly and efficiently with one of the patient's feet elevated on a well-supported footstool and the examination gown lifted slightly to expose the genital region. For POPQ staging, dorsal lithotomy can be used, because studies have shown that results obtained in this position are highly correlated with results obtained in the standing position.[41]

The traditional speculum examination of the vagina should be supplemented with a site-specific evaluation using a Sims retractor or the lower blade of a Graves speculum. Systematic examinations of the apical, anterior, and posterior compartments of the vagina as well as the perineal body and the perineum are important, particularly when the nature of a prolapse is unclear. Because multiple sites of defects can occur simultaneously, an examination of this kind will allow these defects to be identified before surgery, thus helping to facilitate concomitant repairs of all defects and, therefore, minimizing the chance of treatment failure. It is also important to palpate the thickness of the underlying endopelvic fascia.

Vaginal apex   For the examination of apical defects, a bivalve speculum is used to visualize the cervix or vaginal apex, and, with the patient straining maximally, the speculum is withdrawn slowly while observing any descent of the cervix or vaginal cuff. The anterior and posterior fornices are inspected at rest and during Valsalva maneuvers. If the anterior and posterior fornices of the vagina bulge down significantly when the patient strains, detachments of the pubocervical and rectovaginal fasciae as well as the cardinal–uterosacral ligament complex from the pericervical ring are expected. Because of these detachments, the cervix demonstrates wide lateral mobility.

After inspections with the speculum, digital examination is performed. With gentle traction on the cervix along the longitudinal axis of the vaginal canal, the thick and firm uterosacral ligaments can normally be palpated as they insert onto the posterolateral aspect of the pericervical ring. These ligaments can also be appreciated during a gentle rectal examination, with cervical traction, as well as examination under anesthesia. When uterosacral ligaments become detached from the pericervical ring in patients with uterine or vaginal vault prolapse, a thin, empty line is felt in the examination. In vaginal vault prolapse, the pubocervical and rectovaginal fasciae are detached from each other and the underlying support feels very thin with no intervening visceral fascia. The overlying vaginal epithelium is smooth and without rugae. Vaginal vault prolapse usually involves apical enterocele.

Anterior vaginal wall   The anterior vaginal wall is examined with the patient in maximal straining, while the posterior wall is retracted, to allow optimal visualization of the bulging. Anterior compartment defects usually involve bladder descent with or without urethral protrusion. Scarring, tenderness, and rigidity of the urethra from previous vaginal surgeries or pelvic trauma should be noted. A bulging down of the vaginal apex and loss of anterior fornix may occur together with anterior compartment prolapse. Anterolateral sulci going from the mid-vagina back toward the ischial spines should be visualized, unless lateral defects are present. Palpation of the bulging tissues for their thickness is also important in assessment of the prolapse.

If cystocele is observed, midline defects should be distinguished from paravaginal defects. One simple way to do this is to support the lateral walls with a ring forceps. With an opened ring forceps inserted over the speculum blade until the tips are against the bilateral ischial spines, the anterior vaginal wall is observed with maximal straining. If the cystocele resolves, the defect is paravaginal. If the cystocele persists, the defect is midline, existing either in isolation or with a paravaginal defect. The next maneuver is to relieve the lateral support and use a closed ring forceps to support the midline of the anterior wall. If the cystocele resolves while the patient is maximally straining, the defect is most likely midline. If the cystocele persists, a combination of central and paravaginal defects may be present. Usually, loss of rugae of the anterior wall in a well estrogenized vagina is suggestive of a central defect, and collapsing side walls during bivalve speculum examination with maximal straining is suggestive of a paravaginal defect. With maximal straining, a paravaginal defect can also be detected by observing the absence of one or both anterolateral sulci, while in the central defect these sulci are usually well preserved. Because most midline defects occur around the bladder neck and urethra, placing a small and well lubricated dilator in the urethra can help to feel the thinness of the involved tissues.

In a transverse defect caused by detachment of the pubocervical fascia from the anterior margin of the pericervical ring, a distinct bulging out of the anterior vaginal fornix is observed. If the transverse defect is caused by detachment of the uterosacral ligament from the pericervical ring, a significant cervical or vaginal vault descensus can be observed, with no uterosacral ligaments being palpable near the pericervical ring. The bulging in a transverse defect normally has poor rugations due to the loss of underlying pubocervical fascia. It should be noted that an anterior enterocele due to prolapse of the upper anterior vaginal wall can mimic a cystocele on physical examination. After inspection, the anterior vaginal wall, bladder, and urethra should be palpated for tenderness or masses.

Posterior vaginal wall   The posterior vaginal wall is examined for defects while the anterior wall is retracted and the patient is in maximal straining. Sometimes, the lateral walls need to be supported in order to provide a better view for these examinations. Rectocele is

suspected by the observation of posterior vaginal wall bulging and confirmed with an anterior displacement of the rectal wall on rectovaginal examination. On inspection of the lateral vaginal walls in a woman without pelvic prolapse, the anterolateral and posterolateral sulci travel together from the ischial spines to the mid-vagina where they begin to separate. The anterolateral sulcus travels toward the pubic arch, while the posterolateral sulcus, which represents the line of attachment of the rectovaginal fascia to the arcus tendineus fasciae rectovaginalis, courses down toward the perineal body. In patients with posterior vaginal wall prolapse, the disappearance of these sulci suggests lateral defects and the loss of rugations indicates central defects. The upper part of the posterior vaginal wall should be checked with a rectovaginal examination for an enterocele, especially in patients who have undergone hysterectomy. Rectovaginal examination is useful to demonstrate a rectocele, by palpating the thickness and mobility of the rectovaginal fascia, and to distinguish it from an enterocele. Occult enterocele in the cul-de-sac can also be palpated between the thumb and forefinger during a rectovaginal examination while the patient is in maximal straining.

The size and muscle tone of the pubococcygeus and puborectalis muscles are examined by placing one or two fingers within the lower third of the vaginal canal. The medial edge of the pubococcygeus muscle is usually felt at the level of the hymen ring. The patient is then asked to tighten the levator ani muscles around the examining fingers in order to grade the strength and quality of pelvic floor contractions.

Anorectal canal and perineal body   Finally, the anorectal canal and external sphincter tone are assessed with a rectal examination. The strength and position of the levator plate should also be assessed. When contracted, the levator plate can be easily palpated with an impressive strength against the examining finger, and it should be almost horizontal in the standing position. However, in the dorsal lithotomy position, the levator plate presents in a more vertical fashion. If the levator plate is weak and inclined downward, the levator hiatus is widened, thus predisposing to POP (Figure 17.2). This also increases the shear stress on the intact visceral pelvic support structures, especially the cardinal–uterosacral ligament complex.

The perineal body can be palpated as the examining finger moves through the anal canal toward the rectum. The apex of the perineal body is usually at the level of the mid-vagina. An intact perineal body is attached to the rectovaginal fascia, which connects to the uterosacral ligament bilaterally, and makes the perineum concave in appearance. Any significant break in these connections will result in a descent and bulging of the perineal body that can be felt by rectal examination. Such examination can also detect perineal rectocele if the rectal muscularis is in direct contact with the perineal skin without any underlying fascia. Perineal rectocele occurs secondary to disruptions in the integrity of the perineal body and the involved muscles, such as the superficial transverse perinei, the pubocavernosus, and the levator ani. Significant bulging of a perineal rectocele can be demonstrated with a Valsalva maneuver, and the covering skin is usually smooth and stretched.

Potential incontinence   Potential incontinence (or masked incontinence) refers to the stress urinary incontinence that develops only after reduction of the prolapse. POP, particularly prolapse of the apical and anterior vaginal walls, can kink the urethra and, therefore, mask the incontinence. In the preoperative evaluation of patients with POP for surgical treatment, potential incontinence must always be ruled out.

To test for potential incontinence, the patient should have a full bladder. If necessary, the bladder can be filled to maximum capacity (at least 300 ml) with sterile water or normal saline while reducing the prolapse with an appropriately fitted pessary in the vagina. The patient is then asked to cough or perform a Valsalva maneuver. If urinary leakage is observed, potential incontinence is confirmed and urodynamic studies should be performed to determine whether the incontinence is secondary to bladder neck hypermobility or intrinsic sphincter deficiency. This determination is important because intrinsic sphincter deficiency requires a different type of surgical treatment than bladder neck hypermobility. Urodynamic studies also help to rule out detrusor overactivity, which is often caused by bladder outlet obstruction secondary to the prolapse. Other ancillary tests, such as cotton swab testing for bladder neck mobility and the measurement of post-void residual volume, are also very useful (Chapter 15).

Other investigations   Other diagnostic tests may be needed in addition to a careful history and physical examination. In patients with complaints of urinary frequency, urgency, or incontinence, urinalysis should be performed to rule out urinary tract infection. Cervical cultures are indicated in patients who present with ulcerations or purulent discharge. A Pap smear, endometrial biopsy, or biopsy of the ulceration may be necessary in rare cases of suspected carcinoma. Patients who present with vaginal bleeding or spotting should also have an endometrial biopsy. Although rarely

needed, cystourethroscopy can allow examination inside the urethra, urethrovesical junction, bladder walls, and ureteral orifices to determine bladder stones, malignancies, diverticula, or sutures from previous surgery. Cystourethroscopy is usually reserved for patients with confounding factors such as microscopic or macroscopic hematuria, bladder pain on palpation, suburethral mass, or persistent urinary tract infections despite adequate therapy.

Imaging studies including ultrasonography, computed tomography (CT) scan, and magnetic resonance imaging (MRI) are useful in the determination of POP. The CT scan and sector, real-time, or three-dimensional ultrasonography have been employed to provide anatomic details of the pelvic floor support. MRI is an emerging technique for the study of pelvic floor dysfunction and holds promise due to its excellent ability to differentiate soft tissues.[42] However, their use is currently limited to research rather than clinical practice due to the cost and lack of standardized criteria for the diagnosis of POP.

It is also important to measure quality of life in women with pelvic floor disorders when planning treatment and evaluating the efficacy of a particular therapy. Two instruments, the Pelvic Floor Distress Inventory (PFDI) and the Pelvic Floor Impact Questionnaire (PFIQ), have been developed and validated for these purposes.[43,44] These questionnaires allow the inclusion of the patient's perception of POP into the overall assessment. They can be administered in the clinic or office setting.

NON-INVASIVE TREATMENT

Generally, patients with asymptomatic or mild POP do not require treatment. Treatments for symptomatic POP include conservative management and surgical intervention. The patient's baseline functions and medical conditions as well as the severity of the prolapse, rather than age alone, should be the guidelines in selecting treatment.

Although surgery has long been considered the mainstay of treatment for POP, non-surgical interventions can alleviate or improve symptoms for a substantial number of patients. Unless extenuating circumstances exist, it is recommended that non-surgical therapies should be attempted first, particularly with patients who are poor candidates for surgery. The cure rate of non-surgical treatments is lower than that of surgical approaches; however, their costs, risks, and morbidities are low, while patient satisfaction can be quite high. Non-surgical interventions include conservative measures, pelvic muscle exercises, and the use of pessaries.

Conservative measures

Prophylactic measures include diagnosis and treatment of chronic respiratory diseases, correction of constipation and other disorders that may cause a chronic increase in intra-abdominal pressure, and administration of topical estrogen to postmenopausal women. Significant medical problems such as obesity, asthma, and long-term steroid use may contribute to POP. These problems should be corrected before any surgical intervention because recurrences of the prolapse may be more likely if such conditions are not addressed.

Topical estrogen is an important adjunct in the conservative management of patients with POP. Estrogen therapy may improve the quality of the pelvic tissues to better support the pelvic organs. In postmenopausal women or elderly patients with marked vaginal atrophy, topical estrogen can be used for 4–6 weeks to restore prominent rugae before examination to determine the underlying endopelvic fascia. The preoperative use of topical estrogen for 4–6 weeks can improve the quality of the vaginal epithelium, endopelvic fascia, and other pelvic tissues at the time of surgery, thus contributing to a better outcome. Although rare, ulcerations of the prolapsing tissues may be complicated by infection, and antibiotic therapy is indicated.

Pelvic muscle exercises

Pelvic muscle exercises (Kegel exercises) may improve the strength and tone of the pelvic floor musculature. However, their effectiveness in the treatment of POP is unclear because there is no evidence to indicate that an improvement of pelvic floor muscle strength can lead to the regression of POP. Most of the investigations examining the benefits of pelvic floor exercises have been focused on the treatment of urinary incontinence. Recently, a prospective, randomized, and controlled study of 60 patients (30 with therapy and 30 controls) who underwent surgery for POP and urinary incontinence showed that pre- and postoperative physical therapies significantly improve urinary incontinence, pelvic floor muscle strength, and quality of life, although the postoperative follow-up was only 3 months.[45]

Nevertheless, Kegel exercises may strengthen the levator ani muscles to provide better support for the pelvic organs and enhance the patient's ability to retain a pessary in the vagina.[46,47] It is believed that POP develops when the pelvic floor muscles are weakened, thus compromising their ability to provide adequate support to the pelvic organs. The rationale behind Kegel exercises for POP is that they help to recover the pelvic muscle function, which may reverse mild cases and/or prevent progression of the prolapse. Because these exercises have practically no side-effects and no contraindications, they can also be incorporated into routine health maintenance for postmenopausal women to prevent the development of POP.

Kegel exercises for POP are similar to exercises for the management of urinary incontinence as described in Chapter 15. Verbal and written forms of instruction alone are not effective for these exercises in many women. It was shown that up to 40% of women who received verbal instructions were unable to perform Kegel contractions sufficiently.[48] Furthermore, up to 30% of women are unable to perform pelvic muscle exercises correctly at their first attempt. Contractions of other muscle groups, such as the abdominal, gluteal, and hip abductor muscles, are the common errors. Identifying the correct muscles is a critical part, and this can be best achieved by using feedback from a digital palpation. A perineometer provides accurate information on the strength of pelvic muscle contractions and visual feedback to the patients regarding their progress. In some patients, follow-up with repeated evaluations over several months may be necessary to ensure that the exercises are performed correctly. Several studies demonstrated that biofeedback techniques, such as perineometer or vaginal cones, could enhance the success rate of pelvic floor exercises.[49,50] However, in a prospective, randomized study comparing supervised exercises with vaginal cone biofeedback and vaginal electrical stimulation, supervised exercises were found to have the highest success rate (78% with supervised exercises, 30% with vaginal cone, and 13% with electrical stimulation).[51]

Pessaries

Pessaries are designed to restore and maintain the pelvic organs in their normal position. Although they are an effective alternative to surgery, physicians and patients are usually reluctant to use pessaries for the management of POP due to lack of familiarity and concerns regarding discomfort with the device.

Indications and contraindications

Pessaries can be used for relieving symptoms associated with the prolapse permanently as a final therapy or temporarily when undertaking activities or waiting for surgery. These devices can also be used when the patient is medically unfit for surgery, during pregnancy and the postpartum period, and to promote the healing of ulcerated tissues before surgery. Pessaries may also be employed preoperatively for several weeks in order for the patient to have a realistic expectation of whether surgical reduction of the prolapse will resolve her symptoms of pelvic pain, backache, urinary problems, and voiding dysfunction.

Contraindications to pessary use are few, including acute pelvic inflammatory disease and pain after insertion. Recurrent vaginitis is a relative contraindication and may require removal of the pessary. Prior hysterectomy and current sexual activity have also been considered as relative contraindications; however, the majority of clinicians have not found these conditions to be contraindications for the use of pessaries.[52] Wu and co-workers[53] reported that previous surgery, including hysterectomy, does not appear to affect the success rate of pessary fitting.

Type of pessary

The selections of pessary for POP are suggested in Table 17.5. These selections are based on experience rather than scientific data because formal evaluations of different types of pessaries for different kinds of prolapse have not been conducted. The choice of pessary depends on its efficacy for the management of POP and its acceptability by the patient. Although several types of pessary are available, the less expensive and user-friendly device should be tried first.

Ring, cube, and Gellhorn are the most common types of pessary for POP (Figure 17.3). The ring pessary with or without a supportive membrane is the most versatile type because it can be folded in half for easy insertion, is less likely to sequester vaginal secretions, and works for most patients with different types and degrees of prolapse.[52,53] When the ring type fails, a second line of pessaries, such as the Gellhorn, cube, and donut, can be used.[53] The gellhorn pessary is the second most common choice and has been successfully employed in grade 3 or 4 prolapse of the anterior vaginal wall, the vaginal cuff, or the uterus.[52,54] For patients with concomitant prolapse and stress urinary incontinence, a pessary with ring support and knob can be a successful choice. For patients with significant uterine prolapse and a large introital diameter who have not obtained relief with other pessaries, the Gehrung type should be tried. For patients with a well-defined pubic notch and adequate vaginal width, the Smith–Hodge can be attempted. It should be noted that some patients may not tolerate pessary use, and the more severe forms of POP are usually not relieved by placement of these devices.

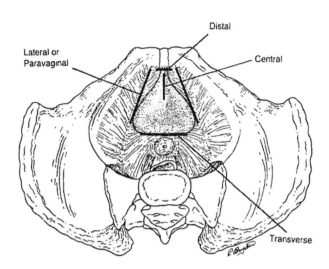

Figure 17.3 Paravaginal, central, and transverse defects. (Reproduced from Contemporary Ob/Gyn, 1990; 35: 100–9.)

Pessary insertion

Pessary fitting is far from an exact science, and a trial and error approach is the rule. The depth and width of the vagina determine the size of the first pessary, and a proper match, which may require several attempts, will avoid compression of the vaginal mucosa, resulting in abrasion, bleeding, and erosion. The properly fitted pessary will also make the patient feel more comfortable. Ring pessary sizes 3, 4, or 5 are usually employed and can be successfully fitted in 70% of patients.[53]

Pessary insertion is a simple technique; however, it is usually overlooked. Women with an atrophic vagina, or any sign of hypoestrogenism, are pretreated locally with estrogen cream for 3–6 weeks. Lubricant is placed on the vaginal introitus and the ring pessary, which has already been folded in half, is inserted with pressure maintained on the posterior vaginal wall while the labia minora are held separated. Once the pessary is inside the vagina, the index finger of the predominant hand is used to direct its leading edge into the posterior fornix and to ensure that the device lies parallel to the vaginal axis with its diaphragm supporting the cervix. The pessary should not too tight in the vagina and it should easily slide up and down along the vaginal sidewall. However, a properly fitted and well supported pessary should not be visible when the labia are separated, and should not fall out or descend to the introitus with a Valsalva maneuver or cough. The patient should then be re-examined in the standing position to confirm the pessary support. If the device falls out with a Valsalva maneuver or cough, a larger size should be tried.

Pessary fitting should be carried out with a moderately full bladder to allow testing of its efficacy in

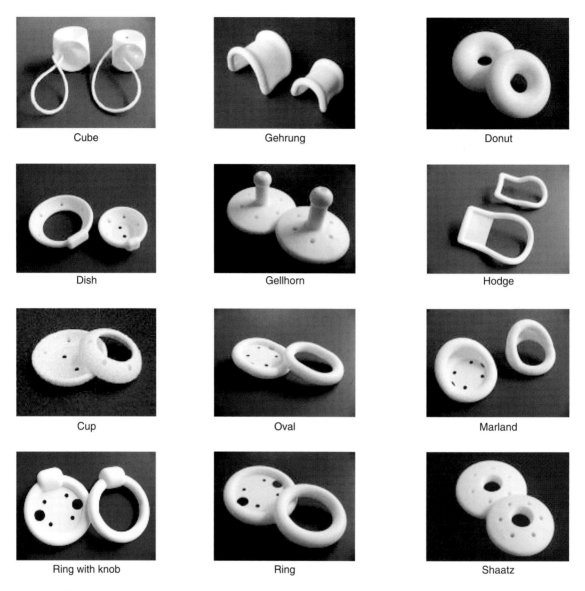

Cube	Gehrung	Donut
Dish	Gellhorn	Hodge
Cup	Oval	Marland
Ring with knob	Ring	Shaatz

Figure 17.4   Different types of vaginal pessaries. (Photo courtesy of Bioteque America Inc., Fremont, California)

improving voiding dysfunction and to see whether reduction of the prolapse is accompanied by urinary incontinence. Also, the patient needs to void comfortably with the pessary in place before being sent home. Patients are also instructed to perform normal activities such as walking, running, jumping, or straining, in the clinic, to ensure that the device is best fitted and patients are comfortable with it. With all of these precautions, however, approximately 25% of patients will return for another fitting.

For pessary removal, index fingers of both hands are placed above and below the leading edge of the device to hook it, and tractions are applied along the vaginal axis to bring it down toward the introitus. In order to avoid discomfort, pressure should be placed on the posterior introitus. Speculum examination is then performed to inspect the vaginal wall for any evidence

of abrasions or erosion. The pessary is rinsed with Betadine®, washed with water, and then dried before reinsertion. Patients should be taught to remove and insert the pessary themselves.

Although a variety of recommendations are found in the literature, we usually schedule a follow-up visit at 2 weeks to examine the vagina for any inflammation, adjust the type and size of pessary if needed, and teach the patient again about insertion and removal of the device. In the first year, follow-up visits are scheduled every 3 months, and after the first year, every 6 months. This schedule is similar to other recommendations.[53] At these visits, the pessary should be removed, inspected, and cleaned. Most silicone pessaries can be used for up to 2 years, although it should be replaced when becoming stiff or coated with thick secretion. The vagina is examined by speculum at every visit to ensure absence of abrasion or erosion. In some women, vaginal accommodation may occur, and increasing the pessary size at the time of follow-up visits may become necessary. For those patients who can remove and insert the pessary themselves, weekly overnight removal and cleansing with soap and warm water is recommended. For patients who are unable to care for their pessary themselves, home care nurses are valuable for visiting the patient once a week, to remove the pessary in the evening, clean it, and return in the morning to replace it.

Side-effects

Modern pessaries are made from silicone, an inert and durable material, and produce a low incidence of troublesome symptoms in patients. Although pessaries may cause vaginal irritation and ulceration, these adverse outcomes are rare if a patient is able to remove and reinsert the pessary on her own at least once a week. Any excessive foul-smelling discharge, abnormal vaginal bleeding, experience of pelvic pain, or leaking of urine indicates the need for medical follow-up. Failure to do so may result in serious consequences, including infections, impaction, and fistula formation by erosion into the bladder or rectum. These complications can also occur with a long-forgotten pessary. If patients complain of vaginal bleeding secondary to abrasion, the pessary should be removed and left out for several weeks to allow the vaginal epithelium to heal. Local estrogen can be given to atrophic epithelium.

Cube pessaries may cause abrasions and erosion more often than the ring type, and they should be inspected more regularly. In advanced degrees of POP, urinary leakage may occur after placing the pessary due to unkinking of the urethra. In these cases, the ring pessary with support and knob can be used to manage both the prolapse and urinary incontinence. Cervical and vaginal malignancies have been reported in association with the use of pessaries, with a mean interval between insertion and cancer diagnosis of 18 years (ranging from 1 to 41 years).[55] It is therefore important to follow patients with speculum examinations and maintain the regular schedule of Pap smears.

REFERENCES

1. Hill K. The demography of the menopause. Maturitas 1996; 23: 113–27.
2. Rogers RM Jr. Anatomy of pelvic support. In: Bent AE, Ostergard DR, Cundiff GW, Swift SE, eds. Ostergard's Urogynecology and Pelvic Floor Dysfunction, 5th edn. Philadelphia: Williams Lippincott & Wilkins, 2003: 19–33.
3. DeLancey JOL, Delmas V. Gross anatomy and functional anatomy of the pelvic floor. In: Bourcier AP, McGuire EJ, Abrams P, eds. Pelvic Floor Disorders. Philadelphia: Elsevier Saunders, 2004: 3–6.
4. DeLancey JO. Anatomic aspects of vaginal eversion after hysterectomy. Am J Obstet Gynecol 1992; 166: 1717–24; discussion 1724–8.
5. Nichols DH, Milley PS, Randall CL. Significance of restoration of normal vaginal depth and axis. Obstet Gynecol 1970; 36: 251–6.
6. Abrams P, Cardozo L, Fall M et al. The standardisation of terminology of lower urinary tract function: report from the Standardisation Sub-committee of the International Continence Society. Neurourol Urodyn 2002; 21: 167–78.
7. Baden WF, Walker T. Fundamental, symptoms, and classification. In: Baden WF, Walker T, eds. Surgical Repair of Vaginal Defects. Philadelphia: JP Lippincott, 1992.
8. Walters MD. Description and classification of lower urinary tract dysfunction and pelvic organ prolapse. In: Walters MD, Karram MM, eds. Urogynecology and Reconstructive Pelvic Surgery, 2nd edn. St Louis: Mosby, 1999: 35–42.
9. Bump RC, Mattiasson A, Bo K et al. The standardization of terminology of female pelvic organ prolapse and pelvic floor dysfunction. Am J Obstet Gynecol 1996; 175: 10–17.
10. Beecham CT. Classification of vaginal relaxation. Am J Obstet Gynecol 1980; 136: 957–8.
11. Hall AF, Theofrastous JP, Cundiff GW et al. Interobserver and intraobserver reliability of the proposed International Continence Society, Society of Gynecologic Surgeons, and American Urogynecologic Society pelvic organ prolapse classification system. Am J Obstet Gynecol 1996; 175: 1467–70; discussion 1470–1.
12. Samuelsson EC, Victor FT, Tibblin G, Svardsudd KF. Signs of genital prolapse in a Swedish population of women 20 to 59 years of age and possible related factors. Am J Obstet Gynecol 1999; 180: 299–305.
13. Tegerstedt G, Maehle-Schmidt M, Nyren O, Hammarstrom M. Prevalence of symptomatic pelvic organ prolapse in a Swedish population. Int Urogynecol J Pelvic Floor Dysfunct 2005; 16: 497–503.
14. Brown JS, Waetjen LE, Subak LL et al. Pelvic organ prolapse surgery in the United States, 1997. Am J Obstet Gynecol 2002; 186: 712–16.
15. Bland DR, Earle BB, Vitolins MZ, Burke G. Use of the Pelvic Organ Prolapse staging system of the International Continence Society, American Urogynecologic Society, and Society of Gynecologic Surgeons in perimenopausal women. Am J Obstet Gynecol 1999; 181: 1324–7; discussion 1327–8.
16. Swift SE. The distribution of pelvic organ support in a population of female subjects seen for routine gynecologic health care. Am J Obstet Gynecol 2000; 183: 277–85.
17. Hendrix SL, Clark A, Nygaard I et al. Pelvic organ prolapse in the Women's Health Initiative: gravity and gravidity. Am J Obstet Gynecol 2002; 186: 1160–6.
18. Nygaard I, Bradley C, Brandt D. Women's Health Initiative. Pelvic organ prolapse in older women: prevalence and risk factors. Obstet Gynecol 2004; 104: 489–97.
19. Kim S, Harvey MA, Johnston S. A review of the epidemiology and pathophysiology of pelvic floor dysfunction: do racial differences matter? J Obstet Gynaecol Can 2005; 27: 251–9.
20. Moalli PA, Shand SH, Zyczynski HM, Gordy SC, Meyn LA. Remodeling of vaginal connective tissue in patients with prolapse. Obstet Gynecol 2005; 106: 953–63.
21. Jackson SR, Avery NC, Tarlton JF et al. Changes in metabolism of collagen in genitourinary prolapse. Lancet 1996; 347: 1658–61.
22. Norton PA, Baker JE, Sharp HC, Warenski JC. Genitourinary prolapse and joint hypermobility in women. Obstet Gynecol 1995; 85: 225–8.

23. McIntosh LJ, Stanitski DF, Mallett VT et al. Ehlers-Danlos syndrome: relationship between joint hypermobility, urinary incontinence, and pelvic floor prolapse. Gynecol Obstet Invest 1996; 41: 135–9.

24. Tetzschner T, Sorensen M, Jonsson L, Lose G, Christiansen J. Delivery and pudendal nerve function. Acta Obstet Gynecol Scand 1997; 76: 324–31.

25. Peschers UM, Schaer GN, DeLancey JO, Schuessler B. Levator ani function before and after childbirth. Br J Obstet Gynaecol 1997; 104: 1004–8.

26. Swift SE, Pound T, Dias JK. Case-control study of etiologic factors in the development of severe pelvic organ prolapse. Int Urogynecol J Pelvic Floor Dysfunct 2001; 12: 187–92.

27. Smith AR, Hosker GL, Warrell DW. The role of partial denervation of the pelvic floor in the aetiology of genitourinary prolapse and stress incontinence of urine. A neurophysiological study. Br J Obstet Gynaecol 1989; 96: 24–8.

28. Allen RE, Hosker GL, Smith AR, Warrell DW. Pelvic floor damage and childbirth: a neurophysiological study. Br J Obstet Gynaecol 1990; 97: 770–9.

29. MacLennan AH, Taylor AW, Wilson DH, Wilson D. The prevalence of pelvic floor disorders and their relationship to gender, age, parity and mode of delivery. BJOG 2000; 107: 1460–70.

30. Patel DA, Xu X, Thomason AD et al. Childbirth and pelvic floor dysfunction: an epidemiologic approach to the assessment of prevention opportunities at delivery. Am J Obstet Gynecol 2006; 195: 23–8.

31. Gurel H, Gurel SA. Pelvic relaxation and associated risk factors: the results of logistic regression analysis. Acta Obstet Gynecol Scand 1999; 78: 290–3.

32. Olsen AL, Smith VJ, Bergstrom JO, Colling JC, Clark AL. Epidemiology of surgically managed pelvic organ prolapse and urinary incontinence. Obstet Gynecol 1997; 89: 501–6.

33. Benson JT, Lucente V, McClellan E. Vaginal versus abdominal reconstructive surgery for the treatment of pelvic support defects: a prospective randomized study with long-term outcome evaluation. Am J Obstet Gynecol 1996; 175: 1418–21; discussion 1421–2.

34. Shull BL, Capen CV, Riggs MW, Kuehl TJ. Preoperative and postoperative analysis of site-specific pelvic support defects in 81 women treated with sacrospinous ligament suspension and pelvic reconstruction. Am J Obstet Gynecol 1992; 166: 1764–8; discussion 1768–71.

35. Symmonds RE, Williams TJ, Lee RA, Webb MJ. Posthysterectomy enterocele and vaginal vault prolapse. Am J Obstet Gynecol 1981; 140: 852–9.

36. Richter K. Massive eversion of the vagina: pathogenesis, diagnosis, and therapy of the 'true' prolapse of the vaginal stump. Clin Obstet Gynecol 1982; 25: 897–912.

37. Thakar R, Sultan AH. Hysterectomy and pelvic organ dysfunction. Best Pract Res Clin Obstet Gynaecol 2005; 19: 403–18.

38. Nygaard IE. Does prolonged high-impact activity contribute to later urinary incontinence? A retrospective cohort study of female Olympians. Obstet Gynecol 1997; 90: 718–22.

39. Jorgensen S, Hein HO, Gyntelberg F. Heavy lifting at work and risk of genital prolapse and herniated lumbar disc in assistant nurses. Occup Med (Lond) 1994; 44: 47–9.

40. Handa VL, Garrett E, Hendrix S, Gold E, Robbins J. Progression and remission of pelvic organ prolapse: a longitudinal study of menopausal women. Am J Obstet Gynecol 2004; 190: 27–32.

41. Swift SE, Herring M. Comparison of pelvic organ prolapse in the dorsal lithotomy compared with the standing position. Obstet Gynecol 1998; 91: 961–4.

42. Hoyte L, Jakab M, Warfield SK et al. Levator ani thickness variations in symptomatic and asymptomatic women using magnetic resonance-based 3-dimensional color mapping. Am J Obstet Gynecol 2004; 191: 856–61.

43. Barber MD, Walters MD, Bump RC. Short forms of two condition-specific quality-of-life questionnaires for women with pelvic floor disorders (PFDI-20 and PFIQ-7). Am J Obstet Gynecol 2005; 193: 103–13.

44. Barber MD, Walters MD, Cundiff GW. PESSRI Trial Group. Responsiveness of the Pelvic Floor Distress Inventory (PFDI) and Pelvic Floor Impact Questionnaire (PFIQ) in women undergoing vaginal surgery and pessary treatment for pelvic organ prolapse. Am J Obstet Gynecol 2006; 194: 1492–8.

45. Jarvis SK, Hallam TK, Lujic S, Abbott JA, Vancaillie TG. Perioperative physiotherapy improves outcomes for women undergoing incontinence and or prolapse surgery: results of a randomised controlled trial. Aust NZ J Obstet Gynaecol 2005; 45: 300–3.

46. Bo K. Can pelvic floor muscle training prevent and treat pelvic organ prolapse? Acta Obstet Gynecol Scand 2006; 85: 263–8.

47. Boyington AR, Dougherty MC. Pelvic muscle exercise effect on pelvic muscle performance in women. Int Urogynecol J Pelvic Floor Dysfunct 2000; 11: 212–18.

48. Bump RC, Hurt WG, Fantl JA, Wyman JF. Assessment of Kegel pelvic muscle exercise performance after brief verbal instruction. Am J Obstet Gynecol 1991; 165: 322–7; discussion 327–9.

49. Burgio KL, Robinson JC, Engel BT. The role of biofeedback in Kegel exercise training for stress urinary incontinence. Am J Obstet Gynecol 1986; 154: 58–64.

50. Peattie AB, Plevnik S, Stanton SL. Vaginal cones: a conservative method of treating genuine stress incontinence. Br J Obstet Gynaecol 1988; 95: 1049–53.

51. Bo K, Talseth T, Holme I. Single blind, randomised controlled trial of pelvic floor exercises, electrical stimulation, vaginal cones, and no treatment in management of genuine stress incontinence in women. BMJ 1999; 318: 487–93.

52. Cundiff GW, Weidner AC, Visco AG, Bump RC, Addison WA. A survey of pessary use by members of the American Urogynecologic Society. Obstet Gynecol 2000; 95: 931–5.

53. Wu V, Farrell SA, Baskett TF, Flowerdew G. A simplified protocol for pessary management. Obstet Gynecol 1997; 90: 990–4.

54. Sulak PJ, Kuehl TJ, Shull BL. Vaginal pessaries and their use in pelvic relaxation. J Reprod Med 1993; 38: 919–23.

55. Schraub S, Sun XS, Maingon P et al. Cervical and vaginal cancer associated with pessary use. Cancer 1992; 69: 2505–9.

18 Conservative management of endometrial hyperplasia and early endometrial cancer

Hetal Kothari, Farzana Martin and Giuseppe DelPriore

INTRODUCTION

Endometrial hyperplasia refers to excessive proliferation of endometrial glands. It is characterized by variation in the size and shape of glands and a potential for cytological atypia, which may progress to malignancy. Treatment options for endometrial hyperplasia include hormones, dilatation and curettage (D&C), endometrial ablation, or hysterectomy.

The most significant aspect of the management of endometrial hyperplasia is the knowledge that it is a premalignant condition and needs active surveillance and management. Endometrial hyperplasia is classified into simple and complex based on histology. Simple hyperplasia is characterized by dilated glands with occasional outpouchings, while complex hyperplasia presents with numerous endometrial glands and luminal outpouchings. Each of these two types can be further termed as atypical hyperplasia based on the presence of atypical cells and mitotic activity.

A study was conducted in Italy to determine the risk of developing endometrial cancer in patients with endometrial hyperplasia. In this study, the incidence of endometrial adenocarcinoma was 3.87% in atypical hyperplasia and 0.81% in other forms; the authors concluded that cellular atypia is the most important predictor of malignant transformation.[1]

In another study published in the United States in 2005, the authors aimed to determine the prevalence of endometrial cancer among patients diagnosed with atypical endometrial hyperplasia who subsequently underwent hysterectomy.[2] Endometrial adenocarcinoma was detected in 48% of these hysterectomy specimens; hence, knowledge of the type of hyperplasia is vital in the management of endometrial hyperplasia because women with atypical hyperplasia need more aggressive management, such as hysterectomy, while conservative management may be preferred in hyperplasia without atypia.

Endometrial adenocarcinoma is the most common gynecologic malignancy and the fourth most frequent site of malignancy in females in North America and Europe. Despite being a common malignancy, it is not a leading cause of cancer deaths. This is due to early presentation, with 75–80% presenting with stage I disease. The prognosis in stage I disease is good, with 5-year overall and cancer specific survival rates of 80–85% and 90–95%, respectively.[3] According to the National Cancer Institute (NCI) approximately 37 000 cases are diagnosed in the United States and about 6000 women die from the disease each year.

The incidence of uterine cancer increases after the menopause, and approximately 75% of cases are diagnosed in postmenopausal patients. Most cases of endometrial cancer occur between the ages of 60 and 70 years, while 15% may occur before age 40. The average age at diagnosis is about 60 years. In the United States, Caucasian women are at higher risk for endometrial cancer and African-American women are at higher relative risk for uterine sarcoma.[4]

RISK FACTORS

The number of menstrual cycles during a woman's lifetime is associated with the risk of endometrial hyperplasia and cancer. During pregnancy, the hormonal milieu reflects progesterone dominance. Therefore, having many pregnancies reduces endometrial cancer risk as there is less unopposed estrogen action. By the same mechanism, infertility increases the risk for endometrial hyperplasia and cancer (Table 18.1).

Hormonal therapy such as the use of tamoxifen, which is an antiestrogen drug that is used to treat breast cancer and to reduce the risk of breast cancer in women who are at a high risk of developing the disease, is a risk factor for endometrial cancer. This is because, although tamoxifen is classified as an antiestrogen, it acts like an estrogen in the uterus and can cause the uterine lining to grow, increasing the risk of endometrial cancer. Similarly, estrogen therapy in postmenopausal women to decrease symptoms such as hot flashes and prevent osteoporosis without the use of progestins is a significant risk factor for endometrial cancer, and can increase the risk to up to five times.[5] Modern low dose regimens of estrogen replacement do

Table 18.1   Risk factors for endometrial hyperplasia/cancer[5]

History of endometrial hyperplasia, polyps, or other benign
    growths of the uterine lining
Estrogen replacement therapy
Tamoxifen
Nulliparity
Early menarche
Nulliparity
Menopause after age 50
Infertility
Diabetes
Obesity
Hypertension
Polycystic ovarian disease
Caucasian race

not increase the risk of hyperplasia. For instance, daily unopposed conjugated equine estrogen 0.3 mg/day and vaginal estrogen rings have not been associated with increased risk of cancer or hyperplasia. Some conditions associated with elevated and/or unopposed serum estrogen, such as granulosa–theca cell tumors that make estrogen, and polycystic ovarian syndrome, may also result in an increased risk of endometrial cancer.

Endometrial cancer also tends to run in some families, and although the exact mechanism is not very well understood, its association with hereditary non-polyposis colon cancer is well known. Women who have had breast cancer or ovarian cancer may have an increased risk of developing endometrial cancer due to the overlap in some of the risk factors.[5]

Obesity, which leads to higher levels of endogenous estrogens due to peripheral conversion of androgens to estrogens, is a well-known risk factor for endometrial hyperplasia. Concentrations of leptin, a hormone secreted by white adipose tissue, correlate strongly with body mass. Leptin interacts with several other hormones, modifies the activities of some enzymes and proinflammatory cytokines, participates in hematopoiesis, thermogenesis, and angiogenesis, and is involved in the control of carbohydrate and lipid metabolism. A study was undertaken to determine whether serum concentrations of leptin in obese patients with endometrial hyperplasia and cancer deviate from values in patients with normal endometrium. Significantly higher concentrations of leptin were noted in every body mass index (BMI) subgroup of patients with endometrial pathology in comparison to controls. It was concluded that leptin promotes proliferation of the endometrium and may contribute to the increased risk of endometrial hyperplasia and cancer associated with obesity.[6]

Feldman et al developed a model based on four risk factors, including age greater than 70 years, diabetes, nulliparity, and postmenopausal status. They estimated an 87% risk of endometrial neoplasia for women with postmenopausal bleeding with all four factors and a risk of 2.6% in women with none.[7]

Although it is commonly accepted that endometrial hyperplasia may result from chronic and unopposed estrogen stimulation, not all females respond in the same manner to estrogen stimulation. Extensive research has been conducted to determine the molecular mechanisms that predispose women to develop endometrial hyperplasia. In one such study, Ashton-Sager et al showed that GLUT-1 (a glucose transporter) is preferentially expressed in complex hyperplasia with atypia and in adenocarcinoma, and that GLUT-1 immunostaining is useful in distinguishing benign hyperplasia from hyperplasia associated with malignancy.[8] Balmer et al showed that steroid receptor coactivator AIB1 levels are higher in non-carcinoma-associated normal and hyperplastic endometrium compared to carcinoma-associated complex atypical hyperplasia.[9] Another study speculated that CYP1A1 genetic polymorphism might be a susceptibility factor for endometrial hyperplasia and endometrial carcinoma.[10]

Another interesting risk factor for developing endometrial hyperplasia is renal transplant. A high rate of endometrial hyperplasia has been observed among female kidney allograft recipients. The immunosupression in transplant patients is believed to be the risk factor.[11]

Phytoestrogens are used for the prevention of hot flashes. A double-blind placebo-controlled trial involving about 300 women and lasting 5 years showed that phytoestrogens were associated with an increase in the incidence of endometrial hyperplasia.[12] This suggests that there is no estrogen replacement therapy that is safe. All have a dose–response effect which, if acknowledged, can be used to avoid hyperplasia. Similarly, as discussed later, withdrawal of estrogen therapy usually results in the spontaneous resolution of hyperplasia.

CLINICAL PRESENTATION

The most common symptom of endometrial hyperplasia or cancer is abnormal uterine bleeding, while most women with these disorders are asymptomatic. Abnormal uterine bleeding may present as menorrhagia, metrorrhagia, menometrorrhagia, or postmenopausal vaginal bleeding or spotting. Other associated symptoms include lower abdominal pain or pelvic cramping, white or clear vaginal discharge after menopause, painful or difficult urination, and pain during intercourse. Pain symptoms usually correlate to the development of hematometra or pyometra.

A pelvic examination is frequently normal, especially in the early stages of disease. Changes in the size, shape, or consistency of the uterus or its surrounding, supporting structures may be seen when the disease is more advanced. A routine Pap smear with atypical endometrial cells is suspicious for a uterine neoplasm and must be investigated. Even completely normal endometrial cells on a Pap in a postmenopausal woman need follow-up.

DIAGNOSIS

Transvaginal ultrasonography

There is no screening policy as yet for endometrial cancer. The most commonly used tool for diagnosis of endometrial hyperplasia is ultrasound.[13] Ultrasonography can be used to measure the thickness of the endometrium. A combination of transabdominal and transvaginal ultrasound (TVUS) is used.

The endometrial features measured with TVUS consist of three areas: the two opposing layers of the basal layer of the endometrium and the reflective midline stripe termed the endometrial stripe. Because endometrial biopsy can be uncomfortable, and most women with bleeding do not have cancer, TVUS has been studied for the initial screening of women with postmenopausal vaginal bleeding. However, there is also evidence that women have died due to overreliance on the sonogram.[14]

In a consensus statement on the evaluation of women with postmenopausal bleeding, the Society of Radiologists in Ultrasound concluded that in the presence of a normal-appearing endometrium measuring 5 mm or less, the risk of endometrial cancer is low and endometrial biopsy is not necessary.[15] A repeat sonogram is recommended in 3–6 months to ensure stability.

However, alternative cut-off values for endometrial thickness have also been proposed. A study conducted in Japan involved 1400 postmenopausal women in whom endometrial thickness was measured with TVUS, and correlated with the histopathological diagnosis of endometrial specimens. The prevalence of endometrial disease in asymptomatic and symptomatic cases was 2.3% and 21%, respectively. In symptomatic cases, at a cut-off limit of 3 mm or less for endometrial thickness, the sensitivity for detecting

endometrial disease was 94%, while the specificity and positive predictive value were 70% and 46%, respectively. With an endometrial thickness 3 mm or less, the probability that endometrial disease would be overlooked was 2.5%. In asymptomatic cases, the corresponding figures at a cut-off limit of 3 mm were 90%, 84%, 12%, and 0.3%. The study recommended a normal cut-off level for endometrial thickness of 4 mm in symptomatic postmenopausal Japanese women.[16] However, given the low pre-test prevalence of hyperplasia or cancer, TVUS has limited value as a screening test in the general population. In contrast, the estimated lifetime risk for endometrial carcinoma in hereditary non-polyposis colorectal cancer syndrome (HNPCC) is 32–60%, thus supporting surveillance. A study was conducted in Finland to determine the efficacy of the use of TVUS alone or in combination with endometrial biopsy for early diagnosis of endometrial pathology in patients with HNPCC, and concluded that TVUS is more effective when combined with endometrial biopsy.[17]

Sonohysterography

Sonohysterography or saline infusion sonography (SIS) is TVUS with instillation of fluid into the uterine cavity to outline intrauterine pathology. SIS may help to differentiate polyps, hyperplasia, and carcinoma. This improves the specificity of TVUS in differentiating endoluminal masses from diffuse endometrial thickening.[3] Office biopsy is still a useful adjunct even with SIS. If SIS or any other imaging is relied on as the only test used, it must be repeated in approximately 3 months to ensure stability.

Magnetic resonance imaging

Imaging may assist in preoperative assessment and surgical planning by predicting the depth of myometrial invasion, cervical involvement, distant spread, and lymph node involvement. Preoperative knowledge of these factors is highly important, as patients at high risk of extrauterine spread and lymph node metastases may have pre/postoperative radiotherapy, chemotherapy, and lymphadenectomy. Importantly, preoperative magnetic resonance imaging (MRI) may decrease the number of unnecessary lymph node dissections.[3]

MRI is considered the most accurate imaging technique for the preoperative assessment of endometrial cancer due its excellent soft-tissue contrast resolution.

Table 18.2 Methods of taking tissue sample in endometrial hyperplasia/cancer

- The most common technique uses a thin, pliable instrument (such as a manual aspirator) to suction a small amount of endometrial tissue from the uterus. This method is faster and causes less discomfort than other methods
- Another method uses an instrument called a curette, with a manual suction device attached. A sample of the endometrium is removed by scraping and collecting it into a syringe or other container
- Vaginal aspiration removes a tissue sample from the uterine lining with an electric suction device (aspirator). This technique can be uncomfortable
- Endometrial washing uses a spray of liquid (jet irrigation) to wash off some of the tissue that lines the uterus
- A small endometrial brush may be used to remove some of the endometrium

Overall staging accuracies have been reported at 83–92%. In comparative studies between computed tomography (CT), MRI, and TVUS, TVUS is considered more accurate than CT for the assessment of myometrial invasion but less accurate than MRI.[3] In patients considering conservative management of an early cancer, in situ lesion, or even atypical complex hyperplasia, MRI may further assure that there is no invasion. MRI should be done in most cases of endometrial neoplasm treated medically.

Endometrial biopsy

Endometrial biopsy is a useful tool for the evaluation of endometrial pathology. There are several methods for obtaining an endometrial biopsy sample (Table 18.2).[18] Histopathological diagnosis and tumor grade can be determined either by outpatient clinic endometrial biopsy or by hysteroscopic assessment. When sampling is sufficient, detection rates for endometrial cancer are up to 99%. False-negative rates of office-based endometrial biopsy and of D&C are 5–15% and 2–6%, respectively. Sampling errors occur when a focal abnormality is not sampled or the sample is insufficient. Up to 28% of endometrial biopsies are non-diagnostic/insufficient.[3] This can be reduced by using appropriate techniques. Either a combined or individual sampling devices, designed for combined cytology and histology testing, is a feasible method to diagnose endometrial pathology, with a very low false-negative rate.[19]

Both office endometrial biopsy and hysteroscopic biopsy have equivalent accuracy in determining tumor grade.[3] About 25% of pre-hysterectomy biopsies overestimate the degree of differentiation compared to final pathology grading of the hysterectomy specimen; for example, D&C can be reported as grade 1, well differentiated, but on final pathology the uterus contains grade 2, moderately differentiated, tumor.

It has been determined that even in the face of a good hysteroscopic view for endometrial hyperplasia and cancer, the histologic study is mandatory with the presence of any lesion in patients with abnormal uterine bleeding. While it has been suggested that a hysteroscopic-guided biopsy may be better than a blind biopsy in terms of accuracy of tissue diagnosis,[20] this is likely to be inaccurate, as the entire endometrium expresses a field effect for the clinically significant diagnoses, e.g. hyperplasia or cancer. Therefore, even if directed biopsies are performed during hysteroscopy, global sampling must also be done, i.e. D&C.

The 2001 Bethesda System (TBS 2001) introduced a new diagnostic category – normal endometrial cells in women aged 40 years or older (EM ≥ 40). The objective of one of the recent studies was to determine whether there was any significant increase in the frequency with which this diagnosis was reported after the implementation of TBS 2001 and the clinical significance of this diagnosis. The study concluded that a significant increase in the incidence of EM ≥ 40 was observed with the implementation of TBS 2001. However, there was no difference in the proportion of patients who underwent endometrial tissue sampling. In addition, the incidence of clinically significant endometrial lesions associated with such a diagnosis was very low. The authors recommend that women aged 40 years or older with benign endometrial cells on Pap tests should undergo endometrial biopsy only when additional clinical indicators are identified.[21]

With advances in science and technology, there is currently great emphasis on assessing the cytoarchitecture of cells in cases of endometrial hyperplasia as a tool for surveillance and follow-up of cases and to predict the risk of malignant changes.[22] These methods might even prove to be more cost-effective. A report suggested that the study of cell cycle kinetics by flow-cytometry might help in picking up, among all women with endometrial hyperplasia, the group of patients who need further close, strict follow-up by endometrial pathologic study. This is going to minimize the cost and invasiveness of surveillance of patients with various grades of endometrial hyperplasia.[23]

It is necessary to be familiar with all the preceding discussions to quantitate the risk to the patient for the non-surgical management of endometrial neoplasm. There is no single algorithm that can be applied to all patients. Instead, an individual assessment must be made using risk factors, biopsy data, imaging, and patient values.

MANAGEMENT

Early endometrial cancer can be treated medically to preserve the uterus for future fertility. However, for patients trying to preserve fertility, medical therapy should be limited to stage IA, i.e. no myometrial invasion, or a very early stage IB with only superficial invasion on histology and MRI. Since endometrial hyperplasia should have no invasion, all of these patients are candidates for non-surgical treatment provided that repeat sampling is done to exclude occult cancer. Patients who are too ill for surgery may also benefit from medical options.

Endometrial hyperplasia represents a continuum of the pre-invasive neoplastic process of endometrial cancer. Oral contraceptive pills, cyclic progestins, continuous progestins, gonadotropin releasing hormone (GnRH) agonists, aromatase inhibitors, intrauterine progestins or danazol, endometrial curettage, and hysteroscopic endometrial resection/ablation are options for treatment.[24]

Hormonal therapy is usually the first-line treatment for simple endometrial hyperplasia without atypia, while hysterectomy is usually the treatment of choice for women with complex hyperplasia and cellular atypia. This is because of the elevated risk of simultaneous occult cancer and the future risk of developing cancer. However, fertility preserving options such as hormonal treatment can be used in certain cases of complex atypical hyperplasia.

Progestins

Progestins are the hormonal treatment of choice for endometrial hyperplasia because of their inhibitory effect on epithelial proliferation (Table 18.3). They act by reducing estrogenic receptors and increasing their catabolism, stimulating the 17β-hydroxyesteroid dehydrogenase and sulfotransferase enzymes and thereby diminishing the estrogenic activity in the environment.[25]

Progestins are effective whether given systemically or locally. Use of local progestogens delivered by intrauterine devices is a common treatment of endometrial hyperplasia. A study was conducted in Norway to determine the efficacy of intrauterine progestogen devices. Perimenopausal and postmenopausal women

Table 18.3 Hormonal therapy of endometrial hyperplasia

Simple hyperplasia
Medroxyprogesterone 5–10 mg per day × 14 days every month for 3 months OR
Oral contraceptive pills for 3 months

Complex hyperplasia
Medroxyprogesterone 5–10 mg per day for 3 months OR
Oral contraceptive pills for 3 months

Simple hyperplasia with atypia
Megace® 40–160 mg per day for 3 months

Complex hyperplasia with atypia
Megace 160–320 mg per day for 3 months

There are a wide variety of acceptable doses depending on the physician and patient in all categories of endometrial hyperplasia
Progesterone IUD is useful and effective in all types of endometrial hyperplasia
GnRH agonists (e.g. triptorelin) and aromatase inhibitors (e.g. anastrozole 1 mg/day) are also useful and can be used as an adjunct or primary therapy

had a baseline endometrial biopsy and were then divided into three groups, namely those who underwent hormonal therapy with a progestin-impregnated intrauterine device (IUD; n=21), those who received cyclic oral progestins (n=28), and those who had surveillance only (n=22). All three groups had follow-up biopsies. All groups had a similar proportion of latent pre-cancers at intake but differed after therapy. The IUD group had the highest rate of regression, with a 62% pre-therapy and a 5% post-therapy rate of latent pre-cancers. Hence, the study suggests the beneficial role of the delivery of high doses of progestins locally to the endometrium by IUD.[26]

Systemic progestin therapy is also an effective therapy for endometrial hyperplasia. Successful treatment of endometrial hyperplasia with progestins is commonly accompanied by the finding of an inactive or suppressed endometrium after therapy. A study suggested that after 3 months of cyclic progesterone treatment, hyperplasia was reversed in all patients and proliferation was decreased significantly. This difference between pre- and post-treatment is due to the antiproliferative effect of progestins, and it is suggested that progestins decrease the proliferative index of simple endometrial hyperplasia without atypia to proliferative index values of the normal secretory endometrium.[27] Several studies indicate that megestrol acetate inhibits the recurrence of adenomatous and atypical hyperplasia as well as adenocarcinoma in situ. These diseases, when left untreated, often progress to invasive adenocarcinoma. Additional studies show that megestrol acetate is effective in the treatment of endometrial adenocarcinoma in inoperable patients and increases survival in patients with recurrent endometrial cancer.[28] Initially, there were concerns that the use of Megace® in the treatment of endometrial pathology could have some adverse effects including lipid abnormalities and hyperglycemia. However, several studies have shown that the short-term use of megestrol acetate, 160–320 mg/day, in the treatment of endometrial pathology is an effective method without marked harmful effects on the serum lipid profile or glucose levels, but is associated with weight gain.[27]

Progestins have been linked with adverse outcomes in patients with endometrial neoplasms if used for extended periods of time. In a study using a progestin as adjuvant therapy in advanced endometrial cancer, patients receiving progestins had a greater overall mortality than did patients not exposed to the hormone. Some progestins when given for years have also been associated with secondary cancers, specifically breast cancer.[29] However, these concerns should not prevent a suitable candidate trying to preserve fertility from using progestins for short-term treatment.

Aromatase inhibitors

At menopause, serum levels of estrogen and progesterone decrease, but there is increased production of androgens by the ovaries. The androgens are converted into estrogens by the enzyme aromatase, mainly in the adipose tissue. This is further accentuated in obesity in which there is increased androgen production by the ovaries as well as an increase in adipose tissue. Aromatase inhibitors, such as anastrozole, are treatment options used for endometrial hyperplasia especially in obese postmenopausal women.

In a study conducted in Greece in 2004, anastrozole was administered for 12 months to 11 obese postmenopausal women with high operative risk, in order to treat endometrial hyperplasia (four simple, five complex, and two atypical). Endometrial thickness and histology became normal in all cases. Follow-up biopsies revealed atrophic endometrium after treatment and after an additional mean follow-up of 10.2 months. The safety and tolerance profile was satisfactory. This study points to the potential increased use of aromatase inhibitors in the future.[30]

In patients who fail progestin therapy, aromatase inhibitors can be added to progestins or replace them. Sequential therapy alternating any of these medical treatments may be better. Theoretically, altering treatment each month may allow receptors to replenish, making the neoplasm more sensitive.

Gonadotropin releasing hormone agonists

Recent studies have also revealed that GnRH agonists could affect endometrial cell proliferation not only indirectly, through the hormonal axis, but also directly, by acting on the GnRH receptors. In 2003, Agorastos et al investigated the response of the various hyperplastic disorders of the endometrium to prolonged treatment with leuprolide acetate, a gonadotropin releasing hormone agonist combined with tibolone, as add-back therapy. Histopathologic evaluation of endometria revealed regression of endometrial hyperplasia in all women after 12 months of treatment; however, during the first 2 years of follow-up, endometrial hyperplasia reappeared in four women (4/21, 19%). The study concluded that the combined GnRH agonist/tibolone treatment in women with endometrial hyperplasia is a potent alternative, so far as endometrial status and clinical course of the disease are concerned, whereas tibolone appears to act sufficiently as add-back therapy to prolonged GnRH agonist treatment. The probability of relapse of the disease during the follow-up period makes close monitoring of the endometrium after cessation of the treatment absolutely necessary.[31]

Another study evaluated the efficacy of a diferent GnRH agonist in women with endometrial hyperplasia. Fifteen women with a mean age of 48.5 years with the histopathological diagnosis of simple hyperplasia were treated with triptorelin for 3 months. After therapy, all patients underwent transvaginal ultrasonography and endometrial biopsy. Atrophic endometrium was observed in all women after 3 months of therapy. The thickness of the endometrium decreased from 10.21±3.2 mm to 3.94±1.56 mm. Hence, it was concluded that the efficacy of the therapy for simple hyperplasia in women with GnRH agonist was 100%.[32]

Other hormonal approaches

Tibolone is a synthetic steroid with both estrogenic and progestogenic effects. During tibolone treatment, it is thought that the progestogenic properties of tibolone stimulate cell differentiation, which may counteract the estrogenic properties of tibolone. However, cases developing endometrial cancer while using tibolone have been reported. In addition, a recent study from the United Kingdom that evaluated a large number of postmenopausal women from whom information about hormone replacement therapy and personal details were collected suggests that both estrogens and tibolone increase the risk of endometrial cancer.

A Japanese study used a danazol-releasing intrauterine device to treat 20 endometrial hyperplasia patients; 16 patients with simple or complex hyperplasia had a regression, while only 25% atypical hyperplasia regressed. Hence, further research is needed before some therapies are used extensively, especially in cases with atypical hyperplasia.[24]

Another study was conducted to evaluate the effects of a non-prescription red clover extract on selected sex hormones and the endometrium in postmenopausal women. The study demonstrated that supplementation with MF11RCE (verum), in contrast to placebo, significantly increased plasma testosterone levels and decreased endometrial thickness. The observed reduction of endometrial thickness provides support for a safe role for isoflavones in terms of endometrial hyperplasia.[33]

Other conservative approaches

Endometrial ablation is one of the newer modalities of treatment for these neoplasms. There are reports of complex endometrial hyperplasia with atypia treated by microwave endometrial ablation (MEA) at a frequency of 2.45 GHz as an alternative to hysterectomy. This approach is still under study, but has the potential to replace hysterectomies in the future, and hence reduce the morbidity associated with surgery.[34]

Transcervical resection of the endometrium is another invasive procedure that can be used in patients in whom hysterectomy is contraindicated due to other medical reasons. A study was conducted in the United States in which five cases underwent transcervical resection due to medical contraindications to hysterectomy. These cases were followed for 3 years and the thickness of endometrium was no more than 5 mm in all these cases at the end of follow-up. This is a useful procedure that can be performed in patients in whom hysterectomy is a contraindication.[35]

Selection of treatment modality

Clark et al analyzed the current practices in the treatment of endometrial hyperplasia and put forth some interesting facts.[36] Complex hyperplasia without atypia accounted for more than half of cases of endometrial hyperplasia. The malignant potential of complex hyperplasia is thought to be low (1–3%). Despite this, the indication for hysterectomy was 'fear of disease progression' in half of the cases. Moreover, this traditional approach to management may no longer be

justifiable given the availability of non-invasive surveillance methods (e.g. outpatient endometrial biopsy, hysteroscopy, and transvaginal ultrasound) and new options in medical treatment. In this study, four out of five women treated conservatively avoided hysterectomy within the study duration. The small numbers of women within each treatment subgroup and incomplete follow-up limit conclusions regarding the relative efficiency of different conservative approaches. Overall, the available data suggest that persistent or progressive disease can be found in one-third of conservatively managed cases (i.e. those treated medically or with surveillance alone).

Endometrial hyperplasia is an important disease that affects women of all ages. We support the view that women with atypical endometrial hyperplasia should be managed by hysterectomy because of its malignant potential and the significant possibility of diagnostic under-call. However, for those women with pressing fertility considerations or medical factors precluding surgery, close disease surveillance and medical therapy can still be an option.[36]

Endometrial cancers are not uncommonly associated with ovarian tumors. This is a very significant aspect, considering that in premenopausal women with endometrial cancer ovarian preservation may be a consideration. Among 102 young women (aged 24–45 years) who underwent hysterectomy for endometrial cancer, 26 (25%) were found to have coexisting epithelial ovarian tumors. Hence, careful preoperative and intraoperative assessment of the adnexa is mandatory in young women with endometrial cancer. Those who desire ovarian preservation should be counseled regarding the high rate of coexisting ovarian malignancy.[37]

Endometrial cancer is usually diagnosed at an early stage. The 1-year survival rate is about 94%. The 5-year survival rate for endometrial cancer that has not spread is 96%. If the cancer has spread to distant organs, the 5-year survival rate drops to 25%. However, these statistics are for surgically staged cancers. It is not possible to determine the exact spread of disease unless a patient has a hysterectomy, oophorectomy, pelvic washings, and lymph node dissection.

Pretreatment assessment including MRI, hysteroscopy, multiple endometrial biopsies, Pap smear, and CA125 can provide useful information, but they are all limited. If all these parameters indicate low risk, or no spread of cancer, then medical therapy can be considered. However, occult disease can be missed by these non-surgical diagnostic tests. Patients have died from cancer after receiving only medical therapy, and should be warned of this risk. Medical therapy is still a reasonable option despite these risks for the select patient.

Prevention

In the current era of chemoprevention, extensive research is being conducted to develop effective strategies for the prevention of endometrial hyperplasia and cancer. In one such study it was found that aromatase inhibitors used by women with breast cancer did not result in endometrial thickening. In addition, when administered after tamoxifen withdrawal, aromatase inhibitors may reverse tamoxifen-associated endometrial thickening. Hence, their use for prophylaxis against endometrial neoplasms for high-risk women may be a possibility in the future.[38]

CONCLUSION

Endometrial hyperplasias can be divided into two categories based on the presence or absence of cytological atypia and further classified as simple or complex according to the extent of architectural abnormalities. They are usually diagnosed because of irregular bleeding in postmenopausal women. Ultrasound is usually the initial investigation of choice. Hysteroscopy with a biopsy gives a more accurate diagnosis than transvaginal ultrasonography, but is an invasive procedure. Some type of biopsy must be done. Endometrial hyperplasias with no cytological atypia, regarded as a response to unopposed endogenous estrogenic stimulation, are normally treated with progestins. The intrauterine route may more effective and better tolerated than the oral route. Either conservative surgery (endometrial resection, thermal ablation) or radical surgery (hysterectomy) in the case of other genital diseases is performed in women who do not respond to medical treatment.

The absence of management protocols in the literature offers various treatment options and indications. Gonadotropin-releasing hormone agonists, danazol, or aromatase inhibitors are effective, but have adverse effects and are expensive. Endometrial ablation can be performed as first-line therapy in women suffering from bleeding related to hyperplasia without cytological atypia. Medical treatment may be offered to young women suffering from hyperplasia with cytological atypia and desiring pregnancy.[39]

The patient and her physician must consider all the information available and decide whether medical therapy is warranted. Hysterectomy may be the standard, but that does not mean it is the only option for every patient. In fact, for women desiring fertility preservation, a short course of medical therapy actually appears to be very prudent. Even if not successful, this approach may give the patient closure before she gives up on her reproductive options.

REFERENCES

1. Novac L, Grigore T, Cernea N, Niculescu M, Cotarcea S. Incidence of endometrial carcinoma in patients with endometrial hyperplasia. Eur J Gynaecol Oncol 2005; 26: 561–3.
2. Shutter J, Wright TC Jr. Prevalence of underlying adenocarcinoma in women with atypical endometrial hyperplasia. Int J Gynecol Pathol 2005; 24: 313–18.
3. Barwick TD, Rockall AG, Barton DP, Sohaib SA. Imaging of endometrial adenocarcinoma. Clin Radiol 2006; 61: 545–55.
4. Oncology Channel. Endometrial Cancer. 2006. Available at: http://www.oncologychannel.com/endometrialcancer/. Accessed 12/11, 2006.
5. American Cancer Society. Risk Factors for Endometrial Cancer. 2006. Available at: http://www.cancer.org/docroot/cri/content/cri_2_4_2x_what_are_the_risk_factors_for_endometrial_cancer.asp? sitearea=cri. Accessed 12/07, 2006.
6. Cymbaluk A, Chudecka-Glaz A, Rzepka-Gorska I. Leptin levels in serum depending on Body Mass Index in patients with endometrial hyperplasia and cancer. Eur J Obstet Gynecol Reprod Biol 2006 Sep 26; [Epub ahead of print]
7. Feldman S, Cook EF, Harlow BL, Berkowitz RS. Predicting endometrial cancer among older women who present with abnormal vaginal bleeding. Gynecol Oncol 1995; 56: 376–81.
8. Ashton-Sager A, Paulino AF, Afify AM. GLUT-1 is preferentially expressed in atypical endometrial hyperplasia and endometrial adenocarcinoma. Appl Immunohistochem Mol Morphol 2006; 14: 187–92.
9. Balmer NN, Richer JK, Spoelstra NS et al. Steroid receptor coactivator AIB1 in endometrial carcinoma, hyperplasia and normal endometrium: correlation with clinicopathologic parameters and biomarkers. Mod Pathol 2006; 19: 1593–605.
10. Esinler I, Aktas D, Alikasifoglu M, Tuncbilek E, Ayhan A. CYP1A1 gene polymorphism and risk of endometrial hyperplasia and endometrial carcinoma. Int J Gynecol Cancer 2006; 16: 1407–11.
11. Bobrowska K, Kaminski P, Cyganek A et al. High rate of endometrial hyperplasia in renal transplanted women. Transplant Proc 2006; 38: 177–9.
12. Phytoestrogens and endometrial hyperplasia. Prescrire Int 2006; 15: 62–3.
13. Marchetti M, Vasile C, Chiarelli S. Endometrial cancer: asymptomatic endometrial findings. Characteristics of postmenopausal endometrial cancer Eur J Gynaecol Oncol 2005; 26: 479–84.
14. Del Priore G. Cost effectiveness of treatment of early endometrial cancer. Gynecol Oncol 2000; 76: 142–3.
15. McFarlin BL. Ultrasound assessment of the endometrium for irregular vaginal bleeding. J Midwifery Womens Health 2006; 51: 440–9.
16. Tsuda H, Nakamura H, Inoue T et al. Transvaginal ultrasonography of the endometrium in postmenopausal Japanese women. Gynecol Obstet Invest 2005; 60: 218–23.
17. Renkonen-Sinisalo L, Butzow R, Leminen A et al. Surveillance for endometrial cancer in hereditary nonpolyposis colorectal cancer syndrome. Int J Cancer 2007; 120: 821–4.
18. Del Priore G, Williams R, Harbatkin CB et al. Endometrial brush biopsy for the diagnosis of endometrial cancer. J Reprod Med 2001; 46: 439–43.
19. Yang GC, Wan LS, Del Priore G. Factors influencing the detection of uterine cancer by suction curettage and endometrial brushing. J Reprod Med 2002; 47: 1005–10.

20. Lasmar RB, Barrozo PR, de Oliveira MA, Coutinho ES, Dias R. Validation of hysteroscopic view in cases of endometrial hyperplasia and cancer in patients with abnormal uterine bleeding. J Minim Invasive Gynecol. 2006; 13: 409–12.

21. Bean SM, Connolly K, Roberson J, Eltoum I, Chhieng DC. Incidence and clinical significance of morphologically benign-appearing endometrial cells in patients age 40 years or older: the impact of the 2001 Bethesda System. Cancer 2006; 108: 39–44.

22. Norimatsu Y, Shimizu K, Kobayashi TK et al. Cellular features of endometrial hyperplasia and well differentiated adenocarcinoma using the Endocyte sampler: diagnostic criteria based on the cytoarchitecture of tissue fragments. Cancer 2006; 108: 77–85.

23. Sherif LS, Totongy M, Tawfeek M, Abdel-Ghafar H, Badawy AM. Can flowcytometric DNA studies forecast the prognosis of endometrial hyperplasia? Eur J Obstet Gynecol Reprod Biol 2005; 122: 104–6.

24. Lai CH, Huang HJ. The role of hormones for the treatment of endometrial hyperplasia and endometrial cancer. Curr Opin Obstet Gynecol 2006; 18: 29–34.

25. Horn LC, Schnurrbusch U, Bilek K, Hentschel B, Einenkel J. Risk of progression in complex and atypical endometrial hyperplasia: clinicopathologic analysis in cases with and without progestogen treatment. Int J Gynecol Cancer 2004; 14: 348–53.

26. Orbo A, Rise CE, Mutter GL. Regression of latent endometrial precancers by progestin infiltrated intrauterine device. Cancer Res 2006; 66: 5613–17.

27. Bese T, Vural A, Ozturk M et al. The effect of long-term use of progesterone therapy on proliferation and apoptosis in simple endometrial hyperplasia without atypia. Int J Gynecol Cancer 2006; 16: 809–13.

28. Wentz WB. Progestin therapy in lesions of the endometrium. Semin Oncol 1985; 12 (Suppl 1): 23–7.

29. WHO 2002.

30. Agorastos T, Vaitsi V, Pantazis K et al. Aromatase inhibitor anastrozole for treating endometrial hyperplasia in obese postmenopausal women. Eur J Obstet Gynecol Reprod Biol 2005; 118: 239–40.

31. Agorastos T, Vaitsi V, Paschopoulos M et al. Prolonged use of gonadotropin-releasing hormone agonist and tibolone as add-back therapy for the treatment of endometrial hyperplasia. Maturitas 2004; 48: 125–32.

32. Radowicki S, Skorzewska K. Treatment of hyperplasia endometrium with GNRH agonists. Ginekol Pol 2003; 74: 836–9.

33. Imhof M, Gocan A, Reithmayr F et al. Effects of a red clover extract (MF11RCE) on endometrium and sex hormones in postmenopausal women. Maturitas 2006; 55: 76–81.

34. Kanaoka Y, Kato M, Tokuyama O, Ishiko O. A case of complex endometrial hyperplasia with atypia treated by microwave endometrial ablation. Gan To Kagaku Ryoho 2005; 32: 1652–3.

35. Sui L, Xie F, Cao B. Management of abnormal uterine hemorrhage with atypical endometrial hyperplasia by transcervical resection of endometrium. Int J Gynecol Cancer 2006; 16: 1482–6.

36. Clark TJ, Neelakantan D, Gupta JK. The management of endometrial hyperplasia: an evaluation of current practice. Eur J Obstet Gynecol Reprod Biol 2006; 125: 259–64.

37. Walsh C, Holschneider C, Hoang Y et al. Coexisting ovarian malignancy in young women with endometrial cancer. Obstet Gynecol 2005; 106: 693–9.

38. Garuti G, Cellani F, Centinaio G et al. Prospective endometrial assessment of breast cancer patients treated with third generation aromatase inhibitors. Gynecol Oncol 2006; 103: 599–603.

39. Brun JL, Descat E, Boubli B, Dallay D. Endometrial hyperplasia: a review. J Gynecol Obstet Biol Reprod (Paris) 2006; 35: 542–50.

19 Preventive strategies and non-invasive treatment options for cervical pre-invasive and invasive disorders

Stacey A South and Kunle Odunsi

INTRODUCTION

The incidence of cervical cancer has decreased significantly in the United States over the past 50 years. Between 1955 and 1992, the number of deaths attributed to cervical cancer dropped by 74%. The incidence continues to decline by nearly 4% a year. In 2006, approximately 9710 new cases of cervical cancer were diagnosed, with 3700 deaths.[1] Despite these advances in the United States, cervical cancer remains a worldwide epidemic. In 2000, over 471 000 new cases of cervical cancer were diagnosed globally, with 288 000 deaths, making it the second most common cancer among women worldwide.[2]

The advent of the Pap smear is responsible for the decreased incidence and mortality of cervical cancer in developed countries. Screening programs allow early detection and prevention of cervical cancer by detecting pre-cancerous cervical intraepithelial lesions (CIN). As a result, the incidence of CIN has risen in the United States. In 1980, the incidence of CIN3 was 27/100 000; by 1990 it rose to 45/100 000.[3] This increase could also be attributed to the mounting prevalence of human papillomavirus (HPV) infection, a virus known to cause CIN and cervical cancer.[4,5]

HPV is the most common sexually transmitted disease in the United States; up to 75% of sexually active women and men contract HPV at some point in their lives,[6] mostly between the ages of 15 and 24 years.

Most infections are asymptomatic and transient, resulting in no cervical abnormalities. Within 1 year, approximately 70% of HPV infections resolve spontaneously, increasing to 90% by 2 years.[7] Persistent infections occur in 10% of cases and are a major risk factor for the development of CIN and cervical cancer.[8,9] Most persistent infections are associated with high-risk HPV types, mainly 16, 18, 31, 33, 39, 45, 52, 58, and 69,[5] with HPV 16/18 associated with approximately 70% of cervical cancer cases.[4] The spontaneous regression rate of CIN is depicted in Table 19.1.[10,11] Although only a small percentage of cases progress to cervical cancer, the current ability to predict patients who will progress is limited.

Surgery remains the mainstay of treatment, with complete response rates ranging from 65 to 98% depending on the patient's risk factors.[12,13] However, surgery is associated with increased risks of pregnancy complications.[14,15] As a result, therapeutic options are evolving to include non-invasive and medical alternatives enabling the preservation of reproductive and sexual abilities. More important, we now understand the pathogenesis of CIN and cervical cancer along with the role of HPV (Figures 19.1 and 19.2), enabling the development of new medical treatments as well as preventive strategies targeting these molecular mechanisms and pathways. In this chapter, we will discuss preventive and non-invasive therapeutic modalities in detail, focusing on efficacy, toxicities, and applicability.

Table 19.1 Natural history of cervical intraepithelial neoplasia (CIN). Based on data from reference 11

	Regression (%)	Persistence (%)	Progression to CIS (%)	Progression to invasive cancer (%)
CIN1	57	32	11	—
CIN2	43	35	22	—
CIN3	32	56	12	—
Overall all grades of CIN	—	—	—	1.7

CIS, carcinoma in situ

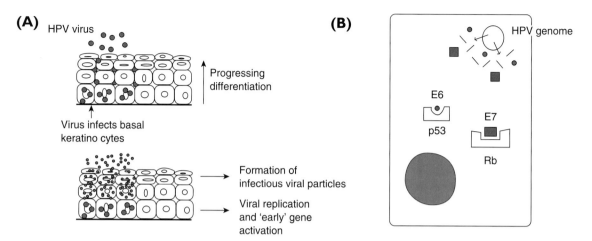

Figure 19.1   Pathogenesis of human papillomavirus (HPV) infection of the cervical epithelium. (A) HPV first penetrates the epithelial layer, usually via microlesions, to infect the basal keratinocytes. Early proteins (E1, E2, E5, E6, and E7) are expressed leading to viral replication. As the basal keratinocytes differentiate toward the surface and undergo terminal differentiation, the 'late' proteins (L1 and L2) are expressed, allowing assembly of infectious viral particles. In carcinoma, terminal differentiation does not occur and thus late proteins are not synthesized. (B) E6 and E7 are the proteins mainly responsible for abnormal cell proliferation and transformation to neoplastic cells. E6 binds p53, while E7 binds retinoblastoma (Rb), causing increased degradation of p53 and Rb with loss of cell cycle control and resistance to apoptosis. HPV integration into the host chromosome is required for the development of invasive cancer

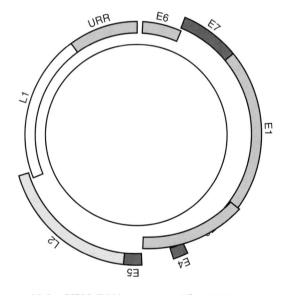

Figure 19.2   HPV DNA structure. The HPV genome is divided into eight open reading frames encoding six 'early' (E) and two 'late' (L) functions, as depicted

INTERFERONS

It is well established that HPV plays an intricate role in the development of CIN and cervical cancer,[5] due mainly to local deficiencies of cellular immunity. Therefore, manipulation of the immune system is another potential avenue for medical therapy of cervical abnormalities. Interferons (IFNs) are naturally occurring proteins with a broad spectrum of antiviral, antiproliferative, and immunoregulatory activities. These proteins are classified into three main categories: interferon α (IFN-α), interferon β (IFN-β), and interferon γ (IFN-γ).[16] IFNs are the body's first line of defense against viral diseases, produced by most cell types in response to viral infections. IFNs induce uninfected neighboring cells to produce enzymes which either destroy the virus upon cell entry or inhibit viral protein synthesis making the cells resistant to infection. IFNs also play a role in cancer cell growth and differentiation. They demonstrate direct and indirect antiproliferative properties against tumor cells by increased activation of the immune system, allowing enhanced tumor cell recognition and killing.[16] The exact mechanisms are not well known. Given the antiviral properties of IFNs, researchers have studied their efficacy in the treatment of several viral diseases, including those caused by HPV. Rockley and Tyring[17] in 1995 wrote a thorough review of studies using IFNs in the treatment of HPV-associated infections of the genital tract. We will summarize the key studies and review more recent studies when applicable.

Interferon α

IFN-α was the first to be studied in the treatment of cervical abnormalities, specifically cervical cancer. Ikic et al[18] treated 15 patients with stage IA (two patients), IB (10 patients), or IIB (three patients) squamous cell carcinoma of the cervix with natural IFN-α given topically only or both topically and intramuscularly followed by surgical resection. Six patients received 2 000 000 IU daily applied via a contraceptive pessary for 21 days, and the remaining patients received the same treatment plus 1 000 000 IU given intramuscularly daily for 21 days. Clinically, tumors regressed by about 30% on average for all patients. The surgical specimens of three patients showed no remaining cancer cells, while two patients regressed to CIN with no evidence of invasion. There was no appreciable difference between the two IFN treatment regimens. Similar benefit was noted by Vasilyev et al[19] in the treatment of cervical cancer using intralesional injections of IFN-α once or twice daily for 10 days. They found a dose-dependent response, with the greatest efficacy at dosages between 1 000 000 and 3 000 000 IU. These studies show a potential role of IFN-α as neoadjuvant therapy in early stage cervical cancer, but additional studies are needed.

Studies assessing the efficacy of IFN-α in the treatment of CIN show varying results, limited by small sample size and no control groups. Several placebo-controlled trials are available, but also with disappointing results. Byrne et al[20] treated 26 patients with CIN2/3 using either placebo or topical IFN-α at 400 000 IU twice weekly applied to the cervix for 24 hours via a cervical cap for 12 treatments. No biopsies were performed at follow-up, only cytology and colposcopy, as the authors stated that biopsies could alter the natural course of CIN. Therapy with IFN-α showed no effect compared to placebo (response rate of 23% vs 15%, respectively). At study initiation, 10 patients were HPV-16 positive, with nine still positive at study completion. Similarly, no effect was noted in another placebo-controlled trial[21] using intralesional injections of recombinant IFN-α2b (Intron® A) at 2 000 000 IU twice weekly for 5 weeks in patients with CIN. These patients also had high infection rates with HPV-16/18. We can conclude that IFN-α is ineffective in the treatment of CIN and high-risk HPV infections. As IFN-α is effective in treating condyloma acuminatum typically caused by HPV-6/11,[22] several authors speculate that the lack of efficacy of IFN-α in CIN may be related to insufficient activity against oncogenic HPV types, especially HPV-16/18.

Other routes of administration for IFN-α were investigated for treating CIN. These data are summarized by Rockley and Tyring.[17] Basically, efficacy was noted in the therapy of condyloma acuminatum but not in CIN, especially when analyzing placebo-controlled trials. The main side-effect in all the studies using intralesional or systemic administration of IFN-α was flu-like symptoms in up to 70% of patients. Symptoms occurred 3–4 hours after each treatment and lasted about 6 hours, but did not require therapy discontinuation. Topical administration caused no significant adverse reactions.

Upon further review of the literature, only one laboratory has published data showing a significant response of CIN to IFN-α therapy. Jach et al[23] enrolled women with CIN1/2 to receive either no treatment (31 patients) or Intron A (30 patients) injected intracervically twice a week for 3 months. After 1 year, biopsies showed complete responses in 24 cases (80%) from the IFN-α group, which was significantly higher than in controls and previously reported response rates to IFN-α therapy. HPV clearance was also greater in the treatment group compared to controls. There are two main differences between this study and the others: the population studied by Jach et al had less severe dysplasia and the duration of IFN-α therapy was doubled. These data indicate a potential role for IFN-α in the management of CIN and HPV infection. However, these data need to be confirmed and an optimal treatment regimen devised before this therapy can be considered in clinical practice.

Given the known mechanism of IFNs as antiviral agents aiding in the prevention of viral infection of uninfected neighboring cells, Gostout et al[24] studied whether systemic IFN-α could prevent recurrence of CIN after conventional therapy. Sixty-three patients with CIN1–3 were randomly treated with either local destructive therapy alone or destructive therapy plus IFN-α at 1 000 000 IU/m^2 subcutaneously three times a week for 10 weeks. IFN-α therapy showed no significant effect on the 2-year recurrence-free survival compared to controls (82% vs 73%, respectively, $p = 0.903$). HPV status was not assessed in this study. These data continue to show limited clinical efficacy of IFN-α in CIN. This therapy cannot be recommended at this time.

Interferon β

The role of IFN-β for the treatment of CIN shows promise. Penna et al[25] treated 41 patients with

HPV-associated CIN, mostly CIN2/3, using 3 000 000 IU of IFN-β injected intralesionally for 3 weeks as follows: daily for 5 consecutive days with 2 days off in week one, then every other day for three doses with 2 days off in weeks two and three. CIN resolution occurred in 33 patients (80%), 3 months after therapy. At 6 months, eight patients (20%) showed persistent CIN and underwent excisional procedures. Recurrences occurred in three patients at 12 months, two patients at 24 months, and one patient at 36 months for an 18% recurrence rate. These response rates are similar to those in other studies using IFN-β to treat CIN.[17] The main side-effects again were flu-like symptoms in 65–70% of patients. This study and others in the literature[17] show that IFN-β has reasonable efficacy, with a recurrence rate comparable to that of surgical inventions.[12,13]

Moreover, Gonzalez-Sanchez et al[26] studied the ability of systemic IFN-β to eliminate recurrent HPV infections of the cervix. Recurrent HPV disease was defined as the histologic reappearance of HPV at least 12 months after prior successful medical or surgical therapy for HPV infection. A total of 122 patients received intramuscular injections of either placebo or IFN-β at 3 000 000 IU daily for 5 days followed by 2 days off for 3 weeks. The IFN-β group showed improved clearance of HPV compared to placebo at 6 months (79% vs 54%, respectively, $p=0.001$) and 12 months (70% vs 43%, respectively, $p=0.002$). Theoretically, decreased HPV infections would result in less CIN; however, the authors did not mention the incidence of CIN in the two groups. Flu-like symptoms were the most common side-effect in the IFN-β group (36%) compared to only 5% in the placebo group. These data indicate promising potential for IFN-β administered either intralesionally or systemically in the treatment of CIN.

Interferon γ

A few investigators assessed IFN-γ in the treatment of CIN. Most recently, Sikorski and Zrubek[27] treated 17 women with 6 000 000 IU (0.02 mg) of IFN-γ 1b injected intracervically divided over four treatments at 2-day intervals. All patients were positive for high-risk HPV and CIN1/2. After 2 months, repeat biopsies and HPV testing showed that 9/17 patients (53%) were negative for CIN and HPV. However, three of these responders developed recurrent CIN1, ranging from 1 to 2.5 years later.[28] An additional three patients tested negative for HPV at 2 months with eventual resolution

of CIN at 9 months.[28] One patient initially with CIN2 displayed a partial response, developing persistent CIN1 and HPV infection. Clearance of HPV is a predictor of CIN recurrence rates after therapy. Chua and Hjerpe[8] found HPV in 96% of CIN recurrences after surgical therapy, while no HPV was detected in complete responders. Unfortunately, Sikorski and Zrubek[28] did not mention the HPV status at the time of recurrence for the three complete responders who relapsed after 1 or more years. It is possible that these patients were not treatment failures, but became re-infected with HPV and developed new lesions. The recurrence rate of 33% (3/9) and overall complete response rate of 71% (12/19 at 9 months) are comparable to rates reported in the literature after surgical excision.[12,13] Although these data need to be confirmed by other researchers, intracervical administration of IFN-γ with close monitoring is a reasonable alternative to surgical intervention with similar efficacy to surgical excision.

Moreover, Schneider et al[29] directly compared conventional laser therapy with topical IFN-γ therapy in CIN2/3. Twenty-four patients were randomly assigned to topical administration of IFN-γ1b while nine patients received laser therapy. At 6 months, the cure rate for IFN-γ therapy was 42% compared to 89% for laser therapy ($p=0.02$). This study using topical IFN-γ shows a significantly lower response rate than the previous study using intracervical administration. Additional studies are needed to optimize a treatment regimen.

IMIQUIMOD

Imiquimod (Aldara®) functions as an immune modulator promoting cell-mediated immune responses.[30] Imiquimod is Food and Drug Administration (FDA)-approved for the treatment of external genital warts caused by HPV. As a result, some clinicians have used imiquimod for the treatment of other HPV-associated lesions of the genitalia. Diaz-Arrastia et al[31] published their limited experience using imiquimod in the treatment of recurrent high-grade intraepithelial neoplasia of the genitalia, including vagina, vulva, and cervix. Eight patients who failed previous standard therapy were offered imiquimod 5% cream self-applied to the lesion at bedtime three times weekly for 6–16 weeks. For the purpose of our discussion, we will focus on the two patients with CIN, both positive for HIV and at high risk for recurrence. One patient responded after 16 weeks of therapy, but developed recurrent CIN1 3 months later. She was re-treated with the same regimen and achieved a complete response again. The other patient had an initial improvement to CIN1, but then progressed again to CIN2/3. No significant toxicities were noted. Given the limited data available, imiquimod remains experimental. Theoretically, imiquimod could be effective in the treatment of CIN, but additional studies are needed.

CIDOFOVIR

Given the proven role of HPV in CIN (see Figure 19.1), antiviral agents such as cidofovir are potential medical therapies. Cidofovir and its metabolites are acyclic nucleoside phosphonates capable of inhibiting certain viral DNA polymerases. Even though HPV does not encode a DNA polymerase, cidofovir showed in vitro and in vivo activity against HPV and its associated lesions. Several researchers demonstrated that cidofovir is able to restore p53 function inducing apoptosis and cell death.[32,33] Cidofovir is approved by the FDA for intralesional treatment of laryngeal papillomas, another HPV-associated disease usually caused by low-risk types. The use of this drug in HPV-associated cervical disease is still under investigation.

Cidofovir induces apoptosis and inhibits cell proliferation of cervical cancer cell lines in vitro.[32,33] A review of the literature uncovered only one clinical trial using cidofovir to treat CIN.[34] Snoeck et al[34] treated 15 women with CIN3 using 1% cidofovir in gel applied topically to the cervix three times every other day. A cervical conization was performed 1 month later to assess treatment response. Complete response was noted in 7/15 patients (47%), which is slightly higher than the reported spontaneous regression rate for high-grade dysplasia (35%).[10] No toxicity was reported. This is the only study to date using cidofovir in CIN. In theory, this drug and its mechanism of action pose an interesting approach to the treatment CIN, potentially altering viral control of the cell and restoring normal cellular physiology and phenotype. Additional studies are needed to explore this drug before it can be used in routine clinical practice.

VACCINES

HPV consists of a double-stranded DNA genome (see Figure 19.2) enclosed within a non-enveloped nucleocapsid. The late proteins (L1 and L2) encode the nucleocapsid proteins which can self-assemble to form virus-like particles (VLPs).[35] There are numerous strains of HPV, distinguished by the DNA sequences

of L1, E6, and E7.[36] Carcinogenesis of cervical cancer is initiated by infection of the cervical epithelium with HPV (see Figure 19.1). Research shows very poor immune responses (humoral and cell-mediated) to HPV infection.[37] Thus, extensive research exists in studying the ability to boost the immune system using vaccines to combat HPV infection and the associated CIN/cervical cancer. Two general approaches for vaccines have been explored: one is therapeutic and the other is prophylactic. The therapeutic approach requires activation of cell-mediated immunity as the virus is located within cells. The prophylactic approach requires activation of humoral immunity as the virus is extracellular. Each of these approaches will be discussed in detail below.

Therapeutic HPV vaccines

The basic concept of the therapeutic approach is enabling cell-mediated cytotoxic T lymphocytes (CTLs) to recognize infected cells that express HPV viral proteins on their cell surface and target them for destruction (see Figure 19.3).[39] Surgical excision targets dysplastic cells, leaving behind normal-appearing cells potentially infected with HPV and at risk for neoplastic transformation. However, approaches targeting HPV directly or indirectly can treat and eradicate HPV-infected cells, whether dysplastic or normal-appearing, preventing recurrent disease.

Therapeutic vaccines target HPV early proteins, as only these proteins are expressed once the virus infects cells. E6 and E7 are the best targets, as they are strictly foreign viral proteins found only in infected cells and are required for transformation to malignant phenotype, targeting cells with oncogenic potential. Most studies focus on E7 because it is more abundantly expressed by infected cells, is better characterized immunogenically,[36] and contains more conserved sequences among different HPV types than E6 to confer broader coverage.[40,41] Several different vaccine strategies have been studied, each with advantages and disadvantages: viral vectors, fusion proteins, DNA, or dendritic cell-based therapies. We will discuss each in detail.

Viral vector vaccines

The use of viral vectors to deliver antigenic material carries several advantages: they are highly immunogenic, are not human leukocyte antigen (HLA) restricted, and allow inclusion of several antigens. However, disadvantages are the potential safety concerns treating patients with infectious agents and limitation of pre-existing viral

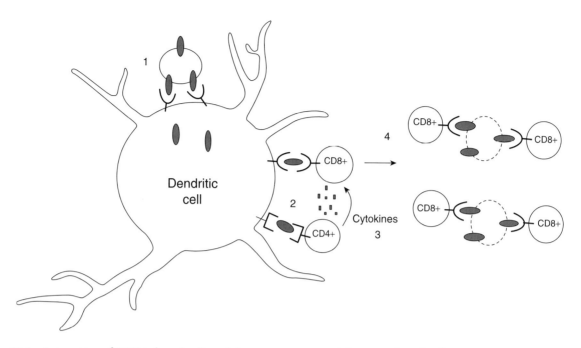

Figure 19.3   Interaction of HPV-infected cells and the immune system. (1) HPV-infected cells process HPV viral proteins and present them in their cell surface. These viral proteins are recognized by dendritic cells. (2) The dendritic cells process the viral proteins and present them for recognition by CD4+ and CD8+ cells. (3) The CD4+ cells subsequently release cytokines facilitating activation of CD8+ cells. (4) The activated CD8+ cells (also called cytotoxic T lymphocytes) proliferate and search the body for infected cells. Cytotoxic T lymphocytes will attack and kill any cell displaying the target proteins. Thus infected or cancerous cells are eliminated from the body while sparing normal cells. Modified from reference 38

immunity from other vaccinations or previous illness. We will discuss the two main vaccinia virus vaccines, TA-HPV and MVA E2.

TA-HPV is a live vaccinia virus engineered to express a fusion protein of E6 and E7 from both HPV-16 and -18. These oncogenic proteins were altered rendering them inactive: E6 at the terminal codon and E7 by a mutation in the retinoblastoma-binding site.[42] The European Organization for Research and Treatment of Cancer[42] conducted a phase II trial administering one dose of TA-HPV by dermal scarification to eight immunocompetent patients with locally advanced or recurrent cervical cancer. This trial established the safety and immunogenicity of the vaccine. No major adverse effects were recorded, only minor local site reactions. Three patients developed antibodies to HPV-18 E7 and one patient to HPV-16 E7. CTLs specific for HPV-18 E6/E7 developed by 9 weeks post-vaccination in one of three patients tested, but were lost by 14 weeks. The authors did not assess tumor response. Kaufmann et al[43] confirmed the above findings, noting a marginal immunological response to vaccine. Twenty-nine patients with early stage cervical cancer (IB or IIA) were given two doses of TA-HPV by scarification: the first dose 2 weeks before radical hysterectomy and the second dose 4–8 weeks after surgery. Four patients

demonstrated HPV-specific CTLs after one vaccination, while eight patients showed HPV-specific serological responses. Again no clinical efficacy was assessed. Davidson et al[44] conducted the only study assessing the clinical efficacy of TA-HPV. After 18 patients with vulvar dysplasia were treated, 13 demonstrated an immune response to HPV-16 after one dose. Eight patients showed a partial response with >50% reduction in lesion volume, and 12 reduced or cleared HPV viral infection.

Another potential HPV early protein target for HPV therapy is E2. E2 negatively regulates E6 and E7 expression. E2 expression is lost when the viral genome integrates into the cellular genome, allowing increased expression of E6 and E7 and potential malignant transformation. Restoration of E2 may be effective therapy for CIN and cervical cancer. Previous studies demonstrated that bovine papillomavirus E2 protein represses different promoters of HPV, inducing downregulation of E6 and E7 expression and apoptosis in human cancer cells.[45] This effect does not appear to be limited to specific HPV types. The exact mechanisms are unknown.

One laboratory developed a vaccinia vaccine containing bovine papillomavirus E2 gene (MVA E2). Corona Gutierrez et al[46] studied this vaccine in a phase I/II trial for the treatment of HPV-16/18-associated CIN1/2. Thirty-six patients between the ages of 25 and 49 received 10^7 viral particles of MVA E2 weekly in 2% lidocaine injected in all four quadrants of the cervix over 6 weeks. Forty-two patients received cryosurgery as a control. Biopsies taken at 6 weeks (completion of vaccination) showed CIN resolution in 18/36 patients (50%), which increased to 31/36 (87%) after 3 more weeks. The remaining five patients showed regression of disease to CIN1 or koilocytosis only. Cyrosurgery resulted in an 80% cure rate (37/42 patients) by 9 weeks, with koilocytes remaining in the other five patients. By 7 weeks, all vaccinated patients developed serologic antibodies against E2 and CTLs directed against tumor cells, which were not present prior to study initiation or in patients who received cryosurgery. Vaccination eliminated HPV infection in 50% of patients (equal rates for HPV-16/18), and significantly reduced viral loads (>90%) for the remaining 50%. Cryosurgery eradicated only 38% of HPV infections. No major adverse events were noted, with flu-like symptoms occurring in 42% of patients. This same laboratory then treated patients with CIN3 using either MVA E2 (34 patients) or conization (20 patients) using the same protocol as above.[47] By 9 weeks from study initiation, repeat biopsies showed a 56% (19/34 patients) cure rate in the vaccine group compared to 80% for the control group. A partial response was noted in 13/34 patients (38%). HPV was eliminated in 56% of the patients. At 1 year of follow-up, no recurrences were noted in the vaccine group versus three recurrences of CIN3 in the control group. These results show that MVA E2 is safe, immunogenic, and equally effective at treating CIN1/2 as cryosurgery. However, MVA E2 is slightly less effective in the treatment of CIN3. MVA E2 shows the most promise of the viral vector vaccines for the therapy of CIN, but these studies need to be confirmed by other laboratories.

Protein vaccines

Protein vaccines have the advantage of being non-infectious, but are only weak activators of cell-mediated immunity. Several different fusion protein vaccines have been studied. TA-CIN fusion protein, which contains a recombinant fusion protein L2/E6/E7 from HPV-16, was studied by two laboratories as reviewed by Kahn and Bernstein[35] in non-cervical high-grade anogenital intraepithelial neoplasia. These studies found the vaccine to be safe and immunogenic. However, clinical efficacy was limited, as only 20% of

patients responded completely to treatment. Another fusion protein, PD-E7, shows a similar lack of efficacy. PD-E7 contains a mutated E7 protein fused to the amino-terminal end of *Hemophilus influenzae* protein D. Hallez et al[48] treated seven patients with high-risk HPV-associated CIN1 or- 3 with 200 µg of PD-E7 in 0.5 ml adjuvant injected intramuscularly at 0, 2, and 4 weeks. Three patients with CIN1 were given placebo infections of normal saline as controls. By 8 weeks, all treated patients developed specific E7 and PD-specific immunoglobulin G (IgG) antibodies, while controls did not. Five of the treated patients developed systemic PD-E7-directed T cell responses. However, these immunological responses did not correlate with clinical responses. Two patients in each group (all with CIN1) had disappearance of disease upon conization 4 weeks after vaccination was completed. Of the five treated patients with CIN3, no viral clearance or lesion regression was noted. Again, this study shows limited clinical efficacy of the PD-E7 vaccination. The lack of vaccine effect shown in these studies could be due to study design. Many of these studies allowed very short intervals from completion of vaccination to biopsies/surgery. It is possible that the vaccines are effective given longer follow-up periods and different vaccination schedules. Additional studies are needed to answer these questions.

Other researchers took a slightly different approach to the development of therapeutic vaccines by utilizing the functions of heat shock proteins (hsps). Hsps are involved in activating the immune system in response to stressors, infections, or certain diseases, especially cancer,[49] causing activation of antigen-presenting cells and promoting antigen-specific T and B cell responses. Numerous hsps are known, with varying abilities to stimulate immune responses. A fusion protein containing heat shock protein 65, which possesses potent immunostimulatory properties, fused to E7 of HPV-16 (HspE7) was created and studied. Theoretically, hsps would increase the presentation efficiency of E7 to antigen-presenting cells, increasing the immune response.[49] The combined fusion protein generates a greater immune response than either protein alone.[49] Einstein et al[50] studied HspE7 for the treatment of CIN3. Thirty-two patients received three monthly subcutaneous injections of 500 µg HspE7. All patients underwent conization 4 months after study entry. A preliminary review of the results (11 patients still receiving vaccination) showed complete responses in 10/21 patients (48%) with partial responses (decrease in size of lesion >50%) in 4/21 patients (19%). The clearance of HPV-16 had no significant impact on clinical response as only half of the complete and partial responders eliminated the presence of HPV-16. However, HspE7 was studied in other disease processes, such as genital warts[49] and recurrent respiratory papillomatosis,[51] generally caused by low-risk HPV types. Higher response rates (80–90%) were noted in patients treated with HspE7, suggesting that this vaccine is not specific to the treatment of HPV-16 only but is also effective against other HPV types. Given the documented abilities of HspE7 to treat HPV-associated diseases, the Gynecologic Oncology Group conducted a randomized phase II trial (#197) using HspE7 for the treatment of HPV-16-associated CIN3. Enrollment finished December 2005, but data analysis is not yet available. HspE7 shows promising efficacy in the treatment of CIN and additional clinical studies are under way.

DNA vaccines

DNA vaccines are advantageous as they provide sustained antigenic expression and are easy to produce, store, and transport. However, they are weakly immunogenic and HLA-restricted.[36] The vaccine particles are engulfed by antigen-presenting cells, bound to major histocompatability complex (MHC) molecules, and presented on the cell surface, causing activation of the immune system. There are numerous different MHC–HLA types present in each person. These vaccines are particular to certain HLA types which all people will not express. At this time, this phenomenon cannot be overcome. However, the weak immunogenicity of the DNA vaccines can be enhanced by encapsulating the DNA, resulting in increased uptake into antigen-presenting cells.[52]

Sheets et al[52] created a DNA vaccine called ZYC101, composed of plasmid DNA encoding a portion of HPV-16 E7 protein encapsulated in biodegradable poly(lactide-co-glycolide) microparticles and restricted to HLA-A2 haplotype. In a phase I dose-escalating study, Sheets et al[53] administered 50 μg, 100 μg, or 200 μg of ZYC101 subcutaneously or intramuscularly every 3 weeks for a total of three injections to women with HLA-A2 and HPV-16-associated CIN2/3. All patients underwent a conization at 10 weeks (4 weeks after the last injection) and were followed for an additional 4 months. The drug was well tolerated, with 33% noting injection site pain independent of dose. Five of 15 patients (33%) completely responded to therapy (four received 100 μg intramuscularly). All of the complete responders developed systemic HPV-specific CTL activity after vaccination, which was gone by the 4-month follow-up. However, six of the 10 non-responders also showed that CTL activity, indicating CTL activity did

not correlate with response. However, response did correlate with elevated levels of IgA specific for HPV-16 E2 protein in cervical secretions: 4/5 complete responders were positive verses 0/10 non-responders. The authors hypothesize that HPV-infected cells undergoing apoptosis and lysis would liberate the E2 protein, stimulating the immune system. They suggest that assessment of cervical secretions for HPV antibodies may serve as a surrogate marker for response to therapy.

This study led to the development of a double-blind, randomized, placebo-controlled trial by Garcia et al[54] using a modified version of ZYC101, termed ZYC101a. The DNA sequences encoded by ZYC101a were expanded to incorporate segments of E6 and E7 of both HPV-16 and -18. One hundred and twenty-seven patients with CIN2/3 and positive HPV were randomized to placebo, 100 μg DNA, or 200 μg DNA administered intramuscularly, once every 3 weeks for three total doses. All patients underwent conization 6 months after study entry. Again the drug was well tolerated with only local injection site reaction. There was no significant difference between the two treatment groups and placebo as a whole (43% vs 27%, $p=0.05$). However, when the treatment groups were divided into certain age groups, <25 years vs ≥25 years, a difference was noted. Patients <25 years old receiving vaccine had a much higher response rate than the placebo group (70% vs 23%, $p=0.007$). However, patients 25 years or older had no significant response compared to placebo (29% vs 29%). This effect in the younger age group was irrespective of HPV type. Patients infected with HPV-16/18 had a cure rate of 64% vs 73% for other subtypes. Again, the systemic immune response did not correlate with clinical response to therapy. Antibodies in cervical secretions were not tested. ZYC101 and ZYC101a both had nominal response rates as a whole. However, ZYC101a was effective in patients <25 years old, raising the question: why does this difference exist?

One conclusion from most of these vaccine studies is that HPV-specific immunological responses do not seem to correlate with clinical response. Obviously, a clinical response to these vaccines involves a very complex sequence of cellular events beyond just the development of specific HPV cellular immune responses. A greater understanding of these mechanisms should allow significant advances in the treatment of HPV, CIN, and cervical cancer.

Dendritic cell-based vaccines

Dendritic cell-based vaccines are highly immunogenic, but difficult to produce and biodeliver.[36] Dendritic cells (DCs) are the most important antigen-presenting cells of the immune system. Immature DCs are highly effective at capturing antigens, although they cannot effectively present them. In contrast, mature DCs cannot phagocytose antigens well, but are able to effectively present antigens and activate T cell responses.[55] The maturation of DCs occurs upon stimulation with certain inflammatory cytokines. Dendritic cell-based vaccines are created as follows: autologous immature DCs are separated out of peripheral blood, cultured, pulsed with antigen, and treated with inflammatory cytokines, and then the mature DCs are re-administered to patients. Two laboratories have performed this procedure using recombinant E7 from HPV-16/18 as an antigen. Ferrara et al[56] treated 15 HPV-16/18-positive patients with locally progressive or recurrent cervical cancer refractory to standard treatment using 1–4 vaccines every 2–3 weeks containing an absolute number of DCs ranging from 2×10^4 to 2×10^6. The vaccine was well tolerated, with only two patients documenting a headache or flu-like symptoms. No objective clinical responses of the tumors were noted. Two weeks after the last vaccination, 3/11 patients noted a specific serological response while 4/11 patients had documented specific cellular responses. Santin et al[57] noted similar results in the same study population. However, this study differed slightly from the former: a constant but significantly greater number of DCs were injected (1×10^7); all patients received injections twice daily of interleukin 2 (IL-2) for 3–7 days postvaccination; and more injections were given, ranging from 6 to 12. Despite the increased dosing and augmentation with IL-2, no objective clinical responses were noted in the four patients enrolled. Two of the four patients demonstrated a positive delayed-type hypersenstivity (DTH) test after 6 vaccinations, while the other two patients did not. These latter two patients developed progression of disease and died within 5 months from vaccine initiation, while the former two patients died 13 months from starting vaccine therapy. These same patients also demonstrated a significant increase in specific HPV antibody titers and cellular immunity compared to pre-vaccination levels. However, the two patients with rapidly progressive disease had no significant change in antibody titers or cellular immunity. Adverse events were increased in this study, as most patients noted significant flu-like symptoms associated with IL-2 injections. These studies show that DC-based vaccinations are safe and can induce immune responses in some patients receiving vaccine therapy. The clinical responses are obviously poor, but could be related to the study populations. Additional studies are being done in earlier stage cervical cancer patients to assess clinical efficacy.

Prophylactic HPV vaccines

Prophylactic vaccine development has focused on strategies inducing antibody-mediated neutralization of HPV.[38] This was initiated with the observation that HPV nucleocapsid proteins (L1 and L2) could spontaneously form virus-like particles (VLPs) resembling the native viruses.[58] These are highly immunogenic, creating high titers of serum neutralizing antibodies. Given that HPV infects mucosal surfaces, protection from infection would require neutralizing antibodies to reach these areas. Nardelli-Haefliger et al[59] found significant titers of neutralizing antibodies in the cervical secretions of patients treated with HPV-16 VLPs. These initial studies led to the development of several prophylactic HPV vaccines summarized by Mahdavi and Monk.[36] We will discuss the two main vaccine therapies noted in the literature, a bivalent vaccine and a quadrivalent vaccine.

The bivalent vaccine is directed against the L1 VLPs of HPV-16/18, associated with 70% of all cervical cancers. A randomized, double-blind, placebo-controlled trial was conducted by Harper et al[60] who investigated the efficacy and safety of this vaccine in the prevention of CIN. The study enrolled 1113 women aged 15–25 with the following inclusion criteria: no history of abnormal Paps, < 6 lifetime sexual partners, seronegative for HPV-16/18, and negative by polymerase chain reaction (PCR) for high-risk HPV types 16, 18, 31, 33, 35, 39, 45, 51, 52, 56, 58, 59, 66, and 68. The participants received either vaccine consisting of 20 μg of each HPV-16/18 L1 VLPs in 500 μg aluminum hydroxide and 50 μg 3-deacylated monophosphoryl lipid A, or placebo containing only 500 μg aluminum hydroxide. Drugs were administered intramuscularly at 0, 1, and 6 months. By according-to-protocol analysis, vaccine efficacy was 91.6% (95% confidence interval (CI) 64.5–98%) against incident HPV infection and 100% effective against persistent HPV-16/18 infection. Using intention-to-treat analysis, vaccine efficacy was 95.1% against persistent HPV-16/18 infections (four cases in vaccine group verses 31 in the placebo group) and 92.9% effective against cytological abnormalities associated with HPV infection (two low-grade lesions in vaccine group verses 26 low-grade lesions and one high-grade in the placebo group). After three injections in the vaccine group, 100% of patients became seropositive for HPV-16 and 99.7% converted to HPV-18 positive, which increased to

100% by 18 months. Antibody titers were generally 80–100 times greater than antibodies induced after natural infection with HPV-16/18. These titers remained elevated to 10–16 times higher than natural infection titers at 18 months, but obviously had decreased significantly. The vaccine was well tolerated, with mainly local injection site issues and fatigue noted equally in both placebo and vaccine groups. It would be important to follow-up these patients to assess them for antibody levels and HPV infection. The duration of protection from these vaccines is unknown. This vaccine has not been submitted to the FDA for approval as yet.

Another laboratory developed a quadrivalent vaccine (also containing L1 VLPs), targeting not only HPV-16 and -18, but also HPV-6 and -11, which are responsible for 90% of genital warts. Villa et al[61] conducted a randomized double-blind placebo-controlled trial to assess the efficacy of this vaccine to prevent HPV infection and associated cervical abnormalities. A total of 552 women were enrolled, aged 16–23 years. Similar inclusion criteria were used as the prior study: no history of abnormal Paps and <5 lifetime sexual partners. However, this study did not exclude participants with previous HPV infections. These patients received either vaccine containing 20 μg HPV-6 L1 VLPs, 40 μg HPV-11 L1 VLPs, 40 μg HPV-16 L1 VLPs, and 20 μg HPV-18 L1 VLPs in 225 μg aluminum adjuvant, or placebo given intramuscularly, at day 1, month 2, and month 6. Using according-to-protocol analysis, the incidence of persistent HPV infection with one of the targeted HPV types or associated genital disease was decreased by 90% (95% CI 71–97%) in the vaccine group compared to placebo. Intention-to-treat analysis showed an 89% (95% CI 73–96%) decrease in the incidence of HPV infection or associated disease in the vaccine group compared to placebo. Six patients in the vaccine group developed an infection with HPV-16/18, with three of these occurring at the last visit (36 months). No disease occurred in the vaccine group compared to 11 occurrences in the placebo group, seven CIN, and four genital warts during the 30 months of follow-up. All patients in the vaccine group developed an antibody response to all four HPV types ranging on average from 60 to 120 times greater than placebo antibody levels. Again, these titers significantly decreased by completion of the study (36 months) to as low as 10 times placebo levels. The significance of this is unknown. However, three patients in the vaccine group developed HPV infection at 36 months: could this be due to waning antibody titers?

Villa et al[62] attempted to answer this question by publishing 5-year follow-up data for this trial. A subset of patients (n=241) were initially enrolled for 60 months of follow-up. The patients were treated the same as already stated above. According-to-protocol analysis demonstrated that the vaccine was 95.8% (95% CI 83.8–99.5%) effective at preventing persistent HPV infection with one of the target HPV types or associated disease, compared to placebo. Intention-to-treat analysis showed a similar efficacy of 93.7% (95% CI 83–98.3%). A total of four HPV infections were noted in the vaccine group (three HPV-16 and one HPV-18), with no associated lesions, compared to 58 HPV infections (22 HPV-6, four HPV-11, 34 HPV-16, and 12 HPV-18) in the placebo group, with 11 associated lesions (seven patients with genital warts and four cases with CIN). These results are similar to the 36-month follow-up data summarized above. Antibody titers were also assessed at 60 months. The antibody titers had again decreased on average from the levels measured at 36 months. When considering the confidence intervals, only HPV-16 levels were still significantly greater than placebo at 60 months (395.4 vs 16.0, respectively). Antibody titers for HPV-6 and -18 were not significantly different from those in the placebo group, while HPV-11 titers were lower in the vaccine group compared to placebo. The authors did not discuss the return of antibody titers to 'normal' levels at 5 years as this may pertain to their immune response and long-term protection. It is possible that the patients are still protected due to memory effector cells. However, this may indicate the need for booster injections.

In addition, a phase III trial[63] is in progress using this same vaccine in over 18 000 women with similar preliminary results after 2 years of follow-up, which was presented at The American Society for Microbiology meeting in December 2005. These studies have led to the approval of this quadrivalent vaccine by the FDA on June 8, 2006. This is the first vaccine for the prevention of cervical cancer and certain types of genital warts. The Advisory Committee on Immunization Practices (ACIP) voted to recommend administration of the vaccine to girls aged 11–12 years, ideally before the onset of sexual activity. They recommend extending the age range to 9–26 years old for those who have not been vaccinated. As noted above, typical ages of study participants were 15–26 years old, ages when HPV infection is greatest. Block et al[64] showed similar antibody responses after vaccination in boys and girls aged 9–15. The vaccine provides no therapeutic benefit to persons already infected with one or more of the target HPV strains. HPV typing is clinically unavailable and not necessary prior to vaccination, as patients will still obtain benefit from the vaccine in preventing infection with other types. Patients must continue routine cervical cancer screening protocols, as this vaccine will prevent at most 70% of cervical cancers (those caused by HPV-16/18) if it is 100% effective. These recommendations have been adopted by the Centers for Disease Control.

Certain issues remain unclear. A couple of the studies reviewed above suggest that the antibody titers in the serum return close to baseline by 5 years. The significance of this is unknown. Antibody titers in the cervical mucosa or secretions may better reflect the ability to prevent HPV infection. Moreover, memory effector cells may cause a natural boost in the immune system when re-infection occurs, conferring continual protection. Another major issue which has been raised is whether boys should be vaccinated. A review of the literature by Dunne et al[65] found that the prevalence of HPV in men ranges from 1.3 to 72.9%. However, men develop minimal sequelae of HPV infection, except transmitting it to their female sexual partners. Since the goal is universal female vaccination, male vaccination would provide no significant benefit, but a much greater cost.[36] Direct studies to answer this question are under way.

PHOTODYNAMIC THERAPY

Photodynamic therapy (PDT) involves the administration of a photosensitizer followed by laser illumination of the affected area. Briefly, the photosensitizer accumulates intracellularly and generates highly reactive oxygen intermediates upon illumination with visible light at a specific wavelength.[66] These molecules cause irreversible cell damage, leading to cell death and tissue necrosis. Studies show that this tissue damage is confined to the superficially treated epithelium, preserving the underlying subepithelial collagen and elastin, as well as the adjacent normal tissues.[67]

PDT is an appealing alternative to surgical treatment of CIN due to the preservation of underlying stromal tissues, with less impact on future fertility. Much work was conducted by Japanese investigators leading to Photofrin® (PHE, polyhematoporphytrin ether/ester) approval in Japan for the treatment of CIN. Yamaguchi et al[68] published the largest study to date, enrolling 105 patients with CIN, mostly CIN3. PHE was administered intravenously at 2 mg/kg, and after 48–60 hours phototherapy was performed using

an excimer dye laser or YAG–OPO laser (yttrium aluminum garnet–optical parametric oscillator) with an energy of $100 J/cm^2$ at a wavelength of 630 nm. Biopsies performed at 3 months showed a complete response in 90% of patients, which increased to 98% by 6 months. Three patients, despite normal histology at 3 months, developed recurrent disease: two developed CIN3 at 645 and 717 days, and one developed stage IB1 cervical cancer at 895 days after therapy. HPV testing was also performed in 69 of these patients before and after therapy. Sixty-four (93%) patients initially tested positive, with 30 patients infected with HPV-16/18. After 3 months, 47/63 (73%) were HPV-negative. Thirteen of the 17 HPV-positive patients had a change in the HPV type present, suggesting re-infection. The patient who developed cancer became infected with new HPV types. The other two recurrences were negative for HPV. No cervical abnormalities were detected at 3 months in the 17 HPV-positive patients. The main toxicity was cutaneous photosensitivity in 50 patients, despite hospitalization in a dark room for 3 weeks after therapy. No significant impact on sexual function or fertility was identified. These authors demonstrate the effectiveness of PDT using intravenous PHE in treating CIN and associated HPV infections. One major pitfall to intravenous photosensitizers is incorporation of the drug within cutaneous tissues, making patients extremely photosensitive for several weeks. This has led additional researchers to study the efficacy of localized photosensitizer administration.

The main photosensitizer studied for topical administration to the cervix is 5-aminolevulinic acid (5-ALA). Keefe et al[69] showed that topical 5-ALA resulted in selective uptake by dysplastic cells compared to normal epithelium and underlying stroma. However, fluorescence micrographs depicted in this paper showed variable penetration of the drug to the basal layer; this was not specifically measured or commented upon by the authors. This observation is important, as HPV initially infects the cells of the basal layer[70] where the earliest changes (i.e. CIN1) occur and progress toward the epithelial surface. Effective treatment of CIN must reach these deepest cells. Anderson and Hartley[71] assessed 343 conization specimens and found that 95% of dysplastic cells reached a depth of 3 mm, with some penetrating to 5 mm. No studies have directly measured the depth of photosensitizer penetration in cervical epithelium after topical or intravenous administration. A study in squamous cell carcinoma of the oral cavity showed that the depth of tissue necrosis after photodynamic therapy using intravenous PHE ranged from 1.1 to 4.1 mm below the surface, with a mean of 2.1 mm[67] Even though these findings place doubt on the theoretical ability of PDT to appropriately penetrate the cervical epithelium and effectively treat CIN, encouraging clinical results are documented.

Bodner et al[72] in a case–control study compared cold knife conization to PDT using topical 5-ALA. Twenty-two HPV-positive women with CIN2 were treated, 11 in each group. The cervix was exposed to 5 ml of 12% 5-ALA in normal saline using a vacuum-sealed cervical adapter for 8 hours followed by phototherapy using a halogen lamp, including lens system, to provide a broadband red light (580–800 nm) delivering 100 J/cm^2 to the superficial portio. The endocervical canal was separately treated with a KTP (potassium titanyl phosphate):YAG laser delivering 50 J/cm^2 of energy at a wavelength of 652 nm. All procedures were performed as an outpatient without anesthesia. Both PDT and conization were equally effective at eliminating HPV infection at 3 months (8/11 patients). At 1 year, biopsies showed a complete response rate of 100% in the conization group and 91% (10/11) in the PDT group. The one PDT failure had persistent HPV infection with a documented CIN1 at 6 months. Conization was performed, with normal subsequent follow-up. No systemic toxicities or local scarring was noted.

However, other studies have shown minimal efficacy of PDT using topically applied 5-ALA. The only randomized double-blind placebo-controlled trial assessing the role of PDT in the treatment CIN was conducted by Barnett et al.[73] Twenty-five patients with CIN, predominantly CIN1 (22/25), were randomized to placebo versus 5-ALA. Twelve patients received 10 g of 3% 5-ALA in gel administered topically over 4 hours using a contraceptive cervical cap, while the remaining 13 patients received placebo (gel alone). The cervix was exposed to 100 J/cm^2 at a wavelength of 635 nm from a diode laser. Three months later, all patients underwent LLETZ (large loop excision of the transformation zone). No difference in response rates was noted between the treatment and placebo groups, 33% vs 31%, respectively. The 33% response rate of this study was significantly less than the 91% response rate[72] noted above, despite the former study enrolling patients with higher grade dysplasia. The reasons for this are probably multifactorial, as the two laboratories used different lasers with different settings, different concentrations of 5-ALA, and different durations of exposure to 5-ALA. These are issues which continuously plague comparisons of

efficacy between different PDT trials. Even though the data are conflicting, we believe that PDT is a viable alternative for patients trying to avoid surgical procedures. Additional well-designed studies are needed before PDT is routinely included in the standard management of CIN.

RADIATION AND CHEMOTHERAPY

Cervical cancer is extremely sensitive to radiation, providing a non-invasive alternative to surgery. However, radiation to the pelvis destroys ovarian function and is associated with a higher rate of sexual dysfunction than surgery. The advantage of radiation as a non-invasive alternative applies to patients considered inoperable due to problems such as comorbid medical issues, or large-volume or multifocal disease requiring extensive surgical resection. Nag et al[74] summarize the recommendations of the American Brachytherapy Society, and Einhorn et al[75] provide a systemic review of radiation uses in cervical cancer. Given the potential for early spread of cervical cancer, studies have investigated the role of chemotherapy. We will review these studies in more detail.

CIN3 and stage IA1 cervical cancer are primarily treated by conization or simple hysterectomy. However, several studies show that radiation is effective in this setting. Grigsby and Perez[76] treated 21 patients with CIN3 using one dose of intracavitary radiation to an average dose of 4600 cGy at point A. No failures were noted, with a mean follow-up of 10 years. Kolstad and Klem[77] followed 1121 patients with CIN3 and found that patients treated with intracavitary radiation versus conization or hysterectomy developed similar rates of invasive carcinoma (1.8% vs 0.9% or 2.1%, respectively). For stage IA invasive carcinoma, Grigsby and Perez[76] treated 34 patients with either intracavitary radiation alone (13 patients) for two doses or external pelvic radiation plus intracavitary radiation (21 patients). The average dose of radiation in patients receiving intracavitary radiation alone was 5570 cGy to point A. Patients who received both external and intracavitary radiation received an average of 1400 cGy to the whole pelvis, with 2350 cGy boost to the parametria plus an additional 5200 cGy to point A via intracavitary radiation. Only one recurrence (3%) occurred in a patient receiving combination therapy. Moreover, patients treated with combination therapy had more complications, developing two bowel obstructions. These findings were confirmed by Kolstad,[78] who noted no recurrences in 136 patients with stage IA1 cervical cancer treated with only intracavitary radiation. Based on these data, intracavitary radiation alone is an effective alternative to surgery for the treatment of CIN3 and early stage cervical cancer.

Stage IA2–IIA cervical cancer can be treated with either radical surgery or definitive radiotherapy, as equivalent disease-free and overall survivals are achievable.[75] However, surgery should be avoided in patients with high-risk factors for recurrence (i.e. tumor >4 cm in diameter, evidence of lymphovascular space invasion on histology, positive lymph nodes), as these patients require radiation to reduce the risk of recurrence. Studies reveal a significant increase in toxicity when surgery is followed by radiation.[74]

Bulky stage IB and stage IIB–IV respond best to definitive radiotherapy.[74] The role of neoadjuvant chemotherapy prior to radiation is limited. A meta-analysis by the Neoadjuvant Chemotherapy for Cervical Cancer Meta-analysis Collaboration[79] analyzed about 2000 women with stage II–III cervical cancer from 18 trials and showed a marginal benefit using cisplatin-based chemotherapy at cycle lengths of ≤ 14 days hazard ratio (HR) 0.83, 95% CI 0.69–1.00, $p=0.046$) administered prior to radiotherapy. However, cycle lengths >14 days were detrimental (HR 1.25, 95% CI 1.07–1.46, $p=0.005$). In addition, dosages of cisplatin <25 mg/m^2 were harmful (HR 1.35, 95% CI 1.11–1.14, $p=0.002$). The benefit of chemotherapy in a neoadjuvant setting is unproven at this time and may even be harmful in certain circumstances.

However, chemotherapy given together with radiation is beneficial according to two meta-analyses conducted by separate authors. Green et al[80] analyzed 11 trials with about 3600 patients treated with platinum verses non-platinum chemotherapy concurrently with radiation for stages I–IV cervical cancer. Concomitant chemoradiation improved disease-free and overall survival compared to radiation alone. The greatest survival advantage occurred with administration of platinum chemotherapy (HR 0.70, 95% CI 0.61–0.80, $p<0.0001$) versus non-platinum chemotherapy (HR 0.81, 95% CI 0.56–1.16, $p=0.2$). Patients receiving platinum chemoradiation had a 20–39% reduction in the chance of death compared to patients treated with radiation alone. Moreover, patients with earlier stage disease obtain the most benefit from chemoradiation versus radiation alone: studies with $\geq 70\%$ stage I and II patients had a hazard ratio of 0.56 (95% CI 0.44–0.70) compared to 0.80 (95% CI 0.69–0.93) for studies with <70% stage I and II patients.

Lukka et al[81] confirmed these findings, as they assessed eight trials administering concurrent cisplatin-based chemotherapy plus radiation in the treatment of cervical cancer. Again, concomitant cisplatin chemoradiation improved the overall survival (HR 0.74, 95% CI 0.64–0.86, $p<0.0001$) compared to radiation alone. These authors too noted that patients with high-risk early stage disease benefited the most (HR 0.56, 95% CI 0.41–0.77). These studies resulted in a new standard of care for all stages of cervical cancer whereby cisplatin chemotherapy is now administered concurrently with radiation. However, the true role of this regimen in locally advance disease (stages IIB–IV) is unknown.

INDOLE-3-CARBINOL

Indole-3-carbinol (I3C) occurs naturally in cruciferous vegetables, including cabbage, broccoli, and brussels sprouts. Aggarwal and Ichikawa[82] summarize the numerous activities of I3C (i.e. increased apoptosis, decreased metastasis, inhibition of tumor cell proliferation and tumorigenesis). Several investigators examined the potential role of I3C for treating CIN. Jin et al[83] conducted in vivo experiments treating HPV-16 transgenic mice with estrogen alone (control) or estrogen plus I3C. These mice develop cervical cancer upon exposure to estrogen. Of 25 control mice, 19 (76%) developed cervical cancer, while only 2/24 mice (8%) given I3C and estrogen developed cancer, suggesting that I3C can prevent cervical cancer. Bell et al[84] performed a randomized placebo-controlled trial of I3C in the treatment of CIN. Twenty-seven patients with CIN2/3 were randomly assigned to either placebo or 200 or 400 mg/day of oral I3C for 12 weeks. Biopsies performed at 12 weeks showed that the two treatment groups had similar response rates, 4/8 (50%) for the 200-mg group and 4/9 (44%) for the 400-mg group. The placebo group had no complete responses. No adverse events were noted. Given the limited data available, I3C is still experimental in the treatment of CIN. Larger studies with longer follow-up are needed to prove its efficacy.

GENE THERAPY

High-risk HPV can cause cell transformation and immortalization via certain oncoproteins responsible for viral-induced carcinogenesis.[5] The HPV genome encodes six different early proteins and two late proteins (see Figure 19.2). Early protein 6 (E6) and early protein 7 (E7) are the main genes with oncogenic properties. As depicted in Figure 19.1, E6 can bind p53, a tumor suppressor gene, rendering p53 inactive. p53 serves many functions within cells, including DNA repair and regulation of apoptosis. Dysfunction of p53 places cells at risk for mutations and tumorigenesis[5] Loss of functional proteins or genes is the basis for gene therapies, whereby a lost protein or gene is reintroduced in an attempt to restore normal cellular mechanisms. For a thorough review of gene therapies and strategies, see reference 85. Brooks and Mutch give a general review of different therapies studied in gynecologic malignancies, including CIN and cervical cancer.[85] However, none of these therapies have progressed into clinical trials. Therefore, we will discuss only a few key studies utilizing the p53-mediated pathway, as this pathway is heavily related to HPV carcinogenesis.

Given the dysfunction of p53 in HPV-infected cells, replacing p53 in these cells via gene therapy may restore function. Ahn et al[86,87] studied effects of recombinant adenovirus-p53 gene transfer on human cervical cancer cells in vitro and in vivo. Cell lines known to be positive for HPV-16 (CaSki and SiHa) and HPV-18 (HeLa and HeLaS3) were transfected with a recombinant adenoviral vector containing human wild-type p53 gene (AdCMVp53). Gene transfer of these cells lines resulted in a dose-dependent inhibition of cell proliferation in vitro. The same effect was evident in vivo as tumors generated from cancer cell-xenografted nude mice grew significantly slower in mice given AdCMVp53 versus placebo. However, the inhibition of tumor growth was lost by day 23 after treatment with AdCMVp53. Gene expression studies found reduced levels of E6 and increased p53 expression in transfected cells, but this effect was lost by 21 days post-transfection, about the same time tumor growth returns to normal. These data suggest that gene transfer of p53 using adenoviral vectors can inhibit cervical cancer cell proliferation in vitro and in vivo, but the effect is short-lived, as the viral production of E6 quickly overwhelms the expression of wild-type p53. Repeated injections of AdCMVp53 may be able to counteract this effect; however, this was not studied.

Another laboratory transfected cells with a different gene, p73, which does not interact with E6. Theoretically, continued expression of E6 should not affect the activity of p73. p73 is a member of the p53 gene family, encoding proteins functionally and structurally similar to proteins encoded by p53. p73 is felt to play a role in p53-mediated apoptosis. Das and Somasundaram[88] assessed the role of p73 gene transfer in cervical cancer cells. The authors generated an adenoviral vector containing p73 (Ad-p73) and transfected cancer cells containing HPV E6 and control cells. They also transfected the same cells with an adenovirus containing p53 (Ad-p53). Cell lines which contained E6 were significantly inhibited by Ad-p73, but only minimally inhibited by Ad-p53, compared to controls. Cell lines without E6 were equally inhibited by both p73 and p53. Therefore, adenoviral vectors containing p73 may be more appropriate for the treatment of cervical cancer, as p73 expression is not affected by viral oncoproteins and bypasses the viral control of intracellular processes.

CONCLUSIONS

Significant knowledge concerning the biology of HPV and the pathogenesis of CIN and cervical cancer has been gained over the last 20 years. This has led to the development of new medical therapies for the treatment of CIN and cervical cancer. However, none of these methods have become part of standard of care. Yet, several of these therapies have gained enough support in the literature to warrant consideration as non-invasive alternatives to surgery in select patient populations. These therapies include PDT, IFN-β, and IFN-γ. Moreover, significant advances have been made in developing vaccination strategies against HPV. The most promising therapeutic vaccines are MVA E2, HspE7, and ZYC101a. Yet, the greatest accomplishment in the management of cervical abnormalities since creation of the Pap test is the development of a prophylactic vaccine against HPV-6, -11, -16, and -18. This vaccine will not eradicate cervical cancer, but should significantly decrease the incidence of CIN and cervical cancer. The next main challenge in the fight against cervical cancer is improved access of these technological advances for all women, including underdeveloped countries, where cervical cancer is epidemic.

ACKNOWLEDGMENTS

REFERENCES

1. American Cancer and Society. Cancer Facts & Figures 2006. Atlanta, GA: ACS, 2006.
2. Pecorelli S, Favalli G, Zigliani L, Odicino F. Cancer in women. Int J Gynaecol Obstet 2003; 82: 369–79.
3. Jones HW 3rd. Impact of the Bethesda System. Cancer 1995; 76 (Suppl): 1914–18.
4. Munoz N, Bosch FX, de Sanjose S et al. Epidemiologic classification of human papillomavirus types associated with cervical cancer. N Engl J Med 2003; 348: 518–27.

5. zur Hausen H. Papillomaviruses causing cancer: evasion from host-cell control in early events in carcinogenesis. J Natl Cancer Inst 2000; 92: 690–8.

6. Koutsky L. Epidemiology of genital human papillomavirus infection. Am J Med 1997; 102: 3–8.

7. Ho GY, Bierman R, Beardsley L, Chang CJ, Burk RD. Natural history of cervicovaginal papillomavirus infection in young women. N Engl J Med 1998; 338: 423–8.

8. Chua KL, Hjerpe A. Human papillomavirus analysis as a prognostic marker following conization of the cervix uteri. Gynecol Oncol 1997; 66: 108–13.

9. zur Hausen H. Papillomaviruses and cancer: from basic studies to clinical application. Nat Rev Cancer 2002; 2: 342–50.

10. Melnikow J, Nuovo J, Willan AR, Chan BK, Howell LP. Natural history of cervical squamous intraepithelial lesions: a meta-analysis. Obstet Gynecol 1998; 92: 727–35.

11. Oster G. Natural history of cervical intraepithelial neoplasia: a critical review. Int J Gynecol Pathol 1993; 12: 186–92.

12. Dietrich CS 3rd, Yancey MK, Miyazawa K, Williams DL, Farley J. Risk factors for early cytologic abnormalities after loop electrosurgical excision procedure. Obstet Gynecol 2002; 99: 188–92.

13. Gonzalez DI Jr, Zahn CM, Retzloff MG et al. Recurrence of dysplasia after loop electrosurgical excision procedures with long-term follow-up. Am J Obstet Gynecol 2001; 184: 315–21.

14. Klaritsch P, Reich O, Giuliani A et al. Delivery outcome after cold-knife conization of the uterine cervix. Gynecol Oncol 2006; 103: 604–7.

15. Sadler L, Saftlas A, Wang W et al. Treatment for cervical intraepithelial neoplasia and risk of preterm delivery. JAMA 2004; 291: 2100–6.

16. Baron S, Tyring SK, Fleischmann WR Jr et al. The interferons. Mechanisms of action and clinical applications. JAMA 1991; 266: 1375–83.

17. Rockley PF, Tyring SK. Interferons alpha, beta and gamma therapy of anogenital human papillomavirus infections. Pharmacol Ther 1995; 65: 265–87.

18. Ikic D, Krusic J, Kirhmajer V et al. Application of human leucocyte interferon in patients with carcinoma of the uterine cervix. Lancet 1981; 1: 1027–30.

19. Vasilyev RV, Bokhman JaV, Smorodintsev AA et al. An experience with application of human leucocyte interferon for cervical cancer treatment. Eur J Gynaecol Oncol 1990; 11: 313–17.

20. Byrne MA, Moller BR, Taylor-Robinson D et al. The effect of interferon on human papillomaviruses associated with cervical intraepithelial neoplasia. Br J Obstet Gynaecol 1986; 93: 1136–44.

21. Frost L, Skajaa K, Hvidman LE, Fay SJ, Larsen PM. No effect of intralesional injection of interferon on moderate cervical intraepithelial neoplasia. Br J Obstet Gynaecol 1990; 97: 626–30.

22. Wiley DJ, Douglas J, Beutner K et al. External genital warts: diagnosis, treatment, and prevention. Clin Infect Dis 2002; 35 (Suppl 2): S210–24.

23. Jach R, Basta A, Szczudrawa A. [Role of immunomodulatory treatment with Iscador QuS and Intron A of women with CIN1 with concurrent HPV infection]. Ginekol Pol 2003; 74: 729–35. [in Polish]

24. Gostout BS, Hartmann LC, Suman VJ et al. A randomized trial of interferon-alpha in cervical dysplasia. Int J Gynaecol Obstet 2001; 74: 207–10.

25. Penna C, Fallani MG, Gordigiani R et al. Intralesional beta-interferon treatment of cervical intraepithelial neoplasia associated with human papillomavirus infection. Tumori 1994; 80: 146–50.

26. Gonzalez-Sanchez JL, Martinez-Chequer JC, Hernandez-Celaya ME, Barahona-Bustillos E, Andrade-Manzano AF. Randomized placebo-controlled evaluation of intramuscular interferon beta treatment of recurrent human papillomavirus. Obstet Gynecol 2001; 97: 621–4.

27. Sikorski M, Zrubek H. Recombinant human interferon gamma in the treatment of cervical intraepithelial neoplasia (CIN) associated with human papillomavirus (HPV) infection. Eur J Gynaecol Oncol 2003; 24: 147–50.

28. Sikorski M, Zrubek H. Long-term follow-up of patients treated with recombinant human interferon gamma for cervical intraepithelial neoplasia. Int J Gynaecol Obstet 2003; 82: 179–85.

29. Schneider A, Grubert T, Kirchmayr R et al. Efficacy trial of topically administered interferon gamma-1 beta gel in comparison to laser treatment in cervical intraepithelial neoplasia. Arch Gynecol Obstet 1995; 256: 75–83.

30. Stanley MA. Imiquimod and the imidazoquinolones: mechanism of action and therapeutic potential. Clin Exp Dermatol 2002; 27: 571–7.

31. Diaz-Arrastia C, Arany I, Robazetti SC et al. Clinical and molecular responses in high-grade intraepithelial neoplasia treated with topical imiquimod 5%. Clin Cancer Res 2001; 7: 3031–3.

32. Andrei G, Snoeck R, Schols D, De Clercq E. Induction of apoptosis by cidofovir in human papillomavirus (HPV)-positive cells. Oncol Res 2000; 12: 397–408.

33. Abdulkarim B, Sabri S, Deutsch E et al. Antiviral agent Cidofovir restores p53 function and enhances the radiosensitivity in HPV-associated cancers. Oncogene 2002; 21: 2334–46.

34. Snoeck R, Noel JC, Muller C, De Clercq E, Bossens M. Cidofovir, a new approach for the treatment of cervix intraepithelial neoplasia grade III (CIN III). J Med Virol 2000; 60: 205–9.

35. Kahn JA, Bernstein DI. Human papillomavirus vaccines and adolescents. Curr Opin Obstet Gynecol 2005; 17: 476–82.

36. Mahdavi A, Monk BJ. Vaccines against human papillomavirus and cervical cancer: promises and challenges. Oncologist 2005; 10: 528–38.

37. Tindle RW. Immunomanipulative strategies for the control of human papillomavirus associated cervical disease. Immunol Res 1997; 16: 387–400.

38. www.nventacorp.com/immunotherapeutic_science/cellular_immunity.htm.

39. Roden RB, Ling M, Wu TC. Vaccination to prevent and treat cervical cancer. Hum Pathol 2004; 35: 971–82.

40. Ahn WS, Bae SM, Kim TY et al. A therapy modality using recombinant IL-12 adenovirus plus E7 protein in a human papillomavirus 16 E6/E7-associated cervical cancer animal model. Hum Gene Ther 2003; 14: 1389–99.

41. Jochmus-Kudielka I, Schneider A, Braun R et al. Antibodies against the human papillomavirus type 16 early proteins in human sera: correlation of anti-E7 reactivity with cervical cancer. J Natl Cancer Inst 1989; 81: 1698–704.

42. Borysiewicz LK, Fiander A, Nimako M et al. A recombinant vaccinia virus encoding human papillomavirus types 16 and 18, E6 and E7 proteins as immunotherapy for cervical cancer. Lancet 1996; 347: 1523–7.

43. Kaufmann AM, Stern PL, Rankin EM et al. Safety and immunogenicity of TA-HPV, a recombinant vaccinia virus expressing modified human papillomavirus (HPV)-16 and HPV-18 E6 and E7 genes, in women with progressive cervical cancer. Clin Cancer Res 2002; 8: 3676–85.

44. Davidson EJ, Boswell CM, Sehr P et al. Immunological and clinical responses in women with vulval intraepithelial neoplasia vaccinated with a vaccinia virus encoding human papillomavirus 16/18 oncoproteins. Cancer Res 2003; 63: 6032–41.

45. Dowhanick JJ, McBride AA, Howley PM. Suppression of cellular proliferation by the papillomavirus E2 protein. J Virol 1995; 69: 7791–9.

46. Corona Gutierrez CM, Tinoco A, Navarro T et al. Therapeutic vaccination with MVA E2 can eliminate precancerous lesions (CIN 1, CIN 2, and CIN 3) associated with infection by oncogenic human papillomavirus. Hum Gene Ther 2004; 15: 421–31.

47. Garcia-Hernandez E, Gonzalez-Sanchez JL, Andrade-Manzano A et al. Regression of papilloma high-grade lesions (CIN 2 and CIN 3) is stimulated by therapeutic vaccination with MVA E2 recombinant vaccine. Cancer Gene Ther 2006; 13: 592–7.

48. Hallez S, Simon P, Maudoux F et al. Phase I/II trial of immunogenicity of a human papillomavirus (HPV) type 16 E7 protein-based vaccine in women with oncogenic HPV-positive cervical intraepithelial neoplasia. Cancer Immunol Immunother 2004; 53: 642–50.

49. Neefe JR, Chu NR, Mizzen L. CoVal fusions: a therapeutic vaccine platform using heat shock proteins to treat chronic viral infection and cancer. Dev Biol (Basel) 2004; 116: 193–200; discussion 229–36.

50. Einstein MH, Kadish AS, Burke RD. Heat shock protein (HSP)-based immunotherapy (HSPE7) for the treatment of CIN III. Gynecol Oncol 2005; 96: 912a–13a.

51. Derkay CS, Smith RJ, McClay J et al. HspE7 treatment of pediatric recurrent respiratory papillomatosis: final results of an open-label trial. Ann Otol Rhinol Laryngol 2005; 114: 730–7.

52. Hedley ML, Curley J, Urban R. Microspheres containing plasmid-encoded antigens elicit cytotoxic T-cell responses. Nat Med 1998; 4: 365–8.

53. Sheets EE, Urban RG, Crum CP et al. Immunotherapy of human cervical high-grade cervical intraepithelial neoplasia with microparticle-delivered human papillomavirus 16 E7 plasmid DNA. Am J Obstet Gynecol 2003; 188: 916–26.

54. Garcia F, Petry KU, Muderspach L et al. ZYC101a for treatment of high-grade cervical intraepithelial neoplasia: a randomized controlled trial. Obstet Gynecol 2004; 103: 317–26.

55. Santin AD, Bellone S, Roman JJ et al. Therapeutic vaccines for cervical cancer: dendritic cell-based immunotherapy. Curr Pharm Des 2005; 11: 3485–500.

56. Ferrara A, Nonn M, Sehr P et al. Dendritic cell-based tumor vaccine for cervical cancer II: results of a clinical pilot study in 15 individual patients. J Cancer Res Clin Oncol 2003; 129: 521–30.

57. Santin AD, Bellone S, Palmieri M et al. HPV16/18 E7-pulsed dendritic cell vaccination in cervical cancer patients with recurrent disease refractory to standard treatment modalities. Gynecol Oncol 2006; 100: 469–78.

58. Zhou J, Sun XY, Stenzel DJ, Frazer IH. Expression of vaccinia recombinant HPV 16 L1 and L2 ORF proteins in epithelial cells is sufficient for assembly of HPV virion-like particles. Virology 1991; 185: 251–7.

59. Nardelli-Haefliger D, Wirthner D, Schiller JT et al. Specific antibody levels at the cervix during the menstrual cycle of women vaccinated with human papillomavirus 16 virus-like particles. J Natl Cancer Inst 2003; 95: 1128–37.

60. Harper DM, Franco EL, Wheeler C et al. Efficacy of a bivalent L1 virus-like particle vaccine in prevention of infection with human papillomavirus types 16 and 18 in young women: a randomised controlled trial. Lancet 2004; 364: 1757–65.

61. Villa LL, Costa RL, Petta CA et al. Prophylactic quadrivalent human papillomavirus (types 6, 11, 16, and 18) L1 virus-like particle vaccine in young women: a randomised double-blind placebo-controlled multicentre phase II efficacy trial. Lancet Oncol 2005; 6: 271–8.

62. Villa LL, Costa RL, Petta CA et al. High sustained efficacy of a prophylactic quadrivalent human papillomavirus types 6/11/16/18 L1 virus-like particle vaccine through 5 years of follow-up. Br J Cancer 2006; 95: 1459–66.

63. Sattler C; for the FUTURE I Investigators. Efficacy of a prophylactic quadrivalent human papillomavirus (HPV) (Types 6, 11, 16, 18) L1 virus-like particle (VLP) vaccine for the prevention of cervical dysplasia and external genital lesions. Abstract presented at 45th Interscience Conference on Antimicrobial Agents and Chemotherapy, 16–19 December, 2005; Washington, DC, abstr LB-8a.

64. Block SL, Nolan T, Sattler C et al. Comparison of the immunogenicity and reactogenicity of a prophylactic quadrivalent human papillomavirus (types 6, 11, 16, and 18) L1 virus-like particle vaccine in male and female adolescents and young adult women. Pediatrics 2006; 118: 2135–45.

65. Dunne EF, Nielson CM, Stone KM, Markowitz LE, Giuliano AR. Prevalence of HPV infection among men: a systematic review of the literature. J Infect Dis 2006; 194: 1044–57.

66. Peng Q, Berg K, Moan J, Kongshaug M, Nesland JM. 5-Aminolevulinic acid-based photodynamic therapy: principles and experimental research. Photochem Photobiol 1997; 65: 235–51.

67. Grant WE, Speight PM, Hopper C, Bown SG. Photodynamic therapy: an effective, but non-selective treatment for superficial cancers of the oral cavity. Int J Cancer 1997; 71: 937–42.

68. Yamaguchi S, Tsuda H, Takemori M et al. Photodynamic therapy for cervical intraepithelial neoplasia. Oncology 2005; 69: 110–16.

69. Keefe KA, Chahine EB, DiSaia PJ et al. Fluorescence detection of cervical intraepithelial neoplasia for photodynamic therapy with the topical agents 5-aminolevulinic acid and benzoporphyrin-derivative monoacid ring. Am J Obstet Gynecol 2001; 184: 1164–9.

70. Doorbar J. The papillomavirus life cycle. J Clin Virol 2005; 32 (Suppl 1): S7–15.

71. Anderson MC, Hartley RB. Cervical crypt involvement by intraepithelial neoplasia. Obstet Gynecol 1980; 55: 546–50.

72. Bodner K, Bodner-Adler B, Wierrani F et al. Cold-knife conization versus photodynamic therapy with topical 5-aminolevulinic acid (5-ALA) in cervical intraepithelial neoplasia (CIN) II with associated human papillomavirus infection: a comparison of preliminary results. Anticancer Res 2003; 23: 1785–8.

73. Barnett AA, Haller JC, Cairnduff F et al. A randomised, double-blind, placebo-controlled trial of photodynamic therapy using 5-aminolaevulinic acid for the treatment of cervical intraepithelial neoplasia. Int J Cancer 2003; 103: 829–32.

74. Nag S, Chao C, Erickson B et al. The American Brachytherapy Society recommendations for low-dose-rate brachytherapy for carcinoma of the cervix. Int J Radiat Oncol Biol Phys 2002; 52: 33–48.

75. Einhorn N, Trope C, Ridderheim M et al. A systematic overview of radiation therapy effects in cervical cancer (cervix uteri). Acta Oncol 2003; 42: 546–56.

76. Grigsby PW, Perez CA. Radiotherapy alone for medically inoperable carcinoma of the cervix: stage IA and carcinoma in situ. Int J Radiat Oncol Biol Phys 1991; 21: 375–8.

77. Kolstad P, Klem V. Long-term followup of 1121 cases of carcinoma in situ. Obstet Gynecol 1976; 48: 125–9.

78. Kolstad P. Follow-up study of 232 patients with stage Ia1 and 411 patients with stage Ia2 squamous cell carcinoma of the cervix (microinvasive carcinoma). Gynecol Oncol 1989; 33: 265–72.

79. Coen M, Lenz EM, Nicholson JK et al. An integrated metabonomic investigation of acetaminophen toxicity in the mouse using NMR spectroscopy. Chem Res Toxicol 2003; 16: 295–303.

80. Green JA, Kirwan JM, Tierney JF et al. Survival and recurrence after concomitant chemotherapy and radiotherapy for cancer of the uterine cervix: a systematic review and meta-analysis. Lancet 2001; 358: 781–6.

81. Lukka H, Hirte H, Fyles A et al. Concurrent cisplatin-based chemotherapy plus radiotherapy for cervical cancer– a meta-analysis. Clin Oncol (R Coll Radiol) 2002; 14: 203–12.

82. Aggarwal BB, Ichikawa H. Molecular targets and anticancer potential of indole-3-carbinol and its derivatives. Cell Cycle 2005; 4: 1201–15.

83. Jin L, Qi M, Chen DZ et al. Indole-3-carbinol prevents cervical cancer in human papilloma virus type 16 (HPV16) transgenic mice. Cancer Res 1999; 59: 3991–7.

84. Bell MC, Crowley-Nowick P, Bradlow HL et al. Placebo-controlled trial of indole-3-carbinol in the treatment of CIN. Gynecol Oncol 2000; 78: 123–9.

85. Brooks RA, Mutch DG. Gene therapy in gynecological cancer. Expert Rev Anticancer Ther 2006; 6: 1013–32.

86. Ahn WS, Bae SM, Lee JM et al. Anti-cancer effect of adenovirus p53 on human cervical cancer cell growth in vitro and in vivo. Int J Gynecol Cancer 2004; 14: 322–32.

87. Ahn WS, Bae SM, Lee KH et al. Recombinant adenovirus-p53 gene transfer and cell-specific growth suppression of human cervical cancer cells in vitro and in vivo. Gynecol Oncol 2004; 92: 611–21.

88. Das S, Somasundaram K. Therapeutic potential of an adenovirus expressing p73 beta, a p53 homologue, against human papilloma virus positive cervical cancer in vitro and in vivo. Cancer Biol Ther 2006; 5: 210–17.

20 Vulvar pre-malignant and malignant disorders: non-surgical and minimally invasive options

Chad A Hamilton and Jonathan S Berek

VULVAR INTRAEPITHELIAL NEOPLASIA

Though vulvar cancer incidence ranks only fourth among gynecologic cancers, its precursor lesions occur more commonly and impose a significant burden on the healthcare system.[1] The disease incidence is increasing and impacting on younger women,[2,3] highlighting the need to refine or replace traditional management. Though treatment for invasive vulvar cancer remains surgical, with few minimally invasive options,[4] vulvar intraepithelial neoplasia (VIN) may respond to less aggressive approaches, providing an opportunity to arrest the process in its pre-malignant state. Unfortunately no single treatment, surgical or otherwise, stands clearly superior, and indeed, most treatments have significant shortcomings. Not surprisingly, defining optimal treatment remains elusive.

CLASSIFICATION AND TERMINOLOGY

Inconsistent classification and terminology for VIN hampers establishment of an optimal treatment strategy. Historically, names such as Bowen's disease, erythroplasia of Queyrat, carcinoma in situ simplex, bowenoid papulosis, and leukoplakia were used to describe various forms of severe squamous epithelial atypia. The International Society for the Study of Vulvar Disease (ISSVD) adopted the term VIN in 1986, mirroring the classification of cervical intraepithelial neoplasia (CIN).[5] As with CIN, VIN was classified on a three-grade system (VIN1–3), as well as a low-grade/high-grade schema. The ISSVD vulvar oncology subcommittee felt that these systems, as well as others, had significant shortcomings due to important differences from CIN. To reflect this, the ISSVD modified its terminology in 2004 (Table 20.1).[6]

The 2004 modification discards the VIN1 classification and consolidates VIN2 and -3 into a single category termed VIN. This change avoids inappropriate parallels with CIN implied by similar grading.

Table 20.1 Squamous vulvar intraepithelial neoplasia (VIN), 2004 modified terminology[6]

VIN, usual type
  warty
  basaloid
  mixed (warty/basaloid)
VIN, differentiated type
VIN, unclassified type

Specifically, there is insufficient evidence supporting a biologic continuum from VIN1–3 or that VIN1 is a cancer precursor. Additionally, VIN2 like VIN1 lacks reproducibility, and investigators achieve good histologic agreement only by combining VIN2 with VIN3.[6,7]

The ISSVD further classifies the unified category of VIN as usual type and differentiated type, based on differing morphology, biology, and clinical features. VIN, usual type subdivides into warty, basaloid, or mixed subtype. These lesions are associated with human papillomavirus (HPV), and in particular high-risk types such as HPV-16. Usual type is more common in younger women. Differentiated VIN derives its name from its highly differentiated histologic features. In contrast to usual type VIN, it is HPV-negative and found in older women. Clinicians typically diagnose differentiated VIN in association with keratinizing squamous cell carcinomas or during surveillance after treatment of vulvar carcinoma. It is also associated with squamous cell hyperplasias and long-standing lichen sclerosis,[7] though emerging evidence may make this more controversial.[8] A final category of VIN, unclassified type, may be applied in cases that cannot be characterized as usual or differentiated type. One may appropriately place a rare VIN of pagetoid type in this category.[5–7]

CLINICAL PROFILE

The clinical features of VIN vary, but generalizations may be made for both usual type and differentiated type. Because VIN, usual type, is HPV related, it significantly impacts on the trends of increasing VIN incidence and decreasing age. Patients typically present with an abnormal Pap smear or other HPV-related pathology at the time of diagnosis, and cigarette smoking, immune suppression, and a history of sexually transmitted diseases are commonly associated cofactors. VIN, usual type is only occasionally found in an asymptomatic patient and less likely to present with pruritus. It tends to form discrete lesions that have sharp margins, and in many cases may be multifocal.[5,7,9]

The typical clinical profile of differentiated VIN sharply contrasts with that described for usual type. These patients tend to be older, and in many cases are symptomatic for months or years. Differentiated lesions tend to itch or burn and are usually unifocal, appearing often in a field of lichen sclerosis or planus.[9]

NATURAL HISTORY

Characterizing the natural history of VIN proves challenging due to the spectrum of pathology as well as treatments reported. Two recent studies shed light on this subject.[10,11] Jones and co-workers from New Zealand reported experience with 405 cases of warty, basaloid, or mixed VIN over a 40-year period. Sixty-three women received no treatment, of whom 10 (16%) progressed to invasion while 47 (75%) regressed before treatment.[10] van Seters and co-workers systematically reviewed 3322 reported cases of VIN focusing on natural history. In their study, 9% of patients progressed when left untreated or with gross residual VIN. These patients were drawn from 10 studies reporting on 88 untreated women.[11]

Jones et al reported that half of the patients treated for VIN, most by excisional or ablative techniques, required additional treatment.[10] They felt that the term *recurrence* could represent either recurrent or persistent disease and therefore chose *additional treatment* instead. This proportion receiving additional treatment dropped to 15% in those with negative margins.[10] Recurrence rates in the systematic review ranged from 19 to 23% in lesions excised or ablated. With positive margins, recurrence increased to 47%.[11] Modesitt et al's report from North Carolina closely mirrored these numbers, with 46% vs 17% recurrence in those with and without positive margins, respectively,[12] though others have found less of a relationship.[13]

Of most concern are patients found to have occult cancer after excision of suspected VIN, or who progress

Table 20.2   Characteristics of an ideal VIN treatment

- Prevents progression to cancer
- Relieves symptoms
- Excludes occult carcinoma
- Prevents recurrence
- Painless
- Spares normal tissue
- Retains normal anatomy

to cancer after treatment of VIN. While the van Seters review reported only a 3.2% rate of occult carcinoma,[11] four other groups report consistently higher rates of 15–22% with occult cancer found in a total of 51 out of 260 cases (20%).[12,14–16] The available data on progression to invasive cancer, again mostly from excisional or ablative experiences, are surprisingly consistent, with most groups reporting around a 3–5% progression rate.[10,11,13]

TREATMENT

Todd and Luesley comment in their excellent review of medical management of VIN that 'if a large number of treatment options exist for a particular condition, then it is likely that none of those treatments provides an ideal solution to the problem'.[17] This indeed appears to be the case regarding treatment options, both invasive and non-invasive, for pre-malignant vulvar disease. Table 20.2 lists characteristics of an ideal treatment, the most important of which are preventing progression and relieving symptoms. Though most treatments fulfill these criteria to a degree, they often have significant shortcomings.

There is substantial blurring, particularly as one moves through the spectrum of ablative and topical treatments, of what is considered non-invasive. For the purposes of this chapter, we arbitrarily define those procedures typically conducted in an operating theater or with significant anesthesia as invasive, and will briefly review them for contextual purposes. We consider those treatments typically administered in an office setting or self-administered as non-invasive, and will discuss them in depth. Several such treatments are only of historical interest, while a few have current therapeutic implications. A number are investigative or exploratory in nature, requiring further evaluation and validation (Table 20.3).

Non-invasive treatments for VIN clearly require refining and advancing. Treatments are needed which minimize morbidity, provide a durable response or cure, and allow rapid resumption of activity as the disease incidence rises and affects increasingly younger women. It will be reasonable to target HPV and HPV-related VIN as it is likely this portion of the disease spectrum that is driving the epidemiologic shifts. It is important to highlight, as one considers non-invasive management, that accurate diagnosis is essential. In the context of a significant occult malignancy rate,[17] we advocate extensive pretreatment biopsying when taking a non-invasive approach, and surveillance must be the same or greater than would be planned after excisional therapies.

Excisional or ablative treatments

Surgical treatments for VIN may include excision with a scalpel, laser, or diathermy, though cavitational ultrasonic surgical aspiration has been described in one report.[18] There has been a trend to limit the extent of resection, and most surgeons have replaced vulvectomy with wide local excision or perhaps superficial ('skinning') vulvectomy for extensive disease. Case series and reviews demonstrate similar long-term cure rates for various methods, but most have not been directly compared in adequately powered prospective trials.[19–21] Excision often relieves symptoms, prevents progression, and allows pathologic assessment to rule out occult invasive disease. These techniques do not always prevent recurrence, as evidenced by the

Table 20.3 Treatment strategies for vulvar intraepithelial neoplasia

Strategy	Treatment
Surgical	Superficial vulvectomy[b]
	Local excision[b]
	Laser or diathermy excision[b]
	Cavitational ultrasonic surgical aspiration[c]
Destructive	Laser ablation[b]
	Photodynamic therapy[c]
Cytotoxic chemotherapy	5-Fluorouracil[a]
	Bleomycin[a]
Immune modulation	Dinitrochlorobenzene[a]
	Interferons[a]
	Imiquimod[c]
Vaccination	Prophylactic[c]
	TA-HPV, TA-CIN[c]
Other therapies	Retinoids[a,c]
	Cidofovir[c]
	Indole-3-carbinol[c]

[a]Largely of historical interest
[b]Considered a standard treatment
[c]Considered investigational or requires further validation

numbers previously cited for patients with and without positive margins. Furthermore, surgical excision often requires anesthesia and operating theater support. Depending on the extent of excision, surgery may be disfiguring, with some using the term mutilating. A number of reports have found significant psychological and psychosexual distress in patients undergoing vulvar surgery for pre-invasive disease.[22–24]

Laser excision and ablation provide an alternative to scalpel excision and vulvectomy, particularly in cases of extensive, multifocal disease. In laser treatment, the patient derives cosmetic benefits, as the low thermal tissue effect induces minimal scarring. Laser excision requires considerable expertise, but has cure rates comparable to those with knife excision, and also provides a pathologic specimen. Cure rates for vaporization may be slightly inferior to those obtained by excisional techniques. Pain is common with laser therapy, and cosmetic benefit may be lost in cases where deeper vaporization is required, such as hair-bearing areas.[9,25]

Photodynamic therapy

Photodynamic therapy (PDT) is a newer treatment modality that may provide an alternative to traditional management of VIN. In this approach, the treating physician administers a topical or systemic photosensitizing agent which preferentially accumulates in neoplastic tissue. Following variable application time, the patient exposes the affected area to non-thermal light at wavelengths absorbed by the photosensitizer, resulting in oxygen-induced cell death. 5-Aminolevulinic acid (5-ALA) is a precursor in the heme biosynthetic pathway and is commonly used in PDT. Exogenous administration of 5-ALA bypasses the rate-limiting step in heme biosynthesis. Heme and porphyrins then accumulate primarily in dysplastic or malignant tissue, making them vulnerable to light-induced cell death. PDT has proven quite effective in the treatment of non-melanoma skin cancers and pre-malignant lesions of the oral cavity.[26,27]

The few published studies of PDT for vulvar dysplasia used 5-ALA most commonly as the photosensitizing agent (Table 20.4). It is difficult to draw conclusions based on these series, as trial results have been mixed and treatments and outcome measures have varied.[32] Martin-Hirsch et al reported the first use of PDT for VIN in 18 patients in 1998,[32] and Abdel-Hady et al updated that group's experience in 2001. After PDT, lesions in 10 of 32 patients regressed to normal histology at 12-week biopsy. Patients with unifocal

Table 20.4 Reports using photodynamic therapy to treat vulvar intraepithelial neoplasia: all studies were prospective observational

Study lead author	VIN grade	Number of patients	Response (%)			Recurrence in CR group	Follow-up (months)
			CR	PR	<PR or LFU		
Hillemanns[26]	VIN2/3	22	10 (45)	9 (41)	3 (14)	NS	NS
Abdel-Hady[28]	VIN3	32	10 (31)	NS	22 (69)	NS	NS
Kurwa[29]	VIN3	6	0 (0)	NS	6 (100)	—	6
Fehr[30]	VIN3	15	11 (73)	4 (27)	0 (0)	3 (27)	32
Campbell[31,a]	VIN3	6	6 (100)	0 (0)	0 (0)	3 (50)	24
Total		81	37 (46)	13 (16)	31 (38)	6/17[b] (36)	20.6 (SEM 7.7)

CR, complete response; PR, partial response; LFU, lost to follow-up; NS, not specified
[a]Photosensitizing agent systemic meta-tetrahydroxyphenylchlorin (mTHPC)
[b]Denominator is number of patients with CR in reports containing recurrence data

lesions were most responsive to PDT, while hyperkeratinized, pigmented, and scarred lesions were resistant. Additionally, these investigators correlated a diminished response to PDT with the presence of HPV infection, human leukocyte antigen (HLA) class 1 loss, and diminished numbers of infiltrating immune cells.[28] Hillemanns and colleagues used a 20% 5-ALA solution rather than cream, and documented complete remission in 13 of 25 patients (52%).[26] They noted a particularly poor response rate of 27% in 15 patients with multifocal disease. Patients with pronounced pigmentation or hyper/parakeratosis were also noted to be poor responders. In a positive study using 10% 5-ALA gel, Fehr et al documented histologic resolution after PDT in 11 of 15 patients with VIN.[30] In multivariate analysis, multifocal disease was the only variable associated with reduced disease-free survival. The recurrence rate was 40.5%, with a mean follow-up of 32 months. Campbell and colleagues administered intravenously the systemic photosensitizing agent meta-tetrahydroxyphenylchlorin (mTHPC) to six patients.[31] All had complete (clinical) responses to PDT. At 6 months, two patients recurred and were retreated. At 2 years, all patients were disease free. All patients experienced varying amounts of pain, edema, and ulceration. The investigators admitted one patient for cellulitis and another patient had a severe photosensitivity reaction of the hands after exposing them to daylight in front of a window.[31]

Research continues into PDT. At present, this therapy appears to be more appropriate for those with unifocal, non-pigmented lesions. Pain as well as inflammation and skin changes are somewhat unpredictable and can be severe at times, and may temper enthusiasm for this treatment. If treatments are refined to limit side-effects with a more consistent response rate, PDT may prove a valuable tool in the treatment of VIN.

Cytotoxic chemotherapy

Investigators first used cytotoxic chemotherapeutic agents as non-surgical alternatives to treat VIN over half a century ago,[33] with modern efforts focusing on topical 5-fluorouracil (5-FU) and topical or intradermal bleomycin.[33,34] Because of side-effects and lack of consistent efficacy, these agents have largely fallen out of favor, except in women declining or unable to undergo other therapies.

5-Fluorouracil

5-FU is a pyrimidine analog taken up efficiently by neoplastic and dysplastic cells and converted to cytotoxic metabolites. These metabolites inhibit thymidilate synthase as well as incorporate into RNA and DNA, impairing their function.[35] Ten years after its synthesis as a novel cytotoxic agent, Jansen and co-workers investigated 5-FU to treat VIN.[36] 5-FU is most commonly supplied as a cream containing 5% fluorouracil. Depending on the frequency and duration of application, patients commonly experience early erythema and edema, which may proceed to a severe inflammatory response by approximately 2 weeks. Prolonged use may lead to blistering, ulcers, necrosis, and pain, requiring local and systemic analgesics. These side-effects commonly limit patient compliance or ability to continue therapy for recommended durations.[37]

Though used intermittently for decades now, rigorous testing of 5-FU in the setting of VIN is meager. Sillman et al reviewed 68 patients with VIN3 in 15 studies treated with topical 5-FU; 34% of patients could be characterized as complete responders while another 7% had partial responses. Therapy failed in 59% of patients.[33] Krebs described maintenance in a trial of

90 patients with vulvar or vaginal dysplasia randomized after ablative or excisional therapy. 5-FU was administered in the maintenance group as a single dose applied twice a week for at least 6 months. Thirteen per cent of those treated with maintenance 5-FU recurred, versus 38% ($p < 0.01$) of controls during a mean follow-up of 14 months, suggesting a possible role in this setting.[38] Recently, Downs et al found that 5-FU when used in a sequential manner after the immune response modulator imiquimod provided no additional benefit compared to the few studies of imiquimod alone.[39] In short, 5-FU used topically for VIN demonstrates inconsistent response rates and sometimes severe side-effects, and should be used very selectively if at all.

Bleomycin

Because of its activity against other squamous neoplasms, bleomycin is a second cytotoxic agent that was investigated in hopes of finding a non-invasive treatment alternative for VIN. It is an antitumor antibiotic originally isolated from *Streptomyces verticillus*, which produces its cytotoxic effect by inducing single-strand breaks in DNA. After promising results using topical bleomycin for extramammary Paget's disease of the vulva, in which four of seven patients experienced a complete response,[40] Roberts et al treated twelve patients with VIN with topical bleomycin. Because of their dismal results in which only two patients demonstrated improvement while five progressed to invasive cancer, topical or intradermal bleomycin has been relegated to historical interest only for VIN.[32]

Local immune stimulation

Agents that promote a localized immune response fulfill a number of criteria characteristic of an ideal treatment for VIN. Some of the earliest investigations used dinitrochlorobenzene (DNCB) and interferons. Current trials are under way exploring the immune response modifier imiquimod, with promising results.

Dinitrochlorobenzene

DNCB is a potent contact allergen, and induces a local hypersensitivity reaction. It has been used therapeutically to treat a number of cutaneous disorders, and has been noted to induce involution of viral warts.[41] Weintraub and Lagasse treated six women with marked bowenoid vulvar atypia with DNCB, noting complete responses in two who remained disease free at 6 months. They did not comment on side-effects.[42] Foster

and Woodruff also treated six women with vulvar carcinoma in situ, recurrent after excision and/or topical 5-FU. Four women cleared their disease with recurrence in two. Of note, in this group some patients experienced 'extensive' and 'apparently intolerable' reactions.[43] Though DNCB continues to be used in a number of dermatologic conditions,[41] we could find no reports on the use of DNCB for VIN in the past two decades.

Interferons

Interferons, and specifically interferon α (IFN-α), inhibit viral replication and neoplastic cell proliferation while stimulating innate immunity. They can be administered systemically, intralesionally, or topically. After remissions were reported using INF-α to treat genital condyloma and squamous cell neoplasms of the cervix, investigators initiated pilot studies in patients with VIN.[44,45] The largest study to date reported 21 patients with VIN3 treated topically with INF-α gel with or without nonoxynol-9 (used to possibly enhance absorption). Overall, 50% of patients had a complete response lasting at least 1 year, while 28% had partial responses. Side-effects were minimal, consisting primarily of mild pain or pruritus. Of note, investigators found invasive cancer in two patients after initial enrollment, highlighting the need for caution and precise diagnosis when non-excisional techniques are used.[46] Except isolated case reports of failed interferon treatment for VIN,[47,48] we could find no further reports since the publication of the Stanford trial.[46]

Imiquimod

Imiquimod, available commercially as Aldara® (3M Pharmaceuticals, St Paul, MN), is approved for the treatment of actinic keratoses, superficial basal cell carcinoma, and external genital and perianal warts/condyloma acuminata. Investigators demonstrated its efficacy in treating condyloma in a number of randomized controlled trials, with results often superior to and with fewer recurrences than with conventional treatments.[49–51] Based on these data, both clinicians and researchers are treating VIN with imiquimod, though published experience thus far is limited to case series and small single-institution trials.

In its commercial form, imiquimod is supplied in single-use packets containing 250 mg of 5% cream. Each gram of cream contains 50 mg of imiquimod. For condyloma, patients apply a thin layer of the cream over the intended area three times per week, prior to normal sleeping hours. They should wash off the cream after 6 hours, and treatment continues until clearance of lesions or for a maximum of 16 weeks.

Table 20.5   Reports using imiquimod to treat vulvar intraepithelial neoplasia

Study lead author	Study design and VIN grade	Number of patients	Response (%)			Recurrence in CR group	Mean follow-up (months)
			CR	PR	<PR or LFU		
Davis[53]	Case series, VIN3	4	4 (100)	0 (0)	0 (0)	2 (50)	12
Diaz-Arrastia[54]	Case series, HG VIN	4	2 (50)	1 (25)	1 (25)	1 (50)	31
Petrow[55]	Case report, VIN3	1	1 (100)	0 (0)	0 (0)	0 (0)	18
Todd[17]	Prospective, VIN3	15	3 (20)	1 (7)	11 (73)	3 (100)	5
Travis[56]	Case report, VIN3	1	1 (100)	0 (0)	0 (0)	0 (100)	2
van Seters[57]	Prospective, VIN2/3	15	4 (27)	9 (60)	2 (13)	NS	NS
Jayne[58]	Case series, VIN2/3	13	8 (61)	4[a] (31)	1 (8)	NS	5.5
Richter[59]	Case report, VIN3	1	1 (100)	0 (0)	0 (0)	0 (0)	18
Campagne[60]	Case report, VIN2/3	1	1 (100)	0 (0)	0 (0)	0 (0)	18
Marchitelli[61]	Prospective, VIN2/3	8	6 (75)	2 (25)	0 (0)	0 (0)	22
Wendling[62]	Prospective, undiff VIN	12	3 (25)	4 (33)	5 (42)	0 (0)	9.7 CR, 20.3 PR, 16.5 <PR
Le[63]	Prospective, VIN2/3	17	9 (53)	5 (29)	3 (18)	NS	NS
Total		92	43 (47)	26 (28)	23 (25)	6/22[b] (27)	14.7 (SEM 2.78)

HG, high grade; undiff, undifferentiated
[a]2 patients diagnosed with invasive squamous carcinoma
[b]Denominator is number of patients with CR in reports containing recurrence data

Most reports describe similar dosing when imiquimod is used to treat VIN.

Imiquimod belongs to a class of compounds known as immune response modifiers. Direct antiviral activity *in vitro* is absent, and its mechanism in animals is likely due to immune stimulation. Specifically, the imidazoquinolones, of which imiquimod is the best known, stimulate macrophages and dendritic cells to produce proinflammatory cytokines such as IFN-α, which promote a T-helper cell type 1 (T_H1) adaptive immune response. The randomized controlled trial in condyloma patients reported by Tyring and co-workers supports this as contributing to the in vivo mechanism. These investigators demonstrated significantly increased mRNA levels for IFN-α and IFN-γ, while HPV viral load, and HPV E7 and L1 mRNA expression, fell after treatment with imiquimod.[51,52]

The body of evidence supporting a role for imiquimod in the treatment of VIN continues to grow (Table 20.5). To date 92 patients have been reported,

with a response rate of 75%, and 47% complete responders. Patients frequently experience dose-limiting vulvar skin reactions, and optimal dosing remains unknown. Le and colleagues used a dose-escalating protocol of once-weekly application for 2 weeks, followed by twice-weekly application for 2 weeks, to three times weekly for the remainder of their study period. Only eight of 17 patients required dose reduction, all at the three times per week dosing, and all were able to return to three times per week dosing to complete the study period after the dose reduction. Interestingly, the need for dose reduction was significantly associated with improved response. This group, as well as others, also noted equivalent response rates between unifocal and multifocal disease, suggesting a field effect to the local immune stimulation.[62,63]

Treating VIN with imiquimod avoids the morbidity of invasive approaches and can be administered at home, reducing costs and inconvenience to the patient. At this time, imiquimod has not been compared directly to standard treatments in a rigorous trial, and data on recurrence rates are insufficient. As data accumulate, imiquimod will likely be an appealing option or at least play a role in either primary treatment or as adjunctive therapy for VIN.

Other topical strategies

Retinoids

Retinoids are natural or synthetic derivatives of vitamin A with antiproliferative properties in cancer treatment and chemoprevention studies. For pre-invasive and invasive cervical disease, retinoids inhibit HPV viral proteins E6 and E7, which promote degradation of tumor suppressors p53 and Rb (retinoblastoma), respectively. Inhibition of E6 and E7 restores the regulatory function of p53 and Rb. Because of this activity directly related to HPV pathogenesis and by inducing apoptosis, growth arrest, and differentiation, retinoids may have a role in treating vulvar pre-invasive and invasive disease.[64]

Data on the use of retinoids to treat VIN are minimal. Markowska et al treated 16 patients with 'leukoplakia' with 13-cis-retinoic acid, and reported 50% complete responders with manageable side-effects.[65] In a more recent report of two patients, 13-cis-retinoic acid in combination with IFN-α led to clinical regression of VIN3, but histologic features remained on post-treatment biopsy.[48] Another report describes a patient in whom VIN persisted with serial treatments of interferon and isotretinoin before her lesion regressed on topical cidofovir.[47]

Cidofovir

Cidofovir is an acyclic nucleoside phosphonate with broad spectrum antiviral activity against DNA viruses. Its activity in HPV-related disease may be through induction of apoptosis in HPV-infected cells and reduction in E6 and E7 expression, allowing tumor suppressor proteins P53 and Rb to exert their cell cycle regulatory functions.[66] Several small series and case reports describe experiences with cidofovir in treating condyloma, and one placebo-controlled study demonstrated superiority over placebo.[67]

Tristram and Fiander recently reported the first trial of treatment of VIN3 using topical application of cidofovir. Patients self-treated with the 1% formulation applied on alternate days for 16 weeks. Twelve patients were recruited, with 10 available for follow-up. Local effects included an intense, sometimes painful, ulcerative reaction limited to the diseased skin. Four complete responders had visual and histologic resolution as well as viral clearance. Three women had partial responses involving a reduction in lesion area by 50%. Two patients failed therapy. One patient with a lesion involving the entire introitus had resolution of the majority of her disease, but biopsy of the remaining lesion showed invasive disease.[66] The only other report of cidofovir used in the treatment of VIN was the aforementioned report of a patient in whom VIN persisted with serial treatments of interferon and isotretinoin before her lesion regressed on topical cidofovir.[47]

Vaccination

A significant proportion of VIN, particularly in younger women, is HPV-related. As such, vaccination becomes an obvious strategy for the management of HPV-induced VIN and vulvar cancer. Vaccination strategies are diverse, but most are either prophylactic, indicating primary prevention of disease, or therapeutic. Vaccination development is costly and time-consuming, requiring rigorous clinical trials. It is unlikely that the societal burden of vulvar disease alone would sufficiently drive the development of vaccines, but with a common oncogenic viral etiology, management of VIN will continue to benefit from gains made in the prevention and treatment of cervical disease.[17]

Preventive vaccination has historically proven the most successful and cost-effective method of disease reduction. With the approval of one HPV vaccine and a second in phase III trials targeting HPV-induced cervical dysplasia and cancer, the impact on cervical disease may be mirrored to some extent in a reduction in VIN and vulvar cancer. Hampl and colleagues recently investigated this potential effect. They first determined the prevalence of HPV DNA in vulvar, vaginal, and anal intraepithelial lesions and vulvar cancer in 241 consecutive women. High-risk HPV type 16 or 18 was detected in 139 of 183 VIN2/3 (76%) samples from 168 women. Additionally, 20 of 48 (42%) vulvar cancer specimens were HPV-16 or -18 positive, with those patients under 56 years of age having a 58% positive rate. Evidence from quadrivalent vaccine trials supports a near 100% prevention rate of genital condyloma, VIN, and vulvar and vaginal carcinoma. Based on this, the authors predicted prevention of approximately one-half of the vulvar carcinomas in women less than 56 years old and two-thirds of the intraepithelial precursor lesions in the lower genital tract.[68]

A therapeutic vaccine approach in which only individuals affected by HPV-related genital tract disease are treated is attractive for several reasons. Such an approach would avoid treating large numbers of unaffected individuals. Additionally, screening is possible for cancer precursor lesions as is analysis to determine whether high-risk HPV DNA is present. Unfortunately, therapeutic vaccines have not demonstrated high-level efficacy in clinical trials.[69]

Most approaches thus far to therapeutic vaccination target the early oncoproteins E6 and E7, which are expressed throughout the spectrum of HPV-associated disease. Two groups evaluated TA-HPV, a live, recombinant vaccinia virus encoding modified versions of E6 and E7, for immunological and clinical response in VIN. TA-HPV previously demonstrated the ability to generate an HPV-directed cell-mediated immune response in cervical cancer,[70,71] Davidson et al treated 18 women with HPV-16 positive high-grade VIN with a single dose of TA-HPV. Thirteen women demonstrated HPV-16 specific immune responses, with eight patients having a partial clinical response in which lesion diameter decreased by 50%. Viral load was reduced or cleared in six of the eight responders but also six of 10 non-responders. The authors concluded that pretreatment local immune infiltration could be a critical factor, as clinical responders had significantly higher levels than non-responders.[71] A second study demonstrated similar clinical and T-cell responses, with 33% partial responders and one of 12 patients showing complete regression of her lesion.[70] Davidson and her colleagues conducted an extension of their TA-HPV study by treating 10 of those women with TA-CIN, a recombinant HPV-16 L2E6E7 fusion protein with the ability to generate T-cell responses in a mouse model and healthy volunteers. All but one patient demonstrated immune responses, but this did not correlate with clinical responses.[72] The reciprocal ordering of the prime-boost immunization strategy with TA-CIN followed by TA-HPV demonstrated a similar lack of correlation between immunological and clinical response.[73]

PAGET'S DISEASE

Extramammary Paget's disease is an uncommon neoplastic condition of apocrine gland-bearing skin. It most commonly affects the vulva, and may be primary cutaneous with or without invasion, or associated with an underlying adenocarcinoma. Patients most commonly present with vulvar pruritus and lesions which may appear as erythematous, well-demarcated plaques. Paget's disease involves the deeper layers of

the epidermis, and frequently epidermal appendages.[33,74] Surgical excision is the most common therapy, but this is plagued to a much greater extent than VIN by positive excision margins and a high recurrence rate, regardless of margin status. In addition to surgical approaches, many of the same non-invasive strategies attempted with VIN have been tried in extramammary Paget's disease.

Non-invasive approaches to vulvar Paget's disease are limited to case reports and small series. Raspagliesi and colleagues provide the most recent experience using PDT in vulvar Paget's. Of seven patients treated, four had complete clinical responses with pathologic confirmation in two cases. Patients developed local edema and mild pain. One patient developed severe pain and a mild local phototoxicity reaction.[75] It is difficult to draw conclusions from this and the few other published reports.[76,77] Groups have also investigated topical or intralesional chemotherapy with both 5-fluorouracil and bleomycin for vulvar Paget's. The utility of 5-FU is limited by its lack of penetration to a necessary skin depth.[33] Watring and co-workers treated seven patients with topical bleomycin and four had complete responses.[34] Side-effects were pain and moist desquamation, and one patient had systemic toxicity. There were no other reports of bleomycin in this setting. Reports of successful treatment of vulvar Paget's are now appearing using imiquimod, and based on these early indications, a pilot study may be of value.[78,79]

VULVAR CANCER

Frankly invasive vulvar cancer remains a surgically treated disease. There has been a dramatic evolution in the extent of surgery over the last half century. With better understanding of the disease process, en bloc radical vulvectomy and bilateral groin and pelvic node dissections have given way to individualized treatments.[80] In many women only radical local excisions are necessary, thus avoiding the significant physical, psychological, and sexual morbidity documented with more extensive resections.[81] Based on promising institutional trials[82] as well as preliminary data from a large European cooperative,[83] we anticipate that sentinel lymph node (SLN) evaluation will further limit morbidity from extensive groin dissections. In the United States, the Gynecologic Oncology Group is also addressing this question in a prospective trial.

A non-surgical approach may be the only option in vulvar cancer patients who are too medically disabled to undergo indicated surgery. In these cases a combination of chemotherapy and radiation can have a dramatic effect.[84] This combination has also proven beneficial preoperatively in limiting the radicality of surgery and avoiding exenteration in advanced vulvar cancer.[85]

Current treatment options for invasive vulvar cancer remain surgery, chemoradiation therapy, or various individualized combinations. As PDT, immunomodulators, and therapeutic vaccines continue to evolve, they may have a role in the treatment of vulvar cancer, and further investigations of these approaches, perhaps at present in an adjuvant setting, are warranted.

REFERENCES

1. Jemal A, Siegel R, Ward E et al. Cancer statistics, 2006. CA Cancer J Clin 2006; 56: 106–30.
2. Joura EA, Losch A, Haider-Angeler MG, Breitenecker G, Leodolter S. Trends in vulvar neoplasia. Increasing incidence of vulvar intraepithelial neoplasia and squamous cell carcinoma of the vulva in young women. J Reprod Med 2000; 45: 613–15.
3. Iversen T, Tretli S. Intraepithelial and invasive squamous cell neoplasia of the vulva: trends in incidence, recurrence, and survival rate in Norway. Obstet Gynecol 1998; 91: 969–72.
4. Tyring SK. Vulvar squamous cell carcinoma: guidelines for early diagnosis and treatment. Am J Obstet Gynecol 2003; 189 (Suppl): S17–23.
5. Hart WR. Vulvar intraepithelial neoplasia: historical aspects and current status. Int J Gynecol Pathol 2001; 20: 16–30.
6. Sideri M, Jones RW, Wilkinson EJ et al. Squamous vulvar intraepithelial neoplasia: 2004 modified terminology, ISSVD Vulvar Oncology Subcommittee. J Reprod Med 2005; 50: 807–10.
7. Scurry J, Wilkinson EJ. Review of terminology of precursors of vulvar squamous cell carcinoma. J Low Genit Tract Dis 2006; 10: 161–9.
8. van Seters M, Ten Kate FJ, van Beurden M et al. In the absence of (early) invasive carcinoma vulvar intraepithelial neoplasia associated with lichen sclerosus is mainly of undifferentiated type: new insights in histology and aetiology. J Clin Pathol 2007; 60: 504–9.
9. Preti M, van Seters M, Sideri M, van Beurden M. Squamous vulvar intraepithelial neoplasia. Clin Obstet Gynecol 2005; 48: 845–61.
10. Jones RW, Rowan DM, Stewart AW. Vulvar intraepithelial neoplasia: aspects of the natural history and outcome in 405 women. Obstet Gynecol 2005; 106: 1319–26.
11. van Seters M, van Beurden M, de Craen AJ. Is the assumed natural history of vulvar intraepithelial neoplasia III based on enough evidence? A systematic review of 3322 published patients. Gynecol Oncol 2005; 97: 645–51.
12. Modesitt SC, Waters AB, Walton L, Fowler WC Jr, Van Le L. Vulvar intraepithelial neoplasia III: occult cancer and the impact of margin status on recurrence. Obstet Gynecol 1998; 92: 962–6.
13. McNally OM, Mulvany NJ, Pagano R, Quinn MA, Rome RM. VIN 3: a clinicopathologic review. Int J Gynecol Cancer 2002; 12: 490–5.
14. Chafe W, Richards A, Morgan L, Wilkinson E. Unrecognized invasive carcinoma in vulvar intraepithelial neoplasia (VIN). Gynecol Oncol 1988; 31: 154–65.
15. Husseinzadeh N, Recinto C. Frequency of invasive cancer in surgically excised vulvar lesions with intraepithelial neoplasia (VIN 3). Gynecol Oncol 1999; 73: 119–20.
16. Thuis YN, Campion M, Fox H, Hacker NF. Contemporary experience with the management of vulvar intraepithelial neoplasia. Int J Gynecol Cancer 2000; 10: 223–7.
17. Todd RW, Luesley DM. Medical management of vulvar intraepithelial neoplasia. J Low Genit Tract Dis 2005; 9: 206–12.
18. Miller BE. Vulvar intraepithelial neoplasia treated with cavitational ultrasonic surgical aspiration. Gynecol Oncol 2002; 85: 114–18.
19. Vlastos AT, Levy LB, Malpica A, Follen M. Loop electrosurgical excision procedure in vulvar intraepithelial neoplasia treatment. J Low Genit Tract Dis 2002; 6: 232–8.
20. Ferenczy A, Wright TC, Richart RM. Comparison of CO2 laser surgery and loop electrosurgical excision/fulguration procedure (LEEP) for the treatment of vulvar intraepithelial neoplasia (VIN). Int J Gynecol Cancer 1994; 4: 22–8.
21. Hillemanns P, Wang X, Staehle S, Michels W, Dannecker C. Evaluation of different treatment modalities for vulvar intraepithelial neoplasia (VIN): CO(2) laser vaporization, photodynamic therapy, excision and vulvectomy. Gynecol Oncol 2006; 100: 271–5.
22. Andersen BL, Turnquist D, LaPolla J, Turner D. Sexual functioning after treatment of in situ vulvar cancer: preliminary report. Obstet Gynecol 1988; 71: 15–19.
23. Andreasson B, Moth I, Jensen SB, Bock JE. Sexual function and somatopsychic reactions in vulvectomy-operated women and their partners. Acta Obstet Gynecol Scand 1986; 65: 7–10.
24. Thuesen B, Andreasson B, Bock JE. Sexual function and somatopsychic reactions after local excision of vulvar intraepithelial neoplasia. Acta Obstet Gynecol Scand 1992; 71: 126–8.
25. Sideri M, Spinaci L, Spolti N, Schettino F. Evaluation of CO(2) laser excision or vaporization for the treatment of vulvar intraepithelial neoplasia. Gynecol Oncol 1999; 75: 277–81.
26. Hillemanns P, Untch M, Dannecker C et al. Photodynamic therapy of vulvar intraepithelial neoplasia using 5-aminolevulinic acid. Int J Cancer 2000; 85: 649–53.
27. Peng Q, Warloe T, Berg K et al. 5-Aminolevulinic acid-based photodynamic therapy. Clinical research and future challenges. Cancer 1997; 79: 2282–308.
28. Abdel-Hady ES, Martin-Hirsch P, Duggan-Keen M et al. Immunological and viral factors associated with the response of vulval intraepithelial neoplasia to photodynamic therapy. Cancer Res 2001; 61: 192–6.
29. Kurwa HA, Barlow RJ, Neill S. Single-episode photodynamic therapy and vulval intraepithelial neoplasia type III resistant to conventional therapy. Br J Dermatol 2000; 143: 1040–2.
30. Fehr MK, Hornung R, Schwarz VA et al. Photodynamic therapy of vulvar intraepithelial neoplasia III using topically applied 5-aminolevulinic acid. Gynecol Oncol 2001; 80: 62–6.
31. Campbell SM, Gould DJ, Salter L, Clifford T, Curnow A. Photodynamic therapy using meta-tetrahydroxyphenylchlorin (Foscan) for the treatment of vulval intraepithelial neoplasia. Br J Dermatol 2004; 151: 1076–80.
32. Martin-Hirsch P, Kitchener HC, Hampson IN. Photodynamic therapy of lower genital tract neoplasia. Gynecol Oncol 2002; 84: 187–9.
33. Sillman FH, Sedlis A, Boyce JG. A review of lower genital intraepithelial neoplasia and the use of topical 5-fluorouracil. Obstet Gynecol Surv 1985; 40: 190–220.
34. Roberts JA, Watring WG, Lagasse LD. Treatment of vulvar intraepithelial neoplasia (VIN) with local bleomycin. Cancer Clin Trials 1980; 3: 351–4.
35. Longley DB, Harkin DP, Johnston PG. 5-fluorouracil: mechanisms of action and clinical strategies. Nat Rev Cancer 2003; 3: 330–8.

36. Jansen GT, Dillaha CJ, Honeycutt WM. Bowenoid conditions of the skin: treatment with topical 5-fluorouracil. South Med J 1967; 60: 185–8.

37. Cardosi RJ, Bomalaski JJ, Hoffman MS. Diagnosis and management of vulvar and vaginal intraepithelial neoplasia. Obstet Gynecol Clin North Am 2001; 28: 685–702.

38. Krebs HB. Prophylactic topical 5-fluorouracil following treatment of human papillomavirus-associated lesions of the vulva and vagina. Obstet Gynecol 1986; 68: 837–41.

39. Downs AM, Geraghty JM, Jones C. Fluorouracil does not improve the outcome of imiquimod treatment of vulval intraepethelial neoplasia. Acta Derm Venereol 2005; 85: 368–70.

40. Watring WG, Roberts JA, Lagasse LD et al. Treatment of recurrent Paget's disease of the vulva with topical bleomycin. Cancer 1978; 41: 10–11.

41. Buckley DA, Du Vivier AW. The therapeutic use of topical contact sensitizers in benign dermatoses. Br J Dermatol 2001; 145: 385–405.

42. Weintraub I, Lagasse LD. Reversibility of vulvar atypia by DNCB-induced delayed hypersensitivity. Obstet Gynecol 1973; 41: 195–9.

43. Foster DC, Woodruff JD. The use of dinitrochlorobenzene in the treatment of vulvar carcinoma in situ. Gynecol Oncol 1981; 11: 330–9.

44. De Palo G, Stefanon B, Rilke F, Pilotti S, Ghione M. Human fibroblast interferon in cervical and vulvar intraepithelial neoplasia associated with viral cytopathic effects. A pilot study. J Reprod Med 1985; 30: 404–8.

45. Slotman BJ, Helmerhorst TJ, Wijermans PW, Calame JJ. Interferon-alpha in treatment of intraepithelial neoplasia of the lower genital tract: a case report. Eur J Obstet Gynecol Reprod Biol 1988; 27: 327–33.

46. Spirtos NM, Smith LH, Teng NN. Prospective randomized trial of topical alpha-interferon (alpha-interferon gels) for the treatment of vulvar intraepithelial neoplasia III. Gynecol Oncol 1990; 37: 34–8.

47. Koonsaeng S, Verschraegen C, Freedman R et al. Successful treatment of recurrent vulvar intraepithelial neoplasia resistant to interferon and isotretinoin with cidofovir. J Med Virol 2001; 64: 195–8.

48. Vilmer C, Havard S, Cavelier-Balloy B et al. Failure of isotretinoin and interferon-alpha combination therapy for HPV-linked severe vulvar dysplasia. A report of two cases. J Reprod Med 1998; 43: 693–5.

49. Beutner KR, Spruance SL, Hougham AJ et al. Treatment of genital warts with an immune-response modifier (imiquimod). J Am Acad Dermatol 1998; 38: 230–9.

50. Edwards L, Ferenczy A, Eron L et al. Self-administered topical 5% imiquimod cream for external anogenital warts. HPV Study Group. Human Papilloma Virus. Arch Dermatol 1998; 134: 25–30.

51. Tyring S, Edwards L, Cherry LK et al. Safety and efficacy of 0.5% podofilox gel in the treatment of anogenital warts. Arch Dermatol 1998; 134: 33–8.

52. Stanley MA. Imiquimod and the imidazoquinolones: mechanism of action and therapeutic potential. Clin Exp Dermatol 2002; 27: 571–7.

53. Davis G, Wentworth J, Richard J. Self-administered topical imiquimod treatment of vulvar intraepithelial neoplasia. A report of four cases. J Reprod Med 2000; 45: 619–23.

54. Diaz-Arrastia C, Arany I, Robazetti SC et al. Clinical and molecular responses in high-grade intraepithelial neoplasia treated with topical imiquimod 5%. Clin Cancer Res 2001; 7: 3031–3.

55. Petrow W, Gerdsen R, Uerlich M, Richter O, Bieber T. Successful topical immunotherapy of bowenoid papulosis with imiquimod. Br J Dermatol 2001; 145: 1022–3.

56. Travis LB, Weinberg JM, Krumholz BA. Successful treatment of vulvar intraepithelial neoplasia with topical imiquimod 5% cream in a lung transplanted patient. Acta Derm Venereol 2002; 82: 475–6.

57. van Seters M, Fons G, van Beurden M. Imiquimod in the treatment of multifocal vulvar intraepithelial neoplasia 2/3. Results of a pilot study. J Reprod Med 2002; 47: 701–5.

58. Jayne CJ, Kaufman RH. Treatment of vulvar intraepithelial neoplasia 2/3 with imiquimod. J Reprod Med 2002; 47: 395–8.

59. Richter ON, Petrow W, Wardelmann E et al. Bowenoid papulosis of the vulva-immunotherapeutical approach with topical imiquimod. Arch Gynecol Obstet 2003; 268: 333–6.

60. Campagne G, Roca M, Martinez A. Successful treatment of a high-grade intraepithelial neoplasia with imiquimod, with vulvar pemphigus as a side effect. Eur J Obstet Gynecol Reprod Biol 2003; 109: 224–7.

61. Marchitelli C, Secco G, Perrotta M et al. Treatment of bowenoid and basaloid vulvar intraepithelial neoplasia 2/3 with imiquimod 5% cream. J Reprod Med 2004; 49: 876–82.

62. Wendling J, Saiag P, Berville-Levy S et al. Treatment of undifferentiated vulvar intraepithelial neoplasia with 5% imiquimod cream: a prospective study of 12 cases. Arch Dermatol 2004; 140: 1220–4.

63. Le T, Hicks W, Menard C, Hopkins L, Fung MF. Preliminary results of 5% imiquimod cream in the primary treatment of vulva intraepithelial neoplasia grade 2/3. Am J Obstet Gynecol 2006; 194: 377–80.

64. Abu J, Batuwangala M, Herbert K, Symonds P. Retinoic acid and retinoid receptors: potential chemopreventive and therapeutic role in cervical cancer. Lancet Oncol 2005; 6: 712–20.

65. Markowska J, Janik P, Wiese E, Ostrowski J. Leukoplakia of the vulva locally treated by 13-cis-retinoic acid. Neoplasma 1987; 34: 33–6.

66. Tristram A, Fiander A. Clinical responses to Cidofovir applied topically to women with high grade vulval intraepithelial neoplasia. Gynecol Oncol 2005; 99: 652–5.

67. Snoeck R. Papillomavirus and treatment. Antiviral Res 2006; 71: 181–91.

68. Hampl M, Sarajuuri H, Wentzensen N, Bender HG, Kueppers V. Effect of human papillomavirus vaccines on vulvar, vaginal, and anal intraepithelial lesions and vulvar cancer. Obstet Gynecol 2006; 108: 1361–8.

69. Roden R, Wu TC. How will HPV vaccines affect cervical cancer? Nat Rev Cancer 2006; 6: 753–63.

70. Baldwin PJ, Van Der Burg SH, Boswell CM et al. Vaccinia-expressed human papillomavirus 16 and 18 e6 and e7 as a therapeutic vaccination for vulval and vaginal intraepithelial neoplasia. Clin Cancer Res 2003; 9: 5205–13.

71. Davidson EJ, Boswell CM, Sehr P et al. Immunological and clinical responses in women with vulval intraepithelial neoplasia vaccinated with a vaccinia virus encoding human papillomavirus 16/18 oncoproteins. Cancer Res 2003; 63: 6032–41.

72. Davidson EJ, Faulkner RL, Sehr P et al. Effect of TA-CIN (HPV 16 L2E6E7) booster immunisation in vulval intraepithelial neoplasia patients previously vaccinated with TA-HPV (vaccinia virus encoding HPV 16/18 E6E7). Vaccine 2004; 22: 2722–9.

73. Smyth LJ, Van Poelgeest MI, Davidson EJ et al. Immunological responses in women with human papillomavirus type 16 (HPV-16)-associated anogenital intraepithelial neoplasia induced by heterologous prime-boost HPV-16 oncogene vaccination. Clin Cancer Res 2004; 10: 2954–61.

74. Shepherd V, Davidson EJ, Davies-Humphreys J. Extramammary Paget's disease. BJOG 2005; 112: 273–9.

75. Raspagliesi F, Fontanelli R, Rossi G et al. Photodynamic therapy using a methyl ester of 5-aminolevulinic acid in recurrent Paget's disease of the vulva: a pilot study. Gynecol Oncol 2006; 103: 581–6.

76. Henta T, Itoh Y, Kobayashi M, Ninomiya Y, Ishibashi A. Photodynamic therapy for inoperable vulval Paget's disease using delta-aminolaevulinic acid: successful management of a large skin lesion. Br J Dermatol 1999; 141: 347–9.

77. Zawislak AA, McCarron PA, McCluggage WG et al. Successful photodynamic therapy of vulval Paget's disease using a novel patch-based delivery system containing 5-aminolevulinic acid. BJOG 2004; 111: 1143–5.

78. Cohen PR, Schulze KE, Tschen JA, Hetherington GW, Nelson BR. Treatment of extramammary Paget disease with topical imiquimod cream: case report and literature review. South Med J 2006; 99: 396–402.

79. Wang LC, Blanchard A, Judge DE et al. Successful treatment of recurrent extramammary Paget's disease of the vulva with topical imiquimod 5% cream. J Am Acad Dermatol 2003; 49: 769–72.

80. Farias-Eisner R, Cirisano FD, Grouse D et al. Conservative and individualized surgery for early squamous carcinoma of the vulva: the treatment of choice for stage I and II (T1-2N0-1M0) disease. Gynecol Oncol 1994; 53: 55–8.

81. Andersen BL, Hacker NF. Psychosexual adjustment after vulvar surgery. Obstet Gynecol 1983; 62: 457–62.

82. Levenback C, Coleman RL, Burke TW et al. Intraoperative lymphatic mapping and sentinel node identification with blue dye in patients with vulvar cancer. Gynecol Oncol 2001; 83: 276–81.

83. Van der Zee AGJ, Oonk MH, de Hullu JA et al. On the safety of implementation of the sentinel node procedure in vulvar cancer, an observational study. Abstract presented at 11th Biennial Meeting of the International Gynecologic Cancer Society, 14 October, 2006, Santa Monica, CA.

84. Berek JS, Heaps JM, Fu YS, Juillard GJ, Hacker NF. Concurrent cisplatin and 5-fluorouracil chemotherapy and radiation therapy for advanced-stage squamous carcinoma of the vulva. Gynecol Oncol 1991; 42: 197–201.

85. Moore DH, Thomas GM, Montana GS et al. Preoperative chemoradiation for advanced vulvar cancer: a phase II study of the Gynecologic Oncology Group. Int J Radiat Oncol Biol Phys 1998; 42: 79–85.

Index